ABERNATHY'S
SURGICAL

SECRETS

T0195128

ABERNATHY'S SURGICAL

SECRETS

SEVENTH EDITION

ALDEN H. HARKEN, MD, FACS
Professor and Chair
Department of Surgery
University of California, San Francisco–East Bay;
Chief of Surgery
Department of Surgery
Alameda County Medical Center
Oakland, California

ERNEST E. MOORE, MD, FACS
Distinguished Professor of Surgery
University of Colorado Denver;
Editor, Journal of Trauma;
Department of Surgery
Denver Health Medical Center
Denver, Colorado

ELSEVIER

ELSEVIER

1600 John F. Kennedy Blvd.
Ste 1800
Philadelphia, PA 19103-2899

Notices

Knowledge and best practice in this field are constantly changing. As new research and experience broaden our understanding, changes in research methods, professional practices, or medical treatment may become necessary.

Practitioners and researchers must always rely on their own experience and knowledge in evaluating and using any information, methods, compounds, or experiments described herein. In using such information or methods they should be mindful of their own safety and the safety of others, including parties for whom they have a professional responsibility.

With respect to any drug or pharmaceutical products identified, readers are advised to check the most current information provided (i) on procedures featured or (ii) by the manufacturer of each product to be administered, to verify the recommended dose or formula, the method and duration of administration, and contraindications. It is the responsibility of practitioners, relying on their own experience and knowledge of their patients, to make diagnoses, to determine dosages and the best treatment for each individual patient, and to take all appropriate safety precautions.

To the fullest extent of the law, neither the Publisher nor the authors, contributors, or editors, assume any liability for any injury and/or damage to persons or property as a matter of products liability, negligence or otherwise, or from any use or operation of any methods, products, instructions, or ideas contained in the material herein.

Previous editions copyrighted 2009, 2005, 2003, 2000, 1996, 1991, and 1986.

Library of Congress Cataloging-in-Publication Data

Names: Harken, Alden H., editor. | Moore, Ernest Eugene, editor.
Title: Abernathy's surgical secrets / [edited by] Alden H. Harken, Ernest E. Moore.
Other titles: Surgical secrets | Secrets series.
Description: Seventh edition. | Philadelphia, PA : Elsevier, [2018] | Series:
Secrets series | Includes bibliographical references and index.
Identifiers: LCCN 2017023841 | ISBN 9780323478731 (pbk. : alk. paper)
Subjects: | MESH: Surgical Procedures, Operative | Examination Questions
Classification: LCC RD37.2 | NLM WO 18.2 | DDC 617.0076--dc23 LC record
available at https://lccn.loc.gov/2017023841

Content Strategist: James T. Merritt
Content Development Specialist: Kayla Smull
Publishing Services Manager: Catherine Jackson
Project Manager: Tara Delaney
Design Direction: Bridget Hoette

Printed in India

Last digit is the print number: 9 8 7 6 5 4 3

Working together
to grow libraries in
developing countries

www.elsevier.com • www.bookaid.org

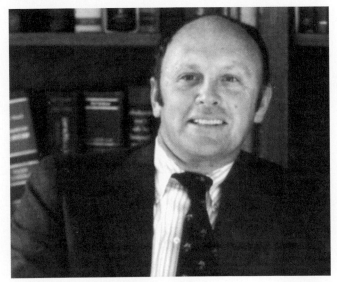

CHARLES M. ABERNATHY, M.D.
1941–1994

CONTRIBUTORS

Shannon N. Acker, MD
General Surgery Resident, Department of Surgery, University of Colorado, Aurora, Colorado

Megan Adams, MD
Transplant Surgery Fellow, Department of Surgery, Division of Transplant, University of Colorado, Aurora, Colorado

Maria B. Albuja-Cruz, MD, FACS
Assistant Professor of Surgery, Department of Surgery, Division of GI, Tumor, and Endocrine Surgery, University of Colorado School of Medicine, Denver, Colorado

Jason Q. Alexander, MD, FACS
Vascular and Endovascular Surgeon, Minneapolis Heart Institute; Associate Professor, University of Minnesota, Minneapolis, Minnesota

Benjamin O. Anderson, MD
Professor of Surgery and Global Health Medicine, Department of Surgery, University of Washington, Seattle, Washington

Sarah Tuttleton Arron, MD, PhD
Associate Professor, Dermatology, University of California, San Francisco, San Francisco, California

Thomas Bak, MD
Associate Professor, Division of Transplant Surgery, University of Colorado Hospital, Denver, Colorado

Carlton C. Barnett, Jr., MD, FACS
Chief, Surgical Oncology Denver VAMC, Professor of Surgery, Department of Surgery–GI Tumor Endocrine–VAMC, University of Colorado, Denver, Colorado

Bernard Timothy Baxter, MD
Professor and Vice-Chairman, Department of General Surgery, University of Nebraska Medical Center, Omaha, Nebraska

Kathryn Beauchamp, MD
Department of Surgery, Division of Neurosurgery, University of Denver Health Medical Center, Denver, Colorado

Taft Bhuket, MD
Chief of Gastroenterology and Hepatology, Director of Endoscopy/Alameda Health System, Highland Hospital, Oakland, California

Walter L. Biffl, MD, FACS
Medical Director, Acute Care Surgery, The Queen's Medical Center; Professor and Associate Chair for Research, John A. Burns School of Medicine, University of Hawaii-Manoa, Honolulu, Hawaii

Natasha D. Bir, MD, MHS
Chair, Department of Surgery, Woodland Memorial Hospital, Woodland, California

Andrea Bischoff, MD
Assistant Director, International Center for Colorectal and Urogenital Care, Children's Hospital Colorado; Associate Professor of Surgery, University of Colorado, Aurora, Colorado

Sarah D. Blaschko, MD
Department of Surgery, Division of Urology, Alameda Health System, Oakland, California

Scott C. Brakenridge, MD, MSCS, FACS
Assistant Professor of Surgery and Anesthesiology, Department of Surgery, University of Florida, Gainesville, Florida

Brooke C. Bredbeck, MD
House Officer, General Surgery, HO I, University of Michigan, Ann Arbor, Michigan

Elizabeth C. Brew, MD
Surgical Specialists of Colorado, Golden, Colorado

Laurence H. Brinckerhoff, MD
Chief, Thoracic Surgery, Department of Thoracic Surgery, Tufts University School of Medicine, Tufts Medical Center, Boston, Massachusetts

Magdalene A. Brooke, MD
General Surgery Resident, Department of Surgery, University of California, San Francisco–East Bay, Oakland, California

Elizabeth E. Brown, BA
Medical Student, Icahn School of Medicine at Mount Sinai, New York, New York

James M. Brown, MD
Associate Professor of Surgery, University of Maryland School of Medicine, Baltimore, Maryland

Jennifer L. Bruny, MD, FACS
Associate Professor of Surgery, Department of Surgery, Division of Pediatric Surgery, Children's Hospital Colorado, University of Colorado, Aurora, Colorado

Eric Bui, MD
Clinical Assistant Professor of Surgery, Department of Surgery, University of California, San Francisco–East Bay, Oakland, California

M. Kelley Bullard, MD
Associate Professor of Clinical Surgery, UCSF Department of Surgery, East Bay Surgery Division, University of California, San Francisco, Oakland, California

Clay Cothren Burlew, MD, FACS
Professor of Surgery, Director, Surgical Intensive Care Unit, Program Director, SCC and TACS Fellowships, Department of Surgery, Denver Health Medical Center, University of Colorado, Denver, Colorado

Kristine E. Calhoun, MD
Associate Professor, Department of Surgery, Division of Surgical Oncology, University of Washington School of Medicine, Seattle, Washington

Eric M. Campion, MD
Assistant Professor of Surgery, Department of Surgery, Denver Health Medical Center, University of Colorado Anschutz School of Medicine, Denver, Colorado

Karel D. Capek, MD
Research and Clinical Fellow, Burns, Reconstruction, and Surgical Critical Care, Department of Surgery, Shriners Hospitals for Children, Galveston, University of Texas Medical Branch, Galveston, Texas

John Chapman, MBA
Chief Administrative Officer, Alameda Health System, Highland Hospital, Oakland, California

Chun W. Choi, MD
Assistant Professor, Department of Cardiac Surgery, Vanderbilt University Medical Center, Nashville, Tennessee

Kathryn H. Chomsky-Higgins, MD, MS
Resident Physician, Department of General Surgery, University of California, San Francisco–East Bay, Oakland, California; Research Fellow, Department of Endocrine Surgery; University of California, San Francisco; San Francisco; California

David J. Ciesla, MD, MS
Professor of Surgery, Director Acute Care Surgery, University of South Florida, Morsani College of Medicine, Tampa, Florida

Joseph C. Cleveland, Jr., MD
Professor of Surgery, Vice-Chair, Faculty Affairs, Department of Surgery, Division of Cardiothoracic Surgery, University of Colorado Anschutz School of Medicine, Aurora, Colorado

Marie Crandall, MD, MPH, FACS
Professor of Surgery, Director of Research, Department of Surgery, Division of Acute Care Surgery, University of Florida College of Medicine Jacksonville, Jacksonville, Florida

Chasen A. Croft, MD, FACS
Assistant Professor of Surgery, Department of Surgery, Division of Acute Care Surgery, University of Florida College of Medicine, Gainesville, Florida

Timothy M. Crombleholme, MD
Surgeon-in-Chief, Children's Hospital Colorado, Department of Surgery, Division of Pediatric General, Thoracic and Fetal Surgery, University of Colorado School of Medicine, Aurora, Colorado

James Cushman, MD, MPH, FACS
Clinical Associate Professor of Surgery, Department of Surgery, University of California, San Francisco–East Bay, Oakland, California

Stephanie N. Davis, MD
General Surgery Resident, Department of Surgery, University of Colorado, Denver, Aurora, Colorado

Rodrigo Donalisio da Silva, MD
Assistant Professor, Department of Surgery, Division of Urology, Denver Health Medical Center, University of Colorado, Denver, Colorado

John C. Eun, MD
Assistant Professor, Department of Surgery, Division of Vascular Surgery and Endovascular Therapy, University of Colorado Anschutz Medical Campus, Aurora, Colorado

Chadrick R. Evans, MD
Assistant Professor, Department of Surgery, University of Illinois College of Medicine at Peoria, Peoria, Illinois

Christina A. Finlayson, MD
Professor, Department of Surgery, Associate Dean, Clinical Affairs, Associate Medical Director, University of Colorado School of Medicine, Aurora, Colorado

Lisa S. Foley, MD
Surgical Resident, Department of Surgery, Denver Health Medical Center, University of Colorado, Denver, Colorado

Charles J. Fox, MD, FACS
Chief of Vascular Surgery, Denver Health Medical Center; Associate Professor of Surgery, University of Colorado School of Medicine, Denver, Colorado

Krister Freese, MD
Pediatric Hand Surgeon, Shriner's Hospital for Children–Portland, Portland, Oregon

David A. Fullerton, MD
Head, Division of Cardiothoracic Surgery,
Department of Surgery, Division of
Cardiothoracic Surgery, University of Colorado
School of Medicine, Aurora, Colorado

*Glenn W. Geelhoed, AB, BS, MD, DTMH, MA, MPH,
MA, MPhil, ScD (honoris causa), EdD, FACS*
Professor of Surgery, Professor of International
Medical Education, Professor of Microbiology,
Department of Immunology and Tropical
Medicine, George Washington University Medical
Center, Washington, D.C.

Jahanara Graf, MD
Surgery Resident, Department of General Surgery,
University of California, San Francisco–East Bay,
Oakland, California

Amanda J. Green, MD
Surgery Resident, Department of Surgery,
University of California, San Francisco–East Bay,
Oakland, California

Richard-Tien V. Ha, MD
Clinical Assistant Professor, Surgical Director,
Mechanical Circulatory Support, Department
of Cardiothoracic Surgery, Stanford University
School of Medicine, Stanford, California

James B. Haenel, RRT
Surgical Critical Care Specialist, Department of
Surgery, Denver Health Medical Center, Denver,
Colorado

David J. Hak, MD, MBA, FACS
Professor, Department of Orthopedic Surgery,
Denver Health Medical Center, University of
Colorado School of Medicine, Denver, Colorado

Aidan D. Hamm, MD
Surgical Resident, Department of Surgery, Denver
Health Medical Center, University of Colorado,
Denver, Colorado

Alden H. Harken, MD, FACS
Professor and Chair
Department of Surgery
University of California, San Francisco–East Bay;
Chief of Surgery
Department of Surgery
Alameda County Medical Center
Oakland, California

Tabetha R. Harken, MD, MPH
Division Director of Family Planning, Associate
Professor of Obstetrics & Gynecology, University
of California, Irvine, California

David N. Herndon, MD, FACS
Professor, Jesse H. Jones Distinguished Chair
in Burn Surgery, University of Texas Medical
Branch; Chief of Staff and Director of Research,
Shriners Hospitals for Children–Galveston,
Galveston, Texas

Brian Hurt, MD, MS
Resident Physician, Department of Surgery,
University of Colorado, Aurora, Colorado

Laurel R. Imhoff, MD, MPH
General Surgeon, Department of General Surgery,
Kaiser Permanente, Santa Rosa Medical Center,
Santa Rosa, California

A. Thomas Indresano, DMD, FACS
T Galt and Lee Dehaven Atwood Professor of
Oral and Maxillofacial Surgery, University of
the Pacific, San Francisco, California; Director,
Division of Oral and Maxillofacial Surgery,
Highland Hospital, Oakland, California

Kyros Ipaktchi, MD, FACS
Chief of Hand Surgery, Department of Orthopedics,
Denver Health Medical Center, Denver, Colorado;
Associate Professor, Department of Orthopedics,
University of Colorado, Aurora, Colorado

Timothy K. Ito, MD
Department of Surgery, Division of Urology,
Alameda Health System, Oakland, California

Ghassan Jamaleddine, MD
Chief Medical Officer, Alameda Health System,
Oakland, California

Jeffrey L. Johnson, MD, FACS
Trauma Medical Director, Henry Ford Hospital,
Detroit, Michigan

Edward L. Jones, MD, MS
Assistant Professor of Surgery, Denver VA Medical
Center & The University of Colorado, Denver,
Colorado

Fernando J. Kim, MD, MBA, FACS
Professor of Surgery/Urology, University of Colorado
Denver; Chief of Urology, Denver Health Medical
Center, Denver, Colorado

Ann M. Kulungowski, MD
Assistant Professor of Surgery, Department of
Surgery, Division of Pediatric Surgery, University
Children's Hospital Colorado, University of
Colorado, Aurora, Colorado

Ramesh M. Kumar, MD
Department of Neurosurgery, University of
Colorado, Aurora, Colorado

Angela R. LaFace, MD
Critical Care Fellow, Research Resident, University of South Florida, Tampa, Florida

Ryan A. Lawless, MD
Trauma/Acute Care Surgeon, Denver Health Medical Center; Assistant Professor of Surgery, University of Colorado, Denver, Colorado

Michael L. Lepore, MD, FACS
Professor Emeritus, Otolaryngology–Head & Neck Surgery, University of Colorado, Denver, Aurora, Colorado

Kathleen R. Liscum, MD
Houston, Texas

Benny Liu, MD
Associate Division Chief, Department of Internal Medicine, Division of Gastroenterology and Hepatology, Highland Hospital, Oakland, California

Jeffrey C. Liu, MD, FACS
Associate Professor of Otolaryngology–Head and Neck Surgery, Department of Otolaryngology, Lewis Katz School of Medicine at Temple University, Philadelphia, Pennsylvania

Karen K. Lo, MD
University of Colorado, Department of Plastic and Reconstructive Surgery, Boulder, Colorado

Ning Lu, MD
Resident, Department of Surgery, University of Hawaii, Honolulu, Hawaii

Stephanie D. Malliaris, MD
Attending Surgeon, Departments of Surgery and Orthopedics, Denver Health Medical Center, Denver, Colorado; Assistant Professor of Plastic & Reconstructive Surgery, University of Colorado, Anschutz Medical Campus, Aurora, Colorado

David W. Mathes, MD, FACS
Professor and Chief of Plastic and Reconstructive Surgery, University of Colorado, Aurora, Colorado

Martin D. McCarter, MD, FACS
Professor of Surgery, Department of Surgery, Division of Surgical Oncology, University of Colorado School of Medicine, Aurora, CO

Robert C. McIntyre, Jr., MD
Professor of Surgery, Department of Surgery, Division of GI Tumor and Endocrine Surgery, University of Colorado, Aurora, Colorado

Logan R. McKenna, MD
Resident, Department of Surgery, University of Colorado, Aurora, Colorado

Daniel R. Meldrum, MD, FACS, FAHA
Professor of Surgery, Michigan State University College of Human Medicine, East Lansing, Michigan

Emily Miraflor, MD
Assistant Clinical Professor, Department of Surgery, University of California, San Francisco–East Bay, Oakland, California

Ernest E. Moore, MD, FACS
Distinguished Professor of Surgery
University of Colorado Denver;
Editor, Journal of Trauma;
Department of Surgery
Denver Health Medical Center
Denver, Colorado

Hunter B. Moore, MD
Trauma Research Fellow, Department of Surgery, University of Colorado, Denver, Colorado

Peter K. Moore, MD
Assistant Clinical Professor, Department of Medicine, Division of Hospital Medicine, University of California San Francisco and San Francisco VA Medical Center, San Francisco, California

Scott M. Moore, MD
Trauma & Acute Care Surgery Fellow, Department of Surgery, Denver Health Medical Center, University of Colorado School of Medicine, Denver, Colorado

Ashley Eleen Morgan, MD
Resident, Department of Surgery, University of California, San Francisco–East Bay, Oakland, California

Tony Nguyen, DO
Vascular and Endovascular Surgery, Kaiser Permanente Central Valley, California

Trevor L. Nydam, MD
Assistant Professor of Transplant Surgery, University of Colorado Anschutz Medical Campus, Aurora, Colorado

Siam Oottamasathien, MD, FAAP, FACS
Associate Professor of Surgery and Pediatric urology, Research Associate Professor of Medicinal Chemistry, Department of Surgery, Division of Urology, Section of Pediatric Urology, University of Utah, Primary Children's Hospital, Salt Lake City, Utah

Douglas M. Overbey, MD
Surgery Resident, Department of Surgery, University of Colorado, Aurora, Colorado

Barnard J. A. Palmer, MD, MEd, FACS
Assistant Clinical Professor of Surgery,
Departments of General and Endocrine Surgery,
University of California, San Francisco-East Bay,
Oakland, California

Chan M. Park, MD, DDS, FACS
Program Director, Oral & Maxillofacial Surgery
Residency, Alameda Health System–Highland
Hospital, Oakland, California; Associate
Professor, Department of Oral and Maxillofacial
Surgery, UOP, Arthur A. Dugoni School of
Dentistry, San Francisco, California

David A. Partrick, MD, FACS, FAAP
Professor of Surgery, Director of Surgical
Endoscopy, Department of Pediatric Surgery,
Children's Hospital Colorado, University of
Colorado School of Medicine, Aurora, Colorado

Nathan W. Pearlman, MD
Department of Surgery, University of Colorado
Health Sciences Center, Aurora, Colorado

Eric D. Peltz, DO, FACS
Assistant Director of Trauma and Acute Care
Surgery, Department of Surgery/GI, Tumor
and Endocrine Surgery, University of Colorado,
Anschutz Medical Campus, Aurora, Colorado

Alberto Peña, MD, FAAP, FACS, FRCS
Director, International Center for Colorectal and
Urogenital Care, Children's Hospital Colorado;
Professor of Surgery, University of Colorado,
Aurora, Colorado

Rodrigo Pessoa, MD
General Surgical Resident, PGY1, University of
Colorado Anschutz Medical Campus, Aurora,
Colorado

Thomas Pshak, MD
Department of Surgery, Division of Transplant
Surgery, University of Colorado, Denver, Colorado

Christopher D. Raeburn, MD, FACS
Associate Professor of Surgery, Department of GI,
Tumor, and Endocrine Surgery, University of
Colorado School of Medicine, Aurora, Colorado

T. Brett Reece, MD
Department of Surgery, Division of Cardiothoracic
Surgery, University of Colorado, Aurora, Colorado

Thomas F. Rehring, MD, FACS
Vice President, Chief Experience Officer, Kaiser
Permanente Colorado Region, Vascular and
Endovascular Surgery, Colorado Permanente
Medical Group, Clinical Associate Professor of
Surgery, University of Colorado Health Sciences
Center, Denver, Colorado

John A. Ridge, MD, PhD
Louis Della Penna Family Professor of Head and
Neck Oncology, Chief, Head and Neck Surgery
Section, Department of Surgical Oncology,
Fox Chase Cancer Center; Professor of
Otolaryngology, Head and Neck Surgery, Lewis
Katz School of Medicine at Temple University,
Philadelphia, Pennsylvania

Jonathan P. Roach, MD
Assistant Professor of Surgery and Pediatrics,
Department of Surgery, Division of Pediatric
Surgery, Children's Hospital Colorado, University
of Colorado School of Medicine, Aurora, Colorado

Thomas N. Robinson, MD, MS
Chief of Surgery, Department of Surgery, Denver VA
Medical Center, Denver, Colorado

Martin D. Rosenthal, MD
Resident, Department of Surgery, University of
Florida, Gainesville, Florida

Craig Selzman, MD, FACS
Professor of Surgery, Chief, Division of
Cardiothoracic Surgery, Surgical Director,
Cardiac Mechanical Support and Heart
Transplantation, University of Utah School of
Medicine, Salt Lake City, Utah

Steven R. Shackford, MD, FACS
Professor Emeritus, Department of Surgery,
University of Vermont, Burlington, Vermont

Erica Shook, DDS
Attending Surgeon, Alameda Health System,
Highland Hospital, Oakland, California; Division
of OMS and Assistant Professor, University of
the Pacific, Dugoni School of Dentistry, San
Francisco, California

David J. Skarupa, MD, FACS
Assistant Professor of Surgery, Department
of Surgery, Division of Acute Care Surgery,
University of Florida College of Medicine–
Jacksonville, Jacksonville, Florida

Stig Sømme, MD, MPH
Department of Surgery, Division of Pediatric
Surgery, University of Colorado School of
Medicine, Aurora, Colorado

Philip F. Stahel, MD, FACS
Professor of Orthopedics and Neurosurgery,
Department of Orthopedics, Denver Health
Medical Center, University of Colorado School of
Medicine, Denver, Colorado

Melissa K. Suh, MD
Department of Surgery, University of Nebraska
Medical Center, Omaha, Nebraska

John M. Swanson, MD
General Surgical Resident, Department of Surgery, University of California, San Francisco–East Bay, Oakland, California

U. Mini B. Swift, MD, MPH, FACP
Associate Chief Medical Officer, Alameda Health System, Oakland, California

Tiffany L. Tello, MD
Department of Dermatology, University of California, San Francisco, San Francisco, California

Robert A. Tessler, MD
Resident, Department of Surgery, University of California San Francisco–East Bay, Oakland, California

Robert J. Torphy, MD
Resident, Department of General Surgery, University of Colorado, Denver, Colorado

Todd F. VanderHeiden, MD
Associate Director of Orthopaedics, Chief of Orthopaedic Spine Surgery, Denver Health Medical Center; Assistant Professor of Orthopaedics, University of Colorado School of Medicine, Denver, Colorado

Erin L. Vanzant, MD
Department of Surgery, General Surgery, University of Florida, Gainesville, Florida

Gregory P. Victorino, MD, FACS
Professor of Clinical Surgery, Chief, Division of Trauma, Department of Surgery, University of California, San Francisco–East Bay, Oakland, California

Priya N. Werahera, PhD
Research Assistant Professor, Department of Pathology, University of Colorado Anschutz Medical Campus, Aurora, Colorado

Jessica L. Williams, MD
Department of Surgery, University of California, San Francisco–East Bay, Oakland, California

Robert Wong, MD, MS
Assistant Clinical Professor of Medicine, Director of Research and Education, Division of Gastroenterology and Hepatology, Alameda Health System–Highland Hospital, Oakland, California

Yuka Yamaguchi, MD
Department of Surgery, Division of Urology, Alameda Health System, Oakland, California

Giorgio Zanotti, MD
Chief Resident, Cardiothoracic Surgery, Division of Cardiothoracic Surgery, University of Colorado, Denver, Colorado

PREFACE

When we refer to a work of art, music, or literature as a "classic," one of the observations that we make is that the work has stimulated a wide variety of treatments and interpretations. Imitation is, of course, the most visible and credible form of flattery. When Charlie Abernathy initially assaulted our surgical clinical comfort zone with a barrage of questions, neither he nor we predicted that his irritating efforts would spawn a whole "Secrets Series" of challenging Abernathyisms in almost all medical disciplines.

But, characteristically, Charlie had his fingers capably placed on the pulse of progress. Casey Stengel famously noted: "In baseball, more games are lost than won." If you are not investigating, learning, or questioning, you are losing. In medicine, and certainly surgery, you cannot stand still. Alfred North Whitehead, the US philosopher, observed: "No man of science could subscribe without qualification ... to all of his own scientific beliefs of ten years ago." We must be flexible, to evolve, to question. Happily, surgeons are almost unique in our ability to be self-critical. We must never march, like a legion of lemmings, into a sea of intellectual acceptance.

This seventh edition of *Surgical Secrets* is again dedicated to Abernathy's irritatingly penetrating series of questions. Charlie never took much stock in the ponderously traditional answer. Intellectually active surgeons should never get too comfortable. Changing your mind proves you've got one. Challenging dogma is good; comfort is bad. Dinosaurs were inflexible and are extinct. Surgeons will never be either.

Alden H. Harken, MD, FACS
Ernest E. Moore, MD, FACS
September 2016

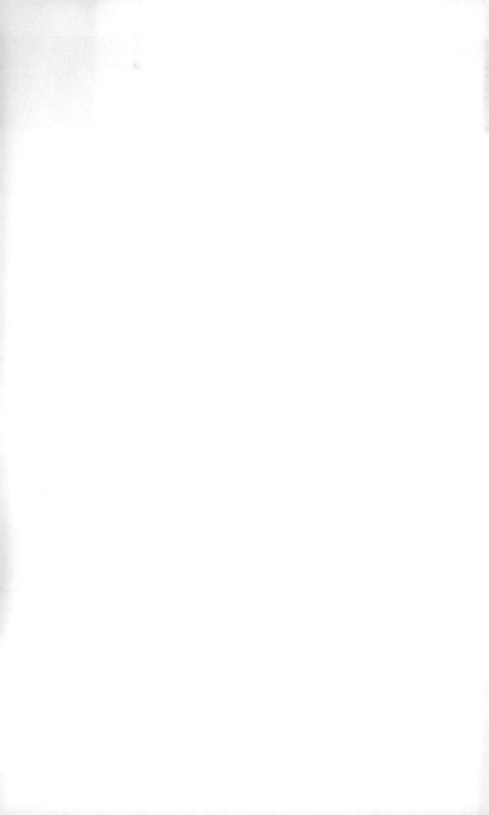

CONTENTS

II TRAUMA

III ABDOMINAL SURGERY

VII VASCULAR SURGERY

VIII CARDIOTHORACIC SURGERY

IX PEDIATRIC SURGERY

ANSWERS TO THE TOP 100 QUESTIONS THAT YOU WILL BE ASKED ON ROUNDS

Emily Miraflor, MD, Barnard J. A. Palmer, MD, MEd, FACS

These top 100 secrets summarize the concepts, principles, and many salient details of surgical practice.

1. The primary goal in treating cardiac dysrhythmias is to achieve a ventricular rate between 60 and 100 beats per minute; the secondary goal is to maintain sinus rhythm.
2. When evaluating hypothermic patients, they are not considered dead until both warm and dead.
3. Clinical determinants of brain death are the loss of papillary, corneal, oculovestibular, oculocephalic, oropharyngeal, and respiratory reflexes for >6 hours. The patient should also undergo an apnea test, in which the PCO_2 is allowed to rise to at least 60 mm Hg without coexistent hypoxia. Breathing is a basic brainstem reflex, and the absence of spontaneous breathing confirms brain death.
4. The estimated risks of hepatitis B virus (HBV), hepatitis C virus (HCV) and human immunodeficiency virus (HIV) transmission by blood transfusion in the United States are 1 in 205,000 for HBV; 1 in 1,935,000 for HCV; and 1 in 2,135,000 for HIV.
5. The most common location of an undescended testicle is the inguinal canal.
6. The most common solid renal mass in infancy is a congenital mesoblastic nephroma, and in childhood, it is a Wilms' tumor.
7. Ogilvie syndrome (colonic pseudo-obstruction) is an acute massive dilation of the entire colon without a mechanical blockage.
8. The most common histologic type of bladder cancer is urothelial cell carcinoma.
9. The most common cause of male infertility is varicocele.
10. The most common nonbacterial cause of pneumonia in transplant patients is cytomegalovirus.
11. Chimerism is leukocyte sharing between the graft and the recipient so that the transplanted graft becomes a genetic composite of both the donor and the recipient and, ultimately, should not require immunosuppression of the host.
12. Mucosa-associated lymphatic tumor is a variant of gastric lymphoma, which can almost always be cured by treating for underlying *H. pylori.*
13. The most common diseases requiring liver transplant in the United States and worldwide are hepatitis C and hepatitis B, respectively.
14. The lung volume at end expiration is termed functional residual capacity.
15. Cystic hygroma (lymphatic malformation) is a congenital malformation with a predilection for the neck. This benign lesion classically presents as a soft mass in the posterior triangle of the left neck.
16. The three most common variants of tracheoesophageal fistula are (1) proximal esophageal atresia with distal tracheoesophageal fistula, (2) isolated esophageal atresia with intact trachea, and (3) tracheoesophageal fistula with esophageal atresia. There is also an "H-type" in which the trachea and esophagus are intact, but with a fistula.
17. Intestinal atresias can occur anywhere in the gastrointestinal (GI) tract—duodenal (50%), jejunoileal (45%), or colonic (5%). Duodenal atresia arises from failure of recanalization during the eighth to tenth week of gestation; jejunoileal and colonic atresias are caused by an in utero mesenteric vascular accident.
18. Ascending aortic dissections (Stanford type A), which begin in the ascending aorta and may continue into the descending aorta, obligate surgical repair with cardiopulmonary bypass. Descending dissections (Stanford type B), which typically begin just distal to the subclavian artery, involve only the descending aorta and are treated with aggressive blood pressure control.
19. The likelihood that a solitary lung nodule is cancer is the same as the age of the patient; thus, a 60-year-old patient's nodule is 60% likely to be cancer.

20. Mediastinal staging (mediastinoscopy) is indicated if (1) the lung nodule is >2 cm, (2) the mediastinum is "wide" as seen on a computed tomography (CT) scan, and (3) the nodule is "kissing" mediastinum. A lung resection is contraindicated if (1) "high" ipsilateral paratracheal nodes are positive, (2) contralateral nodes are positive, or (3) undifferentiated (small cell) histology is identified anywhere.

21. The most common causes of aortic stenosis are bicuspid aortic valve and calcific (degenerative) disease.

22. The indications for coronary artery bypass graft are (1) left main coronary artery stenosis, (1) three-vessel coronary artery disease (CAD) (70% stenosis) with depressed left ventricular (LV) function, (3) two-vessel CAD with proximal left anterior descending involvement, and (4) angina despite aggressive medical therapy.

23. Anticipated patency of a saphenous vein graft in a coronary artery is 70% over 5 years, and 85% for an internal mammary artery.

24. The preferred surgical treatment of medically refractory ulcerative colitis is total proctocolectomy with ileoanal pouch anastomosis.

25. Dieulafoy's ulcer is a gastric vascular malformation with an exposed submucosal artery, usually within 2–5 cm of the gastroesophageal junction. It presents with painless, often massive, hematemesis.

26. Blind subtotal colectomy in the management of massive lower GI bleeding is limited to a small group of patients in whom a specific bleeding source cannot be identified. The procedure is associated with a 16% mortality rate.

27. Patients with colorectal cancer with lymph node involvement (stage III) should receive chemotherapy postoperatively.

28. Goodsall's rule states that the location of the internal opening of an anorectal fistula is based on the position of the external opening. An external opening posterior to a line drawn transversely across the perineum originates from a curvilinear internal opening in the posterior midline. An external opening anterior to this line originates from the nearest anal crypt in a straight radial direction.

29. Structures in the hernia sac of an incarcerated inguinal hernia still have an intact blood supply but are stuck in the sac because of adhesions or a narrow hernia sac neck. Structures in a strangulated hernia have a compromised blood supply because of anatomic constriction at the neck of the hernia.

30. Chvostek's sign is spasm of the facial muscles caused by tapping the facial nerve trunk. Trousseau's sign is carpopedal spasm elicited by occlusion of the brachial artery for 3 minutes with a blood pressure cuff. Both signs indicate hypocalcemia.

31. The only biochemical test routinely needed to identify patients with unsuspected hyperthyroidism is serum thyroid-stimulating hormone concentration.

32. The surgically correctable causes of hypertension are renovascular hypertension, pheochromocytoma, Cushing's syndrome, primary hyperaldosteronism, coarctation of the aorta, and unilateral renal parenchymal disease.

33. The "triple test" or "diagnostic triad" for diagnosing a palpable breast mass includes physical examination, breast imaging, and biopsy.

34. Triple negative breast cancer is a heterogeneous group of more aggressive cancers that do not express the genes for the estrogen receptor, progesterone receptor, and human epidermal growth factor receptor.

35. Sentinel lymph nodes represent the first site of spread for tumor cells metastasizing through lymphatics from a primary tumor.

36. A patient in whom fine-needle aspiration (FNA) of a cervical node reveals squamous cell carcinoma should have examination of the mouth, pharynx, larynx, esophagus, and tracheobronchial tree under anesthesia (triple endoscopy). If no lesion is found, biopsies of the tonsils, nasopharynx, base of tongue, and pyriform sinuses should be performed at the same sitting.

37. The cumulative 10-year amputation rate for claudication with a gangrenous toe is only 10%. Because vascular disease is systemic, many of these patients die of cardiovascular disease prior to amputation.

38. The absolute reduction in risk of stroke is 6% over a 5-year period in asymptomatic patients with >60% stenosis who undergo carotid endarterectomy plus aspirin versus patients treated with aspirin alone (5.1% surgery versus 11% medical treatment). These data derive from the Asymptomatic Carotid Atherosclerosis Study (see Chapter 108).

39. The average expansion rate of an infrarenal abdominal aortic aneurysm (AAA) is 0.4 cm/year. In an otherwise healthy patient, a 5.5 cm AAA is an indication for either open or stent graft.

40. Heparin binds to antithrombin III, rendering heparin more antithrombotic.

41. The patient with suspected intermittent claudication should initially be evaluated by obtaining an ankle brachial index (ABI) or segmental limb pressures at rest. Typically, an ABI of 0.5–0.8 reflects claudication and an ABI of <0.4 reflects limb threat.

42. Fondaparinux and rivaroxaban are anticoagulants that inhibit factor Xa. Dabigatran is an anticoagulant that works as a direct thrombin inhibitor.

43. Nitric oxide is a vasodilator that is synthesized in vascular endothelial cells by constitutive nitric oxide synthase (NOS) and inducible NOS.

44. Basal caloric expenditure is equal to 25 kcal/kg per day with a requirement of approximately 1 g of protein per kilogram per day.

45. Dextrose has 3.4 kcal/g, protein 4 kcal/g, and fat 9 kcal/g; a 20% lipid solution delivers 2 kcal/mL.

46. Refeeding syndrome occurs in moderately to severely malnourished patients (e.g., chronic alcoholism or anorexia nervosa) who, with a large nutrient load, develop clinically significant decreases in serum phosphorus, potassium, calcium, and magnesium levels. Hyperglycemia is common secondary to blunted insulin secretion. Adenosine triphosphate (ATP) production is mitigated, and respiratory failure is common.

47. Fever is caused by activated macrophages that release interleukin-1, tumor necrosis factor, and interferon in response to bacteria and endotoxin. The result is a resetting of the hypothalamic thermoregulatory center.

48. Cardiac output (CO) is equal to heart rate multiplied by stroke volume; normal CO is 5–6 L/min, and cardiac index is 2.4–3.0 L/min/m^2. Systemic vascular resistance (SVR) is equal to mean arterial pressure (MAP) minus central venous pressure (CVP) divided by CO multiplied by 80; it is written as: SVR = (MAP − CVP)/CO × 80. Normal SVR is 800–1200 dyne-s/cm^5.

49. The signs of hypovolemic shock are low CVP, low pulmonary capillary wedge pressure (PCWP), low cardiac output, low mixed venous oxygen saturation (SVO$_2$), and high systemic vascular resistance (SVR). The signs of cardiogenic shock are high CVP, high PCWP, low CO, low SVO$_2$, and typically high SVR. The signs of septic shock are low or normal CVP, low or normal PCWP, high CO initially, high SVO$_2$, and low SVR.

50. Kehr's sign is concurrent left upper quadrant and left shoulder pain, indicating diaphragmatic irritation from a ruptured spleen or left subdiaphragmatic abscess. Anatomically, the diaphragm and the back of the left shoulder enjoy parallel innervation.

51. The five Ws of postoperative fever are wound (infection), water (urinary tract infection), wind (atelectasis, pneumonia), walking (thrombophlebitis), and wonder drugs (drug fevers).

52. Cricothyroidotomy should not be performed on patients <12 years old or on any patient with suspected direct laryngeal trauma or tracheal disruption.

53. The palpable radial (wrist) pulse reflects systolic blood pressure (SBP) >80 mm Hg, palpable femoral (groin) pulse reflects SBP >70 mm Hg, and palpable carotid (neck) pulse reflects SBP >60 mm Hg.

54. Raccoon eyes (periorbital ecchymosis) and Battle's sign (mastoid ecchymosis) are clinical indicators of basilar skull fracture.

55. Cerebral perfusion pressure (CPP) is equal to mean arterial pressure (MAP) minus intracranial pressure (ICP), and it is written as CPP = MAP − ICP. Some debate exists on the minimum allowable CPP, but consensus indicates that a CPP of at least 50–70 mm Hg is necessary.

56. Violation of the platysma defines a penetrating neck wound.

57. Tension pneumothorax is air accumulation in the pleural space eliciting increased intrathoracic pressure with a decrease in venous return to heart and a decrease in cardiac output. This is a hemodynamic, not a respiratory problem, and cannot be diagnosed via x-ray.

58. The most common site of thoracic aortic injury in blunt trauma is immediately distal to the takeoff of the left subclavian artery.

59. The most common manifestation of blunt myocardial injury is an arrhythmia.

60. Indications for thoracotomy in a stable patient with hemothorax include an immediate tube thoracostomy output of 1500 mL or ongoing bleeding of 250 mL/h for 4 consecutive hours.

61. Beck's triad of hypotension, distended neck veins, and muffled heart sounds indicates pericardial tamponade.

62. The hepatic artery supplies approximately 30% of blood flow to the liver, and the portal vein supplies the remaining 70%. Oxygen delivery, however, is similar for both at 50%.

63. The Pringle maneuver, which is used to reduce liver hemorrhage, is a manual occlusion of the hepatoduodenal ligament to interrupt blood flow to the liver.

64. The treatment for intraperitoneal bladder rupture from blunt trauma is operative repair, whereas the treatment for extraperitoneal rupture is Foley catheter bladder decompression and observant management.

65. The earliest sign of leg compartment syndrome is neurologic in the distribution of the deep peroneal nerve with numbness in the first dorsal webspace and weak dorsiflexion. The leg has four separate compartments, each of which can independently exhibit a compartment syndrome.

66. Posterior knee dislocations are associated with popliteal artery injuries and are an indication for angiography.

67. The Parkland formula for burn resuscitation is lactated Ringer's at 4 mL/kg × percentage of total body surface burned (second and third degree only). Infuse 50% of the volume in first 8 hours and the remaining 50% over the subsequent 16 hours.

68. The metabolic rate peaks at 2.5 times the basal metabolic rate in severe burns >50% TBSA.

69. Gallstones and alcohol are the two main causes of acute pancreatitis. Alcohol abuse accounts for 75% of cases of chronic pancreatitis.

70. Isolated gastric varices with hypersplenism indicate splenic vein thrombosis and are an indication for splenectomy.

71. The treatment for gallstone pancreatitis is cholecystectomy during the same hospital stay once the pancreatitis has subsided.

72. Proton pump inhibitors (PPIs) irreversibly inhibit the parietal cell H+/K+ ATP pump.

73. A Cushing's ulcer is a stress ulcer in critically ill patients with central nervous system injury. It is typically single and deep, with a tendency to perforate. A Curling's ulcer is a stress ulcer in critically ill patients with burn injuries. A marginal ulcer is an ulcer near the margin of the gastroenteric anastomosis, usually on the small bowel side. A Marjolin's ulcer is a squamous cell carcinoma arising in chronic wounds.

74. The most common cause of small bowel obstruction is an adhesion due to prior surgery, the second most common cause is a hernia.

75. Charcot's triad, indicative of cholangitis, is right upper quadrant pain, fever, and jaundice. Reynolds' pentad includes Charcot's triad, hypotension, and altered mental status.

76. Bilirubin levels must be >2 mg/dL for jaundice to become apparent.

77. Early jaundice becomes apparent under the tongue and on the palms of the hands.

78. The international normalized ratio (INR) of FFP is about 1.4.

79. One unit of blood will raise the hemoglobin level by 1 g/dL and the hematocrit level by 3%.

80. The macrophage is essential for wound healing.

81. Long-term biliary obstruction can result in coagulopathy due to malabsorption of the fat soluble vitamin K.

82. After abdominal surgery, the small bowel typically gains motility first, followed by the stomach, and then the colon.

83. The borders of the gastrinoma triangle are the common bile duct where it is joined by the cystic duct, the junction of the neck and body of the pancreas, and the junction of the second and third portion of the duodenum.

84. After splenectomy, vaccination against *Streptococcus pneumoniae, Neisseria meningitidis,* and *Haemophilus influenzae* should be given.

85. Child's Pugh score predicts mortality after surgical intervention in cirrhotic patients. The components of the score are encephalopathy, ascites, INR, albumin and bilirubin levels. The Model for End-Stage Liver Disease score is a prognostic system used in liver disease to assess need for liver transplant. Calculation is based on the INR, creatinine, and bilirubin levels.

86. Respiratory quotient is the ratio of CO_2 produced to oxygen consumed. An RQ >1 indicates overfeeding. An RQ <7 indicates starvation.

87. Psoas sign (pain with extension of the leg) indicates a retrocecal appendicitis.

88. Leptin is produced in adipocytes and is an appetite suppressant.

89. Focal nodular hyperplasia is an asymptomatic hypervascular liver mass with a central scar that does not require treatment.

90. Colon cancers demonstrate a predictable sequence of genetic mutations starting with the *APC* gene, *KRAS, DCC,* and finally p53.

91. The presence of a *KRAS* mutation predicts poor response to chemotherapy targeting the epidermal growth factor receptor.

92. Silvadene causes neutropenia; Sulfamylon causes metabolic acidosis; silver nitrate causes electrolyte imbalances.

93. Intraductal papillary mucinous neoplasms (IPMN) can be main-duct or side-duct lesions within the pancreas. Mucinous secretion from the ampulla seen on ERCP is pathognomonic for main duct IPMN. Main-duct IPMNs are more likely to be malignant than side-duct IPMNs.

94. Bleomycin, which is given for lymphoma and reproductive cancers, can cause pulmonary fibrosis.

95. Adriamycin, which is commonly used in breast cancer, can lead to cardiac dysfunction.

96. The criteria for acute respiratory distress syndrome are bilateral infiltrates seen on chest x-ray and a PaO_2/FiO_2 ratio of <300 that cannot be explained by cardiac failure or fluid overload.

97. The hard signs of vascular injury mandating operative exploration are hemorrhage, loss of pulse, expanding or pulsatile hematoma, distal ischemia, and bruit.

98. Motilin is the hormone that regulates the migrating motor complex of the gut.

99. A small bowel obstruction with air seen in the biliary tree should prompt an evaluation for gallstone ileus.

100. Bloody nipple discharge is most likely due to an intraductal papilloma.

ABERNATHY'S SURGICAL

SURGICAL

SECRETS

I

GENERAL TOPICS

CHAPTER 1

ARE YOU READY FOR YOUR SURGICAL ROTATION?

Tabetha R. Harken, MD, MPH, U. Mini B. Swift, MD, MPH, FACP, Alden H. Harken, MD, FACS

Surgery is a participatory, team, and contact sport. Present yourself to patients, residents, and attendings with enthusiasm (which covers a multitude of sins), punctuality (type A people do not like to wait), and cleanliness (you must look, act, and smell like a doctor).

1. **Why should you introduce yourself to each patient and ask about his or her chief complaint?**
   Symptoms are perception, and perception is more important than reality. To a patient, the chief complaint is not simply a matter of life and death; it is much more important. Patients routinely are placed in compromising, uncomfortable, embarrassing, and undignified predicaments. Patients are people, however, and they have interests, concerns, anxieties, and a story. As a student, you have an opportunity to place your patient's chief complaint into the context of the rest of his or her life. This skill is important, and the patient will always be grateful. You can serve a real purpose as a listener and translator for the patient and his or her family.

   Patients want to trust and love you. This trust in surgical therapy is a formidable tool. The more a patient understands about his or her disease, the more the patient can participate in getting better. Recovery is faster if the patient helps.

   Similarly, the more the patient understands about his or her therapy (including its side effects and potential complications), the more effective the therapy is (this principle is not in the textbooks). You can be your patient's interpreter. This is the fun of surgery (and medicine).

2. **What is the correct answer to almost all questions?**
   Thank you. Gratitude is an invaluable tool on the wards.

3. **Are there any simple rules from the trenches?**
   a. **Getting along with the nurses.** The nurses do know more than the rest of us about the codes, routines, and rituals of making the wards run smoothly. They may not know as much about pheochromocytomas and intermediate filaments, but about the stuff that matters, they know a lot. Acknowledge that, and they will take you under their wings and teach you a ton!
   b. **Helping out.** If your residents look busy, they probably are. So, if you ask how you can help and they are too busy even to answer, asking again probably would not yield much. Always leap at the opportunity to grab x-rays, track down lab results, and retrieve a bag of blood from the bank. The team will recognize your enthusiasm and reward your contributions.
   c. **Getting scutted.** We all would like a secretary, but one is not going to be provided on this rotation. Your residents do a lot of their own scut work without you even knowing about it. So if you feel like scut work is beneath you, perhaps you should think about another profession.
   d. **Working hard.** This rotation is an apprenticeship. If you work hard, you will get a realistic idea of what it means to be a resident (and even a practicing doctor) in this specialty. (This has big advantages when you are selecting a type of internship.)
   e. **Staying in the loop.** In the beginning, you may feel like you are not a real part of the team. If you are persistent and reliable, however, soon your residents will trust you with more important jobs.
   f. **Educating yourself, and then educating your patients.** Here is one of the rewarding places (as indicated in question 1) where you can soar to the top of the team. Talk to your patients about everything (including their disease and therapy), and they will love you for it.

g. **Maintaining a positive attitude.** As a medical student, you may feel that you are not a crucial part of the team. Even if you are incredibly smart, you are unlikely to be making the crucial management decisions. So what does that leave? Attitude. If you are enthusiastic and interested, your residents will enjoy having you around, and they will work to keep you involved and satisfied. A dazzlingly intelligent but morose complainer is better suited for a rotation in the morgue. Remember, your resident is likely following 15 sick patients, gets paid less than $2 an hour, and hasn't slept more than 5 hours in the last 3 days. Simple things such as smiling and saying thank you (when someone teaches you) go an incredibly long way and are rewarded on all clinical rotations with experience and good grades.

h. **Having fun!** This is the most exciting, gratifying, rewarding, and fun profession and is light years better than whatever is second best (this is not just our opinion).

4. What is the best approach to surgical notes?
Surgical notes should be succinct. Most surgeons still move their lips when they read. See Table 1.1.

HOSPITAL DISCHARGE

5. What is a care transition?
It is a fancy word for any change in a clinical care setting. Examples include from hospital to home, from home to emergency department (ED), and from nursing home to home.

6. What is one of the most dangerous things that you can do to your patient?
Discharge them from the hospital.

7. Why is a hospital discharge a dangerous procedure?
Hospitals are designed for maximal support. Procedures are managed; diet is controlled; and even the increasingly obligate polypharmacy is orchestrated such that each pill is swallowed with metronomic precision. Then, much like a baby eaglet, the patient is unceremoniously "pushed out" of this federally regulated inpatient nest. And again, like the baby eaglet, we expect that patient to take flight at home.

8. What would improve safety at discharge?
Follow through on the "last sign out." Sign out to your patient, their family members, and the next doctor who is going to take care of them in the nursing home or clinic.

9. What are the most important elements of the final sign out (discharge summary)?
Discharge summaries should include:
- Primary and other diagnoses
- Pertinent medical history and physical findings
- Dates that they were hospitalized and brief hospital course (assume that the doctor on the outside knows how to treat hyperkalemia)
- Results of procedures
- Abnormal lab tests
- Recommendations of the specialists that you consulted
- Information that you gave to the patient and family
- Discharge medications
- Details of follow-up arrangements
- To-do list of appointments, pending tests, or procedures to be scheduled or checked
- Name and contact information of the inpatient doctor

The idea that a hospital discharge is a risky business, but the risk can be reduced by a conscientious physician or medical student, comes from Kripalani et al.

Table 1.1 Best Approach to Surgical Notes

Admission Orders

Admit to 5 West (attending's name)

Condition:	Stable
Diagnosis:	Abdominal pain; r/o appendicitis
Vital signs:	q 4 h
Parameters:	Please call HO for:
	T >38°C; HR >140

Table 1.1 Best Approach to Surgical Notes *(Continued)*

Diet:	NPO
Fluids:	1000 LR w 20 mEq KCl @ 100 mL/h
Med[ication]s:	ASA 650 mg PR PRN for T >38.5°C
	Thank you.

Sign your name/leave space for resident's signature (your beeper number)

History and Physical Examination (H&P)

Mrs. O'Flaherty is a 55 y/o w♀ [white woman] admitted with a cc [chief complaint]: "My stomach hurts." Pt [patient] was in usual state of excellent health until 2 days PTA [prior to admission] when she noted gradual onset of crampy midepigastric pain. Pain is now severe (7/10; 7 on a scale of 10) and recurring q 5 minutes. Pt described + vomiting (+ bile, − blood) [with bile, without blood].

PMH [past medical history]

Hosp[italizations]:	Pneumonia (2001)
	Childbirth (1982, 1984)
Surg[ery]:	Splenectomy for trauma (1987)
Allergies:	Codeine, shellfish
Social:	ETOH [alcohol]
Tobacco:	1 ppd [pack per day] x 25 years
ROS [review of systems]	
Resp[iratory]:	Productive cough
Cardiac:	ō chest pain
	ō MI [myocardial infarction]
	[ō = not observed, noncontributory, or not here]
Renal:	ō dysuria, ō frequency
Neuro[logic]:	WNL [within normal limits]
Physical Examination (PE)	
BP:	140/90
HR:	100 (regular)
RR [respiratory rate]:	16 breaths/min
Temp:	38.2°C

WD [well developed], WN [well nourished], mildly obese, 55 y/o female; in moderate abdominal distress

HEENT [head, eyes, ears, nose, and throat]:	WNL
Resp:	Clear lungs bilat[erally]
	ō wheeze, rales
Heart:	ō m [murmur]
	RSR [regular sinus rhythm]
Abdomen:	Mildly distended
	High-pitched rushes that coincide with crampy pain
	Tender to palpation (you do not need to hurt the patient to find this out)
	ō rebound
Rectal:	(Always do; never defer the rectal exam on your surgical rotation)
	Hematest stool—negative for blood

No masses, no tenderness

Pelvic:	No masses
	No adnexal tenderness
	No cervical motion tenderness or chandelier sign; if quick motion of cervix makes your patient hit the chandelier → nonspecific peritoneal sign, possibly pelvic inflammatory disease (PID; gonorrhea)
Extremities:	Full ROM [range of motion]
	ō edema
	Bounding (3+) pulses

Continued on following page

Table 1.1 Best Approach to Surgical Notes *(Continued)*

Imp[ression]:	Abdominal pain
	r/o SB [small bowel] obstruction 2° [secondary] to
	adhesions
Rx:	NG [nasogastric] tube
	IV fluids
	Op[erative] consent
	Type and hold (Blood Bank)

[Signature]

Notes on the surgical H&P

- A surgical H&P should be succinct and focused on the patient's problem.
- Begin with the chief complaint (in the patient's words).
- Is the problem new or chronic?
- PMH: always include prior hospitalizations and medications.
- ROS: restrict review to organ systems (lung, heart, kidneys, and nervous system) that may affect this admission.
- PE: always begin with vital signs (including respiration and temperature); that is why these signs are vital.
- Rebound means inflammatory peritoneal irritation or peritonitis.

Preop[erative] note

The preoperative note is a checklist confirming that you and the patient are ready for the planned surgical procedure. Place this note in the Progress Notes:

Preop dx [diagnosis]:	SB obstruction 2° to adhesions
CXR [chest x-ray]:	Clear
ECG [electrocardiogram]:	NSR ō ST-T wave changes
Blood:	Type and cross-match x 2 u
Consent:	In chart

Operative note

The operative note should provide anyone who encounters the patient after surgery with all the needed information:

Preop dx:	SB obstruction
Postop dx:	Same, all bowel viable
Procedure:	Exp[loratory] Lap[arotomy] with lysis of adhesions
Surgeon:	Name him or her
Assistants:	List them
Anesthesia:	GEA [general endotracheal anesthesia]
I&O [intake and output]:	In: 1200 mL Ringer's lactate (R/L)
	Out: 400 mL urine
EBL [estimated blood loss]:	50 mL
Specimen:	None
Drains:	None
[Sign your name]	

ASA, Aspirin; *BP*, systolic blood pressure; *BRP*, bathroom privileges; *h*, hour; *HO*, house officer; *HR*, heart rate; *NPO*, nothing by mouth (this includes water and pills); *OOB*, out of bed; *PR*, per rectum; *PRN*, as needed; *q*, every; *r/o*, rule out; *T*, temperature.

Note: You cannot be too polite or too grateful to patients or nurses.

BIBLIOGRAPHY

Kripalani S, LeFevre F, Phillips CO, et al. Deficits in communication and information transfer between hospital-based and primary care physicians: implications for patient safety and continuity of care. *JAMA.* 2007;297:831–841.

CARDIOPULMONARY RESUSCITATION

Peter K. Moore, MD

CHAPTER 2

1. **What is cardiac arrest and sudden cardiac death?**
   Cardiac arrest is the sudden cessation of effective cardiac pumping function. Sudden cardiac death is the unexpected natural death from a cardiac cause within 1 hour of onset of symptoms, in a person without a previous condition that would appear fatal.

2. **What is the most common dysrhythmia encountered during sudden cardiac death and what is its treatment?**
   Ventricular fibrillation (VF) is the predominant rhythm encountered in the first 3–5 minutes after sudden cardiac arrest. Immediate therapy with defibrillation is the only effective treatment for VF and is most effective if performed within 5 minutes of collapse. Initiation of cardiopulmonary resuscitation (CPR) with chest compressions provides a small but critical amount of blood to the heart and brain while waiting for a defibrillator to arrive.

3. **What is the C-A-B approach to the pulseless patient for basic life support (BLS), and why was this changed from A-B-C?**
   The 2010 AHA guidelines for CPR changed the sequence in steps in BLS from A-B-C (airway, breathing, circulation) to C-A-B (circulation, airway, breathing). This change was made because the highest survival is seen among patients with cardiac arrest from pulseless ventricular tachycardia (VT) or VF. The critical initial elements in resuscitation of these patients are chest compressions and early defibrillation. Assessing the airway and delivering mouth-to-mouth breaths delays the critical time to performing defibrillation.

4. **What is the proper method of chest compressions in children and adults?**
   Rescuers should push hard and fast (rate 100–120 compressions per minute). The proper position for the hands during chest compressions in children and adults (about 1 year of age and older) is in the center of the chest at the nipple line. Using the heel of both hands, the rescuer should compress the chest approximately 2–2.5 inches for adults. The same method is used for children; however, one hand is often adequate to compress the chest, and the depth of compression should be one-third to one-half of the depth of the chest. Rescuers should allow complete chest recoil between compressions and minimize interruptions in compressions. Use 30:2 compression to ventilation ratio without an advanced airway or continuous chest compressions with advanced airway.

5. **Is endotracheal intubation mandatory during cardiopulmonary resuscitation?**
   No. Adequate ventilation may be achieved with proper airway positioning, an oropharyngeal or nasopharyngeal airway, and a bag-valve mask attached to an oxygen source. Insertion of an endotracheal tube may be deferred until the patient fails to respond to initial CPR and defibrillation. If an advanced airway is placed (endotracheal intubation or supraglottic airway), this should be performed by an experienced provider and should not interrupt adequate delivery of chest compressions.

6. **How is the airway positioned during a resuscitation attempt?**
   In an unconscious patient, the most common airway obstruction is the patient's tongue, which falls back into the throat when the muscles of the throat and tongue relax. Opening the airway to relieve the tongue from obstruction can be done using the head tilt-chin lift maneuver, or in the patient with suspected cervical spine injury, the jaw-thrust maneuver. If available, an oral airway or nasal trumpet should be inserted. Oral airway is preferred if there is suspicion for basal skull fracture or severe coagulopathy.

7. **What is the rate of ventilation after placement of an advanced airway?**
Delivery of one breath every 6 seconds (or 10 breaths per minute) is recommended while continuous chest compressions are being performed after an advanced airway is in place. It is important not to hyperventilate as this can increase intrathoracic pressure and lead to decreased preload and reduced cardiac output, especially in the setting of hypovolemia or obstructive lung disease. Hyperventilation may also lead to intracranial vasoconstriction, further impeding cerebral blood flow.

8. **What are the two major categories of cardiac arrest?**
Cardiac arrest can be divided into asystole/pulseless electrical activity (PEA) and pulseless VT/VF. PEA arrest was previously called electromechanical dissociation because, while the electrical system of the heart is functioning, there is mechanical dysfunction (which can be caused by a variety of conditions) resulting in inadequate cardiac output to maintain a pulse. In cardiac arrest purely due to VT/VF, inadequate cardiac output is mediated primarily by the rhythm disturbance: In VT, the heart is beating too rapidly to allow adequate filling during diastole, and in VF, there is chaotic rapid depolarization in the ventricle causing the heart to quiver rather than beat effectively.

9. **What are the reversible causes of PEA arrest?**
The potentially reversible causes of PEA arrest are split into "5 Hs and 5 Ts" (Table 2.1).
5 Hs:

> Hypovolemia
> Hypoxia
> Hydrogen ion (acidosis)
> Hyperkalemia (or hypokalemia or hypomagnesemia)
> Hypothermia

5 Ts:

> Toxins
> Tamponade, cardiac
> Tension pneumothorax
> Thrombosis, coronary (massive myocardial infarction)
> Thrombosis, pulmonary (massive pulmonary embolism)
> Trauma is sometimes included as a "sixth T," which causes cardiac arrest through one or more of the other Hs and Ts (hypovolemia, tamponade, tension pneumothorax).

Table 2.1 Scenarios and Treatments of Advanced Cardiac Life Support (ACLS)

CONDITION	CLINICAL SCENARIO	TREATMENT
Hs		
Hypovolemia	Trauma, major burns, GI bleed, diarrhea, diabetes	Fluids, blood products, evaluate for site of fluid/blood loss and treat
Hypoxia	Consider in all patients with cardiac arrest, those with underlying lung pathology, or risk for aspiration	Supplemental oxygen, advanced airway placement, ensure adequate CPR
Hypokalemia	Profound GI losses, diuretic use, diabetes, alcohol use, hypomagnesemia	If <2.5 meq/L give KCl 2 meq/min IV up to 10–15 meq then reassess Evaluate for hypomagnesemia
Hyperkalemia	Renal failure, dialysis patients, metabolic acidosis, massive tissue injury, rhabdomyolysis, hemolysis	CaCl 1 gram IV, NaHCO3 1–2 amps IV, Insulin 10 units IV w/ 1 amp D50, Continuous albuterol nebulizer
Hydrogen ions (acidosis)	Prolonged resuscitation, renal failure, sepsis, diabetes	Ensure adequate CPR and ventilation, NaHCO3 1–2 amp IV

Continued on following page

Table 2.1 Scenarios and Treatments of Advanced Cardiac Life Support (ACLS) *(Continued)*

CONDITION	CLINICAL SCENARIO	TREATMENT
Hypothermia	Burns, CNS disease, homeless, elderly, drowning, endocrinopathy (thyroid/adrenal), exposure	Active internal and external rewarming. Limit defibrillation to three attempts if temp <30°C, then restart usual ACS once temp >30°C Prolonged resuscitation may be appropriate
Ts		
Thrombosis, pulmonary	Hospitalized, recent surgery, pregnant, history of DVT	Consider thrombolytics or urgent ECMO
Thrombosis, coronary	Consider in all patients with cardiac arrest, especially those with known CAD	Consider thrombolytics, emergent cardiac catheterization
Toxins	Alcohol use, intoxication, classic toxidrome	Treat suspected ingestion (naloxone for opioids, $NaHCO_3$ for TCA, consider intravenous lipid emulsion for local anesthetic overdose) Prolonged resuscitation may be appropriate
Tamponade, cardiac	Postcardiac surgery, thoracic trauma, post MI, pericarditis	Administer intravenous fluids, emergent pericardiocentesis, thoracotomy, and pericardial window
Tension Pneumothorax	Trauma, mechanical ventilation, placement of central line, lung disease	Needle thoracostomy, chest tube placement.

10. **What are the causes of pulseless VT/VF?**
    VT/VF is most commonly seen in:
    a. Active myocardial infarction/ischemia;
    b. Structurally abnormal hearts (cardiomyopathy, scar from prior myocardial infarction, infiltrative diseases);
    c. Electrolyte/metabolic disturbance (hypomagnesemia, severe hypokalemia, QT-interval prolonging medications, severe hypothermia);
    d. Rare inherited disorders that affect myocardial conduction (Brugada syndrome, hypertrophic obstructive cardiomyopathy, arrhythmogenic right ventricular dysplasia, long QT syndrome).

11. **Describe the general principles of advanced cardiac life support (ACLS) for a pulseless patient**
    ACLS algorithms have been simplified to aid in adherence to key principles that may help achieve return of spontaneous circulation (ROSC) and improve survival. When a patient is pulseless, CPR should be started immediately and supplemental oxygen delivered. A defibrillator/cardiac monitor should be placed as soon as possible to determine whether the patient has a shockable rhythm (VT/VF) or nonshockable rhythm (PEA/asystole). If the rhythm is shockable, defibrillation with 120–200 J with a monophasic defibrillator (or 360 J if monophasic defibrillator) should be performed immediately followed by resumption of chest compression. In both shockable and nonshockable algorithms, 2 minutes of high quality chest compressions should be performed between each pulse and rhythm check; epinephrine 1 mg should be given every 3–5 minutes; and reversible causes should be treated (Table 2.1). For shockable rhythms refractory to cardioversion, antiarrhythmics can be given. This cycle of defibrillation (if shockable), CPR for 2 minutes, brief pulse/rhythm check is repeated until the patient has ROSC or resuscitative measures are terminated.

12. **What medications and interventions are used in asystole/PEA arrest?**
Epinephrine 1 mg intravenous (IV) or intraosseous (IO) (endotracheal administration if no other access) every 3–5 minutes. This should be given as soon as possible. Observational studies of both in hospital and out of hospital cardiac arrest with nonshockable rhythms have found that earlier epinephrine administration is associated with increased ROSC, survival to hospital discharge, and neurologically intact survival. Treatment guided by the suspected underlying reversible cause of PEA arrest should be given (Table 2.1). Vasopressin and atropine are no longer recommended for treatment of PEA arrest. See question 18 for discussion of corticosteroids in cardiac arrest.

13. **Is there a role for routine fibrinolysis in patients with pulseless electrical activity cardiac arrest?**
No. The results from a large clinical trial failed to show any significant treatment effect when a fibrinolytic agent (tPA) was given to out-of-hospital patients with undifferentiated cardiac arrest unresponsive to initial interventions. Individual patients in cardiac arrest in whom a strong suspicion for PE exists (e.g., immobilized patient, peripartum, deep venous thrombosis [DVT] by history or suggested by physical examination) may benefit from the use of fibrinolytics as a last-ditch, life-saving intervention.

14. **What medications and interventions are used for VT/VF arrest?**
Defibrillation is the mainstay of treatment for pulseless VT/VF. Epinephrine 1 mg IV/IO every 3–5 minutes is the vasopressor of choice in any pulseless cardiac arrest including VT/VF. Amiodarone is administered for VT/VF that is refractory to defibrillation. An initial dose of 300 mg IV or IO is given. A second dose of 150 mg can be given if the patient remains in VT/VF after the first dose. Lidocaine can be given as alternative to amiodarone. The first dose should be 1–1.5 mg/kg IV or IO. Subsequent doses of 0.5–0.75 mg/kg can be given for total of up to 3 mg/kg. Magnesium should be administered if polymorphic ventricular tachycardia (torsades de pointes) is seen on the cardiac monitor or is suspected. There is no benefit to routine administration of magnesium in VT/VF that is not mediated by torsades de pointes. Vasopressin is no longer recommended for treatment of pulseless VT/VF.

15. **What options are available for medication delivery during cardiac resuscitation?**
During cardiac arrest, access can be obtained with large-bore peripheral intravenous (IV) catheters, central venous catheters, or intraosseous (IO) cannulation. IO access is being used more frequently when peripheral IV access cannot be obtained expediently. Epinephrine can be given through an endotracheal tube, if IV or IO access has not been obtained.

16. **What physiologic parameters can be monitored to assess for adequacy of CPR?**
Animal studies have demonstrated that end-tidal CO_2 (ETCO$_2$), arterial relaxation pressure, and central venous oxygen saturation (SCVO$_2$) correlate with cardiac output during CPR. While no clinical study has evaluated titrating to specific goals, the current AHA guidelines state that it is reasonable to follow physiologic measures of cardiac output to monitor/optimize CPR and to detect ROSC. These measures include quantitative waveform capnography (if intubated), invasive arterial pressure monitoring (if arterial catheter is in place), central venous oxygen saturation (if central venous catheter with SCVO$_2$ monitoring is in place prior to cardiac arrest). Previous guidelines had set goals of ETCO$_2$ >10 mm Hg, diastolic blood pressure >20 mm Hg and SCVO$_2$ >30%. However, there are no longer specific titration parameters in the latest AHA guidelines given lack of evidence for precise numerical targets. An abrupt, sustained increase in ETCO$_2$ >40 mm Hg or spontaneous arterial pressure waves on the intraarterial monitor are suggestive of ROSC.

17. **How can bedside ultrasound assist with CPR?**
Bedside ultrasound can be used during PEA arrest to assess for pericardial effusion, tension pneumothorax, massive PE, and myocardial infarction in the hands of an experienced operator. It is reasonable to use bedside cardiac and noncardiac ultrasound during PEA arrest as long as it does not interfere with adequate delivery of chest compressions. However, one limited small study did not find that ultrasound during PEA arrest had a significant effect on ROSC, and the exact usefulness of bedside ultrasound has yet to be established.

18. **What is the role of corticosteroids in cardiac arrest?**
The exact role of corticosteroids in cardiac arrest is still not fully understood. A modest sized single-center RCT and a subsequent three-center RCT of patients with in-hospital cardiac arrest found survival benefit and improved neurologic outcome with combination therapy of methylprednisolone, vasopressin, and epinephrine during cardiac arrest with hydrocortisone after ROSC compared to epinephrine and placebo. However, in a separate study of out-of-hospital cardiac arrest, administration of dexamethasone was not associated with improvements in ROSC or survival. At this time, the AHA does not recommend for or against the routine use of corticosteroids in cardiac arrest.

19. **What are the initial objectives of postresuscitation support after return of spontaneous circulation (ROSC)?**
There are three main principles around post arrest care: (1) identification and treatment of underlying cause of cardiac arrest, (2) provision of adequate circulatory support while mitigating ischemia-reperfusion injury, (3) prognostication to guide clinical team and inform family when selecting goals of care. If the patient is hypotensive vasopressors should be started with a goal MAP >65 mm Hg. Supplemental oxygen should be supplied and titrated to a goal arterial oxygen saturation of ≥94%. A 12-lead electrocardiogram should be obtained as soon as possible after ROSC. If acute ST elevations are present or cardiac etiology of arrest is suspect, prompt coronary angiography and percutaneous coronary intervention should be performed. In patients unresponsive after cardiac arrest, therapeutic hypothermia should be considered. Prognostication using clinical neurologic examination should be undertaken 72 hours after cardiac arrest or 72 hours after return to normothermia if the patient was therapeutically cooled. The prognostication exam may be performed later if the exam is thought to be confounded by the residual effects of sedative or paralytic medications.

20. **What is postresuscitation targeted temperature management (therapeutic hypothermia)?**
Postresuscitation induction of hypothermia for comatose patients with return of spontaneous circulation has been shown to lead to improved neurologic outcome in patients with cardiac arrest. Initial studies cooled patients to 32°C–34°C, but a recent well-designed study noted no difference in outcomes between goal temperature of 33°C and 36°C. Consequently, guidelines now recommend targeted temperature management in comatose patients with a constant temperature between 32°C and 36°C for at least 24 hours. Cooling can be achieved using external cooling techniques (e.g., cooling blankets and frequent application of ice bags) or internal cooling techniques (e.g., cold saline, endovascular cooling catheter). Cooling can result in coagulopathy, bradycardia, other cardiac arrhythmias, hypotension, and hyperglycemia. There are few true contraindications to cooling, but the risk is higher in patients with documented intracranial hemorrhage, severe hemorrhage, hypotension refractory to vasopressors, or pregnancy. Hyperthermia should be avoided in all patients after cardiac arrest.

21. **What are the common causes for cardiac arrest resulting from anaphylaxis?**
Life-threatening anaphylaxis is seen with reactions to antibiotics (especially parenteral penicillins and other b-lactams), aspirin and nonsteroidal antiinflammatory drugs, and IV contrast agents. Certain foods, including nuts, seafood, and wheat, are associated with life-threatening anaphylaxis from bronchospasm and asphyxia.

22. **What advanced cardiac life support modifications are required in patients with cardiac arrest resulting from anaphylaxis?**
Cardiac arrest from anaphylaxis is a result of acute airway obstruction coupled with profound venous vasodilation leading to cardiovascular collapse. Early endotracheal intubation, prolonged CPR, aggressive volume administration (typically between 4 and 8 L of isotonic crystalloid), and adrenergic drugs are the cornerstones of therapy. Patients with full cardiac arrest may receive high-dose epinephrine (i.e., escalating from 1 mg to 3 mg to 5 mg over 5 minutes). Surgical or needle cricothyrotomy is indicated if airway edema precludes endotracheal intubation.

23. **What advanced cardiac life support modifications are required in patients with cardiac arrest associated with trauma?**
Basic and advanced life support for the trauma patient is fundamentally the same as that for the patient with a primary cardiac arrest. Hypovolemia, tension pneumothorax, and pericardial tamponade must be quickly evaluated and addressed during resuscitation. Surgical management of these conditions, including bedside thoracotomy and resuscitative endovascular balloon occlusion of the aorta (REBOA), are discussed in the trauma chapter.

24. **Should all patients in cardiac arrest receive cardiopulmonary resuscitation?**
No. Legitimate reasons to withhold CPR include:
    a. The patient has a valid do not resuscitate (DNR) order.
    b. The patient has signs of irreversible death (e.g., rigor mortis, decapitation, decomposition, or dependent lividity).
    c. No physiologic benefit can be expected because vital functions have deteriorated despite maximal therapy (e.g., progressive septic or cardiogenic shock).

25. When should resuscitative efforts be terminated?

The decision to terminate resuscitative efforts rests with the treating physician in the hospital and is based on consideration of many factors, including time to CPR, time to defibrillation, comorbid disease, prearrest state, and initial arrest rhythm. $ETCO_2$ <10 mm Hg after 20 minutes of CPR is associated with poor outcomes and can assist in the decision to terminate resuscitation. None of these factors alone or in combination is clearly predictive of outcome. Reports indicated that prolonged CPR could be effective in cardiac arrest resulting from hypothermia, drug overdose, and anaphylaxis.

26. Can family members be present during resuscitation of a loved one?

Yes. Not only do the majority of family members surveyed prior to a resuscitation state that they would like to be present during a resuscitation attempt, many family members say that it is comforting to be at the side of their loved one and eases the grief associated with a sudden or expected loss.

BIBLIOGRAPHY

1. Link MS, Berkow LC, Kudenchuk PJ, et al. Part 7: adult advanced cardiovascular life support. *Circulation.* 2015;132(18):S444–S466. (suppl 2).
2. Mentzelopoulos SD, Malachias S, Chamos C, et al. Vasopressin, steroids, and epinephrine and neurologically favorable survival after in-hospital cardiac arrest. *JAMA.* 2013;310(3):270–279.
3. Neumar RW, Shuster M, Callaway CW, et al. Part 1: executive summary. *Circulation.* 2015;132(18):S315–S368. (suppl 2).
4. Nielsen N, Wetterslev J, Cronberg T, et al. Targeted temperature management at 33°C versus 36°C after cardiac arrest. *N Engl J Med.* 2013;369(23):2197–2206.
5. Scirica BM. Therapeutic hypothermia after cardiac arrest. *Circulation.* 2013;127(2):244–250.

HOW TO TREAT ALL CARDIAC DYSRHYTHMIAS

Ashley Eleen Morgan, MD, Alden H. Harken, MD, FACS

CHAPTER 3

1. **Are all cardiac dysrhythmias clinically important?**
   Most are not. Many of us have isolated premature ventricular contractions (PVCs) or premature ventricular depolarizations (PVDs) all the time. Superbly conditioned athletes frequently exhibit resting heart rates in the 30s. A clinically important cardiac dysrhythmia is a rhythm that bothers the patient. As a rule, if the patient's ventricular rate is 60–100 beats per minute (regardless of mechanism), cardiac rhythm is not a problem.

2. **State the goals in the treatment of cardiac dysrhythmias**
   The primary goal is to control ventricular rate between 60 and 100 beats per minute, and the secondary goal is to maintain sinus rhythm.

3. **How important is sinus rhythm?**
   It depends on the patient's ventricular function. Induction of atrial fibrillation in a medical student volunteer causes no measurable hemodynamic effect. Your ventricular compliance is so good that you do not need an atrial "kick" to fill the ventricle completely.
   Conversely, the worse (the stiffer) the older patient's heart, the more you should try to maintain sinus rhythm. We observed a patient with a 7% left ventricular (LV) ejection fraction (EF) whose cardiac output (CO) decreased by 40% when he postoperatively developed atrial fibrillation.

4. **Do you need to be ankle deep in electrocardiogram paper and be personally acquainted with Drs Mobitz, Lown, and Ganong to treat cardiac dysrhythmias in the intensive care unit (ICU)?**
   No.

5. **When you are called by the ICU nurse to see a patient with any dysrhythmia, what questions do you ask yourself?**
   a. *Does the patient really exhibit a dysrhythmia?* What is the patient doing? Is the stuff that looks like ventricular fibrillation (VF) really just the patient brushing his or her teeth? Or is the rhythm strip that looks like asystole really just a loose lead?
   If you still think that the patient has a cardiac rhythm problem, ask yourself the following questions:
   b. *Does the arrhythmia require intervention?* Isolated PVCs usually can be ignored safely. Similarly, a resting bradycardia in a triathlete is normal. This is the occasion to launch into your "2-second physical exam." Is the patient sweaty and confused or alert and happy?
   c. *What is a 2-second physical exam?* You look into the patient's eyes, hoping to determine whether he or she is perfusing his or her brain. If the patient looks back at you, you have some time.
   If the patient requires therapy, ask yourself the following question:
   d. *How soon is therapy required?* At this point, the patient becomes (paradoxically) irrelevant. The most robust indicator dictating velocity of intervention is not how sick the patient is but how frightened you are. You must determine rapidly whether delay in therapy is likely to put the patient at risk. If the cardiac arrhythmia is likely to inflict psychopathologic (hypoxemic) consequences not only on the patient but also, by extension, on his or her extended (societal) family, you should be frightened.
   If you are frightened, you must ask yourself:
   e. *What is the safest and most effective therapy?*

6. **If the patient requires antiarrhythmic therapy, what is the safest and most effective strategy?**
   Therapy for cardiac arrhythmias is simple and comprises three comprehensible concepts:
   a. If the patient is hemodynamically unstable (the sole determinant of instability is whether you are frightened), cardiovert with maximum J. (For lower energy, see Chapter 2.)

    b. If the patient has a wide-complex tachycardia, cardiovert with maximum J.

    c. If the patient has a narrow-complex tachycardia, infuse an atrioventricular (AV) nodal blocker intravenously (IV). If at any time the patient becomes unstable, proceed with cardioversion.

7. **In assessing a cardiac impulse, how do you distinguish supraventricular from ventricular origin?**

Supraventricular origin: When an impulse originates above the AV node (supraventricular) it can access the ventricles only through the AV node. The AV node connects with the endocardial Purkinje system, which conducts impulses rapidly (2–3 m/sec). A supraventricular impulse activates the ventricles rapidly (<0.08 seconds, 80 msec, or two little boxes on the electrocardiogram [ECG] paper), producing a narrow-complex beat.

Ventricular origin: When an impulse originates directly from an ectopic site on the ventricle, it takes longer to access the high-speed Purkinje system. A ventricular impulse activates the entire ventricular mass slowly (>0.08 seconds, 80 msec, or two little boxes on the ECG paper), producing a wide-complex beat (Fig. 3.1).

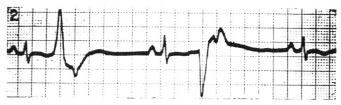

Fig. 3.1 Wide-complex beats are of ventricular origin. Narrow-complex beats are of supraventricular origin.

8. **Extra credit: Correlate the ECG with cardiomyocyte membrane ion flux. (Fig. 3.2)**

9. **Do all wide-complex beats derive from the ventricles?**

No, but most do. An impulse of supraventricular origin that is conducted with aberrancy through the ventricle can take enough time to make it a wide-complex beat. In one study, 89% of 100 patients presenting to an emergency department (ED) with a wide-complex tachycardia eventually proved to exhibit ventricular tachycardia, whereas 11% were diagnosed with supraventricular tachycardia with aberrancy.

10. **What do you do if you cannot tell whether a ventricular complex is wide or narrow?**

Acutely and transiently (for 5 seconds) block the AV node by giving 6 mg of adenosine IV; if the ventricular complex persists, it is ventricular. If the ventricular complex stops, it was supraventricular.

11. **To prevent lots of supraventricular impulses from getting to the ventricles, how do you block the atrioventricular node pharmacologically?**

In seconds: Give 6 mg adenosine IV push.

In minutes: Draw up 20 mg Diltiazem (calcium channel blocker), and infuse as IV over 2 minutes. If necessary, start continuous IV infusion of 5–10 mg/hr immediately following IV bolus. (For IV infusion, do not exceed 15 mg/hr and the drug should not be infused for more than 24 hours.)

In hours: Put 0.5 mg digoxin in 100 mL of Ringer's lactate and infuse by IV drip over 30 minutes.

In days: Give amiodarone 200 mg orally every day.

KEY POINTS: CHARACTERIZATION OF CARDIAC DYSRHYTHMIAS

1. Supraventricular origin: When an impulse originates above the AV node, it can access the ventricles only through the AV node to reach the Purkinje system, which conducts and activates the ventricles rapidly, producing a narrow-complex beat (<2 small boxes on ECG).

2. Ventricular origin: When an impulse originates from an ectopic site on the ventricle, it takes longer to access the high-speed Purkinje system. A ventricular impulse activates the entire mass, slowly producing a wide-complex beat (>2 small boxes on ECG).

3. Not all wide-complex beats are ventricular in origin.

4. To distinguish ventricular from supraventricular tachycardia, transiently block the AV node with adenosine intravenous push. If ventricular complex persists, it is ventricular tachycardia; if the complex stops, it is supraventricular tachycardia.

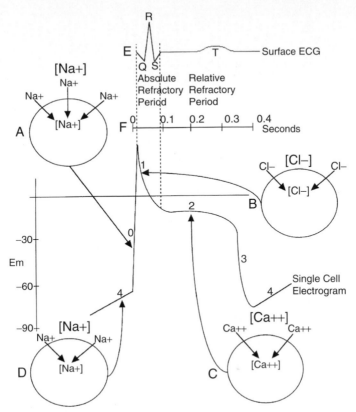

Fig. 3.2 Typical action potential of a cardiac myocyte, the ionic shifts responsible for each phase, and correlation with the surface ECG. **A,** Phase 0 = rapid depolarization, characterized by rapid influx of sodium (Na+) through the voltage-gated Na+ channels. **B,** Phase 1 = brief repolarization, characterized by transient influx of chloride (Cl-). **C,** Phase 2 = plateau phase, characterized by a rapid rise in calcium (Ca2+) permeability through L-type Ca2+ channels. Phase 3 = repolarization with potassium (K+) exiting the cell. **D,** Slow depolarization of pacemaker cells caused by slow influx of Na+. *(From Meldrum DR, Cleveland JC, Sheridan BC, et al. Cardiac surgical implications of calcium dyshomeostasis in the heart.* Ann Thorac Surg *1996;61:1273–1280.)*

12. **Why give digoxin?**
    Digoxin is an effective AV nodal blocker, but it makes cardiomyocytes more excitable. By giving digoxin, you make supraventricular impulses more likely, but by blocking the AV node, you render these impulses less dangerous.

13. **Why infuse digoxin over 30–60 minutes intravenously?**
    Studies indicate that a big pulse of digoxin (IV push) concentrates in the myocardium, making the myocytes hyperexcitable. Digoxin infused more slowly avoids this problem.

14. **List the steps in calling a dysrhythmia by name**
    Bradycardia: <60 beats per minute
    Tachycardia: 100–250 beats per minute
    Flutter: Atrial or ventricular rate 250–400 beats per minute
    Fibrillation: Atrial or ventricular rate >400 beats per minute

BIBLIOGRAPHY

Harken AH. Cardiovascular pharmacology. In: Cameron JL, Cameron AM, eds. *Current Surgical Therapy.* 12th ed. Philadelphia: Elsevier; 2017.

CHAPTER 4

HOW TO THINK ABOUT SHOCK

Kathryn H. Chomsky-Higgins, MD, MS, Alden H. Harken, MD, FACS

1. **Define shock**
   Shock is:
   - Not just low blood pressure
   - Not just decreased peripheral perfusion
   - Not just limited systemic oxygen delivery

   Ultimately, shock is decreased tissue respiration. Shock is suboptimal consumption of oxygen and excretion of carbon dioxide (CO_2) at the cellular level.

2. **Is shock related to cardiac output?**
   Yes. A healthy medical student can redistribute blood flow preferentially to vital organs. After a 3- to 4-unit bleed, your typical young gunslinger can still think and can tell you, "Four dudes jumped me." From this history you have no idea what happened to him, but you do know that he is still perfusing his brain.

3. **Is organ perfusion democratic?**
   No. Limited blood flow always is redirected toward the carotid and coronary arteries. Peripheral vasoconstriction steals blood initially from the mesentery, then skeletal muscle, and then kidneys and liver.

4. **Is this vascular autoregulatory capacity uniform in all patients?**
   No. With age and atherosclerosis, patients lose their ability to redistribute limited blood flow. A 20% decrease in cardiac output (CO), or a fall in blood pressure to 90 mm Hg, can be life-threatening to a Supreme Court justice, whereas it may be undetectable in a triathlete.

5. **For diagnostic and practical therapeutic purposes, can shock be classified?**
   Yes. See Table 4.1.
   a. Hypovolemic shock mandates volume resuscitation.
   b. Cardiogenic shock mandates cardiac stimulation (pharmacologic and eventually mechanical).
   c. Peripheral vascular collapse shock mandates pharmacologic manipulation of the peripheral vascular tone (and direct attention to the cause of the vasodilation—typically sepsis).

6. **Is it advisable to treat all shock in the same sequential fashion?**
   Ultimately, yes. Whether a cigar-chomping banker presents with a big gastrointestinal (GI) bleed (hypovolemic shock) or crushing substernal chest pain (cardiogenic shock), the surgeon should take the following steps in order:
   a. Optimize volume status; give volume until further increase in right-sided (central venous pressure [CVP]) and left-sided (pulmonary capillary wedge pressure [PCWP]) preload confers no additional benefit for CO or blood pressure (BP). (This step is Starling's law; place the patient's heart at the top of the Starling curve.)
   b. If CO, BP, and tissue perfusion remain inadequate despite adequate preload, the patient has a pump (cardiogenic shock) problem. Infuse cardiac inotropic drugs (β-agonist) to the point of toxicity (typically cardiac ectopy), which will have lots of frightening premature ventricular contractions. For pharmacologically refractory cardiogenic shock, insert an intraaortic balloon pump (IABP).
   c. If the patient exhibits a surprisingly high CO and a paradoxically low BP (such unusual loss of vascular autoregulatory control is associated typically, but not always, with sepsis), infuse a peripheral vasoconstrictor drug (α-agonist).

7. **What is the preferred access route for volume infusion?**
   Flow depends on catheter length and radius. Volume may be infused at twice the rate through a 5-cm, 14-gauge peripheral catheter as through a 20-cm, 16-gauge central line. Assessment of CVP (and left-sided filling pressure) is necessary if the patient fails to respond to initial volume resuscitation.

Table 4.1 Shock Types

SHOCK TYPE	CO	CVP/PCWP	SVR
Hypovolemic	↓	↓	↑
Cardiogenic	↓	↑	↑
Peripheral vascular collapse (septic)	↑	↑	↓

CO, Cardiac output; CVP, central venous pressure; PCWP, pulmonary capillary wedge pressure; SVR, system
vascular resistance.

8. **Should one infuse crystalloid, colloid, or blood?**
   If the goal is only to improve preload and to repair CO and BP, crystalloid solution should be sufficient. It is controversial whether infused colloid remains in the vascular compartment. If the goal is to augment systemic oxygen delivery, red blood cells bind much more oxygen than plasma (see Chapter 7). Crystalloid should enhance flow, and blood should augment oxygen delivery.

9. **When cardiac preload is adequate, which inotropic agents are useful?**
   Dobutamine, epinephrine, and norepinephrine are the chocolate, vanilla, and strawberry of the 32 flavors of cardiogenic drugs. These three drugs are all that the surgeon really needs.

10. **Is dopamine the same as dobutamine?**
    No. Dopamine stimulates renal dopaminergic receptors and may be useful in low doses (2 mcg/kg per minute) to counteract the renal arteriolar vasoconstriction that accompanies shock. Dopamine has no place as a primary cardiac inotropic agent.

11. **Discuss the use of dobutamine, epinephrine, and norepinephrine**
    See Table 4.2.

12. **When is an intraaortic balloon pump indicated?**
    Mechanical circulatory support is indicated when the preload to both ventricles (CVP and PCWP) has been optimized and further cardiac stimulatory drugs are limited by frightening runs of premature ventricular contractions. Do not be afraid to resort to mechanical support.

KEY POINTS: SUMMARY OF ADRENERGIC AGENTS

1. Dobutamine: β1 agonist (cardiac inotrope) with mild-to-moderate β2 effects (peripheral vasodilation).
2. Epinephrine: Combined β and α adrenergic agent, with the β effects predominating at lower doses and progressive vasoconstriction accompanying increased doses.
3. Norepinephrine: Combined β and α adrenergic agonist, with the α effects predominating at all doses.

---

13. **What does an intraaortic balloon pump do?**
    It provides diastolic augmentation and systolic unloading.

14. **What is diastolic augmentation?**
    A soft 40-mL balloon is inserted percutaneously through the common femoral artery into the descending thoracic aorta. The balloon is not occlusive (it should not touch the aortic walls). When it is inflated, it displaces 40 mL of blood and is exactly like acutely transfusing 40 mL of blood into the aorta, augmenting each left ventricular stroke volume by 40 mL. Balloon infusion is triggered by the QRS complex from a surface ECG (any lead). The balloon is always inflated during diastole to increase diastolic blood pressure (DBP) and augment coronary blood flow (CBF). Eighty percent of CBF occurs during diastole.

Use of Dobutamine, Epinephrine, and Norepinephrine

...ne is a β1 agonist ...c inotrope), but it ...has some β2 effects ...ipheral vasodilation).	*Start at:* 5 mcg/kg per minute and increase to the point of toxicity (cardiac ectopy).	*Note:* Infuse to desired effect (do not stick rigidly to a preconceived dose). Because dobutamine has some vasodilating effects, it may be frightening to infuse into typically hypotensive patients in shock.
Epinephrine is a combined β and α adrenergic agonist, with the β effects prevailing at lower doses and progressive vasoconstriction accompanying increased doses.	*Start at:* 0.05 mcg/kg per minute and increase to point of toxicity (cardiac ectopy).	*Note:* As with dobutamine, infuse to desired effect.
Norepinephrine is a combined α and β adrenergic agonist, with the α effects prevailing at all doses.	*Start at:* 0.05 mg/kg per minute and increase to point of toxicity (cardiac ectopy).	*Note:* Relatively pure peripheral vasoconstriction rarely is indicated and should be used only to modulate the peripheral vascular tone in peripheral vascular collapse shock.

KEY POINTS: INTRAAORTIC BALLOON PUMP

1. Indicated for cardiogenic shock refractory to pharmacologic manipulation.
2. Triggered by QRS complex of surface ECG; inflates during diastole (T wave) and deflates on systole (R wave or at dicrotic notch on aortic pressure curve).
3. Eighty percent of CBF occurs during diastole.
4. Mechanistically results in diastolic augmentation and systolic unloading (afterload reduction).

15. What is systolic unloading?

Balloon deflation is an active (not a passive) process. Helium abruptly is sucked out of the balloon, leaving a 40-mL empty space in the aorta. The left ventricle can eject the first 40 mL of its stroke volume into this empty space at dramatically reduced workload. An intraaortic balloon increases CBF during diastole, while decreasing cardiac oxygen consumption just presystole.

16. Name the contraindications to intraaortic balloon pump

The two main contraindications to an IABP are aortic insufficiency and atrial fibrillation. In the case of aortic insufficiency, diastolic augmentation distends and injures the left ventricle. An IABP is contraindicated in atrial fibrillation because balloon inflation and deflation cannot be appropriately timed.

BIBLIOGRAPHY

1. Rivers E, Nguyen B, Havstad S, et al. Early Goal-Directed Therapy Collaborative Group. Early goal-directed therapy in the treatment of severe sepsis and septic shock. *N Engl J Med.* 2001;345:1368–1377.
2. Investigators ProCESS, Yealy DM, Kellum JA, Huang DT, et al. A randomized trial of protocol-based care for early septic shock. *N Engl J Med.* 2014;370:1683–1693.

CONGESTIVE HEART FAILURE (CHF) AND PULMONARY INSUFFICIENCY

Magdalene A. Brooke, MD, Alden H. Harken, MD, FACS

CHAPTER 5

1. **What is congested in CHF?**
   The lungs.

2. **Why the lungs?**
   When cardiac output falls, the kidney releases renin. Renin converts angiotensinogen to angiotensin I in the liver. Angiotensin I is converted to angiotensin II by angiotensin-converting enzyme (ACE) in the lung. Angiotensin II stimulates release of aldosterone from the adrenal and antidiuretic hormone (ADH) from the posterior pituitary. Both aldosterone and AHD collaborate to increase blood volume. As the left ventricle fails, blood is backed up in the lungs. As the pulmonary vasculature fills, intravascular hydrostatic pressure pushes fluid into the pulmonary extravascular space, "congesting" the lungs. Lung congestion prevents ventilated alveoli (Va) from matching up with pulmonary capillary blood flow (Q).

3. **What is Va/Q?**
   The ratio of alveolar ventilation to perfusion.

4. **What should Va/Q be?**
   Equal, or one.

5. **What is the alveolar-capillary surface area of a healthy pair of lungs?**
   About the size of a singles tennis court.

6. **What is it called when alveoli are not ventilated (Va = 0) but are perfused?**
   A shunt.

7. **What is it called when alveoli are ventilated but are not perfused?**
   Dead space.

8. **What is functional reserve capacity (FRC)?**
   The volume of air left in your lungs when you stop exhaling after a normal breath.

9. **What is closing volume?**
   As we exhale down below FRC toward residual volume (RV), we reach a point at which we close off terminal airways so that alveoli are no longer ventilated but are perfused, creating a shunt. Closing volume (CV) is the minimum volume required to keep airways from collapsing.

10. **Why is closing volume important in CHF?**
    As our patients go into CHF their FRC decreases below the CV, so that alveolar collapse and the corresponding shunt become prominent during normal tidal breathing.

11. **Do we see this in the inpatient setting?**
    Yes, it is common in the ICU.

12. **Can we do anything about it?**
    Yes. If we raise positive end-expiratory pressure (PEEP) to a ventilator, we prevent full exhalation, thus increasing FRC above closing volume. This prevents terminal airways from collapsing, which avoids Va/Q mismatch, which avoids shunting.

13. **How much energy is expended in the work of breathing?**
A healthy medical student expends about 3% of total oxygen consumption (energy use) on work of breathing. After injury, particularly a large burn, patients may increase fractional energy expenditure of breathing to 20% of their total energy use.

14. **Which surgical incisions most significantly compromise a patient's vital capacity?**
Intuitively, an extremity incision or injury influences vital capacity least, followed sequentially by a lower abdominal incision, median sternotomy, thoracotomy, and upper abdominal incision. An upper abdominal incision is worse than a thoracotomy!

15. **Is a chest radiograph helpful in assessing respiratory failure?**
Yes, it can help identify the cause and severity of respiratory failure in many cases. A negative chest radiograph in respiratory failure also helps rule out obvious etiologies.

16. **What should you look for on the chest radiograph of a patient with impending respiratory failure?**
    a. Are the endotracheal and other tubes in proper position?
    b. Are both lungs fully expanded?
    c. Are there localized areas of infiltrate, atelectasis, or consolidation?
    d. Are there generalized areas of infiltrate, atelectasis, or consolidation?

17. **What is acute respiratory distress syndrome?**
ARDS is diffuse respiratory failure that cannot be explained purely by cardiac failure or fluid overload. It typically occurs in patients who are critically ill and significantly increases a patient's chances of death.

18. **How does ARDS compromise lung function?**
ARDS is a diffuse, multilobar capillary transudation of fluid into the pulmonary interstitium that dissociates the normal concordance of Va with Q. Strictly speaking, the pulmonary artery hydrostatic pressure (PAP) must also be below 18 mm Hg. This distinguishes pure left ventricular failure (with a high PAP) from "leaky" pulmonary endovasculature characteristic of ARDS. This buildup of alveolar fluid leads to impaired oxygenation, decreased lung compliance, and secondary inflammatory damage to the alveoli. ARDS patients often require mechanical ventilation.

19. **What causes ARDS?**
ARDS is caused by injury to the alveoli, either direct or indirect. Direct causes would include alveolar damage through infection (pneumonia), chemical trauma (aspiration, smoke inhalation), or physical trauma (pulmonary contusions). Indirect injury to lung tissue occurs through generalized inflammatory states such as in patients suffering from sepsis, severe trauma, significant burns, or transfusion reactions.

KEY POINTS: CLINICAL FEATURES OF ACUTE RESPIRATORY DISTRESS SYNDROME

1. Severe hypoxemia refractory to increased inspired oxygen concentration
2. Diffuse pulmonary infiltrates
3. Low lung compliance (a stiff lung requires higher peak inspiratory pressure in order to ventilate the patient)
4. Large ventilation/perfusion (V/Q) mismatch

---

20. **What governs fluid flux across pulmonary capillaries into the interstitium of the lung?**
Starling initially described the balance between intravascular hydrostatic pressure (Pc), which tends to push fluid out of the capillaries, and colloid oncotic pressure (COP), which pulls fluid back in across the capillary endothelial barrier (K).

21. **What is a normal colloid oncotic pressure (COP)?**
It is 22 mm Hg.

22. **What produces colloid oncotic pressure?**
There are hundreds of proteins floating around in our blood, but 75% of the COP is created by serum albumin and globulins.

23. **What is pulmonary capillary wedge pressure (PCWP)?**
The PCWP reflects the pulmonary capillary hydrostatic pressure that conceptually pushes fluid out into the lung interstitium. Measurement requires floating a pulmonary artery (Swan-Ganz) catheter and blowing up the balloon to "wedge" it into the pulmonary capillaries. We don't use these catheters much anymore, but they can be useful in assessing left ventricular "preload."

24. **Define low-pressure ARDS**
Low-pressure ARDS is a redundant term. To make the diagnosis of ARDS, the PCWP must be <18 mm Hg.

25. **How can the pulmonary capillaries leak if the COP exceeds the PCWP?**
The current concept involves a septic expression of neutrophil CD11 and CD18 adhesion receptors, which stick to pulmonary vascular endothelial intercellular adhesion molecules (ICAM). Septic stimuli provoke the adherent neutrophils to release intravascular proteases and oxygen radicals. Resultant endovascular damage permits leakage, even at low PCWP.

26. **What is a "Lasix sandwich"?**
This refers to a technique often used by surgeons when they are concerned that a patient is depleted of intravascular fluid (hypotensive with low urine output) but overloaded with extravascular fluid (chest x-ray [CXR] showing "wet" lungs or known severe CHF). Generally, a colloid such as albumin is given followed in 20 minutes by a diuretic such as furosemide (Lasix). The concept is that albumin will pull fluid from a water-logged lung by increasing intravascular oncotic pressure. The Lasix then promotes diuresis of this extra fluid. This therapeutic concept probably works only in patients who are not very sick. The sicker the patient, the faster the infused albumin leaks and equilibrates across the damaged endovascular endothelial barrier.

27. **List the goals of therapy for ARDS**
    a. Reduce lung edema (typically with a diuretic).
    b. Reduce oxygen toxicity (inspired oxygen concentration <60% is safe).
    c. Limit lung barotrauma (avoid peak inspiratory pressure in >40 cm H_2O).
    d. Promote matching of V and Q; frequently positive end-expiratory pressure (PEEP) is useful.
    e. Maintain systemic oxygen delivery (arterial oxygen content × cardiac output [CO]).

28. **What governs the distribution of lung perfusion?**
Primarily gravity. The dependent portions of the lung always are better perfused.

29. **Discuss hypoxic pulmonary vasoconstriction (HPV)**
Most students believe that after dedicating the entire second year of medical school to pheochromocytoma and hypoxic pulmonary vasoconstriction (HPV), both entities may be safely forgotten. At least in the case of HPV, this is not true. A patient who has just undergone carotid endarterectomy (CEA) illustrates the relevance of HPV. As the patient awakens from anesthesia, the blood pressure (BP) is 220/120 mm Hg and arterial partial pressure of oxygen (PO_2) with 100 % oxygen is 400 mm Hg. So that the patient will not blow the carotid anastomosis, the surgeon urgently infuses nitroprusside. In 20 minutes, the blood pressure is 120/80 mm Hg, but PO_2 (still with 100% oxygen) has dropped to 125 mm Hg!

Did the lab technician screw up the blood gas analysis? No. This is an example of the clinical significance of HPV, which directs pulmonary arteriolar delivery of deoxygenated blood toward ventilated alveoli and away from poorly ventilated lung regions. The patient was using HPV to attain a PO_2 of 400 mm Hg. All antihypertensive agents (e.g., nitroprusside) and most general anesthetics block HPV. The PO_2 increment from 125 to 400 mm Hg is a result of HPV, which steered perfusion toward ventilated areas of the lung.

30. **What governs the distribution of ventilation in lung?**
A large pleural pressure gradient (more negative at the top of the lung by 20 cm H_2O) squeezes gas primarily out of the dependent lung during each exhaled breath. The regional compliance of dependent lung is much better than that of lung apex, which still is distended with gas at the end of exhalation. Thus, in both instances, the dependent lung is preferentially both ventilated and perfused, optimizing Va/Q matching.

KEY POINTS: THERAPEUTIC GOALS IN ACUTE RESPIRATORY DISTRESS SYNDROME

1. Reduce lung edema
2. Reduce oxygen toxicity (FiO_2 <60%)
3. Minimize barotraumas (keep peak inspiratory pressure <40 cm H_2O)
4. PEEP to promote V/Q matching
5. Maintain systemic oxygen delivery (arterial oxygen content × CO)

31. **When may the patient come off mechanical ventilation and be extubated safely?**
    This is a controversial question, and many hospitals have their own specific stepwise method of identifying patients in whom extubation is likely to be successful. Studies have shown that it is important for intubated patients to undergo daily "spontaneous breathing trials" either using a T-piece or pressure support without ventilator-generated breaths. Specific extubation criteria often depend on the patient's disease process. However, there are certain general, widely-accepted criteria the patient should meet. The patient should be conscious and responsive, able to follow directions and maintain their airway. They should be able to complete a spontaneous breathing trial without tachycardia, hypotension, tachypnea, severe agitation, or desaturation. Several other factors including cough strength, secretion quantification, negative inspiratory force, and rapid shallow breathing index are used to help predict success or failure of expiration, but the literature is currently divided on the "best" metric on which to rely.

32. **What is a rapid shallow breathing index (RSBI)?**
    A patient in respiratory distress tends to take rapid shallow breaths. To quantify this, you divide the respiratory rate (BPM) by the tidal volume (L). An RSBI of 105 or lower has become an accepted cutoff for extubation. A patient with an RSBI of above 105 is more likely to fail extubation.

BIBLIOGRAPHY

1. Bartlett R. *Pulmonary insufficiency.* Surgery WebMD Corporation: New York American College of Surgeons; 2006.
2. Chetta A, Tzani P, Marangio E, et al. Respiratory effects of surgery and pulmonary function testing in the preoperative evaluation. *Acta Biomed.* 2006;77(2):69–74.
3. Davidson TA, Caldwell ES. Reduced quality of life in survivors of acute respiratory distress syndrome compared with critically ill control patients. *JAMA.* 1999;281(4):354–360.
4. Gust R, McCarthy TJ. Response to inhaled nitric oxide in acute lung injury depends on distribution of pulmonary blood flow prior to its administration. *Am J Respir Crit Care Med.* 1999;159(2):563–570.
5. Pesenti A, Fumagalli R. PEEP: blood gas cosmetics or a therapy for ARDS? *Crit Care Med.* 1999;27(2):253–254.
6. Wang T, Tagayun A, Bogardus A, et al. How accurately can we predict forced expiratory volume in one second after major pulmonary resection? *Am Surg.* 2007;73(10):1047–1051.
7. Westwood K, Griffin M. Incentive spirometry decreases respiratory complications following major abdominal surgery. *Surgeon.* 2007;5(6):339–342.
8. Torchio R, Gulotta C, Greco-Lucchina P, et al. Closing capacity and gas exchange in chronic heart failure. *Chest.* 2006;129(5):1330–1336.
9. Berg KM, Lang GR, Salciccioli JD, et al. The rapid shallow breathing index as a predictor of failure of noninvasive ventilation for patients with acute respiratory failure. *Respir Care.* 2012;57(10):1548–1554.
10. ARDS Definition Task Force. Acute respiratory distress syndrome: the Berlin definition. *JAMA.* 2012;307(23):2526–2533.
11. Fanelli V, Vlachoe A. Acute respiratory distress syndrome: new definition, current and future therapeutic options. *J Thorac Dis.* 2013;5(3):326–334.

CHAPTER 6

MECHANICAL VENTILATION

Scott M. Moore, MD, Jeffrey L. Johnson, MD, FACS,
James B. Haenel, RRT

1. **Why do patients need mechanical ventilation?**
   There are three basic categories of need when it comes to mechanical ventilation (MV): (1) inadequate respiratory drive; (2) inability to maintain adequate alveolar ventilation; and (3) hypoxia. The decision to provide MV should be based on clinical examination and assessment of gas exchange by arterial blood gas (ABG) analysis as needed. It is an individualized decision because arbitrary cutoff values for the partial pressure of oxygen (PO_2), partial pressure of carbon dioxide (pCO_2), or acid-base balance (pH) may not be germane to all patients. Common derangements necessitating the need for MV include primary parenchymal disorders, such as pneumonia, pulmonary edema, or pulmonary contusion, and systemic disease that indirectly compromises pulmonary function, such as sepsis or central nervous system (CNS) dysfunction.

2. **Does mechanical ventilation make the lung better?**
   Not really. In the setting of respiratory failure, the aim is to support gas exchange while the underlying disease process is reversed. Certain techniques can be used to recruit more airspace for gas exchange, but overall it is much easier to hurt the lung with a ventilator (i.e., ventilator induced lung injury [VILI]) than to fix it.

3. **How many modes of ventilation can you name?**
   Common modes include controlled mechanical ventilation (CMV), assist-control ventilation (ACV), intermittent mandatory ventilation (IMV), synchronized IMV (SIMV), pressure-controlled ventilation (PCV), pressure-support ventilation (PSV), inverse ratio ventilation (IRV), airway pressure release ventilation (APRV), mandatory minute ventilation (MMV), high-frequency oscillatory ventilation (HFOV), and dual control modes, such as pressure regulated volume control (PRVC). The most basic difference between these modes of ventilation is based on whether they deliver *mandatory breaths* (whether inspiration is machine triggered or machine cycled) versus *spontaneous breaths* (whether inspiration is patient triggered and patient cycled).

4. **What three elements can characterize all of the aforementioned mechanical ventilation modes?**
   Each mode can be described by how a breath is *triggered* (by the patient or by the machine), how it is *cycled* (switches from inhalation to exhalation), and how it is *limited* (for example by time, by pressure, or by flow).

5. **What are the most commonly used modes of positive-pressure ventilation?**
   ACV, IMV, SIMV, and PSV, which all differ primarily in how the breaths are triggered and cycled.

6. **How does assist-control ventilation work?**
   The ACV mode delivers a set minimum number of machine triggered breaths and also allows the patient to trigger a breath. Every breath (mandatory or patient triggered spontaneous) is *cycled* when a preset volume has been delivered at a preset flow rate. Because the patient receives a full tidal volume with every breath, even when tachypneic, ACV may result in respiratory alkalosis more often and may promote auto-positive end-expiratory pressure (PEEP).

7. **How does intermittent mechanical ventilation differ from assist-control ventilation?**
   Like ACV, the ventilator provides a preset number of machine triggered breaths at a preset tidal volume and flow rate in the IMV mode. Unlike ACV, however, the patient-triggered breaths are not cycled at a preset volume. Rather, spontaneous breaths are cycled based on the patient's own respiratory efforts (usually by sensing the end of patient effort as the flow rate falls). IMV may allow a decreased mean airway pressure (P_{aw}) and possibly less barotrauma because not every breath is a full positive-pressure breath.

23

8. **Compare intermittent mechanical ventilation with synchronized intermittent mechanical ventilation**
SIMV prevents "stacking" of breaths by deferring a machine-triggered breath if it would occur in the middle of a spontaneous breath. It is therefore easier to synchronize the patient's effort with the ventilator in the SIMV mode. In practice, most IMV is delivered as SIMV. Both modes involve additional work of breathing on the patient's part. Pressure support can be added during the spontaneous breaths to alleviate this work. It may be advantageous to relieve as much work of breathing as possible in the early part of respiratory failure.

9. **What are the pressure-limited types of ventilation?**
PSV, PRVC, HFV, and PCV. PSV is a mode of ventilation used in spontaneously breathing patients to decrease the imposed work of breathing from the endotracheal tube and to overcome resistance in the breathing circuit. It is often used to "wean" or determine the readiness of a patient to discontinue MV. PSV is a pure assisted form of ventilation. The patient must always trigger the breath (not the machine). This causes the ventilator to deliver a clinician-determined preset pressure, augmenting the tidal volume (V_T). PEEP or continuous positive airway pressure (CPAP) may be added. PCV is a machine-triggered mode (based on time) in which a set pressure (limit) is applied. It is cycled based on a preset amount of *time*, regardless of the size of the breath that was delivered during that time.

10. **Summarize the advantages and limitation of pressure-controlled ventilation**
Advantages include (1) limiting of peak pressure and theoretical prevention of overdistention and (2) better matching of patient flow requirement than with a set flow rate. Potential limitations include variation in delivered volumes as a result of increased airway resistance, decreased pulmonary compliance, and decreased patient effort.

11. **What are phase variables?**
There are four basic phase variables: pressure, volume, flow, and time. These are the same variables incorporated by the ventilator to detect the end of the inspiratory flow phase of a breath, (i.e., pressure cycled, volume cycled, flow cycled, and time cycled). Phase variables may be controlled either by the patient or by the ventilator.

12. **What are trigger variables?**
Trigger variables describe how a ventilator initiates inspiration. One or more of the phase variables may be used: time, pressure, flow, or volume. For example, in the CMV mode, time is the only trigger option available; no matter what the patient does, they cannot trigger a breath. In the ACV or SIMV mode, the patient may receive a breath based on time; however, a patient-generated decrease in baseline pressure (pressure-triggered) or patient-generated gas flow (flow-triggered) can also initiate a breath.

13. **What are limit variables?**
The limit variables (pressure, volume, and flow) are parameters that cannot be exceeded during inspiration. During an inspiration the pressure, flow, and volume will rise, and if they do not exceed a preset value, a breath is said to be limited by the primary variable.

14. **What are the goals of mechanical ventilation in patients with acute respiratory failure?**
In patients with acute respiratory failure (ARF), the goals are to preserve or improve arterial oxygenation and ventilation, to optimize lung mechanics, and to promote patient comfort while preventing VILI. Complications may arise from elevated alveolar pressures or persistently high inspired concentrations of oxygen (FiO_2).

15. **What are the initial ventilator settings in acute respiratory failure?**
There are lots of possibilities and styles, but generally a mode that provides full support is desired. Evidence from the ARDS-Net trial is centered on ACV, which ensures delivery of a preset volume; this mode is simply most well studied. Pressure-cycled modes are acceptable but probably offer only theoretical advantage. In any mode, the FiO_2 begins at 1.0 and is titrated downward as tolerated. High FiO_2 in the face of acute lung injury results in worsening of intrapulmonary shunt, possibly as a result of absorption atelectasis. Tidal volume is based on ideal body weight (IBW) and the pathophysiology of lung injury. Volumes of 8–10 mL/kg of IBW are probably acceptable if the plateau pressure is within a safe range. However, in the setting of acute respiratory distress syndrome (ARDS) or acute lung injury (ALI), large pressures or volumes may exacerbate the underlying lung injury. Therefore, smaller volumes ($\leq$6 mL/kg IBW) are delivered at a higher frequency.

16. **Which ventilator variables control the inspiratory/expiratory (I/E) ratio?**

The inspiratory/expiratory (I/E) ratio is the net effect of four ventilator settings: the respiratory rate (RR), Vt, peak flow, and the waveform setting. The peak flow rate is the maximal flow rate delivered by the ventilator during the inspiratory part of the respiratory cycle. An initial flow rate of 50–80 L/min is usually satisfactory. In a volume-cycled mode (e.g., ACV), then, a higher flow rate means a shorter inspiratory time, and a lower I/E ratio. An I/E ratio of 1:2–1:3 is reasonable in most situations. Patients with chronic obstructive pulmonary disease (COPD) may require longer expiratory times to allow adequate exhalation. This can be accomplished by increasing flow, thus decreasing the I/E ratio. High flow rates may increase airway pressures and worsen gas distribution in some cases; slower flow rates may reduce airway pressures and improve gas distribution by increasing the I/E ratio. The ventilator waveform (e.g., square versus decelerating) will also effect the I/E ratio. Without changing the peak flow setting the square waveform results in a higher peak airway pressure and longer E time than the selection of a decelerating waveform.

17. **What is positive end-expiratory pressure?**

PEEP is an elevation of the baseline pressure above atmospheric pressure at end exhalation.

18. **What does positive end-expiratory pressure do?**

PEEP prevents alveolar collapse, recruits atelectatic alveoli, increases functional residual capacity, and reverses hypoxemia. In all patients early in the course of their respiratory failure, PEEP probably needs to be manipulated in response to periods of desaturation (after common causes for hypoxemia have been ruled out, such as mucous plugging and barotrauma) to assess for recruitment potential.

19. **What is intrinsic or auto-positive end-expiratory pressure?**

Intrinsic PEEP (PEEPi) is the development of positive pressure and continued flow within the alveoli at end expiration without application of extrinsic PEEP (PEEPe). Patients with high minute ventilation requirements or patients receiving high I/E ratios are at risk for PEEPi. In healthy lungs during MV, if the respiratory rate is too rapid or the expiratory time is too short, there is insufficient time for full exhalation, resulting in stacking of breaths and generation of positive airway pressure at end exhalation. Small-diameter endotracheal tubes may also limit exhalation and contribute to PEEPi. Patients with increased airway resistance and decreased pulmonary compliance are at high risk for PEEPi. Such patients have difficulty in exhaling gas because of small airway obstruction or collapse and are prone to development of PEEPi during spontaneous ventilation and MV. PEEPi has the same side effects as PEEPe, but detecting it requires more vigilance.

Failure to recognize the presence of auto-PEEP can lead to inappropriate ventilator changes. The only way to detect and measure PEEPi is to occlude the expiratory port at end expiration while monitoring airway pressure. Decreasing rate or increasing inspiratory flow (to decrease I/E ratio) may allow time for full exhalation. Consider administering bronchodilator therapy in the setting of bronchospasm.

20. **What are the side effects of positive end-expiratory pressure?**

- Barotrauma may result from overdistension of alveoli.
- Cardiac output (CO) may be decreased as a result of intrathoracic pressure, producing an increase in transmural right atrial pressure and a decrease in venous return. PEEP also increases pulmonary artery pressure, potentially decreasing right ventricular output. Dilation of the right ventricle may cause bowing of the interventricular septum into the left ventricle, thus impairing filling of the left ventricle, decreasing CO, especially if the patient is hypovolemic.
- Incorrect interpretation of cardiac filing pressures: Pressure transmitted from the alveolus to the pulmonary vasculature may falsely elevate the readings. A rule of thumb is to subtract one-half of the PEEP applied over five from the pulmonary artery occlusion pressure.
- Overdistension of alveoli from excessive PEEP decreases blood flow to these areas, increasing dead space volume (V_D).
- Work of breathing may be increased with PEEP because the patient is required to generate a larger negative pressure to trigger flow from the ventilator. This problem has been mostly eliminated in modern ventilators, which are "PEEP compensated" and automatically adjust the pressure (or flow) trigger based on the PEEP setting.
- Increase in intracranial pressure (ICP) and fluid retention.
- Increase in lung water.

21. **What is a ventilator bundle?**

    The term *ventilator bundle* encompasses several preventative measures that virtually all ventilated patients should receive. Use of such bundles can minimize the incidence of ventilator associated pneumonia (VAP) and other complications. Simple bedside techniques such as oral care and elevating the head of bed, for example, have been shown to decrease VAP. The need for prolonged MV also places the patient at risk for gastrointestinal (GI) bleeding and deep venous thrombosis (DVT), and therefore prophylaxis from stress ulceration and DVTs should be initiated as part of the ventilator bundle.

22. **What is controlled hypoventilation with permissive hypercapnia?**

    Controlled hypoventilation (or permissive hypercapnia) is a pressure- or volume-limiting, lung-protective strategy whereby pCO_2 is allowed to rise, placing more importance on protecting the lung than on maintaining eucapnia. The set V_T is lowered to a range of approximately 4–6 mL/kg of IBW in an attempt to keep the alveolar pressure (static pressure) <30 cm H_2O. Several studies in ARDS and status asthmaticus have shown a decrease in barotrauma, intensive care days, and mortality using this approach. The pCO_2 is allowed to rise slowly to a level up to 80–100 mm Hg. If cardiovascular instability results as the pH falls, then the addition of intravenous sodium bicarbonate may be necessary. Alternatively, one may wait for the normal kidney to retain bicarbonate in response to the hypercapnia. Permissive hypercapnia is usually well tolerated. Potential adverse effects include cerebral vasodilatation, which can lead to increased ICP and exacerbate intracranial hypertension, and is the only absolute contraindication to permissive hypercapnia. Increased sympathetic activity, pulmonary vasoconstriction, and cardiac arrhythmias may occur but are rarely significant. Depression of cardiac contractility may be a problem in patients with underlying ventricular dysfunctions. In cases of ARF, worsening of acid-base may preclude or limit aggressive permissive hypercapnia.

23. **What is a lung recruitment maneuver?**

    The goal of a lung recruitment maneuver (LRM) is to reexpand collapsed alveoli, which have a smaller diameter than open alveoli and, according to the law of Laplace, have a higher opening pressure. Depletion of surfactant likely also plays a role. This is also why simply increasing the PEEP by several cm H_2O will not recruit collapsed alveoli to any significant degree. Alveolar recruitment is accomplished in practice by applying a relatively large amount of PEEP over a short duration of time.

    An example of a recruitment maneuver would be to place a patient on pressure control ventilation and increase the PEEP to 25 cm H_2O with peak pressure set at 40 cm H_2O. Pressures are then incrementally increased by 5 cm H_2O for every five breaths up to a maximum PEEP of 45 cm H_2O and peak inspiratory pressure of 55–60 cm H_2O. Following the LRM, which typically lasts 2–3 minutes, the patient is placed on elevated PEEP settings to keep the alveoli open. Because of the hemodynamic effects of elevated PEEP, not all patients will tolerate these aggressive maneuvers.

24. **What is the open lung concept?**

    The term *open lung* was first coined in the early 1990s and generally refers to a ventilation strategy in ARDS that makes use of a LRM to reexpand atelectatic alveoli, followed by use of PEEP to prevent re-collapse. Theoretical advantages of this approach include the requirement for lower P_{aw} to maintain alveoli in the open state, which should reduce the incidence of ventilator-induced lung injury as a result of less barotrauma and atelectrauma (the latter refers to the injury induced by shear forces that occur when alveoli are repeatedly collapsed and reopened). Proponents of this strategy have historically combined this approach with so-called alternative modes of ventilation (i.e., airway pressure release ventilation—APRV, high frequency oscillatory ventilation—HFOV), though conventional modes can also be used in the open lung approach.

25. **What is airway pressure release ventilation (APRV) and how is it used?**

    APRV is a type of pressure control mandatory ventilation that is characterized by a prolonged inspiratory phase interspersed with a brief expiratory phase, while also allowing unrestricted spontaneous breathing throughout the cycle. The latter promotes patient comfort and may lead to less need for sedation and neuromuscular blockade than conventional modes with an inverse I:E ratio. The operator sets the high pressure (P_{high}—typically obtained from the plateau pressure with patient on conventional volume control mode and not >30 cm H_2O), the low pressure (P_{low}—almost always set at 0 cm

H_2O), the time in the inspiratory phase (T_{high}—usually 4–6 seconds), and the time in the expiratory phase (T_{low}—usually 0.4–0.6 seconds, and adjusted so that expiratory flow never drops below 25% of the peak expiratory flow rate). The respiratory rate is not set directly and is determined instead by the length of T_{high} and T_{low}. Note that the expiratory phase is intentionally shortened to prevent full exhalation, which generates PEEPi. The net effect of this intentional auto-PEEP and inverse I:E ratio is a higher P_{aw} than is typically achieved with a conventional mode, while peak airway pressures are usually lower. For this reason, many practitioners prefer APRV for managing ARDS over conventional modes, and in some centers APRV is the only mode of mechanical ventilation used.

Though the theoretical benefits are attractive, no trials to date have convincingly shown a mortality benefit for ARDS using APRV or any of the other alternative modes of ventilation. At the same time, the mortality benefits of lung protective ventilation are quite convincing. This suggests that the specific mode of ventilation is probably less important as long as efforts are focused on minimizing plateau pressure (<30 cm H_2O), delivering low tidal volumes (≤6 mL/kg IBW), and providing adequate PEEP to maintain alveolar recruitment. Finally, it should be stressed that certain patients require a prolonged expiratory phase for adequate ventilation— that is, status asthmaticus, severe COPD—these patients will often fail APRV and any other mode with an inverse I:E ratio.

26. **What is compliance? How is it determined?**
    Compliance is a measure of distensibility and is expressed as the change in volume for a given change in pressure. Determination of compliance involves the interrelationship between pressure, volume, and resistance to airflow. The two relevant pressures that must be monitored during MV are peak and static (or plateau) pressures.

27. **How is peak pressure measured?**
    Peak pressure is measured during the delivery of airflow at the end of inspiration. It is influenced by the inflation volume, airway resistance, and elastic recoil of the lungs and chest wall and reflects the dynamic compliance of the total respiratory system.

28. **How is static pressure measured?**
    Static or plateau pressure (P_{plat}) is measured during an end-inspiratory pause, during a no-flow condition, and reflects the static compliance of the respiratory system, including the lung parenchyma, chest wall, and abdomen.

29. **How is compliance calculated?**
    Both dynamic and static compliance should be calculated as a routine part of ventilator monitoring. Dynamic compliance is calculated as V_T / (P_{aw} − total PEEP), and static compliance is V_T / (P_{plat} − total PEEP). Normal values for both dynamic and static compliance are 60–100 mL/cm H_2O. A decrease in dynamic compliance without a change in the static compliance suggests an acute increase in airway resistance and can be assessed further by comparing peak pressure and plateau pressure. The normal gradient is approximately 10 cm H_2O. A gradient >10 cm H_2O may be secondary to endotracheal tube obstruction, mucous plugging, or bronchospasm. If volume is constant, acute changes in both dynamic and static compliance suggest a decrease in respiratory system compliance that may be caused by worsening pneumonia, ARDS, atelectasis, or increasing abdominal pressures.

    Compliance is a global value and does not describe what is happening regionally in the lungs with ARDS, in which diseased regions are interspersed with relatively healthy regions. Compliance values of 20–40 cm H_2O are common in advanced ARDS. Decreased lung compliance reflects the compliance of the lung that is participating in gas exchange, not the collapsed or fluid-filled alveoli. As a general rule, when static compliance is <25 mL/cm H_2O, ventilator weaning may be difficult secondary to tachypnea during spontaneous breathing trials.

30. **Is ventilation in the prone position an option for patients who are difficult to oxygenate?**
    Absolutely! PaO_2 improves significantly in approximately two-thirds of patients with ARDS when they are placed prone. The mechanisms include (1) recruitment of collapsed dorsal lung fields by redistribution of lung edema to ventral regions; (2) increased diaphragm motion enhancing ventilation; (3) elimination of the compressive effects of the heart on the inferior lower lung fields, thus improving regional ventilation; (4) maintenance of dorsal lung perfusion in the face of improved dorsal ventilation, which leads to improved ventilation/perfusion (V/Q) matching; and (5) a change in the pleural pressure gradient from the ventral to dorsal regions of the lung.

31. **What are the indications for prone ventilation?**

    Indications for prone ventilation are not clearly established. We initiate a prone trial in any patient who remains hypoxemic or requires high FiO_2 concentrations after the performance or recruitment/PEEP maneuvers. The best predictor of improved outcome during prone ventilation may be a decrease in the $PaCO_2$ and not improved oxygenation.

32. **Does prone positioning improve outcomes in ARDS?**

    Early trials of proning for hypoxemic respiratory failure and ARDS failed to show any significant mortality benefit with prone positioning, despite improvements in oxygenation. However, these trials suffered from inclusion of patients with a wide variation in severity of illness, and either implemented prone positioning late in the course of disease (>48–72 hours from intubation) or for short durations (7–8 hours per day). The PROSEVA trial demonstrated that proning early (within 36 hours of intubation), for long duration (>16 hours per day), and using specific selection criteria (PaO_2:FiO_2 ratio <150) improves mortality and that this benefit appears to be independent of effects on oxygenation. This study included mostly medical ICU patients, and whether the results can be extended to trauma and surgical ICU patients is not known. Also, proned patients have been shown by multiple trials to have increased rates of pressure ulcers and ET tube complications, which highlights the need for training and familiarity among ICU personnel before implementing this potentially risky procedure.

33. **Junior O'Flaherty is "fighting the ventilator." What do I do?**

    Initially, the potential causes are separated into ventilator (machine, circuit, and airway) problems and patient-related problems. Patient-related causes include hypoxemia, secretions or mucous plugging, pneumothorax, bronchospasm, infection (pneumonia or sepsis), pulmonary embolus, myocardial ischemia, GI bleeding, worsening PEEPi, and anxiety. The ventilator-related issues include system leak or disconnection; inadequate ventilator support or delivered FiO_2; airway-related problems, such as extubation, obstructed endotracheal tube, cuff herniation, or rupture; and improper triggering sensitivity or flows. Until the problem is identified, the patient should be ventilated manually with 100% O_2. Breath sounds and vital signs should be immediately checked. ABG analysis and portable chest radiograph are valuable, but if a tension pneumothorax is suspected, immediate decompression precedes the chest radiograph.

34. **Should neuromuscular blockage be used to facilitate mechanical ventilation?**

    Neuromuscular blocking agents (NMBAs) are commonly used to facilitate MV during ARDS, but despite wide acceptance, there are few data and as yet no consensus available for when these agents should be used. Gainnier and colleagues were the first to report the effects of a 48-hour NMBA infusion on gas exchange in patients with early ARDS. All patients were ventilated according to the ARDSnet protocol. Significant improvements in oxygenation and ability to lower PEEP occurred in the NMBA group and were sustained beyond the 48-hour infusion period. Although it remains to be elucidated why muscle paralysis improves oxygenation, NMBAs are thought to decrease oxygen consumption, promote patient-ventilator interface, and increase chest wall compliance.

    Muscle paralysis may also be of benefit in specific situations, such as intracranial hypertension or unconventional modes of ventilation (e.g., IRV or extracorporeal techniques). Drawbacks to the use of these drugs include loss of neurologic examination, abolished cough, potential for prolonged paralysis, diaphragmatic atrophy, and death associated with inadvertent ventilator disconnects. Use of NMBAs must not be taken lightly. Adequate sedation should be attempted first; if deemed absolutely necessary, use of NMBAs should be limited to 24–48 hours to prevent potential complications.

35. **When is a patient ready to be removed from the ventilator?**

    Some patients can be liberated from mechanical ventilation as soon as the offending factor that mandated ventilator support is removed or corrected (i.e., general anesthetic, drug overdose, pulmonary edema), whereas others have multifactorial requirements for mechanical ventilation and demand more experience and scrutiny. In general, an appropriate candidate for extubation fulfills the following criteria:

    - Hemodynamically stable, no evidence for sepsis or neuromuscular disease, and has normal intracranial pressure
    - Not a risk for airway compromise or aspiration (audible cuff leak, able to clear secretions)
    - Adequate oxygenation and ventilation (P_aO_2:FiO_2 ratio ≥200 on FiO_2 ≤0.5 and PEEP ≤10; pCO_2 normal or at baseline)
    - Appropriate mental status (follows commands)
    - Sufficient strength and respiratory drive (forced vital capacity [FVC] >10–15 mL/kg, negative inspiratory force [NIF] >20 cm H_2O, rapid shallow breathing index [RSBI] = RR/V_T <105, minute ventilation [V_e] of 5–13 L/min, able to lift head off of pillow)

A simple mnemonic for remembering these criteria is *S-O-A-P*, which stands for *s*ecretions, *o*xygenation/ventilation, *a*irway/alertness, and *p*arameters.

36. What is a spontaneous breathing trial (SBT)?

In an effort to quickly identify patients that can be removed from mechanical ventilation, SBTs are a method for determining how a patient will tolerate unassisted breathing without removing the endotracheal tube. The most common method is to keep the patient on the ventilator but eliminate all mandatory breaths and only provide 5 cm H_2O of pressure support ventilation, which is meant to only offset the resistance of the ventilator circuit. An alternative approach is to remove the patient from the ventilator entirely, and attach a T-shaped adapter ("T-piece") to the ET tube that allows for delivery of high-flow O_2 while also preventing rebreathing of CO_2. The main disadvantage of the latter method is that tidal volumes are more difficult to measure and require a special devise called a Wright spirometer. Failure of an SBT is signified by a RR >35 for over 5 minutes, a minute ventilation >20 L/min, SpO_2 <90%, SBP >180 or <90 mm Hg, or signs of respiratory distress (HR >120% of baseline for >5 minutes, marked use of accessory muscles, paradoxical abdominal breathing, diaphoresis, marked subjective dyspnea, or apnea).

KEY POINTS: MECHANICAL VENTILATION

1. Inadequate alveolar ventilation, hypoxia, and impaired respiratory drive are the three reasons patients may need MV.
2. All modes of ventilation can be described based on how a breath is triggered, cycled, and limited.
3. Initial ventilator settings for ARF should provide full support. ACV mode is the most studied.
4. Hypoventilation and letting pCO_2 rise is permissible—and beneficial—if it allows the physician to limit alveolar pressure and stretch (permissive hypercapnia).
5. When a patient appears to be "fighting" the ventilator, the first step is to remove the ventilator and manually ("bag") ventilate the patient. This allows you to eliminate ventilator variables as a cause and assess patient variables that may need urgent treatment (e.g., tension pneumothorax).
6. If considering placing a patient prone because of hypoxemic respiratory failure, use it early and for long duration in order to derive the most benefit.
7. The most important principles of ventilator management in ARDS are to use low tidal volumes (≤6 mL/kg), keep plateau pressures low (<25–30 cm H_2O), and apply adequate PEEP to prevent alveolar collapse.
8. All patients being considered for removal from mechanical ventilation should fulfill certain criteria, which can be easily remembered using the SOAP mnemonic.

BIBLIOGRAPHY

1. Burger CD, Resar RK. "Ventilator bundle" approach to prevention of ventilator-associated pneumonia. *Mayo Clin Proc.* 2006;81(6):849–850.
2. Bein T, Grasso S, Moerer O, et al. The standard of care of patients with ARDS: ventilatory settings and rescue therapies for refractory hypoxemia. *Intensive Care Med.* 2016;42(5):699–711.
3. Campbell RS, Davis BR. Pressure-controlled versus volume-controlled ventilation: does it matter? *Respir Care.* 2002;47(4):416–424.
4. Daoud EG, Farag HL, Chatburn RL. Airway pressure release ventilation: what do we know? *Respir Care.* 2012;57(2):282–292.
5. Gainnier M, Roch A, Forel JM. Effect of neuromuscular blocking agents on gas exchange in patients presenting with acute respiratory distress syndrome. *Crit Care Med.* 2004;32(1):113–119.
6. Guérin C, Reignier J, Richard J-C, et al. Prone positioning in severe acute respiratory distress syndrome. *N Engl J Med.* 2013;368(23):2159–2168.
7. Lachmann B. Open up the lung and keep the lung open. *Intensive Care Med.* 1992;18(6):319–321.
8. Levine S, Nguyen T, Taylor N, et al. Rapid disuse atrophy of diaphragm fibers in mechanically ventilated humans. *N Engl J Med.* 2008;358(13):1327–1335.
9. Meade MO, Cook DJ, Guyatt GH, et al. Ventilation strategy using low tidal volumes, recruitment maneuvers, and high positive end-expiratory pressures for acute lung injury and acute respiratory distress syndrome: a randomized controlled trial. *JAMA.* 2008;299(6):637–645.
10. Mercat A, Richard JM, Vielle B, et al. Positive end-expiratory pressure setting in adults with acute lung injury and acute respiratory distress syndrome. *JAMA.* 2008;299(6):646–655.
11. Pierson DJ. Indications for mechanical ventilation in adults with acute respiratory failure. *Respir Care.* 2002;47(3):249–262.
12. Thille AW, Cortés-Puch I, Esteban A. Weaning from the ventilator and extubation in ICU. *Curr Opin Crit Care.* 2013;19(1):57–64.

CHAPTER 7

WHY GET ARTERIAL BLOOD GASES?

Kathryn H. Chomsky-Higgins, MD, MS, Alden H. Harken, MD, FACS

1. **Is breathing really overrated?**
   It may be. A Japanese yoga master survived just fine breathing once per minute for 1 hour (see reference 1). But, when medical students and residents prioritize activities that they really enjoy, year after year, "breathing" consistently ranks very high.

2. **Mr. O'Flaherty has just undergone an inguinal herniorrhaphy under local anesthesia. The recovery room nurse asks permission to sedate him. She says that he is confused and unruly and keeps trying to get out of bed. Is it safe to sedate Mr. O'Flaherty?**
   No. A confused, agitated patient in the recovery room or surgical intensive care unit (SICU) must be recognized as acutely hypoxemic until proved otherwise. This is really important!

3. **Mr. O'Flaherty is moved to the SICU, and at 2:00 a.m. the SICU nurse calls to report that he has a partial pressure of oxygen (pO_2) of 148 mm Hg on facemask oxygen. Is it okay to roll over and go back to sleep?**
   No. More information is needed.

4. **You glance at the abandoned cup of coffee sitting on your well-worn copy of *Surgical Secrets*. What is the pO_2 of that cup of coffee?**
   It is 148 mm Hg.

5. **How can Mr. O'Flaherty and the coffee have the same pO_2?**
   The abandoned coffee presumably has had time to equilibrate completely with atmospheric gas. At sea level, the barometric pressure is 760 mm Hg. To obtain the pO_2 in the coffee, subtract water vapor pressure (47 mm Hg) and multiply by the concentration of oxygen (20.8%) in the atmosphere:
   $pO_2 = (760 - 47) \times 20.8\% = 148$ mm Hg

6. **What is the difference between Mr. O'Flaherty's and the coffee's pO_2?**
   Nothing. Both represent the partial pressure of oxygen in fluid. A complete set of blood gases is necessary.

7. **What constitutes a complete set of blood gases?**
   - pO_2
   - pCO_2
   - pH
   - O_2 Sat
   - Hgb concentration

8. **If Mr. O'Flaherty and the coffee have the same pO_2, how would Mr. O'Flaherty do if he were exchange-transfused with coffee?**
   Badly.

9. **Why?**
   Although the oxygen tensions are the same, the amount of oxygen in blood is vastly greater.

10. **How does one quantify the amount of oxygen in blood?**
    Arterial oxygen content (CaO_2) is quantified as mL of oxygen/100 mL of blood. (Watch out: Almost all other concentrations traditionally are provided per mL or per L and not per 100 mL.) Because mL of oxygen is the volume of oxygen in 100 mL of blood, these units frequently are abbreviated as vol %.

11. **Why is blood thicker than coffee (or wine)?**
   Because hemoglobin binds a huge amount of oxygen. A total of 10 g of fully saturated hemoglobin (hematocrit about 30%) binds 13.4 mL of oxygen, whereas 100 mL of plasma at a pO_2 of 100 mm Hg contains only 0.3 mL of oxygen.

12. **Does the position of the oxyhemoglobin dissociation curve make any difference?**
   A little—but not a lot. A shift in the oxyhemoglobin curve to the right does permit oxygen to be released more easily in the tissues. Within physiologic limits, however, Mae West probably said it best: "There is less to this than meets the eye."
   With regular frequency this relationship does surface on multiple-choice examinations. So, each of the following "increases" the right shift of the O_2-Hbg curve:
   a. An increase in pCO_2
   b. An increase in hydrogen ion concentrations (not pH)
   c. An increase in temperature

KEY POINTS: MEDIATORS OF OXYHEMOGLOBIN DISSOCIATION CURVE

Right Shift
1. Increase in pCO_2
2. Increase in $[H]^+$, lower pH
3. Increase in temperature
4. Increase in 2,3-DPG

Left Shift
1. Decrease in $[H]^+$, higher pH
2. Higher altitudes/elevations
3. Decrease in 2,3-DPG (at 4 weeks storage, blood maintains *no* 2,3-DPG.)

---

13. **If CaO_2 or ultimately systemic oxygen delivery (cardiac output × CaO_2) is what the surgeon really wants to know, why does the nurse report Mr. O'Flaherty's pO_2 instead of his CaO_2 at 2:00 a.m.?**
   No one knows.

14. **What is the fastest and most practical method of increasing Mr. O'Flaherty's CaO_2?**
   Transfusion of red blood cells. The patient's CaO_2 is increased by 25% with transfusion from a hemoglobin concentration of 8–10 g/dL. The patient's CaO_2 is affected negligibly by an increase in arterial pO_2 from 100 to 200 mm Hg (hemoglobin is fully saturated in both instances).

15. **What is a transfusion trigger?**
   The hematocrit at which a patient is automatically transfused. This is not a useful concept. The NIH Consensus Conference, drawing data from Jehovah's Witnesses, patients with renal failure, and monkeys, concluded that it is not necessary to transfuse a patient until the hematocrit is 21%. Traditional surgical dogma has long mandated a hematocrit >30%. The Canadian TRICC trial, however, has convincingly concluded that unless a critically ill patient is at risk for cardiac ischemia, the hemoglobin may safely be allowed to drift down to 7 g/dL prior to transfusion.

16. **What is the Transfusion Requirements in Critical Care (TRICC) trial?**
   In 1999, 838 critically ill patients were enrolled who, following three days in an ICU, were deemed to be euvolemic and had an Hbg <9 g/dL. Patients who were allowed to drift along with an Hbg between 7 and 9 g/dL fared better than patients who were transfused up to a target Hbg of 10–12 g/dL (see the Required Reading in Chapter 108).

17. **What's wrong with transfused blood?**
   It's likely not the extra hemoglobin. Indeed, Tour de France elite athletes are convinced that a hematocrit of 50% permits them to ride faster. It's more likely that the red blood cell membrane and activated white cell sludge is the problem. Blood banks now leukodeplete all bags of blood, but some white cells remain. Infectious disease transmission is a persistent worry, but blood banking is now so good that when your patient's Hbg hits 7 g/dL—give blood.

18. What governs respiratory drive?

pCO_2 and pH are inextricably intertwined by the Henderson-Hasselbalch equation. By juggling this equation in the cerebrospinal fluid (CSF) of goats, it is, however, clear that CSF hydrogen ion concentration (not pCO_2) controls respiratory drive. This distinction is not clinically important, however. What is important is that if a person becomes acidotic either with diabetic ketoacidosis (DKA) or by running up a flight of stairs, minute ventilation (VE) is increased. This is respiratory compensation (driving down pCO_2) in response to a metabolic acidosis.

19. How tight is respiratory control? Or, if you hold your breath for 1 minute, how much do you want to breathe?

A lot (unless you are a yoga master approaching nirvana).

20. After 60 seconds of apnea, what happens to your $PaCO_2$?

It increases only from 40 to 47 mm Hg. Tiny changes in pCO_2 (and pH) translate into a huge respiratory stimulus; you want to breathe a lot. Normally, respiratory compensation for metabolic acidosis is tight.

21. Define base excess

Base excess is a poor man's indicator of the metabolic component of acid-base disorders. After correcting the pCO_2 to 40 mm Hg, the base excess or base deficit is touted as an indirect measure of serum lactate. Although many parameters directing volume resuscitation in shock are more practical and direct (see Chapter 4), base deficit has been advertised as helpful. The base excess or deficit is calculated from the Siggaard-Andersen nomogram in the blood gas laboratory. Normally, there is no base excess or deficit. Acid-base status is "just right."

BIBLIOGRAPHY

1. Miyamura M, Nishimura K. Is man able to breathe once a minute for an hour?: the effect of yoga respiration on blood gases. *Jpn J Physiol.* 2002;52(3):313–316.
2. Hébert PC, Wells G, Blajchman MA, et al. A multicenter, randomized, controlled clinical trial of transfusion requirements in critical care. Transfusion Requirements in Critical Care Investigators, Canadian Critical Care Trials Group. *N Engl J Med.* 1999;340(6):409–417.
3. Tada T, Hashimoto F. Study of life satisfaction and quality of life of patients receiving home oxygen therapy. *J Med Invest.* 2003;50(1-2):55–63.
4. Hsia CC, Mahon JL. Use of n-of-1 (single patient) trials to assess the effect of age of transfused blood on health-related quality of life in transfusion-dependent patients. *Transfusion.* 2016;56(5):1192–1200.

CHAPTER 8

FLUIDS, ELECTROLYTES, GATORADE, AND SWEAT

Robert A. Tessler, MD, Alden H. Harken, MD, FACS

1. **What is hypertonic saline?**
   Normal saline is 0.9% sodium chloride. Hypertonic saline is 7.5% sodium chloride (eight times as concentrated as normal saline).

KEY POINTS: ION CONCENTRATIONS IN CRYSTALLOID SOLUTIONS

1. One-half normal saline or 0.45% NaCl: 77 mEq of Na+, 77 mEq of Cl-
2. Normal saline or 0.9% NaCl: 154 mEq of Na+, 154 mEq of Cl-
3. Hypertonic normal saline or 7.5% NaCl: 1283 mEq of Na+, 1283 mEq of Cl-
4. Lactated Ringer's: 130 mEq of Na+, 110 mEq of Cl-, 38 mEq of lactate, 4 mEq of K+, and 3 mEq of Ca+

2. **What is hypertonic saline good for?**
   Resuscitation. The initial hypothesis was that a little hypertonic saline would pull extravascular water into the intravascular compartment, rapidly restoring volume. It now appears that an osmotic jolt (even a transient jump from 140 to 180 mOsm) would pacify circulating neutrophils so that they do not stick to the endovasculature and provoke posttraumatic inflammation.

3. **Is hypertonic saline good for anything else?**
   Pacification of "primed" neutrophils should decrease the risk of posttraumatic multiple organ failure.

4. **How do you convert 1 g of sodium into milliequivalents (mEq)?**
   Divide by the atomic weight of sodium:
   One gram (1 g/1000 mg) of sodium = 43.5 mEq

5. **How many mEq of sodium are in 1 teaspoon of salt?**
   104 mEq (2400 mg).

6. **How many mEq of sodium are in an 8-oz bottle of Gatorade?**
   5 mEq.

7. **How much does a 40-lb block of salt cost?**
   $3.40 at the feed store.

8. **What is the electrolyte content of intravenous fluids?**
   See Table 8.1.

Table 8.1 Electrolyte Content of Intravenous Fluids

SOLUTION (mEq/L)	SODIUM	POTASSIUM	CHLORIDE	BICARBONATE/ LACTATE
Normal saline (0.9% NaCl)	154	—	154	—
Ringer's lactate solution	130	4	109	28[a]
5% dextrose and 1/2 normal saline	77	—	77	—

[a]Lactate is converted immediately to bicarbonate.

9. How do these concentrations relate to body fluid and electrolyte compartments? See Table 8.2.

Table 8.2 Electrolyte Concentrations in Body Fluids

COMPARTMENT (mEq/L)	SODIUM	POTASSIUM	CHLORIDE	BICARBONATE/ LACTATE
Plasma	142	4	103	27
Interstitial fluid	144	4	114	30
Intracellular fluid	10	150	—	10

10. What are the daily volumes (mL/24h) and electrolyte contents (mEq/L) of body secretions for a 70-kg medical student? See Table 8.3.

Table 8.3 Daily Volumes and Electrolyte Contents of Body Secretions

	mL/24H	SODIUM	POTASSIUM	CHLORIDE	BICARBONATE
Saliva	+1500	10	25	10	30
Stomach	+1500	50	10	130	—
Duodenum	+1000	140	5	80	—
Ileum	+3000	140	5	104	30
Colon	-6000	60	30	40	—
Pancreas	+500	140	5	75	100
Biliary	+500	140	5	100	30
Sweat[a]	+1000	50	—	—	—
Gatorade	—	21	—	21	—

[a]See question 11.

11. Are sweat glands responsive to aldosterone? Can they be trained? Yes and yes. Archie Bunker's sweat contains 100 mEq/L sodium, whereas an Olympic marathon runner retains sodium (sweat sodium may be as low as 25 mEq/L).

12. Is Gatorade really just flavored athlete's sweat? Yes.

13. What are the daily maintenance fluid and electrolyte requirements for a 70-kg medical student?

Total fluid volume: 2500 mL
Sodium: 70 mEq (1 mEq/kg)
Potassium: 35 mEq (0.5 mEq/kg)

14. Does the routine postoperative patient require intravenous sodium or potassium supplementation? Routine serum electrolyte testing? No and no.

15. Can a patient with a good heart and kidneys overcome all but the most woefully incompetent fluid and electrolyte management?
Yes.

16. Can one throw a healthy medical student into congestive heart failure by intravenous infusion of 100 mL of 5% dextrose in saline solution per kilogram per hour?
No. One will simply be ankle-deep in urine.

17. What is subtraction alkalosis?
Vigorous nasogastric suction of a patient with a lot of gastric acid eliminates hydrochloric acid, leaving the patient alkalotic.

18. Which electrolyte is most useful in repairing a hypokalemic metabolic alkalosis?
Chloride.

19. List the best indicators of a patient's volume status:
    • Heart rate
    • Blood pressure
    • Urine output
    • Big-toe temperature

20. Does a warm big toe indicate a hemodynamically stable patient?
Most likely. The vascular autoregulatory ability of a young healthy patient is huge. The carotid and coronary circulations are maintained until the bitter end. Conversely, if the patient's big toe is warm and perfused, the patient is stable.

21. What is the minimal adequate postoperative urine output?
It is 0.5 mL/kg per hour.

22. What is a typical postoperative urine sodium?
It is <20 mEq/L.

23. Why?
Surgical stress prompts mineralocorticoid (aldosterone) secretion so that the normal kidney retains sodium.

24. Explain paradoxical aciduria
Postoperative patients, by virtue of nasogastric suction (loss of gastric acid), blood transfusions (the citrate in blood is converted to bicarbonate), and hyperventilation (decreased pCO_2), are typically alkalotic. Patients also are stressed, and their kidneys retain sodium and water. The renal tubules must exchange some other cations for the retained sodium. The kidney chooses to exchange potassium and hydrogen ions. Even in the face of systemic alkalosis, the postoperative kidney absorbs sodium and excretes hydrogen ions, producing a paradoxical aciduria.

25. What is third spacing?
Hypotension and infection prime neutrophils (CD11 and CD18 receptor complexes), promoting adherence to vascular endothelial cells. Subsequent activation of adherent neutrophils spews out proteases and toxic superoxide radicals, blowing big holes in the vascular lining. Water and plasma albumin leak through the holes. The volume pulled out of the vascular space into the third space of the interstitial and hollow viscus (gut) creates relative hypovolemia and requires additional fluid replacement.

26. What is a Lasix sandwich?
It is 25 g albumin followed by 20 mg of furosemide (Lasix) intravenously (IV). If the patient is edematous, the intravenous albumin theoretically sucks water osmotically out of the interstitial third space. As the excessive water enters the vascular compartment, Lasix produces a healthy diuresis. In most patients in the intensive care unit (ICU), however, the infused albumin rapidly equilibrates across the damaged vascular endothelium. No additional water is pulled into the blood volume. Although surgeons often order Lasix sandwiches, they probably work only in healthy patients who do not need them.

BIBLIOGRAPHY

1. Brown MD. Evidence-based emergency medicine. Hypertonic versus isotonic crystalloid for fluid resuscitation in critically ill patients. *Ann Emerg Med.* 2002;40(1):113–114.
2. Bunn F, Roberts I. Hypertonic versus near isotonic crystalloid for fluid resuscitation in critically ill patients. *Cochrane Database Syst Rev.* 2004;(3):CD002045.
3. Dellinger RP, Levy MM, Rhodes A, et al. Surviving Sepsis Campaign Guidelines Committee including the Pediatric Subgroup. Surviving sepsis campaign: international guidelines for management of severe sepsis and septic shock: 2012. *Crit Care Med.* 2013;41(2):580–637.
4. Greaves I, Porter KM. Fluid resuscitation in pre-hospital trauma care: a consensus view. *J R Coll Surg Edinb.* 2002;47(2):451–457.
5. Perel P, Roberts I. Colloids versus crystalloids for fluid resuscitation in critically ill patients. *Cochrane Database Syst Rev.* 2013;28(2):CD000567.

CHAPTER 9

NUTRITIONAL ASSESSMENT, PARENTERAL, AND ENTERAL NUTRITION

Martin D. Rosenthal, MD, Erin L. Vanzant, MD, Scott C. Brakenridge, MD, MSCS, FACS

NUTRITIONAL ASSESSMENT

1. **What does a nutritional assessment include?**

   The **medical and surgical history** determine preexisting conditions, metabolic stress, and alterations in organ function that influence nutritional support. Nutritional status is recently having a resurgence of importance as it can be predictive of morbidity and mortality. Assessment begins with the **physical exam** and evaluates muscle mass, adipose stores, skin integrity, temporal muscle wasting, and clinical signs of micronutrient deficiency or cachexia. **Laboratory data** should include the basic labs, which include serum sodium (Na), potassium (K), carbon dioxide (CO_2), chloride (Cl), blood urea nitrogen (BUN), creatinine, glucose, ionized calcium (Ca), serum phosphate (PO_4), magnesium (Mg), and complete blood count (CBC) with differential. Arterial blood gases (ABGs) to assess acid-base status and CO_2 retention, albumin, transferrin, prealbumin, and urinary nitrogen are useful. Glycosylated hemoglobin (HgbA1C), lipid profile, C-reactive protein (CRP), 25-OH vitamin D, trace elements, and liver function tests (LFTs) may also be valuable. The **drug profile** reveals agents that affect the metabolism of nutrients (insulin, levothyroxine, corticosteroids), alter energy expenditure (β-blockers, propofol), or affect gastrointestinal (GI) function (prokinetic agents, antibiotics). **Anthropometric data** include height, weight, and waist and hip circumference. Skinfold testing with calipers is useful once edema has resolved, but is rarely used in the fat-free acute care setting. **Bioelectrical impedance analysis (BIA)** quantifies adipose reserve, intracellular and extracellular water, and third space fluid in stable surgical patients. Dual energy x-ray absorptiometry (DEXA) is effective for tracking bone mineral density that may be compromised with age, hormonal status, drug therapy, and chronic disease. One of the most versatile questions in assessing nutritional status revolves around **nutritional history.** A simple question, "How have you been eating lately? Have you had any recent weight changes? Can you walk me through a normal day's diet?" could easily reveal information on the nutritional practices of the individual. The **social history** explores economic data, social support network, or substance abuse behaviors and may predict the likelihood of adequate home care and treatment compliance for the patient, once discharged.

2. **Are there any nutritional assessments that can be used in the ICU and be objective?**

   There are assessments that can be utilized to better understand the nutritional deficits among the critically ill ICU patients. (1) The Nutrition Risk in Critically ill (NUTRIC) score is the first nutritional risk assessment tool developed and validated specifically for ICU patients. The recognition that not all ICU patients will respond the same to nutritional interventions was the main concept behind the NUTRIC score, as most other risk scores and assessment tools consider all critically ill patients to be at high nutrition risk. (2) Another assessment tool of malnutrition in ICU is the Nutrition Risk Score-2002 (NRS). It is based on the concept that nutritional support is indicated in patients who are severely ill with increased nutritional requirements, or who are severely undernourished, or who have certain degrees of severity of disease in combination with certain degrees of undernutrition. Degrees of severity of disease and undernutrition were defined as absent, mild, moderate, or severe from data sets in a selected number of randomized controlled trials (RCTs) and converted to a numeric score. After completion, the screening system was validated against all published RCTs known to us of nutritional support versus spontaneous intake to investigate whether the screening system could distinguish between trials with a positive outcome and trials with no effect on outcome.

3. **What are primary malnutrition and secondary malnutrition?**
Primary malnutrition results when the individual consumes inadequate kilocalories, protein, vitamins, or minerals. It may occur as a result of poor food choices, anorexia, poverty, alcoholism, suboptimal support regimens, or after bariatric surgery. Secondary malnutrition occurs even when adequate food is infused or consumed. It may result from organ dysfunction (hypoalbuminemia with cirrhosis), malabsorption (Crohn's disease), immobility (muscle wasting), drug therapy (insulin resistance with corticosteroids), or the inflammatory state (Persistent Inflammatory Immunosuppressed Catabolic Syndrome).

4. **What is the significance of serum visceral proteins in nutritional assessment?**
The most commonly cited and readily available proteins for nutritional assessment are albumin, transferrin, and prealbumin, which are produced in the liver (Table 9.1). All three constitutive proteins plummet shortly after injury or surgery because the liver reprioritizes the production of acute phase proteins. Then, as the stress response resolves, the liver resumes production of constitutive proteins, as it makes the transition from catabolism to anabolism. Meeting protein and nonprotein caloric needs helps to facilitate this process. As a result of shorter half-lives, prealbumin and transferrin are most useful in the intensive care unit (ICU) and should be limited to patients with creatinine clearance >50 mL/min. Prealbumin travels in the circulation bound to retinol binding protein (RBP) and vitamin A. Levels of prealbumin may be elevated in renal failure despite nutritional compromise resulting from decreased catabolism and excretion of RBP. Transferrin is elevated with iron depletion, independent of the effects of nutrition.

5. **How are protein requirements determined?**
Protein need is determined based on patient weight, current stress factors, extraordinary skin losses, and organ function. Although the recommended daily intake (RDI) for protein for healthy individuals is only 0.8 g of protein/kg of body weight, the following guidelines may be used in the surgical patient:

Injury level	Protein requirement
Mild stress/injury	1.2–1.4 g of protein/kg
Moderate stress/injury	1.5–1.7 g of protein/kg
Severe stress/injury	1.8–2.5 g of protein/kg

6. **What is the significance of urinary nitrogen in nutritional assessment?**
Total urinary nitrogen (TUN) is the most reliable indicator of nitrogen use and excretion in the patient who is in the surgical intensive care unit (SICU). However, urinary urea nitrogen (UUN) is more readily available in most hospital laboratories. Although TUN and UUN are nearly equal in healthy ambulatory patients with normal renal and hepatic function, critically ill patients have a poor correlation between the two. A 12-hour urine collection compares well with a 24-hour collection (Graves). Optimal nutrition support promotes a +3 to +5 nitrogen balance. Estimate the protein needs of the patient by adding:

$$[24\ h\ UUN\ (g)\ +\ 2\ g\ N\ insensible\ losses\ +\ 3]\ \times\ 6.25\ =\ required\ amount\ of\ protein\ (g)$$

Remember that 6.25 g of protein yields 1 g of nitrogen. Insensible losses are increased with burns, decubiti, wound vacuums, and large wounds. UUN is not useful as a guide for nutritional prescription in hepatic failure, renal dysfunction (<50 mL/min creatinine clearance), or recent spinal cord injury.

7. **Should protein be severely restricted in the surgical patient with hepatic failure or renal failure?**
Limit protein to 0.6–0.8 g/kg in patients with hepatic encephalopathy; if the encephalopathy produces significant clinical consequences, branched chain amino acids can be considered (though no mortality benefit has been found). However, only about 10% of chronic liver disease patients are protein sensitive; thus, other causes of encephalopathy, such as infection, constipation, and electrolyte disturbance, should be explored. Otherwise, give a more typical postsurgical protein load (1.3–1.5 g/kg).

In injured and acutely ill patients with **renal failure**, withholding protein is now an old recommendation. Giving adequate protein may require more frequent dialysis. Amino acid losses and requirements increase with more intensive hemodialysis (HD) (10–12 g of amino acids removed with each HD, or 5–12 g of amino acids daily with continuous venovenous hemodialysis [CVVHD]).

Table 9.1 Serum Proteins

PROTEIN	SYNTHETIC SITE	CLINICAL SIGNIFICANCE	HALF-LIFE	LIMITATIONS	INTERPRETATION
Albumin	Liver	Relates to outcomes; relates to edema	20–21 days	Best case scenario for hepatic production: 12–25 g/24 hr; dilutional effects; long half-life; used alone, sensitivity poor	Normal <3.5 g/dL Mild depletion 2.8–3.5 g/dL Moderate 2.2–2.8 g/dL Severe <2.2 g/dL
Prealbumin	Liver	Indicates nutritional deficits before albumin	2–4 days	Short half-life	Normal >18 mg/dL Mild depletion 10–18 mg/dL Moderate 5–10 mg/dL Severe <5 mg/dL
Transferrin	Liver	More sensitive than albumin; relatively useful parameter in liver disease compared with albumin; can calculate from total iron binding capacity (TIBC)	8–10 days	Poor marker of early repletion; sensitive to changes in body iron	Mild depletion 150–200 mg/dL Moderate 100–150 mg/dL Severe <100 mg/dL
C-Reactive Protein (CRP)	Liver	Increases abruptly after injury. Early and reliable indicator of disease or injury severity.	48–72 hr	May be increased with obesity and other chronic inflammatory states	Baseline normal <3 mg/dL Bacterial infection 30–35 mg/dL Viral infection <20 mg/dL Peaks 48–72 h post-trauma up to 35 mg/dL

8. **How are kilocalorie needs determined?**
There are numerous methods for setting kilocalorie targets in the surgical patient: (a) prediction equations, (b) kcal/kg estimations or, (c) indirect calorimetry. One common prediction equation, the Harris Benedict (HBE), was developed in 1919 for use on ambulatory, fasted, healthy people but is of limited usefulness in hospitalized patients.
   A number of prediction equations have been developed but most physicians employ a total kcal/kg goal as shown in Table 9.2.

Table 9.2 Kilocalorie Goals in Surgical Patient

PATIENT	FEEDING LEVEL (KCAL/KG)	LEVEL BY INDIRECT CALORIMETRY
Normal weight patients	25–30	REE[a] × 1.0
Underweight patients	30–35	REE × 1.2
Obese patients	20–25[b]	REE × 0.85
Morbidly obese	10–20[b]	REE × 0.75

[a]Basal energy expenditure (BEE) is the number of kilocalories expended at rest, in a fasted state. Resting energy expenditure (REE) is measured in a fed state and is 5%–10% higher than BEE.
[b]Adjusted weight = [(Actual weight − Ideal weight) × 0.25] + Ideal weight

9. **What is indirect calorimetry, and when is it useful?**
Indirect calorimetry is a respiratory test that measures the patient's production of CO_2 and consumption of oxygen for approximately 30 minutes, until steady state is achieved. Results are worked into the modified Weir equation:

$$REE = [(3.796 \times VO_2) + (1.214 \times VCO_2)] \times 1440 \text{ min/day}$$

Where:
   REE = resting energy expenditure (kcal/day)
   VO_2 = oxygen consumption (L/min)
   VCO_2 = CO_2 exhaled (L/min)
The report indicates the number of kilocalories the patient consumes in 24 hours and the respiratory quotient (RQ). RQ = VCO_2/VO_2 and provides information on the type of substrate being used. The RQ for the metabolism of fat, protein, and carbohydrate are 0.7, 0.83, and 1.0, respectively. Overfeeding will result in an RQ >1.0 as a result of increased CO_2 production associated with lipogenesis.
   The test is useful in the patient on mechanical ventilation (MV) once a patient is relatively stable, with a fractional concentration of oxygen in inspired gas (FiO_2) <60% and peak end-expiratory pressure (PEEP) <10. Studies are helpful:
   a. When overfeeding (diabetes mellitus [DM], chronic obstructive pulmonary disease, obesity) is undesirable.
   b. When underfeeding (renal failure, large wounds) is detrimental.
   c. In patients whose physical or clinical factors promote alterations in energy expenditure (spinal cord injury).
   d. When drugs are used that significantly alter energy expenditure (paralytic agents, β-blockers).
   e. In patients who do not respond as expected to calculated regimens.

ENTERAL NUTRITION

10. **When should enteral nutrition be considered?**
Always, but especially when a patient is unlikely to meet >70% of nutritional needs by mouth. Patients who have sustained major head injury (Glasgow Coma Scale <8), major torso trauma, major trauma to the pelvis and long bones, or major chest trauma benefit from enteral nutrition. Approximately 85% of patients (even those undergoing GI surgery) tolerate early enteral feeding within 24 hours postoperatively.

11. **How do you access the gastrointestinal tract for feeding?**
Pursue access by blind placement of a nasogastric (NG) tube or a nasoduodenal tube. Place a nasojejunal tube (NJ) blindly, endoscopically, or fluoroscopically. Achieve gastric

decompression with concurrent nasojejunal feeds with an endoscopic percutaneous gastrostomy/jejunostomy (PEG/PEJ). Alternatively, place a gastrostomy or feeding jejunostomy intraoperatively.

12. **What types of enteral formulas are available?**
Polymeric enteral feedings are soy-based, lactose-free products containing intact protein, carbohydrate, and fat. Most offer 1 kcal/mL and 37–62 g of protein per liter. Special modifications of the standard formulas include dietary fiber or "immune-enhancing" agents, such as fish oil, arginine, glutamine, and nucleotides. "Elemental" formulas contain amino acids, di-, tri-, and quatrapeptides, dextrose, and minimal fat. Several concentrated formulas (2 kcal/mL) are available for use in patients with congestive heart failure (CHF), renal failure, and hepatic failure, but have a higher rate of tube-feed–related diarrhea. In general, products that are "disease-specific" or contain nutrients in elemental form are more expensive than standard products.

13. **Are specialized formulas necessary for the patient with DM who is critically ill?**
No. Formulas with reduced carbohydrate and increased fat loads are marketed as being superior in maintaining glycemic control. These products have not shown superior, clinically significant outcome in hospitalized patients in randomized controlled trials. The use of standard high protein formulas in an isocaloric or hypocaloric load, combined with appropriate insulin therapy, is the most effective treatment for hyperglycemia in the stressed patient with type 2 DM. The level of glycemic control associated with enhanced outcome is best achieved with insulin, as opposed to carbohydrate restriction. Furthermore, gastric feedings with high fat formulas in the diabetic patient with gastroparesis may delay gastric emptying and increase risk of aspiration.

14. **Should specialized "pulmonary" formulas be used on all patients on ventilators?**
No. Specialized, high omega-6 fat formulas have been marketed to reduce CO_2 production in COPD patients who retain CO_2. In theory, these formulas minimize CO_2 production and facilitate weaning. However, avoiding overfeeding is more important for reducing CO_2 production than providing high fat formula. Gastric feeding with these products increases the risk of aspiration.

15. **What complications are related to enteral support?**
Enteral feeding may produce electrolyte abnormalities, hyperglycemia, GI intolerance, pulmonary aspiration, and nasopharyngeal erosions. Surgical complications of enteral access include leaks, tube dislodgement, volvulus, soft tissue infection, and bowel necrosis.

16. **Should one wait for bowel sounds or flatus before beginning enteral feedings?**
No.

17. **Should one delay nutrition support longer in obese patients assuming they have increased reserves?**
No. Obese patients have more fat, but during stress all patients become hypermetabolic and break down endogenous protein stores to mobilize amino acids for gluconeogenesis, protein production, and adenosine triphosphate. As with patients of normal weight, patients who are obese require high protein nutritional supplementation to meet increased nitrogen demands.

18. **Should enteral formulas be diluted for initial presentation?**
No. Dilution delays the attainment of feeding goals and increases the likelihood of bacterial contamination. Solution osmolarity is a relatively minor culprit in producing diarrhea.

19. **How should enteral feeding-related diarrhea be managed?**
Mild diarrhea usually requires no treatment. With moderate to severe diarrhea, consider feeding reduction, antidiarrheal agents, and stool studies for clostridium difficile. Evaluate the medication profile for sorbitol-containing elixirs, laxatives, stool softeners, and prokinetic agents. Monitor sanitation issues related to formula handling. Some success has been reported with soluble fiber or lactobacillus probiotics (yogurt) in antibiotic-associated diarrhea.

20. **During gastric feeding, at what level of gastric residual volume (GRV) should one hold feedings?**
Depends. Recent evidence suggests that we should not check residual volumes in medical ICU patients, but the postoperative surgical patient could benefit from checking. Always use measurements of gastric residual volume (GRV) in tandem with clinical assessment. Increase vigilance at 200–500 mL of GRV and start prokinetic agents. Hold feedings if GRV >500 mL.

21. **Do enteral feedings contain enough water to meet all fluid needs?**

    Most 1 kcal/mL formulas (standard) contain 85% water by volume, whereas 2 kcal/mL formulas contain 70% water. Water is generally not an issue in the patient in ICU receiving multiple intravenous (IV) fluids and drugs. However, post-ICU, or in patients bound for home or extended care facilities, it is essential to write a water prescription with the tube feeding order. General guidelines for the total water needs are shown in Table 9.3.

    For example, if the total calculated need for fluid is 2400 mL for a 60-kg patient and 2400 cc of the tube feeding provides approximately 2000 mL of free water, write an order to give 200 mL of water to the patient twice daily.

Table 9.3 Daily Water Needs in Relation to Age

PATIENT	AGE	DAILY WATER NEEDS
Average adult	25–55 years	35 mL/kg
Young, active adult	16–35 years	40 mL/kg
Adult	>55–65 years	30 mL/kg
Elderly	>65 years	25 mL/kg

22. **How is enteral nutrition infused?**

    Enteral nutrition is infused continuously, in bolus form or cyclically. Continuous infusion is best in the patient who is critically ill requiring postpyloric feedings. Bolus feedings are used in more stable patients with gastric feedings. Cyclic feedings or nocturnal feedings are useful for the patient who is on concurrent oral intake and in transition to full oral support, or for those requiring feeding-free periods for physical therapy or activities of daily living.

23. **Is enteral nutrition better than total parenteral nutrition?**

    Yes. Substrates delivered enterally are better tolerated, are associated with fewer metabolic and hepatic complications, and help preserve normal mucosal integrity. Eighty percent of the body's immune tissue is in the gut and needs local and systemic nutrition. A review of 13 studies describing a total of 856 patients who were critically ill, contrasting total parenteral nutrition (TPN) with enteral nutrition, concluded that enteral nutrition reduces infectious complications and is typically more cost-effective than parenteral nutrition.

24. **Should you discontinue enteral feeding at midnight on all patients undergoing elective surgery with general anesthesia?**

    No. The American Society of Anesthesiologists recommends that healthy adults cease intake of solids for at least 6 hours and liquids for 2 hours before undergoing elective procedures. The guidelines may need to be modified for patients with coexisting diseases that may affect gastric emptying-pregnancy, obesity, DM, hiatal hernia, gastroesophageal reflux disease (GERD), ileus or bowel obstruction, emergency care, or enteral tube feeding. Recent clinical investigation shows enhanced immunologic and functional recovery of the GI tract with decreased perioperative fasting periods.

25. **Is the clear liquid diet mandatory after surgery?**

    No. Clinical outcomes are similar when patients are fasted or given clear liquids until the appearance of flatus or BM as opposed to receiving a regular diet beginning one day postoperatively.

26. **Does preoperative nutrition with immune-enhancing diets improve surgical outcome?**

    Yes. Perioperative immune-enhancing diets (IEDs) can reduce postoperative complications and infections and enhance postoperative immunocompetence in properly selected patients. The consensus recommendations from the US Summit on Immune-Enhancing Enteral Therapy (2001) advise giving IEDs to severely malnourished patients undergoing lower GI surgery 5–7 days before surgery. Emerging data suggest a benefit for patients who are not clinically malnourished. Heyland et al. recently concluded in a metaanalysis, "Immunonutrition may decrease infectious complication rates but it is not associated with an overall mortality advantage."

27. **Should actual, ideal, or adjusted body weight be used in nutrition calculations for the patient with obesity?**
    Studies using an obesity-adjusted weight in kilocalorie calculations [ideal body weight (IBW) + .25 (actual–IBW)] correlate better with measured energy expenditure than when using actual weight.

ENTERAL CONTROVERSIES

28. **What are probiotics, and when are they useful?**
    Probiotics are live microbes that benefit the host. Clinical studies show therapeutic or preventive use of varied probiotic strains for antibiotic-associated diarrhea, rotavirus-associated diarrhea and pouchitis. Results are promising for irritable bowel syndrome, ulcerative colitis, and side-effect reduction in antibiotic therapy for helicobacter pylori.

29. **Which is more important: nitrogen or caloric balance?**
    Ultimately, maintaining positive nitrogen balance may be more important than achieving positive kilocalorie balance.

30. **Are postpyloric feedings superior to gastric feedings?**
    Following major surgery or injury, gastric emptying is impaired for several days. Early enteral feeding, with its known benefits, may not easily occur through a gastric feeding in the early stages of injury. Postpyloric feedings deliver more kilocalories, more timely return to anabolism, and promote a lower rate of infectious complications than continuous gastric feeding.

31. **When should immune-enhancing formulas be used?**
    Rarely. Patients in randomized controlled trials have demonstrated that IEDs improve outcome and reduce septic morbidity in patients prone to intraabdominal sepsis after major torso trauma and after major operative resection of upper GI cancers. The use of IEDs should be restricted to these patients, and duration should be limited because of the increased expense. The IEDs have not been adequately tested in other types of patients, and, when tested in a variety of patients in the ICU, there is some evidence to suggest that they could be harmful. There is controversy that administering arginine in patients with sepsis, who have upregulated expression of inducible nitrous oxide synthase (iNos), will result in excessive nitrous oxide production and resultant exaggerated vasodilation and oxidant stress. This fear is slowly being phased out. Luiking et al. published several reports suggesting that even parenteral arginine is safe. It will take more time to understand its safety and efficacy in the critically ill population, but in sepsis we understand that excessive NO production from arginine supplementation is a misconception.

32. **Should formula with increased fish-oil formula be used in patients who are going into acute respiratory distress syndrome?**
    Two industry-funded, randomized controlled trials demonstrate superior outcome in patients with acute respiratory distress syndrome (ARDS) when provided a high omega-3 fatty acid enteral product as opposed to a high omega-6 "pulmonary" formula. Unfortunately, the control diet, a high omega-6 fatty acid formula, is not the standard of care and may worsen ARDS. High omega-6 fatty acids increase inflammation and produce lipid mediators that worsen ventilation/perfusion (V/Q) mismatch in the lung and worsen oxygenation in ARDS. A randomized controlled trial comparing standard, moderate-fat polymeric formula and a high omega-3 formula is needed. There is, however, on-going controversy as an ARDSnet trial in 2011 studying omega supplementation was stopped short because of futility, as there was not a benefit for the primary endpoint of ventilator free days at 28 days.

PARENTERAL NUTRITION

33. **What is parenteral nutrition?**
    Parenteral nutrition is the provision of protein as amino acids (4 kcal/g), dextrose (3.4 kcal/g), fat (lipid 20% solution delivers 2 kcal/mL), vitamins, minerals, trace elements, fluid, and sometimes insulin through an IV infusion.

34. **What are the indications for parenteral nutrition?**
    Use parenteral nutrition when the GI tract is totally nonfunctional, e.g., major bowel resection, "short gut," peritonitis, intestinal hemorrhage, paralytic ileus, and high volume enterocutaneous fistulae.

35. **What types of access are available for the delivery of parenteral nutrition?**
Central parenteral solutions have osmolarities up to 3000 mOsm/L. These require delivery into a large lumen vein (e.g., subclavian, or, less commonly, a femoral vein). If a multiple-port catheter is used, a "virgin port" should be reserved exclusively for nutrient infusion. When prolonged parenteral nutrition infusion is necessary in the postacute setting, consider a long-term access device such as a Hickman or Broviac catheter. This may not be necessary, however, when the central venous catheter is placed under sterile conditions and the patient and caretakers deliver meticulous care.

36. **Should patients with pancreatitis be exclusively fed parenterally?**
Although patients with pancreatitis have traditionally been given "gut rest" and TPN, studies demonstrate improved outcome with enteral feeding past the ligament of Treitz. Enteral feedings delivered into the jejunum promote decreased infectious morbidity, shorter hospital length of stay, fewer complications, a faster resolution of systemic inflammatory response syndrome (SIRS), and a shorter disease course than parenteral nutrition. If enteral nutrition is not tolerated, parenteral nutrition should be considered no sooner than 7 days into the hospitalization.

37. **Are intravenous lipids contraindicated in pancreatitis?**
In extremely rare instances of pancreatitis caused by congenital hyperlipidemia, lipids should be withheld. However, in most cases of severe pancreatitis where enteral nutrition is not tolerated, it is best to avoid IV lipid emulsions until the inflammatory response has subsided.

38. **What complications are associated with parenteral nutrition?**
Fluid and electrolyte imbalance, altered glucose metabolism, increased LFTs, hepatic steatosis, systemic candidiasis, site infections, and gut atrophy are associated with TPN. Hemothorax or pneumothorax may occur during central line placement. Although rare, air emboli or extravascular placement of central lines occur.

39. **Why do parenterally fed patients often develop hyperglycemia?**
Patients who are fed parenterally may develop hyperglycemia as a result of increased stress and the inflammatory response, limited mobility, concurrent steroid therapy, and excessive kilocalorie intake.

40. **How should hyperglycemia be managed?**
Evaluate information on the home glucose control regimen from the medication history. A continuous insulin infusion is often necessary during critical illness to achieve adequate glycemic control. When insulin requirements are predictable and the patient becomes more stable metabolically and moves outside of the ICU, insulin is added to the TPN. NPH insulin is geared toward patients consuming meals at regular intervals and thus is not appropriate with continuous IV feedings. Glucose infusion rates should not exceed 5 mg/kg per minute.

41. **Why are intravenous fat emulsions used, and when are they contraindicated?**
Theoretically, fat emulsions are employed to prevent essential fatty acid deficiency. In reality, this condition is rare, takes several weeks to develop, and requires only 3%–4% of kilocalories as linoleic acid (or 10% of kilocalories as a standard fat emulsion). Fat emulsions are also used to provide additional kilocalories once glucose delivery exceeds 5 kcal/kg per minute. When delivered in total-nutrient-admixtures (3-in-1 solutions) lipid emulsions are stable for 24 hours. When infused as a sole nutrient, limit hang times to <12 hours to prevent bacterial growth. Avoid fat emulsions with hyperlipidemia-induced pancreatitis and when serum triglycerides are significantly elevated (e.g., >500 mg/dL). Because they are associated with increased mortality early after trauma, and increased infections in critical illness, IV fat emulsion risk outweighs benefit during the early acute-phase response.

42. **What is refeeding syndrome, and how is it managed or prevented?**
Refeeding syndrome occurs when a patient is moderately to severely malnourished and has limited substrate reserves, usually as a result of chronic alcoholism, anorexia nervosa, postbariatric surgery, or chronic starvation. When presented with a large nutrient load, the patient rapidly develops a clinically significant decline in serum K, phosphorus (P), Ca, and Mg because of compartment shifts or increased utilization of these ions. Hyperglycemia is common as a result of blunted basal insulin secretion (see Kraft). Provide ample quantities of K, P, Ca, and Mg with the initial parenteral mixture, within the solubility limits of the solution. Reduce the initial kilocalorie load by 25% of goal by limiting dextrose kilocalories. Monitor blood glucose four times daily, and serum K, P, Ca, and Mg daily for 5 days after initiating feeding, while advancing kilocalories to goal levels.

43. **How should parenteral nutrition be monitored?**
Parenteral nutrition should be monitored daily with serum chemistries (Na, K, Cl, CO_2, glucose, Mg, P, and Ca) during the initial days of therapy in the critical care setting. Check blood glucose every 6 hours. With acceptable fluid and electrolyte balance, reduce frequency to one to two times weekly. The adequacy of the nutrition regimen may be assessed by evidence of proper wound healing, maintenance of hydration status, preservation of body cell mass, and a timely repletion of constitutive protein levels. Overfeeding may present as insulin resistance, hypertriglyceridemia, increased LFTs, and hypercapnia.

44. **What infusion schedules are used for TPN?**
TPN is usually infused continuously. In more ambulatory patients, and those on home therapy, a cyclic or nighttime infusion schedule (12- to 18-hour cycle) increases patient freedom.

45. **How should TPN be discontinued?**
To discontinue TPN, reduce the infusion rate by half for 2 hours, halved again for 2 hours, and then turn it off. This "ramp down" prevents reactive hypoglycemia.

46. **What is the cost of parenteral nutrition?**
Parenteral solution costs vary widely depending on the constituents. The cost of TPN solution components, preparation, access devices, and laboratory monitoring costs up to 10 times that of a standard enteral feeding. Many third-party payers do not provide more reimbursement for parenteral therapy than enteral in the hospital setting.

47. **How much gut is necessary to avoid TPN dependence after small bowel resection?**
The normal adult small bowel is 300–800 cm in length. Loss of more than two-thirds is considered short-bowel syndrome. The condition of the remnant small bowel is important.

PARENTERAL CONTROVERSIES

48. **Should TPN solutions contain the same percentage of fat kilocalories that are recommended in the diet of healthy Americans (i.e., 30 of total kilocalories)?**
The American Heart Association (AHA) recommendations for 30% of total kilocalories as fat are geared toward cardiovascular disease prevention in healthy people and were never intended for IV feeding in individuals who are critically ill. Furthermore, AHA suggests that those kilocalories be distributed among saturated, monounsaturated, and polyunsaturated fat, including omega-3 series fatty acids. Current lipid formulations available in the United States are made from either soybean oil or a mixture of soybean and safflower oil; thus, they are predominately polyunsaturated (omega-6) fat. Glucose kilocalories are the most cost-effective kilocalories, followed by standard amino acid kilocalories, then lipid calories. Lipid infusions exceeding 1 g/kg of body weight are associated with decreased immunocompetence and impaired oxygenation in patients who are critically ill.

49. **Does supplemental glutamine enhance outcome in surgical patients?**
Glutamine, the amino acid found in greatest concentration in muscle and plasma, decreases after surgery, injury, or stress. Thus, it is a conditionally essential amino acid. It plays a role as a metabolic substrate for rapidly replicating cells, maintains the integrity and function of the intestinal barrier, and protects the enterocyte from free radical damage. Glutamine is not included in standard amino acid solutions because of limited solubility and stability. Enteral supplementation may reduce infectious complication rates and decrease hospital stay in surgical patients. The recent REDOX trial showed that parenteral glutamine may actually be deleterious and increase mortality compared to control. Parenteral glutamine should be used cautiously or not at all in the critically ill patients.

50. **Should recombinant growth hormone, glutamine, and a modified diet be used routinely to maximize gut adaptation after intestinal resection?**
Five clinical trials have appeared in the past decade. Three showed negative results, whereas two showed positive results. Positive results are short-lived. Until further research occurs, this expensive therapy should not be routine, and intensive nutrition and pharmacologic management should remain the mainstay of care.

BIBLIOGRAPHY

1. Brady M, Kinn S, Stuart P. Preoperative fasting for adults to prevent perioperative complications. *Cochrane Database Syst Rev.* 2003:CD004423.
2. Heyland DK, Dhaliwal R, Day A, et al. Canadian Critical Care Clinical Practice Guidelines Committee. Canadian clinical practice guidelines for nutrition support in mechanically ventilated, critically ill adult patients. *JPEN J Parenter Enteral Nutr.* 2003;27(5):355–373.
3. Frankenfield D, Hise M, Malone A, et al. Prediction of resting metabolic rate in critically ill adult patients: results of a systematic review of the evidence. *J Am Diet Assoc.* 2007;107(9):1552–1561.
4. Gadek JE, DeMichele SJ, Karlstad MD, et al. Effect of enteral feeding with eicosapentaenoic acid, gamma-linoleic acid, and antioxidants in patients with acute respiratory distress syndrome. *Crit Care Med.* 1999;27(8):1409–1420.
5. Graves C, Saffle J, Morris S. Comparison of urine urea nitrogen collection times in critically ill patients. *Nutr Clin Pract.* 2005;20(2):271–275.
6. Haugen HA, Chan LN, Li F. Indirect calorimetry: a practical guide for clinicians. *Nutr Clin Pract.* 2007;22(4):377–388.
7. KDOQI clinical practice guidelines for nutrition in chronic renal failure. *Am J Kidney Dis.* 2000;35(6 suppl 2):S1–S140.
8. Konstantinides FN, Konstantinides NN. Urinary urea nitrogen: too sensitive for calculating nitrogen balance studies in surgical clinical nutrition. *JPEN J Parenter Enteral Nutr.* 1991;15(2):189–193.
9. Kozar R, McQuiggan M, Moore F. Nutritional support of trauma patients. In: Shikora S, Martindale RG, Schwaitzburg S, eds. *Nutritional Considerations in the Intensive Care Unit.* Silver Springs, MD: ASPEN Publishers; 2002.
10. Kraft MD, Btaiche IF. Review of the refeeding syndrome. *Nutr Clin Pract.* 2005;20(6):625–633.
11. Matarese LE, O'Keefe SJ. Short-bowel syndrome: clinical guidelines for nutrition management. *Nutr Clin Pract.* 2005;20(5):493–502.
12. McClave SA. Nutrition support in acute pancreatitis. *Gastroenterol Clin North Am.* 2007;36(1):65–74.
13. Novak F, Heyland DK. Glutamine supplementation in serious illness: a systematic review of the evidence. *Crit Care Med.* 2002;30(9):2022–2029.
14. Pontes-Arruda A, Aragão AM. Effects of enteral feeding with eicosapentaenoic acid, gamma-linolenic acid, and antioxidants in mechanically ventilated patients with severe sepsis and septic shock. *Crit Care Med.* 2006;34(9):2325–2333.
15. Van den Berghe G, Wouters P, Weekers F, et al. Intensive insulin therapy in critically ill patients. *N Engl J Med.* 2001;345(19):1359–1367.
16. Luiking YC, Poeze M, Deutz NE. Arginine infusion in patients with septic shock increases nitric oxide production without haemodynamic instability. *Clin Sci (Lond).* 2015;128(1):57–67.
17. Luiking YC, Engelen MP, Deutz NE. Regulation of nitric oxide production in health and disease. *Curr Opin Clin Nutr Metab Care.* 2010;13(1):97–104.
18. Luiking YC, Poeze M, Ramsay G, Deutz NE. Reduced citrulline production in sepsis is related to diminished de novo arginine and nitric oxide production. *Am J Clin Nutr.* 2009;89(1):142–152.

CHAPTER 10

WHAT DOES POSTOPERATIVE FEVER MEAN?

Robert A. Tessler, MD, Alden H. Harken, MD, FACS

1. **What is a fever?**
   Normal core temperature varies between 36°C and 38°C. Because humans hibernate a little at night, we are cool (36°C) just before rising in the morning; after revving our engines all day, we are hot at night (38°C). A fever is a pathologic state reflecting a systemic inflammatory process. The core temperature is >38°C but rarely >40°C.

2. **What is malignant hyperthermia?**
   A rare, life-threatening response to inhaled anesthetics or some muscle relaxants. Core temperature rises >40°C. Abnormal calcium metabolism in skeletal muscle produces heat, acidosis, hypokalemia, muscle rigidity, coagulopathy, and circulatory collapse.

3. **How is malignant hyperthermia treated?**
   a. Stop the anesthetic.
   b. Give sodium bicarbonate (2 mEq/kg intravenously [IV]).
   c. Give dantrolene (calcium channel blocker at 2.5 mg/kg IV).
   d. Continue dantrolene (1 mg/kg every 6 hours for 48 hours).
   e. Cool patient with alcohol sponges and ice.

KEY POINTS: MALIGNANT HYPERTHERMIA

1. Rare, familial (autosomal dominant with variable penetrance), catastrophic response to inhaled anesthetics or muscle relaxants
2. Mechanism: Abnormal calcium metabolism in skeletal muscle
3. Clinical manifestations: Core temperature >40°C, trismus, hypercapnia, tachycardia, tachypnea, hypertension, cardiac dysrhythmias, metabolic acidosis, hypoxemia, myoglobinuria, or coagulopathy
4. Management: Halt anesthetic; administer dantrolene over 48 hours, supplemental sodium bicarbonate; actively cool patient

---

4. **What causes fever?**
   Macrophages are activated by bacteria and endotoxin. Activated macrophages release interleukin-1, tumor necrosis factor (TNF), and interferon, which reset the hypothalamic thermoregulatory center.

5. **Can fever be treated?**
   Yes. Aspirin, acetaminophen, and ibuprofen are cyclooxygenase inhibitors that block the formation of prostaglandin E_2 in the hypothalamus and effectively control fever.

6. **Should fever be treated?**
   This is controversial. No evidence suggests that suppression of fever improves patient outcome. Patients are more comfortable, however, and the surgeon receives fewer calls from the nurses.

7. **Should fever be investigated?**
   Yes. Fever indicates that something (frequently treatable) is going on. The threshold for inquiry depends on the patient. A transplant patient with a temperature of 38°C requires scrutiny, whereas a healthy medical student with an identical temperature of 38°C 24 hours after an appendectomy can be ignored.

8. Summarize a fever work-up.
   a. Order blood cultures, urine Gram stain and culture, and sputum Gram stain and culture.
   b. Look at the surgical incisions.
   c. Look at old and current intravenous sites for evidence of septic thrombophlebitis.
   d. If breath sounds are worrisome, obtain a chest x-ray.

9. What is the most common cause of fever during the early postoperative period (1–3 days)?
   The traditional answer is atelectasis. A total pneumothorax does *not* cause fever, however. Why does a little atelectasis cause fever, whereas a lot of atelectasis (pneumothorax) does not? The most likely explanation is that sterile atelectasis (and early postoperative lung collapse typically is not infected) has nothing to do with fever.

10. Do surgical incisions compromise spontaneous breathing patterns?
    Yes. Vital capacity was measured in a large group of patients 24 hours after various surgical procedures. An upper abdominal incision was the worst, followed by lower abdominal incision, then (counterintuitively) thoracotomy, median sternotomy, and extremity incision.

11. Should atelectasis be treated with incentive spirometry?
    Yes, but not to avoid fever.

12. Define a wound infection.
    A wound infection contains >10^5 organisms per gram of tissue. An infected incision appears erythematous (red), edematous (swollen), and tender.

13. Are certain wounds prone to infection?
    Each milliliter of human saliva contains 10^8 aerobic and anaerobic, gram-positive and gram-negative bacteria. All human bite wounds must be considered as contaminated. Animal bite wounds typically are less contaminated. (It is safer to kiss your dog than your partner.)

14. Do incisions become infected early after surgery?
    The incision must be examined in a patient with a fever (39°C) <12 hours after surgery. Look for a foul-smelling, serous discharge in a particularly painful wound (all incisions hurt) with or without crepitus. Gram stain of the serous discharge for gram-positive rods confirms or excludes the diagnosis of clostridial infection.

15. What is the therapy for clostridial gas gangrene?
    a. The wound should be opened immediately, with fluid resuscitation of the patient. The mainstay of therapy is aggressive surgical debridement of necrotic tissue (skin, muscle, and fascia). Make a big hole, and do not worry about closing it.
    b. Give penicillin, 12 million U/day IV for 1 week.
    c. Hyperbaric oxygen is not helpful.

16. Are nonclostridial necrotizing wound infections a cause of concern?
    Hemolytic streptococcal gangrene, idiopathic scrotal gangrene, and gram-negative synergistic necrotizing cellulitis are distinct entities but have been lumped into the single category of necrotizing fasciitis. All require the same initial approach:
    a. Fluid and electrolyte resuscitation.
    b. Broad-spectrum antibiotics ("triples").
    c. Aggressive surgical debridement of all necrotic tissue.

17. What are "Big Gun" antibiotics?
    A shotgun approach to potentially life-threatening infections when the patient is seriously ill and the surgeon is seriously concerned:
    a. Zosyn 3.375 g Q6° IV
    b. Vancomycin 1.0 g IV over 10 minutes
    To avoid overgrowth of yeast and resistant bacteria, focus on the culprit bacteria as soon as the cultures define it.

KEY POINTS: CLOSTRIDIAL VERSUS NONCLOSTRIDIAL NECROTIZING WOUND INFECTIONS

1. Clostridial infection involves underlying muscle resulting in myonecrosis or gas gangrene.
2. Nonclostridial infection involves subcutaneous fascia (also known as necrotizing fasciitis).
3. Similar management: Fluid and electrolyte resuscitation, antibiotics (high-dose penicillin for clostridial infection, broad-spectrum triples for necrotizing fasciitis), and aggressive surgical debridement of necrotic tissue.

18. **Which surgical procedures are predisposed to wound infections?**
    Gastrointestinal (GI) procedures, especially when the colon is opened.

19. **When do wound infections typically occur?**
    They occur between 12 hours and 7 days postoperatively.

20. **How is a wound infection treated?**
    The wound should be opened and completely drained.

21. **Is it necessary to irrigate an infected wound?**
    Tap water irrigation decreases the bacterial load and promotes healing. Alcohol is toxic to tissues. Sodium hypochlorite (Dakin's solution) and hydrogen peroxide kill fibroblasts and slow epithelialization. As a rule of thumb, put nothing into a wound that you would not put in your eye.

22. **Are routine peritoneal fluid cultures during appendectomy justified?**
    No.

23. **When do urinary tract infections occur?**
    The longer the urethral (Foley) catheter is in place, the more likely the urinary tract infection (UTI). Urologic instrumentation at the time of surgery may accelerate the process considerably. Germs crawl up the outside of the urethral catheter, and by 5–7 days after surgery, most patients harbor infected urine.

24. **How is a urinary tract infection diagnosed?**
    A UTI has a urine culture with >10^5 bacteria/mL. White blood cells on urinalysis are highly suspicious.

25. **What are the most common late causes of postoperative fever?**
    Septic thrombophlebitis (from an intravenous line) and occult (usually intraabdominal) abscesses tend to present about 2 weeks after surgery.

BIBLIOGRAPHY

1. Bansal BC, Wiebe RA, Perkins SD, et al. Tap water for irrigation of lacerations. *Am J Emerg Med.* 2002;20(5):469–472.
2. da Luz Moreira A, Vogel JD. Fever evaluations after colorectal surgery: identification of risk factors that increase yield and decrease cost. *Dis Colon Rectum.* 2008;51(5):1202–1207.
3. Helmer KS, Robinson EK. Standardized patient care guidelines reduce infectious morbidity in appendectomy patients. *Am J Surg.* 2002;183(6):608–613.
4. Lewis RT. Oral versus systemic antibiotic prophylaxis in elective colon surgery: a randomized study and meta-analysis send a message from the 1990s. *Can J Surg.* 2002;45(3):173–180.
5. Singer AJ, Quinn JV. Determinants of poor outcome after laceration and surgical incision repair. *Plast Reconstr Surg.* 2002;110(2):429–435.

CHAPTER 11

SURGICAL WOUND INFECTION

M. Kelley Bullard, MD

1. **What is a surgical site infection?**
   Surgical wound infections are now more appropriately referred to as "surgical site infections" (SSIs). There are different types of SSIs, which are classified by depth, timing after surgery, clinical criteria, and symptoms.
   The three categories of SSIs as defined by the Centers for Disease Control and Prevention are:
   a. Superficial incisional
   b. Deep incisional
   c. Organ/deep space
   Superficial incisional infections involve the skin and subcutaneous tissues. These SSIs must occur within 30 days of surgery unless a foreign body (e.g., cardiac pacemaker) is left in situ. In the case of implanted foreign materials, 1 year must pass before surgery can be excluded as the source of an infection.
   Deep incisional infections involve the deep soft tissues, such as fascial and muscle layers. They must occur within 90 days of the operation to be considered a surgical site infection (except in the event of a foreign material as mentioned above).
   Organ/deep space infections involve any part of the body deeper than the fascial/muscle layer that is openly manipulated during an operation. These infections must occur within 90 days of the operation to be considered a surgical site infection.

2. **How common are surgical site infections?**
   Surgical site infections have become the most common healthcare-associated infections (HAIs) in the United States. Surveillance data from the Centers for Disease Control's National Health Safety Network noted that SSIs comprise 31% of all HAIs. Despite advances in critical care and infection control practices, these infections continue to be a substantial cause of morbidity, prolonged hospitalizations, and death. Annual healthcare expenditures related to surgical site infections range from 3.5 billion to 10 billion dollars.

3. **What are the classic signs of surgical infections?**
   Superficial and deep incisional SSIs:
   - Calor (heat)
   - Rubor (redness)
   - Tumor (swelling)
   - Dolor (pain)
   - Purulent drainage
   Organ space SSIs should be suspected in the presence of systemic signs and symptoms:
   - Fever
   - Ileus
   - Shock
   Definitive diagnosis of organ space SSIs may require imaging studies.

4. **What factors increase the risk of surgical site infections?**
   Depth and complexity of the wound, patient factors, procedure related conditions, and microbial factors all contribute to the occurrence of surgical site infections.

5. **How does the complexity of the wound affect surgical site infection?**
   Many organisms found in surgical site infections originate from the epidermis. Intact skin is the most resistant to infection, requiring an inoculum of 8 million bacteria to initiate infection, whereas only 1 million are required if the dermis has been violated. When foreign material is being used, only 100 organisms are required (e.g., mesh in hernia repairs, pacemaker placement, total joint replacement, etc.). An additional source of organisms in surgical site infections is wound contamination from deeper tissues. Organisms in these deeper tissues can arise from sources such as the epithelial

lining of the gastrointestinal tract or the genitourinary tract. Exposure to these organisms occurs after spontaneous perforation or trauma. Organisms in the deep tissues of the operative field can also arise from a systemic source such as septic emboli to the spleen, mediastinitis from an oral infection (a.k.a. Ludwig's angina), or endocarditis from bacteremia.

The wound classification system describes the complexity of the wound and predicts an increased risk for postoperative surgical site infections. (See Table 11.1.)

Table 11.1 Wound Classification System

CLASS	TYPE	DESCRIPTION
I	Clean	Uninfected operative wound in which no inflammation is encountered, and the respiratory, alimentary, genital, or infected urinary tracts are not entered. Clean wounds are primarily closed, if drained, closed drainage must be used for class to remain "clean." Operative incisional wounds after nonpenetrating (i.e., blunt) trauma should be included if it meets the above criteria.
II	Clean-contaminated	Operative wounds in which the respiratory, alimentary, genital, or urinary tracts are entered under controlled conditions and without unusual contamination. For example, operations involving the biliary tract, appendix, vagina, and oropharynx are included in this category, provided no evidence of infection or major break in technique occurs.
III	Contaminated	Open, fresh, traumatic wounds. In addition, operations with major breaks in sterile technique (e.g., open cardiac massage) or gross spillage from the gastrointestinal tract, and incisions in which acute, nonpurulent inflammation is encountered, including necrotic tissue without evidence of purulent drainage (e.g., dry gangrene).
IV	Dirty or infected	Includes old traumatic wounds with retained devitalized tissue and those that involve existing clinical infection or perforated viscera. This definition suggests that organisms causing postoperative infection were present in the operative field prior to the operation.

6. What patient factors increase risk for surgical site infections?
   a. Age
   b. Nutritional status
   c. Smoking
   d. Obesity
   e. Diabetes
   f. Coexistent infections at a remote body site
   g. Colonization with microorganisms
   h. Altered immune response
      i. neutropenic
      ii. receiving corticosteroids or other immunosuppressive agents
   i. Length of perioperative stay
   j. ASA grade 3 or 4
   k. Emergent versus elective presentation
   Antimicrobial prophylaxis may be indicated in high-risk patients regardless of case classification.

7. What preventive operative measures can surgeons take to reduce surgical site infections?
   1. Hand washing
      Since the advent of aseptic technique, hand washing has remained the cornerstone of infection control measures. Adequate techniques for surgeons include a 3-minute hand brushing with povidone-iodine or chlorhexidine gluconate soap solutions, or a 1-minute hand wash with nonantiseptic soap followed by hand rubbing with a liquid aqueous alcoholic solution. Equitable outcomes and better protocol adherence were found with the latter technique.

2. Preoperative skin preparation

 There is persistent controversy over the most effective preoperative skin preparation for reducing surgical site infections. Chlorhexidine gluconate with either alcohol base or aqueous base and iodophor prep solution with either alcohol base or aqueous base are commonly used and compared in clinical studies.

 Alcohol is effective and bactericidal when used for preoperative skin antisepsis; however, its benefit does not persist. For this reason, alcohol is combined with chlorhexidine gluconate or an iodophor to achieve rapid and persistent antisepsis. Either of these agents when combined with alcohol reduce surgical site infections when compared to the agents with an aqueous base. It is important to remember that alcohol poses a fire risk and should not be used in situations where it may pool, or inadequately dry (based on body location such as dense hair-bearing regions). Alcohol is also caustic to certain tissues such as mucosa, corneas, and inner ear and should be avoided in these areas.

3. Perioperative normothermia

 Maintaining a core temperature of 35.5°C or more during the perioperative period can reduce surgical site infections. In addition to impairing neutrophil function, hypothermia also results in subcutaneous vasoconstriction that decreases perfusion to the wound. Additionally, hypothermia causes coagulopathy that can result in need for transfusions and wound hematomas, both factors have been shown to increase surgical site infections.

4. Avoid hair removal

 Do not remove hair unless it interferes with the site of operation. If hair removal is necessary, it should be removed outside of the operating room, using clippers or a depilatory agent. The practice of using razors to remove hair has been shown to increase the risk of surgical site infection because of the abrasion/injury to the epidermal/superficial dermal layers of the skin. This practice has been eliminated in most hospitals. One instance where it is still used is to rapidly shave the skull for emergent craniotomies after traumatic brain injury.

5. Duration of operation

 In the early days of assessing risk for surgical site infections, any operation >2 hours was considered to increase risk of surgical site infection. As outcome tracking has matured, the nationally based outcome surveillance organizations (e.g., United States Centers for Disease Control and Prevention and United Kingdom Centre for Infections) have derived "T" times for operative procedures based on the category of surgical procedure being performed. "T hours" represents the maximum amount of time for a given type of procedure to be performed. It is based on the 75th percentile of distribution for duration of a given procedure. Operations lasting longer than T times are associated with increased surgical site infections.

6. Antimicrobial prophylaxis

 Antimicrobial prophylaxis should be given within 60 minutes of incision time. If the drug requires prolonged infusion, give within 120 minutes of incision time. Obese patients should receive weight-based dosing.

 Redosing should occur if the duration of the case lasts longer than two antibiotic half-lives, or if there is extensive blood loss.

 GOAL: Ensure adequate serum and tissue concentrations throughout the duration of the procedure.

 The surgeon may limit the duration of surgery and follow good surgical principles by eliminating dead space, controlling hemorrhage, minimizing placement of foreign material (including excessive suture), and exhibiting gentle tissue handling. The surgeon should ensure that the patient remains warm during the perioperative period. This simple act of warming was shown in two prospective studies to decrease significantly the incidence of SSIs.

8. **What role do antibiotics play in prevention of surgical site infections? How do I use antibiotics correctly to prevent SSIs?**

 First by knowing what organism you are targeting, then choosing an appropriate antibiotic and delivering it at the appropriate time via the appropriate route. Because you usually will not have a preoperative culture to guide therapy, you need to base your choice of antibiotic on predicted organisms. Staphylococci are the most common skin organism and the most common etiologic agent in SSIs. Cefazolin, a first-generation cephalosporin, is usually the recommended antibiotic for prophylaxis in clean surgical procedures. In circumstances in which known contamination has occurred, initial antibiotics should be tailored based on the violated organ's common flora. If the gut was entered, enterobacteriaceae and anaerobes are common; biliary tract and esophageal incisions yield these organisms plus enterococci. The urinary tract or vagina may contain group D streptococci, *Pseudomonas*, and *Proteus* species.

To a degree, SSIs can be anticipated. Factors that have been shown to have some predictive value to the surgeon are the physical status of the patient as classified by the American Society of Anesthesiologists, results of intraoperative cultures, and duration of preoperative hospital stay. Adequacy of regional blood supply also is important, as evidenced by the low infection rate in facial wounds. The classic description of wounds based on degree of gross contamination also may be of value. This scheme places wounds into one of four categories. (See Table 11.1.)

9. **If antibiotics are used, how and when should they be administered?**
Maximal benefit is obtained when tissue concentrations are therapeutic at the time of contamination. Efficacy is enhanced when prophylactic antibiotics are administered intravenously (IV) <1 hour before surgical incision; late administration is similar to no administration. Multiple-dose regimens have no proven benefit over single-dose regimens. Indiscriminate antibiotic selection outside recommended hospital protocols may increase the incidence of SSIs. In special circumstances, administration routes other than IV may be indicated.

KEY POINTS: WOUND CLASSIFICATION AND INFECTION RATE

1. Clean wound is atraumatic, with no breaks in sterile technique, no entry into respiratory, alimentary, or genitourinary tract. Incidence is 2.1%.
2. Clean-contaminated wound is same as clean wound except entry into respiratory, alimentary, or genitourinary tract. Incidence is 3.3%.
3. Contaminated wound has trauma from a clean source or minor spillage of infected materials. Incidence is 6.4%.
4. Dirty wound is trauma from a contaminated source or spillage of infected materials. Incidence is 7.1%.

---

10. **Name other routes that you would use for prophylactic antibiotic administration.**
In patients with nasal carriage of *Staphylococcus aureus*, intranasal administration of mupirocin ointment may have some efficacy in decreasing nosocomial and SSIs. In elective colon surgery, a metaanalysis of published studies indicated that orally administered antibiotics combined with intravenous antibiotics are superior to intravenous antibiotics alone in preventing surgical site infections.

11. **Does all that pulsatile lavage the surgeon uses in the operating room really do any good?**
Yes. High-pressure pulsatile lavage has been evaluated extensively in soft tissue contamination and shown to be seven times more effective in reducing bacterial load than bulb syringe lavage. The inherent elastic recoil of the soft tissues allows particulate matter to escape between pulses of fluid. The optimal pressure and pulse frequency seems to be 50–70 lb/in^2 and 800 pulses/min. Adding antibiotics to lavage solutions, although commonly practiced, has not been shown definitively to improve outcome.

12. **What can the patient do to help decrease SSIs?**
Stop smoking. Although obesity, poor nutritional status, advanced age, and diabetes are risk factors for SSIs, cigarette smoking is probably the leading preventable patient factor for SSIs, just like it is the leading preventable cause of death and disability in the United States. Half of all people who smoke eventually die from a smoking-related illness. Smoking not only kills but also more than triples that risk of incisional wound breakdown. In one study, smoking increased the incidence of SSIs in clean operative procedures sixfold, from 0.6% to 3.6%. Tobacco use results in decreased blood flow and decreased oxygen delivery to the wound. Toxic tobacco by-products also directly impede all stages of wound healing. Despite this knowledge, surgeons continue to operate electively on smokers, and most smokers continue to smoke up until the day of surgery.

13. **When prevention fails, what do you do for SSIs?**
The first line of therapy in SSIs is drainage. This is established by reopening the wound or, in the case of deep space infections, using techniques that are guided by computed tomography (CT) or ultrasound for drain placement or presurgical planning. Antibiotic therapy is used to control associated cellulitis and generalized sepsis.

14. **What may happen with untreated superficial or deep incisional SSIs?**
Locally, the wound breaks down, and infection dissects through the tissue planes and continues to advance. If the infection progresses rapidly, necrotizing fasciitis may develop. Finally, the strength layers of the wound closure break open (dehisce).

15. **Define wound dehiscence.**
The partial or total disruption of any or all fascial layers of the operative wound.

16. **Define evisceration.**
Rupture of the abdominal wall and extrusion of the abdominal viscera.

17. **What factors predispose to dehiscence?**
Age >60 years, obesity, increased intraabdominal pressure, malnutrition, renal or hepatic insufficiency, diabetes mellitus (DM), use of corticosteroids or cytotoxic drugs, and radiation have been implicated in wound dehiscence. Infection also plays an important role; an infective agent is identified in more than half of wounds that undergo dehiscence. The most important factor in wound dehiscence is the adequacy of closure. Fascial edges should not be devitalized. Ideally, the linea alba sutures should be placed neither too laterally nor too medially. Excessive lateral placement may incorporate the variable blood supply of the rectus abdominis muscle and compromise fascial circulation. Excessive medial placement misses the point of maximal strength at the transition zone between the linea alba and rectus abdominis sheath. In addition, sutures should be tied correctly without excessive tension, and suture material of adequate tensile strength should be chosen.

18. **When does wound dehiscence occur?**
It may occur at any time after surgery; however, it is most common between the fifth and tenth postoperative days, when wound strength is at a minimum.

19. **What are the signs and symptoms of wound dehiscence?**
Normally, a ridge of palpable thickening (healing ridge) extends about 0.5 cm on each side of the incision within 1 week. Absence of this ridge may be a strong predictor of impending wound breakdown. More commonly, leakage of serosanguineous fluid from the wound is the first sign. In some instances, sudden evisceration may be the first indication of abdominal wound dehiscence. The patient also may describe a sensation of tearing or popping associated with coughing or retching.

20. **Describe the proper management of wound dehiscence.**
If the dehiscence is not associated with infection, elective reclosure may be the appropriate therapeutic course. If the condition of the patient or wound makes reclosure unacceptable, however, the wound should be allowed to heal by second intention. An unstable scar or incisional hernia may be dealt with at a later, safer time. Dehiscence of a laparotomy wound with evisceration is a surgical emergency with a reported mortality of 10%–20%. Initial treatment in this instance consists of appropriate resuscitation while protecting the eviscerated organs with moist towels; the next step is prompt surgical closure. Exposed bowel or omentum should be lavaged thoroughly and returned to the abdomen; the abdominal wall should be closed; and the skin wound should be packed open. Vacuum-assisted wound closure may be valuable in select cases.

KEY POINTS: SURGICAL SITE INFECTIONS

1. Surgical site infections (SSIs) are the most common healthcare-associated infections (HAIs) in the United States.
2. Wound classification assessed at the time of surgery predicts risk of postoperative infection.
3. The goal of prophylactic perioperative antibiotics is to have therapeutic tissue concentrations at time of contamination (e.g., time of incision).
4. Patients who stop smoking significantly decrease their risk of surgical site infection.
5. Dehiscence is the separation of the fascial layers resulting in an opening in the abdominal wall.

BIBLIOGRAPHY

1. Anderson DJ, Podgorny K, Berrios-Torres S, et al. Strategies to prevent surgical site infections in acute care hospitals: 2014 update. *Infect Control Hosp Epidemiol.* 2014;35(6):605–627.
2. Bratzler D, Dellinger EP, Olsen KM, et al. Clinical practice guidelines for antimicrobial prophylaxis in surgery. *Am J Health-Syst Pharm.* 2013;70(3):195–283.
3. Leong G, Wilson J, Charlett A. Duration of operation as a risk factor for surgical site infection: comparison of English and US data. *J Hosp Infect.* 2006;63(3):255–262.
4. Yokoe DS, Anderson DJ, Berenholtz SM, et al. A compendium of strategies to prevent healthcare-associated infections in acute care hospitals: 2014 update. *Infect Control Hosp Epidemiol.* 2014;35(8):967–977.
5. National Nosocomial Infections Surveillance (NNIS) System Report, data summary from January 1992 through June 2004, issued October 2004. A report from the NNIS System. *Am J Infect Control.* 2004;32(8):470–485.

CHAPTER 12

PRIORITIES IN EVALUATION OF THE ACUTE ABDOMEN

Alden H. Harken, MD, FACS

1. **What is the surgeon's responsibility when confronted by a patient with an acute abdomen?**
   a. To identify how sick the patient is (treat the patient first and *then* the disease).
   b. To determine whether the patient (1) needs to go directly to the operating room, (2) should be admitted for resuscitation or observation, or (3) can be sent safely home.

2. **What is the most dangerous course in a patient with an acute abdomen?**
   To send the patient home.

3. **Is it important to make the diagnosis in the emergency department?**
   No. Frequently time spent confirming a diagnosis in the emergency department (ED) is lost to in-hospital resuscitation or treatment in the operating room. The only patient who needs a relatively firm diagnosis is a patient who is to be sent home.

4. **If the essential goal is not to make the diagnosis, what should the surgeon do?**
   a. Resuscitate the patient. Most patients do not eat or drink when they are getting sick. Most patients are depleted of at least several liters of fluid. Fluid depletion is worse in patients with diarrhea or vomiting.
   b. Start a big intravenous (IV) line.
   c. Replace lost electrolytes (see Chapter 8).
   d. Insert a Foley catheter.
   e. Examine the patient (frequently).

5. **Are symptoms and signs uniquely misleading in any groups of patients?**
   Yes. Watch out for the following groups:
   • The very young, who cannot talk.
   • Diabetics because of visceral neuropathy.
   • The very old, in whom, much as in diabetics, abdominal innervation is dulled.
   • Patients taking steroids, which depress inflammation and mask everything.
   • Patients with immunosuppression (a heart or kidney transplant patient may act cheerful even with dead or gangrenous bowel).

6. **Summarize the history needed**
   a. **The patient's age.** Neonates present with intussusception; young women present with ectopic pregnancy, pelvic inflammatory disease, and appendicitis; the elderly present with colon cancer, diverticulitis, and appendicitis.
   b. **Associated problems.** Previous hospitalizations, prior abdominal surgery, medications, heart and lung disease? An extensive gynecologic history is valuable; however, it is probably safer to assume that all women between 12 and 40 years old are pregnant.
   c. **Location of abdominal pain.**
      i. *Right upper quadrant:* Gallbladder or biliary disease, duodenal ulcer
      ii. *Right flank:* Pyelonephritis, hepatitis
      iii. *Midepigastrium:* Duodenal or gastric ulcer, pancreatitis, gastritis
      iv. *Left upper quadrant:* Ruptured spleen, subdiaphragmatic abscess
      Right lower quadrant: Appendicitis (see Chapter 39), ectopic pregnancy, incarcerated hernia, rectus hematoma
      Left lower quadrant: Diverticulitis, incarcerated hernia, rectus hematoma
      er, unless it obstructs (colon cancer), and is bleeding (diverticulosis) typically does not hurt.

d. **Duration of pain.** The onset of the pain of a perforated duodenal ulcer or perforated sigmoid diverticulum is sudden, whereas the pain of pyelonephritis is gradual and persistent. The pain of intestinal obstruction is intermittent and crampy.

Note: Although the surgeon is rotating through a gastrointestinal (GI) service, the patient may not know this and may present with urologic, gynecologic, or vascular pathology.

PHYSICAL EXAMINATION

7. Are vital signs important?

   Yes. They are vital. If heart rate (HR) and blood pressure (BP) are on the wrong side of 100 (heart rate >100 beats/min, systolic blood pressure <100 mm Hg), watch out! Tachypnea (respiratory rate >16) reflects either pain or systemic acidosis. Fever may develop late, particularly in the immunosuppressed patient who may be afebrile in the face of florid peritonitis.

8. What is rebound?

   The peritoneum is well innervated and exquisitely sensitive. It is not necessary to hurt the patient to elicit peritoneal signs. Depress the abdomen gently and release. If the patient winces, the peritoneum is inflamed ("rebound tenderness").

9. What is mittelschmerz?

   Mittelschmerz is pain in the middle of the menstrual cycle. Ovulation frequently is associated with intraperitoneal bleeding. Blood irritates the sensitive peritoneum and hurts.

10. What do bowel sounds mean?

    If something hurts (e.g., a sprained ankle), the patient tends not to use it. Inflamed bowel is quiet. Bowel contents squeezed through a partial obstruction produce high-pitched tinkles. Bowel sounds are notoriously unreliable, however.

11. Explain the significance of abdominal distention

    Distention may derive from either intraenteric or extraenteric gas or fluid (worst of all, blood). Abdominal distention is always significant and bad.

12. Is abdominal palpation important?

    Yes. Remember, the patient is (or should be) the surgeon's friend. There is no need to cause pain. Palpation guides the surgeon to the anatomic zone of most tenderness (usually the diseased area). It is best to start palpation in an area that does not hurt. Rectal (test stool for blood) and pelvic examinations localize pathology further.

13. What is Kehr's sign?

    The diaphragm and the back of the left shoulder enjoy parallel innervation. Concurrent left upper quadrant and left shoulder pain indicate diaphragmatic irritation from a ruptured spleen or subdiaphragmatic abscess.

14. What is a psoas sign?

    Irritation of the retroperitoneal psoas muscle by an inflamed retrocecal appendix causes pain on flexion of the right hip or extension of the thigh.

LABORATORY STUDIES

15. How is a complete blood count helpful?

    a. **Hematocrit.** If the hematocrit is high (>45%), the patient is most likely dry or may have chronic obstructive pulmonary disease (COPD). If it is low (<30%), the patient probably has a more chronic disease (associated with blood loss; always do a rectal and test the stool for blood).

    b. **White blood cell count.** It takes hours for inflammation to release cytokines and elevate the white blood cell count. A normal white blood cell count is entirely consistent with significant abdominal trouble.

16. Is urinalysis necessary?

    Yes. White blood cells in the urine may redirect attention to the diagnosis of pyelonephritis or cystitis. Hematuria points to renal or ureteral stones. Because an inflamed appendix may lie directly on the right ureter, red and white blood cells may be found in the urine of patients with appendicitis.

17. **What is a sentinel loop?**
Except in children (who swallow everything, including air), small bowel gas is always pathologic. A single loop of small bowel gas adjacent to an inflamed organ (e.g., the pancreas) may point to the diseased organ.

18. **Is ultrasound valuable?**
Yes, if the working diagnosis is cholecystitis, gallstones, ectopic pregnancy, ovarian cyst, abdominal aortic aneurysm, or intraperitoneal/retroperitoneal fluid.

19. **Is abdominal computed tomography valuable?**
Yes, if the working diagnosis is an intraabdominal abscess (sigmoid diverticulitis), pancreatitis, retroperitoneal bleeding (leaking abdominal aortic aneurysm; this patient should have gone straight to the operating room), or intrahepatic or splenic pathology.
Honors: Air in the biliary system indicates a biliary-enteric fistula; this in association with intestinal air-fluid levels makes the diagnosis of gallstone ileus.

KEY POINTS: RADIOGRAPHIC EVALUATION FOR THE ACUTE ABDOMEN

1. May assist in diagnostic evaluation but should not supplant physical examination in evaluation of an acute abdomen.
2. Upright chest x-ray: Look for free air under the diaphragm, intrathoracic pathology, air-fluid levels, and dilated alimentary canal.
3. Ultrasound: Useful for biliary, ob-gyn, and vascular assessments; may note intraperitoneal or retroperitoneal fluid collections.
4. CT: Increasing use in clinical arena, with excellent visualization of abdominal structures. Drawbacks: Cost, radiation exposure.
5. MRI is preferable to CT in pregnant patients.

20. **What is a double-contrast computed tomography scan?**
The bowel is delineated with barium or Gastrografin. The blood vessels are delineated with an iodinated vascular dye. The CT scan precisely displays the abdominal contents relative to vascular and intestinal landmarks. Contrast CT of pancreatitis is valuable to assess zones of perfusion or necrosis.

SURGICAL TREATMENT

21. **If the patient is sick (and not getting better), what should be done?**
After fluid resuscitation, the patient's abdomen should be explored. An exploratory laparotomy has been touted as the logical conclusion of a complete physical examination.

22. **Is a negative laparotomy harmful?**
Yes, but patients can uncomfortably survive a negative laparotomy, whereas missed bowel infarction (or appendicitis) can be life threatening.

23. **Name the most challenging problem in all of medicine?**
An acute abdomen.

BIBLIOGRAPHY

1. D'Agostino J. Common abdominal emergencies in children. *Emerg Med Clin North Am.* 2002;20(1):139–153.
2. Dhillon S, Halligan S. The therapeutic impact of abdominal ultrasound in patients with acute abdominal symptoms. *Clin Radiol.* 2002;57(4):268–271.
3. Baron KT, Arleo EK. Comparing the diagnostic performance of MRI versus CT in the evaluation of acute nontraumatic pain during pregnancy. *Emerg Radiol.* 2012;9(6):519–525.
4. Gajic O, Urrutia LE. Acute abdomen in the medical intensive care unit. *Crit Care Med.* 2002;30(6):1187–1190.
5. Rozycki GS, Tremblay L, Feliciano DV, et al. Three hundred consecutive emergent celiotomies in general surgery patients: influence of advanced diagnostic imaging techniques and procedures on diagnosis. *Ann Surg.* 2002;235(5):681–688: discussion 688–689.

SURGICAL INFECTIOUS DISEASE

Glenn W. Geelhoed, AB, BS, MD, DTMH, MA, MPH, MA, MPhil, ScD (honoris causa), EdD, FACS

1. **Have modern antibiotic developments controlled many, if not most, of the problems of surgical infection?**
   No. In seriously ill surgical patients in intensive care unit (ICU) settings, the problems of sepsis have increased and remain among the principal causes of death in ICU patients, especially those with multiple organ failure (MOF) and impairments of host defense. Antibiotic treatment may change the biographical sketch of the flora associated with patients' deaths but cannot overcome the multiple causes of failing host resistance to infection that accompany barrier breeches to microbial invasion and the inflammatory and immunologic responses to the "usual suspects."

2. **What kinds of barrier breech allow microbial invasion that may set up surgical site infection?**
   The skin and mucosal linings of the body maintain a barrier between the multifloral outside world and the sterile interior milieu of the tissues and organs (even when the outside world is a tube of heavily populated flora through the middle of usually sterile body cavities, such as the gastrointestinal [GI] tract). It is easy to see the barrier breech when a knife penetrates the skin, carrying exterior flora beneath the skin, or when that knife perforates and spills the contaminated contents of the gut into the abdomen. It is less obvious when the breech is caused by a low-flow state or when inadequate nutrition or toxins impair mucosal immunoglobulins, making the "bug-body barrier" permeable. These polymicrobial communities of organisms may begin to invade through the breech in such barriers, particularly if there are further failures in the third line of defense in humoral and cellular resistance.

3. **What is the difference between contamination and infection?**
   The presence of microorganisms does not an infection make!
   Resident communities of flora on body surfaces do little harm, and gut flora are even beneficial when contained in the gut. It is even possible for bacteria to be transiently present outside their usual commensal residences without constituting an infection in the normally intact host. For example, in vigorously brushing one's teeth, gram-negative bacteria of various kinds that are resident in the oral cavity are introduced into the bloodstream but are probably quickly eliminated by normal defense mechanisms, unless they meet lowered host resistance or seed a prosthetic heart valve.

4. **How can the enormous load of bacteria in the lower gastrointestinal tract be beneficial?**
   Bugs can be beautiful. These are the same bacteria that have lived with and in humans symbiotically for millennia. They synthesize vitamin K—something we literally cannot do without—or crowd out pathogenic organisms by their overwhelming numbers. They also help to metabolize bile salts and play a role in detoxifying some environmental hazards, similar to septic systems.

5. **Whenever intraabdominal bowel spillage is encountered, is it mandatory to culture the fecal contamination and obtain sensitivities of all identified organisms?**
   No. There is a difference between contamination and infection. Therefore, cultures of fecal spillage into the peritoneum will not provide useful information. The contaminant, just because of its change in position with reference to the bowel wall, is not likely to be sterile. When would you like the laboratory to quit? Will you be content to hear a report of *Escherichia coli* and bacteroides, two of the more than 800 species that even the most compulsive laboratory can hardly be competent to identify, given the exposure to air and time lapse until processing on different media? How will information from a sampling error of mixed, community-acquired contaminants change your therapy? If, for instance, no

anaerobes are identified from the fecal specimen, will you be so confident that they are not present as to exclude these species from coverage?

The lesson to be learned is that culture of community-acquired contaminants is expensive, incomplete, and unedifying; the culture of invading microbes in infections, particularly hospital-acquired microbes that persist after treatment, may give critical information and is a more appropriate use of microbiologic resources.

6. **What are preps (e.g., bowel preps)?**

Preps are decontamination procedures, designed to reduce resident flora before an elective invasive procedure. Preps may take the form of a simple process such as an alcohol swab smeared over the skin before a quick prick of the subcutaneous injection or may involve preparation of a larger area of the skin surface for the surgical field of incision (see question 8).

A bowel prep is similarly designed to reduce the resident flora in the gut through (1) mechanical catharsis (i.e., purge); (2) osmotic or volume dilution with large volumes of saline, other electrolyte solutions, or mannitol; or (3) oral administration of nonabsorbed antibiotics. Of these methods, the most important is clearly mechanical catharsis because it purges huge amounts of flora, which may account for up to two-thirds the dry weight of colon contents. One of the most cogent reasons for the choice of certain oral antibiotics in bowel preps (see question 9) is their vigorous cathartic action.

7. **How is the skin or mucosal cavities of a patient sterilized to prepare a sterile field for operative incision?**

There is one way, hardly recommended, by which patients can be "sterilized"; similar to instruments and drapes, they can be placed in an autoclave. But short of this absurd example, the skin is never sterile. Decontamination processes are never perfect, particularly in so complex a tissue with crevices and accessory skin structures in which bacteria reside. Resting gloved hands on a "sterile field" does not include the skin or mucosal surfaces.

At best, we simply reduce the flora to the low-level inoculum that can be handled by most intact host defense systems—as in the example of brushing your teeth—but living tissue surfaces are never sterile. A method that kills all microbial organisms from such surfaces would also devitalize mammalian cells and render them more susceptible to lower-level microbial inocula.

8. **What means can be used to reduce surface resident flora without further injuring the skin or mucosa?**

- **Volume lavage** (for mnemonic value only: dilution is the solution to pollution)
- **Defatting,** which solubilizes the sebaceous oils that may trap flora
- **Microbicidal killing** with a bacteriostatic agent

To an amazing extent, one cheap, simple fluid that may serve as a diluent, fat solvent, and anti-microbial is alcohol. Alcohol is nearly ideal as prepping solution, with the minor disadvantages that it is dehydrating and minimally flammable. Because it vaporizes and disappears, flora may spread from interstices, outside the field, or even via aerosolized fallout onto the field, thus requiring the addition of extended-duration bacteriostasis to the alcohol prep.

Iodine also kills bacteria but with a greater hazard to sensitive mammalian cells (it oxidizes the cell walls of small plants). A lower initial concentration of iodine and a longer duration of action can be achieved by incorporation of an iodophor, a substance in nearly universal use in preps. The application of moisture- and vapor-permeable "incise drapes" or desiccation-preventing "ring drapes" may further retard repopulation of flora over the prepped (but still not sterile) field.

9. **What are "pipe cleaner" antibiotics?**

Pipe cleaners are orally administered antibiotic regimens that reduce the flora in the GI tract, from which they are not well absorbed. They are an almost ideal component of bowel preps because they are potent cathartic agents and accomplish the vast majority of their "pipe cleaning" by mechanical purgative action. The most popular pipe cleaners include a neomycin or erythromycin base.

10. **What is selective gut decontamination? How does it work?**

It does not work. This method used pipe cleaners in patients at high risk for the development of sepsis from MOF with the theoretic aim of reducing the risk involved in barrier breech of the GI tract and inoculation with gut flora. Good experimental evidence indicated that this method should reduce the high mortality rate in seriously ill patients at high risk of surgical sepsis. After prolonged clinical trials, however, it failed to demonstrate a benefit in patient survival. The likely reason is that whereas the laboratory studies were done in intact animal models with functioning host defense systems, failures of defense beyond the barrier breech may explain why selective gut decontamination failed to benefit seriously ill patients. Furthermore, resident hospital flora repopulated the purged gut over time, but with virulent forms of microbes selected by their resistance to the broad-spectrum antibiotics. The method still has some use in patients undergoing procedures such as high-dose chemotherapy or bone marrow transplantation and in some patients isolated in "life islands" (e.g., patients with immunodeficiency diseases or burns).

ANTIBIOTICS

11. **Are antibiotics the classic wonder drugs?**
Only because you wonder if they are going to work, if they are going to cause more harm than good, and if the next generation will be unaffordable or toxic.

Skepticism is healthy with regard to any procedure or agent in healthcare, but especially with regard to antibiotics, which are embraced almost universally as agents that both prevent and cure infections. The primacy of the host defense in this vital process and the potential interference by the very drugs given credit for infection control are overlooked. We must look critically at the limited role that antibiotics should play in healthcare and restrain their overuse, which generates even more harm than unnecessary expense.

12. **What is meant by generations of antibiotics, as in third-generation cephalosporins?**
The earliest antibiotics were bacteriostatic, largely through interference in protein synthesis, so that they might keep a microorganism from reproducing even if they did not kill it. The difference between infestation (presence of living microbes in the host) and infection (replication and spread of microorganisms in the host) may be useful in understanding how previous drugs possibly controlled infection but were less capable of eliminating organisms in any brief period of therapy.

Penicillin changed all that. It may be the first antibiotic with a legitimate claim to the title "wonder drug" because it has the microbicidal capability of eradicating sensitive organisms. Penicillin was the first generation of the beta-lactam antibiotics, joined by the congener first-generation cephalosporins (e.g., cefazolin). They shared beta-lactam structure and had good gram-positive coverage with less range in any effect over gram-negative microbes.

The second-generation beta-lactam antibiotics (e.g., cefoxitin) covered new classes of microbes beyond gram-positive aerobes, such as many of the *Bacteroides* species, but had little effect on gram-negative aerobic microbes. Because the third-generation cephalosporins covered some of the latter microbes, they were touted as single-agent therapy for all principal-risk floras.

As with penicillin, the original wonder drug, the wonderment waned with failures of the new agents because of rapidly induced antimicrobial resistance. The most easily measured and calculated difference in the generations is cost: Wholesale values are about $2.00/g for the first generation, $5.00/g for the second, and $30.00/g for the third. Despite this bracket creep in cost, the higher generations lose some of their potency against the original gram-positive organisms for which the first-generation agents were truly wonderful. Therefore, it takes 2 g of moxalactam to be half as good as 1 g of cefazolin for gram-positive coverage. It does not take a pharmaco-economist to ask, "What have I got in return for this sixty-fold surcharge?"

13. **What is the role of third-generation cephalosporins in surgical prophylaxis?**
None (no more wondering here!). If the principal-risk flora are gram-positive, the first generation is better; if the anaerobic risk is sizable, the second generation is better. And either class is cheaper by far and seems to have generated less resistance than the third-generation cephalosporins, which are unconscionably expensive for use in prophylaxis and rarely as effective as other single-agent therapy for established surgical site infection (SSI). Specific indications, such as pediatric meningitis, hospital-acquired pneumonia, or other specific infections outside the indications of surgical predominance, might use or exclude these agents.

14. **How do enzyme inhibitors combined with antibiotics enhance their antimicrobial spectrum?**
Microorganisms have defense mechanisms of their own, and the strains that have the capacity to make antibiotic-degrading enzymes achieve an unnatural selection advantage with the widespread use of antibiotics. This is what happened to penicillin—penicillinases emerged. But clever pharmaceutical manufacturers closed that loophole for bacterial ingenuity in degrading penicillin

by strategic placement of a methyl group to ruin the survival fitness of penicillinase producers. Methicillin was the result, but the persistence of the microbes means that we now have a plague of methicillin-resistant *Staphylococcus aureus* (MRSA). Besides, microbes outnumber pharmaceutical manufacturers and have a shorter turnaround time than the approval process of the Food and Drug Administration (FDA). Microbes will always be ahead of us in ingenuity, if only because of their numbers.

Newer strategies by the bacteria included the production of beta-lactamases. The response of the pharmaceutical industry was a group of inhibitors of beta-lactamase, such as clavulanic acid or sulbactam. The combination of a beta-lactamase inhibitor with a modified penicillin such as ampicillin should have enhanced activity against bacteria that produce beta-lactamase, provided that they were ampicillin sensitive in the first place. Higher doses of the original agent for a shorter time may accomplish the same effect, often at lower cost, because the combined drugs were developed much more recently and are under patent protection.

15. **What are the most expensive kinds of antibiotic therapy?**
    - Drugs that are given when they are not needed.
    - Drugs that are badly needed but do not work.
    - Drugs that cause more harm than good because of host toxicity, whatever their antibiotic potential.

16. **Can oral antibiotics be given in place of intravenous antibiotics in seriously ill surgical patients?**
    Yes, if only they could take them! These patients almost invariably can take nothing by mouth (NPO), are often unconscious, and are as likely as not to be on a ventilator. In addition, the gut has been put out of commission by nasogastric (NG) suction tubes, laparotomy, and ileus, and primary intraabdominal problems often associated with the need for the antibiotics, such as intraabdominal sepsis and pancreatitis. Usually, such patients are on complete gut rest and are likely to be on parenteral nutrition as well.

    The attempt to use some form of gut-delivered antibiotic is based on the favorable pharmacokinetics and spectrum of quinolones, which can be started intravenously and switched as soon as possible to the oral form when feeding has resumed. Nearly all such patients begin on some form of intravenous (IV) antibiotic program and the start-up of the antibiotic regimen is more important than the form to which patients are tapered before treatment is discontinued.

PROPHYLAXIS

17. **Should systemic antibiotic prophylaxis be used in elective colon resection?**
    Yes, beyond any statistical shadow of a doubt. At least two dozen clinical trials have been carried out using placebo controls against a variety of antibiotics, principally those active against at least the anaerobic-predominant flora, and nearly all have shown a reduction in infectious complications in the antibiotic group. Never again should this point need repeating, and no patient should be placed at risk when systemic antibiotic prophylaxis has been established as the standard of care. No new clinical trials against placebo in this group of patients with known risk can be performed ethically given the confirmed risk reduction.

    Other risk groups (e.g., cesarean section after membrane rupture) besides patients undergoing colon resection have been standardized by trials in large patient populations and have shown similar risk reduction. The benefit of prophylaxis has been demonstrated. In other groups of patients that cannot be standardized because of unusual contamination factors or unique factors of host resistance impairment, guidelines for rational prophylaxis should follow similar principles.

18. **Are two prophylactic doses better than one in preventing infection? Are three doses better still?**
    Only one dose (the dose in systemic circulation at the time of the inoculum) of prophylactic antibiotic can be proved, beyond statistical or clinical doubt, to be efficacious. Whether the dose needs to be repeated one or more times during the 24 hours after the inoculum depends on the blood levels of the drug, which are largely a function of protein binding and clearance rate. We also know for sure that 10 days of the same prophylactic drug that is efficacious if given immediately before the inoculum results in a higher risk of infection than no antibiotic at all.

KEY POINTS: PREOPERATIVE ANTIBIOTIC PROPHYLAXIS

1. Timing of administration is the most important factor.
2. Dose 30 minutes before incision so that antibiotic is circulating before the inoculum.
3. No evidence supports continuation of prophylaxis beyond 24 hours.

19. **What factors determine the timing of antibiotic administration under the criteria of prophylaxis?**
    The most important element in timing of prophylaxis is that the drug be circulating before the inoculum. When should it stop? When the reduction in infection risk is no longer provable and before continued use will defeat the prophylactic purpose (as explained previously). To summarize with an arbitrary rule of thumb: There is no justification for prophylactic antibiotic 24 hours after the inoculum of an invasive procedure.
    What does this rule imply? Should we not continue prophylaxis for weeks to cover the presence of a prosthetic hip joint? Presumably, the prosthetic hip will be in the patient for many years; but surely you do not argue that the antibiotic should continue on a daily basis as long as the hip is in place! What is "prophylaxed" is not the prosthetic hip but the procedure of implantation. And it is not only implantation that poses a risk to the patient with a prosthesis, so does the hemorrhoidectomy done years later, for which prophylaxis is made mandatory by the presence of the hip prosthesis.
    The prosthetic or rheumatic heart valve is a risk, but the indication for the use of prophylactic antibiotics is an invasive procedure; a root canal is an example in which an inoculum is unavoidable. Operations are covered by prophylactic antibiotics; the conditions that are risk factors during the operation are not.

20. **To be safe, why not administer prophylactic antibiotics to all patients undergoing any kind of operation?**
    Can you give me the indication for a prophylactic antibiotic in a patient undergoing a clean elective surgical procedure that implants no prosthesis, such as hernia repair?
    "Sure," one of my brighter students once responded, "the patient who has a serious impairment in host response, such as acute granulocytic leukemia in blast crisis."
    I responded, "Why on earth are you fixing his hernia? That is a clean error (hopefully not a clean kill) in surgical judgment that has nothing to do with antibiotics at all. A patient with that degree of host impairment does not undergo an elective surgical procedure."
    Rule of thumb: If you can provide the indication for a prophylactic antibiotic to cover a clean elective nonprosthetic operation for a patient, you have provided the contraindication for the operation.

MANAGEMENT OF SURGICAL SITE INFECTIONS

21. **What is the drug of choice for the treatment of an abscess?**
    A knife. Surgically drain the abscess. Abscesses have no circulation of blood within them to deliver an antibiotic. The antibiotic, even if injected directly into the abscess, would be worthless because the abscess contains a soup of dead microorganisms and white blood cells (WBCs). Even if the organisms were barely alive, they would not be reproducing and incorporating the antibiotic. The drug most likely would not work at all at the acid-base balance (pH) and pKa conditions of the abscess environment.
    If there is an indication for an antibiotic, it would be in the circulation around the compressed inflammatory edge of the abscess and the cellulitis (at the vascularized "peel of the orange") and uncontaminated tissue planes through which the necessary drainage must be carried out. A focal infection is managed by a local treatment, which is both necessary in all abscesses and sufficient treatment in many. Adjunctive systemic antibiotics are occasionally indicated for protection of the tissues through which drainage is carried out. If it helps to make this fundamental surgical principle clear, here is the rule of thumb for management of abscesses: Where there is pus, let there be steel. Perhaps one of the most gratifying procedures in all of medicine is the drainage of pus with immediate relief of local and systemic symptoms (e.g., a perirectal abscess).

22. **Which abscess treatment is the important one in determining the outcome of a patient with intraabdominal sepsis?**

    It is the drainage of the last abscess that counts. There should be little applause for drainage of a pelvic abscess in the patient who retains a subphrenic abscess. The patient responds dramatically when the last pus is drained.

    This has been an area of significant advance in managing surgical infections because noninvasive scanning capability has facilitated the finding of multiple pockets of pus. Furthermore, such modalities as the computed tomography (CT) scan not only find but also percutaneously direct the fixing of the last abscess. What might have been an indication for an exploratory return trip to the operating room only a decade before (i.e., a failing patient on appropriate therapy should trigger the first response, "Where's the pus?") is now a good indication for a CT scan to find and drain the focal infection.

23. **Which is preferred for draining an intraabdominal abscess, a needle or a knife?**

    Which can be done most expeditiously? The patient with intraabdominal sepsis is quite ill, and the earliest safe drainage is the procedure of choice. There may be advantages to the less invasive CT scanning, which can be repeated and has less morbidity if the results are negative. Surgery, on the other hand, can fix associated conditions that may have caused the abscess, such as the devitalized loop of bowel or the leak in the anastomosis that can be exteriorized. Each method is likely to find multiple collections, and each can leave external drains for lavage and continuing drainage. Whether by needle or by knife, the urgency and adequacy of local treatment of focal infection determine which methods takes precedence.

24. **What is the role of gallium scanning in early finding of abscesses in the abdomen?**

    There is none. Ordering a gallium scan is a temporizing means of self-deception that some progress is being made in finding out what is wrong with the patient. In fact, it merely postpones decisions about intervention in critical illness for several days, often to a point beyond salvage. Gallium scanning involves bowel prepping, a vigorous WBC response from an active bone marrow, and false-positive test results at the sites of tubes and incisions. It is a time-consuming and unreliable test that is the obverse of the principles of early and definitive management. Do not order a gallium scan to satisfy a consultant that "something is being done for this patient."

EXTRA CREDIT QUESTIONS

25. **Should all patients undergoing elective laparotomy receive prophylactic antibiotic coverage?**

    No. Doing so would contribute to driving up the cost of antibiotics and their complication rate and devaluing formerly good drugs by rendering them useless against common flora against which they were once highly potent. Operating room nurses have always classified the kind of operation by its status with respect to microbial exposure—clean, contaminated, or septic. These categories are approximation of the microbial risk exposure, and if additionally are superimposed categories of patient resistance (higher risk associated with aging, obesity or other malnutrition, concomitant drugs, or viral or mycobacterial or neoplastic disease immune compromise), these same strata are called class I, II, and III.

26. **Which abscess is the most important one to be drained?**

    It is the last abscess that counts in drainage because the patient's dramatic response is often only achieved when the last pus is drained. Draining a pelvic abscess, for example, but leaving behind a subphrenic abscess, would not result in the quenching of the inflammatory mediators of the sepsis syndrome.

27. **Is postoperative fever the earliest and most frequent sign of an incisional infection?**

    Postoperative fevers are much more frequent than are wound infections, and the typical wound infection presents far later. The principal sources of postoperative fever are:
    - Wind (atelectasis or pneumonia)
    - Water (urinary tract infection)
    - Walk (get your patient up and around; thrombophlebitis)
    - Wound

28. **Should you begin amphotericin at the first isolation of *Candida* species drawn from any intravenous catheter line?**
   No. Again, remember the distinction between colonization and infection, and the source from which the specimen is taken. The IV lines through which hyperalimentation solutions are infused make colonization possible. The presence of a fungus such as *Candida* species is frequent in patients who do not have an invasive fungal infection or a true candidemia. The latter might be distinguished from catheter colonization by a blood culture drawn from another source, such as a venipuncture. If evidence of any invasive fungal infection is also present (e.g., as endoscopic biopsy of inflammatory mucositis), a choice of antifungal therapies is now indicated.
   Topical fungal solutions (e.g., mycostatin mouthwashes or lavage) may control the local fungal infection and may sometimes be instituted as prophylaxis in high-risk patients (e.g., patients on antirejection therapy for bone marrow or solid organ transplantation).
   Systemic antifungal agents include fluconazole, caspofungin, and amphotericin.

29. **Are antibiotic drug combinations always superior to a single antibiotic agent?**
   Monotherapy is superior to combination antibiotic treatment regimens, but this is provable probably only in the highest-risk patients. With the carbapenem class antibiotic agents, a large multicenter clinical trial proved imipenem therapy superior to aminoglycoside and a macrolide antibiotic, with survival demonstrably superior only in the patients with the highest acute physiology and chronic health evaluation (APACHE) scores. Ertapenem monotherapy was the equivalent of ceftriaxone and metronidazole in a smaller, more recent trial.
   More is not always better, and the R & S on culture reports do not translate directly to the M & M (morbidity and mortality) at the Death and Complications Conference reports. It is not just important that the effective antibiotic regimen kills the bacteria; also important are how this microbicidal effect is carried out and what effect it may have on the patient in quenching or prolonging the systemic inflammatory response.

30. **Is antibody treatment of circulating endotoxin a clinically important tool?**
   Not yet. The neutralization of circulating endotoxin might give a theoretic benefit to patients with sepsis, and animal studies looked promising. But antigen/antibody complexes initiate complement cascade and release of activated leukocyte products such as leukotrienes that may further augment the inflammatory process. The complexes are also filtered in the kidney where they may further impair renal function. To date, no clinical therapeutic benefit has been demonstrated for such mono-clonal antibody therapy.

31. **What is the role of human recombinant activated protein C in patients with sepsis?**
   Of the multiple clinical trials of mediator neutralization or receptor blockade, the evidence to date seems marginally favorable only for a few, and the major response to treatment comes from early and complete control of the focus of sepsis (not the cytokine sequelae).

WEBSITES

www.medscape.com
Search: preoperative antibiotics

BIBLIOGRAPHY

1. Bartlett JG. Intra-abdominal sepsis. *Med Clin North Am.* 1995;79(3):599–617.
2. Bernard GR, Vincent JL, Laterre PF, et al. Efficacy and safety of recombinant human activated protein C for severe sepsis. *N Engl J Med.* 2001;344(10):699–709.
3. Bilik R, Burnweit C. Is abdominal cavity culture of any value in appendicitis? *Am J Surg.* 1998;175(4):267–270.
4. Castaldo ET, Yang EY. Severe sepsis attributable to community-associated methicillin-resistant *Staphylococcus aureus:* an emerging fatal problem. *Am Surg.* 2007;73(7):684–687, discussion 687–688.
5. Christou NV, Turgeon P. Management of intra-abdominal infections. The case for intraoperative cultures and comprehensive broad-spectrum antibiotic coverage. The Canadian Intra-abdominal Infection Study Group. *Arch Surg.* 1996;131(11):1193–1201.

6. Ciftci AO, Tanyei FC. Comparative trial of four antibiotic combinations for perforated appendicitis in children. *Eur J Surg.* 1997;163(8):591–596.

7. Falagas ME, Barefoot L. Risk factors leading to clinical failure in the treatment of intra-abdominal or skin/soft tissue infections. *Eur J Clin Microbiol Infect Dis.* 1996;15(12):913–921.

8. Geelhoed GW. Preoperative skin preparation: evaluation of efficacy, timing, convenience, and cost. *Infect Surg.* 1985;85:648–669.

9. Murray AC, Cran RP. Bowel preparation: are antibiotics necessary for colorectal surgery? *Adv Surg.* 2016;50(1):49–66.

10. Ozdemir S, Gulpinar K, Ozis SE, et al. The effects of preoperative oral antibiotic use on the development of surgical site infection after elective colorectal resections: a retrospective cohort analysis in consecutively operated 90 patients. *Int J Surg.* 2016;25;33(Pt A):102–108.

CHAPTER 14

RISKS OF BLOOD-BORNE DISEASE

Natasha D. Bir, MD, MHS

1. **What infectious diseases are transmissible via blood transfusion?**
   Over 100 million blood donations are collected annually worldwide. Approximately half of these are collected in developed countries. Viruses, parasites, and bacteria and the diseases they transmit have all been found in donated blood. HBV, HCV, HIV 1 and 2, HTLV1 and 2, CMV, Parvovirus B19, Dengue virus, West Nile virus, trypanosomiasis, malaria, and variant Creutzfeldt-Jakob disease can all be transmitted in transfused blood. The most commonly transmitted diseases in developed nations include hepatitis B virus (HBV) and hepatitis C virus (HCV); human immunodeficiency virus (HIV) and cytomegalovirus (CMV) transmission are far less common. Parasites such as malaria *(Plasmodium),* Chagas' disease *(Trypanosoma cruzi),* toxoplasmosis *(Toxoplasma gondii),* and babesiosis *(Babesia)* are only a problem where these diseases are endemic. Lymphomas and leukemias can be caused by human T-cell lymphotropic virus (HTLV-1) and infectious mononucleosis by Epstein-Barr virus (EBV). Viruses such as West Nile were also transmitted prior to instituting testing. The Zika virus is currently under investigation. Bacterial contamination of blood products occurs most often in platelets, which are stored at room temperature. Bacterial contamination can result in sepsis or a toxic shock-like syndrome, or in transmission of syphilis (treponema pallidum).

   Donor screening has nearly eliminated blood-transfusion-transmitted HIV, HTLV, and the hepatitides. However, infection remains a significant risk in less-developed countries, where millions of units of blood are not screened for transmissible pathogens. To date, 25 countries are still not able to screen blood for HIV, HBV, HCV, and syphilis according to WHO recommendations.

2. **What are the estimated risks of HBV, HCV, and HIV transmission by blood transfusion in the United States?**
   Rates of viral disease transmission are lower than ever, particularly after nucleic acid testing for HIV, HBV, and HCV began in 1999. At present, mathematical models are employed to estimate risks of viral transmission in developed countries because the rates are so low.

Disease	Risk of disease per actual unit transfused in the United States
HBV	1/70,000 to 1/2,70,000
HCV	1/103,000 to 1/230,000
HIV	1/1,000,000 to 1/2,000,000
Bacterial transmission; packed red blood cells	0.21/1,000,000
Bacterial transmission; platelets	1/100,000 units

3. **Which blood-borne pathogens pose a risk to surgeons?**
   HIV, HBV, and HCV are diseases of concern to surgeons because of the morbidity and mortality associated with these diseases. There has never been a confirmed case of HIV infection from occupational exposure in a surgeon. As of 2003 (the most recent data available in 2008), only 58 confirmed cases of healthcare-worker HIV infection by patients have been reported, including six physicians (all nonsurgeons). In all cases, the inciting injury involved significant cuts or penetration with large-bore hollow needles, never with solid needlesticks. The hepatitides do remain threats. HBV infection of surgeons has declined with the widespread use of the HBV vaccine (see below). A hollow needlestick can result in HBV transmission in as many as 30% of cases. The risk of HCV in the operating room remains significant because the number of chronically infected patients numbers—2.7 million to 3.9 million in the United States alone.

4. **What is the risk to healthcare workers of exposure to hepatitis B virus?**

Of the 35 million healthcare workers globally, approximately 3 million are exposed percutaneously to blood-borne pathogens every year. This includes 2 million exposures to HBV, 900,000 to HCV, and 170,000 to HIV. More than 90% of documented transmissions are in developing countries. Millions of healthcare workers are exposed to blood or other body fluids annually. Eighty-two percent are exposed through percutaneous injury such as needlesticks, and another 14% through contact with the mucosal membranes of the eyes, mouth, or nose.

Blood, cerebrospinal fluid, synovial fluid, pleural fluid, peritoneal fluid, pericardial fluid, and amniotic fluid all carry a risk for transmitting HBV. Sputum, urine, and vomitus are not considered to be infectious unless they contain blood. HBV is highly infectious and can remain infectious on environmental surfaces for at least 7 days.

Hepatitis B e antigen (HBeAg)—a degradation product of the viral nucleocapsid that represents active replication in the liver—is the marker for HBV replication and viral load. In studies of healthcare personnel who sustained injuries from needles contaminated with HBV, 37%–62% developed serologic evidence of HBV and 22%–31% developed clinical hepatitis. However, if the exposure was to HBsAg-positive, HBeAg-negative blood the risk for serologic evidence of HBV infection was 23%–37%, and 1%–6% will develop clinical hepatitis. Thirty percent of acute HBV cases are clinically occult, and 5% remain chronic carriers for life. About 25% of people with chronic HBV eventually die of hepatic disease.

In the United States, the incidence of HBV has declined sharply over the last 15 years, mainly because of effective vaccination strategies. In 2013 the CDC estimated just fewer than 20,000 new cases. In 2014 the CDC estimated 850,000 persons with chronic HBV in the United States.

5. **What is the risk to healthcare workers of exposure to hepatitis C virus (HCV)?**

HCV is transmitted via blood, and patients at higher risk include injection drug users, patients who received a blood transfusion before 1999, hemophiliacs, patients on hemodialysis, and healthcare workers. Acute HCV infection is asymptomatic in 70% of cases. Approximately 1.8% of needlesticks or sharps exposures result in HCV infection, but one study indicated that only exposure with hollow-bore needles was associated with transmission. After exposure, the rate of seroconversion to HCV is approximately 10%. Fifty percent to 80% of seroconverters develop a persistent chronic HCV infection, and 20% of these advance to hepatic cirrhosis. Recent years have seen the development of new and promising treatment for hepatitis C with a high cure rate; however, success depends on the genotype of the virus and treatments are very expensive.

6. **What is the risk to healthcare workers of exposure to HIV?**

Among healthcare workers only 58 confirmed cases and fewer than 150 "possible" cases (unconfirmed as a result of poor documentation) of HIV transmission have occurred since 1983. The majority of confirmed cases were nurses (n = 24), while six were physicians. None were surgeons. Eighty-four percent of the affected individuals suffered percutaneous routes of transmission—that is, cuts or punctures. The risk of seroconversion to HIV after a percutaneous exposure is 0.3%. After exposure via mucous membrane, the risk of conversion is 0.09%. Since 1999, only one confirmed case of occupationally acquired HIV infection has been reported to the CDC, a lab technician who sustained a needlestick while working with live HIV cultures in 2008.

7. **How well does hepatitis B vaccination protect against the disease?**

An anti-HBsAg level of 10 or more mIU/mL confers a protective efficacy of nearly 100%. Ninety percent of individuals who complete the three-dose immunization series for HBV develop antibody titer levels consistent with immunity. An additional 8% display appropriate titer levels after additional doses. While about half of successfully vaccinated adults demonstrate a decreased or nondetectable titer level within 10 years, a lifelong "immune memory" to the viral antigen persists and people do not require booster doses.

A bivalent vaccine immunizing against both hepatitis A and B was approved in 2001 by the U.S. Food and Drug Administration (FDA) for individuals 18 years of age and older, and it is as successful as the monovalent vaccine in conferring protection against HBV infection with the added benefit of protecting against hepatitis A viral infection. There are also two brands of monovalent recombinant DNA vaccines available.

8. **Are patients at risk of infection from surgeons who are infected with HBV or HCV?**

Some cases of surgeon-to-patient transmission of HBV have been documented. Those with the highest chance of transmitting disease to patients are positive for the e-antigen of hepatitis B. E-antigen positive people generally exhibit a high viral load. However, transmission of disease has been documented even when a surgeon was negative for e-antigen. Only two reported instances of transmission of HCV from surgeon to patient are known.

9. **What is the proper response after percutaneous exposure to a patient with known hepatitis B?**
For practitioners who have been immunized and *demonstrated positive titers*, no additional response is necessary. For these individuals, there is no need to confirm titer levels at the time of exposure—even if titer levels decline over time, immunity is lifelong. People who were not immunized or who had a weak or incomplete response to vaccine should receive a dose of Hepatitis B immunoglobulin (HBIg) and then begin the vaccination series anew. As well, multiple doses of the immune globulin within a week of exposure will confer 75% protection.

10. **What are the recommendations for hepatitis B immunization?**
Vaccination against hepatitis B is strongly encouraged for all healthcare workers, particularly those who perform tasks involving contact with blood or blood-contaminated fluids, other body fluids, or sharps. It is required for surgical trainees. The recommendations of the United States Public Health Service are that all healthcare workers who perform tasks that may involve exposure to blood or body fluids should receive a three-dose series of hepatitis B vaccine at 0-, 1-, and 6-month intervals. They should then be tested for hepatitis B surface antibody (HBsAg) 1–2 months after vaccination, to document immunity. If the anti-HBsAg is at least 10 mIU/mL then the patient is immune. If <10 mIU/mL, the patient remains unprotected; another three-dose series of vaccination should be given and titers should be rechecked 1–2 months. If still <10 mIU/mL, the patient is deemed a nonresponder. They should be considered susceptible to HBV and should maintain strict precautions and be treated with HBIg for any known or probable exposure.

11. **What are the recommendations for hepatitis C immunization?**
The only effective protection against HCV is the rigorous use of universal precautions to prevent exposure to infected body fluids. There is no effective vaccine, and immunoglobulin does not confer protection.

12. **Does laparoscopic surgery minimize the risk of HIV contamination?**
Laparoscopic technique reduces exposure to blood and sharp instruments. However, discharge of pneumoperitoneum can release aerosolized blood and peritoneal fluid into the operating room if not evacuated into a closed system.

13. **Is double gloving an effective method of protection?**
Yes. The contact rates between blood and skin decrease by 70% with the addition of a second pair of gloves. The nondominant index finger is the most common target.

14. **Are nonpercutaneous exposures (eye splash) a major threat to surgeons?**
According to the Centers for Disease Control and Prevention (CDC), the risk of seroconversion after mucocutaneous exposure (eyes, nose, or mouth) is 0.1. Mucocutaneous contact is responsible for 13% of documented HIV transmissions. Among surgeons, eye splash injuries are often overlooked as a major risk for disease transmission. One study of surgical procedures examined the eye shields of 160 surgeons and assistants for operations 30 minutes or greater. Although the surgeons were aware of spray in only 8% of cases, blood splashes were macroscopically visible in 16% of cases, and microscopically positive in 44% of cases. Eye protection is a crucial part of universal barrier precautions.

15. **What is the surgeons' rate of exposure to blood and body fluids?**
Exposure is widely underreported, but percutaneous exposure occurs in an estimated 1%–6% of operative procedures and mucocutaneous exposure in up to 50% of surgical cases. No healthcare worker has ever been infected by exposure through intact skin.

16. **Again, what are the seroconversion rates for HIV, HBV, and HCV exposure?**
Seroconversion rates from a hollow needlestick are 0.3% for HIV, 10% for HCV, and range between 6% and 30% for HBV.

17. **Are there effective methods to reduce the risk of transmission of blood-borne diseases to surgeons?**
Obviously, the most effective way to reduce disease transmission is to limit exposure to infected blood or body fluid and to vaccinate for HBV. For HBV, postexposure immunoglobulin administration reduces infection. For HIV, percutaneous exposure antiretroviral medications can reduce the risk of transmitting HIV.

18. **What is the risk to surgeons in training?**

A recent multicenter survey of surgeons in training noted that needlesticks are frequent and often go unreported. Number of needlesticks increased with each postgraduate year (PGY) in training: PGY-2, 3.7; PGY-3, 4.1; PGY-4, 5.3; and PGY-5, 7.7, and by their final year of training, 99% of residents had at least one needlestick. About half of residents had been exposed to blood from high-risk patients (patients with a history of HIV, HBV, HCV, or injection drug use). The most common reason for not reporting a needlestick was "lack of time." However, protecting oneself from communicable diseases will benefit surgical trainees, their families, and their future patients.

BIBLIOGRAPHY

1. Anonymous. Hepatitis C virus transmission from health care worker to patient. *CDC Weekly*. 1995;5:121.
2. Esteban JI, Gomez J, Martell M, et al. Transmission of hepatitis C virus by a cardiac surgeon. *N Eng J Med*. 1996;334(9):555–560.
3. CDC. Recommendations for identification and public health management of persons with chronic hepatitis B virus infection. *MMWR*. 2008;57. No. RR-8.
4. Update CDC. Human immunodeficiency virus infections in health-care workers exposed to blood of infected patients. *MMWR*. 1987;36:285–289.
5. CDC. Updated CDC recommendations for the management of hepatitis B virus-infected health-care providers and students. *MMWR*. 2012;61. No. RR-3.
6. Jaffray CE, Flint LM. Blood-borne viral diseases and the surgeon. *Curr Probl Surg*. 2003;40(4):195–251.
7. Fry DE. Occupational blood-borne diseases in surgery. *Am J Surg*. 2005;190(2):249–254.
8. Bell DM. Occupational risk of human immunodeficiency virus infection in healthcare workers: an overview. *Am J Med*. 1997;102(suppl 5B):81S–85S.
9. Dodd RY, Notari EP, Stramer SL. Current prevalence and incidence of infectious disease markers and estimated window-period risk in the American Red Cross blood donor population. *Transfusion*. 2002;42(8):975–979.
10. Mast EE, Weinbaum CM, Fiore AE, et al. A comprehensive immunization strategy to eliminate transmission of hepatitis B virus infection in the United States: recommendations of the Advisory Committee on Immunization Practices (ACIP) Part II: immunization of adults. *MMWR Recomm Rep*. 2006;55(RR-16):1–33.
11. Weiss ES, Makary MA, Wang T, et al. Prevalence of blood-borne pathogens in an urban, university-based general surgical practice. *Ann Surg*. 2005;241(5):803–807. discussion 807–809.
12. Klein HG, Spahn DR, Carson JL. Red blood cell transfusion in clinical practice. *Lancet*. 2007;370(9585):415–426.
13. Allain JP, Stramer SL, Carneiro-Proietti AB, et al. Transfusion-transmitted infectious diseases. *Biologicals*. 2009;37(2):71–77.
14. Goodnough LT. Risks of blood transfusion. *Anesthesiol Clin North America*. 2005;23(2):241–252.
15. Makary MA, Al-Attar A, Holzmueller CG, et al. Needlestick injuries among surgeons in training. *N Engl J Med*. 2007;356(26):2693–2699.
16. Kuehnert MJ, Roth VR, Haley NR, et al. Transfusion-transmitted bacterial infection in the united States, 1998 through 2000. *Transfusion*. 2001;41(12):1493–1499.
17. Recommendations for prevention and control of hepatitis c virus (HCV) infection and HCV-related chronic disease. *MMWR Recomm Rep*. 1998;47(RR-19):1–39.
18. Barrie PS, Patchen Dellinger E, Dougherty SH, et al. Assessment of hepatitis B virus immunization status among North American surgeons. *Arch Surg*. 1994;129(1):27–32.
19. Puro V, Petrosillo N. Italian Study Group on Occupational Risk of HIV and Other Bloodborne Infections. Risk of hepatitis C seroconversion after occupational exposure in health care workers. *Am J Infect Control*. 1995;23(5):273–277.
20. Gershon RR, Sherman M, Mitchell C, et al. Prevalence and risk factors for bloodborne exposure and infection in correctional healthcare workers. *Infect Control Hosp Epidemiol*. 2007;28(1):24–30.
21. Koff RS. Hepatitis A, hepatitis B, and combination hepatitis vaccines for immunoprophylaxis: an update. *Dig Dis Sci*. 2002;47(6):1183–1194.
22. Dodd RY, Notari EP, Stramer SL. Current prevalence and incidence of infectious disease markers and estimated window-period risk in the American Red Cross blood donor population. *Transfusion*. 2002;42(8):975–979.
23. Eubanks S, Newman L, Lucas G. Reduction of HIV transmission during laparoscopic procedures. *Surg Laparosc Endosc*. 1993;3(1):2–5.
24. Marasco S, Woods S. The risk of eye splash injuries in surgery. *Aust N Z J Surg*. 1998;68(11):785–787.
25. Stramer SL, Glynn SA, Kleinman SH, et al. Detection of HIV-1 and HCV infections among antibody-negative blood donors by nucleic acid-amplification testing. *N Eng J Med*. 2004;351(8):760–768.
26. United States Public Health Service. Updated U.S. Public Health Service guidelines for the management of occupational exposures to HBV, HCV, and HIV and recommendations for postexposure prophylaxis. *MMWR Recomm Rep*. 2001;50(No. RR-11):1–52.
27. Wasley AM, Kruszon-Moran D, Kuhnert WL, et al. The prevalence of hepatitis B virus infection in the United States in the era of vaccination. *J Infect Dis*. 2010;202(2):192–201.
28. WHO Global database on blood safety 2012.

SEPSIS

M. Kelley Bullard, MD

CHAPTER 15

1. **What is sepsis?**
   Sepsis is a profound host immune response to infection. This systemic process can be accompanied by hypotension and can cause acute organ dysfunction.

2. **What is septic shock?**
   Septic shock is when hypotension secondary to sepsis persists despite adequate fluid resuscitation. A patient in septic shock will have signs of hypoperfusion, such as altered mental status, hypoxemia, acidosis, elevated lactate, tachypnea, and oliguria.

3. **When does sepsis become septic shock?**
   When the septic patient becomes hypotensive—when the mean arterial pressure is below 70 mm Hg or the systolic pressure is <90 mm Hg.

4. **What is the difference between sepsis and systemic infection?**
   Systemic infection means the bacterial or fungal pathogen has entered the bloodstream. Sepsis occurs when an unbalanced immune response causes systemic hypoperfusion and subsequent organ dysfunction. Proinflammatory mediators are usually balanced by antiinflammatory mediators in response to an infection. When this balance is disrupted by additional insults or an upregulated proinflammatory response, the resultant "inflammatory mediator surge or cytokine storm" causes vasodilatory shock, global hypoxia, cellular injury, and organ dysfunction.

5. **Why do some patients in septic shock have warm extremities?**
   The hypoperfusion seen in early septic shock is due to vasodilation of the systemic vasculature caused by inflammatory mediators (e.g., nitric oxide, histamine, and many others). During the early period of septic shock, a patient's extremities may be warm because of the maldistribution of blood to the periphery. In later stages of the shock state this finding is less consistent because of loss of intravascular volume by microvascular leak and third spacing.

6. **What are the priorities in treatment of septic shock?**
   Stabilization (the "A, B, Cs") and diagnosis are the priorities. After confirming that the patient's airway and breathing are okay, the next priority is to establish vascular access and begin aggressive fluid resuscitation. At the time of initial volume replacement, a baseline lactate level is measured to guide ongoing resuscitation. Blood cultures should be obtained as early as possible and prior to the prompt administration of broad-spectrum antibiotics. In the event that blood cultures cannot be obtained within 45 minutes of sepsis recognition, broad-spectrum antibiotics should be started without further delay. For each hour of delay in infusing antibiotics, there is a 4% increase in mortality.

7. **What is early goal directed therapy?**
   Early goal directed therapy (EGDT) is a protocolized approach to diagnosis and treatment of sepsis at time of presentation. When the concept was first introduced over a decade ago, initial data showed a significant decrease in mortality in the group managed by EGDT protocols versus groups managed by "routine care." There is good reason to believe that "routine care" has been influenced by EGDT over the last decade. It is now "routine" to treat patients by aggressive resuscitation practices and slight modifications of EGDT guidelines. Because of the shift in routine care, subsequent trials examining EGDT protocols (and their components) versus routine care have shown less-reductions in mortality and some have shown no benefit. Some degree of controversy exists today as to how strictly EGDT must be followed. Despite these controversies, it is agreed that early volume resuscitation, antibiotics, support with vasopressors, and source control remain the cornerstone of treatment in the septic patient.

8. **Does everyone with bacteremia have sepsis?**
   No. The systemic inflammatory state may exist in the absence of positive blood cultures. Severe sepsis is when infection triggers a robust inflammatory response that compromises perfusion to end organs. Bacteremia alone will not result in such systemic decompensation. It is this immune response that acts in a deleterious manner to cause perfusion abnormalities and subsequent multisystem organ failure.

9. **How much volume is "enough" when resuscitating the septic patient?**
   Early resuscitation goals include a central venous pressure of 8–12. Once this range is reached, vasopressor agents are added to reach a goal mean arterial pressure (MAP) of ≥65 mm Hg.

10. **Is there a preferred vasopressor to use in septic shock?**
    Norepinephrine offers both alpha-adrenergic (vasoconstrictive) and beta-adrenergic (inotropic) support in septic shock. It has been shown to be less arrhythmogenic than dopamine in prospective clinical trials and is the first line recommended vasoactive agent in the surviving sepsis guidelines for treatment of hypotension related to sepsis.

11. **What is systemic inflammatory response syndrome (SIRS)?**
    SIRS is defined by two of the following criteria:
    - Fever >38°C or hypothermia <36°C
    - Tachycardia >90 beats/min
    - Tachypnea >20 breaths/min
    - Leukocytosis >12 × 10 (9th)/L
    - Leucopenia <4 × 10 (9th)

12. **Is the severity of sepsis due to the bacterial burden or type?**
    No, the severity of sepsis is more related to the host response. A fulminate inflammatory response alone can progress to multiple organ dysfunction, organ failure, and death.

13. **Are there different types of sepsis?**
    Sepsis exists on a spectrum of severity. "Sepsis" is defined as infection accompanied by SIRS. "Severe sepsis" is defined as infection ı SIRS + associated organ dysfunction. The inciting infections can be from any focal organ source. Pneumonia is one of the more common sources of sepsis; however, urosepsis and surgical diseases (i.e., perforated viscus, abscesses, diverticulitis, cholecystitis, cholangitis, etc.) can also result in severe septic episodes. The severity of the septic episode is related to the robust nature and imbalance of the host immune response and not the particular type or location of the inciting infection.

14. **Is there a way to predict if someone will survive a septic episode?**
    The sequential organ failure assessment score (SOFA Score) predicts mortality by assessing the degree of dysfunction of six organ systems—lungs, brain, liver, kidney, hematologic (platelets), and hemodynamic.

15. **What is source control?**
    The term *source control* describes finding and eliminating the source of a septic site such as draining an intraabdominal abscess or treating pneumonia.
    Examples of surgical source control:

Pathologic source	Example of source control
Perforated duodenal ulcer	Graham Patch Repair
Diverticulitis	Percutaneous drainage of abscesses, or partial colectomy, colonic diversion
Cholecystitis	Cholecystostomy or cholecystectomy
Cholangitis	Endoscopic sphincterotomy and stent placement, or transhepatic biliary drainage
Appendicitis	Percutaneous drainage or appendectomy

KEY POINTS: SEPSIS

1. Sepsis is caused by the immune system at time of infection.
2. Priorities in treatment of sepsis are the A, B, Cs and resuscitation.
3. Early administration of antibiotics decreases mortality.
4. Profound inflammatory response secondary to infection is known as "sepsis," whereas profound inflammatory response to noninfectious insults is known as systemic inflammatory response syndrome (SIRS).
5. Optimize perfusion to end organs by targeting CVP and MAP goals as early as possible in the treatment of sepsis.

BIBLIOGRAPHY

1. Dellinger RP, Levy MM, Rhodes A, et al. Surviving sepsis campaign: international guidelines for management of severe sepsis and septic shock: 2012. *Crit Care Med.* 2013;41(2):580–637.
2. ARISE Investigators, ANZICS Clinical Trials. Group goal-directed resuscitation for patients with early septic shock. *N Eng J Med.* 2014;371(16):1496–1506.
3. Angus DC, van der Poll T. Severe sepsis and septic shock. *N Eng J Med.* 2013;369(9):840–851.
4. The ProCESS Investigators. A randomized trial of protocol-base care for early septic shock. *N Eng J Med.* 2014;370(18):1683–1693.
5. Hotchkiss RS, Karl IE. The pathophysiology and treatment of sepsis. *N Eng J Med.* 2003;348(2):138–150.

CHAPTER 16

FRAILTY

Douglas M. Overbey, MD, Thomas N. Robinson, MD, MS

1. **What defines a geriatric patient?**
   "Geriatrics" is best described as promoting the health of seniors. There is no specific age at which a patient is prescribed geriatric treatments. The United Nations uses 60+ as the numerical criterion, and most developed countries use 65 years. Currently, 15% of the US population is age 65+; an age group that consumes approximately 40% of healthcare resources.

2. **How do geriatric patients differ physiologically?**
   Older adults have less physiologic reserve and less ability to maintain homeostasis after stressors. This intrinsic vulnerability is sometimes termed *frailty*.

3. **What is the life expectancy by age?**
   Life expectancy is longer as age increases, and tends to be 0–3 years longer for females. Fiftieth percentile life expectancy at age 65 is 17 years for men and 20 years for women. At age 80, life expectancy is 8 years for men and 10 years for women.

4. **What are common causes of death in the geriatric population?**
   Frailty, cancer, organ failure, and advanced dementia.

5. **What is frailty?**
   Frailty is an age-related, multidimensional state of decreased physiologic reserves that results in diminished resiliency, loss of adaptive capacity, and increased vulnerability to stressors. By definition, frailty is associated with poor healthcare outcomes and disability.

6. **What is the pathophysiology of frailty and human aging?**
   Biologic hallmarks clinically express themselves as frailty and include genomic instability, telomere attrition, epigenetic alterations, loss of proteostasis, deregulated nutrient sensing, mitochondrial dysfunction, cellular senescence, stem cell exhaustion, and altered intercellular communication.

7. **Why does frailty matter?**
   Frailty is one of the most critical issues facing healthcare because it is closely related to poor health-care outcomes. Frail older adults are at highest risk for falls, disability, delirium, cognitive decline, iatrogenic complications, social withdrawal, and death following an operation.

8. **What is the comprehensive geriatric assessment?**
   A comprehensive geriatric assessment describes a multidisciplinary, multidimensional evaluation aimed to define high-risk health characteristics of older adults, which will allow individualized inter-vention plans. Common clinical characteristics assessed by a comprehensive geriatric assessment include functional status, mobility, comorbid medical conditions, cognition, psychologic state, social support, nutritional status, and a review of the patient's medications. The interventions recommended following a comprehensive geriatric assessment are typically carried out by a multidisciplinary team.

9. **How can you assess for frailty?**
   There is no single tool that measures frailty. Instead, a variety of measurements have been described, which should be chosen for use based on the clinical situation. Examples of frailty measurement tools include:
   a. Deficit accumulation frailty assessment describes summing abnormal characteristics found in evaluations like the comprehensive geriatric assessment and equating a higher number of abdominal characteristics to increased health risk.
   b. The FRAIL scale is performed by assessing fatigue, resilience, ambulation, illnesses, and loss of weight.
   c. Biologic, or "phenotypic," frailty is measured by assessing walking speed, grip strength, fatigue, weight loss, and activity level.
   d. Brief single item assessment can rapidly and accurately screen for frailty, including the timed up-and-go score (time to get up and walk 10 feet, return to sitting) and gait speed.

10. **What is the significance of frailty in the perioperative period?**
Frailty predicts poor postoperative outcomes in elderly patients. Adverse outcomes related to baseline frailty include 30-day mortality, 1-year mortality, serious complications, prolonged length of stay, and need for postdischarge institutionalization.

11. **How can you treat a patient with frailty?**
Frail patients and their families should be counseled on the patient's increased risk of adverse complications postoperatively, which include the possibility of functional decline leading to postdischarge institutionalization. Prior to elective operations, prehabilitation may be prescribed with the goal of modifying and improving surgical risk. Prehabilitation, intraoperative modifications, and postoperative care can all be used to create a patient-centered realistic treatment plan.

12. **What is prehabilitation?**
Prehabilitation describes an intervention that occurs between the time of diagnosis and the operation, which aims to modify and improve surgical outcomes. Prehabilitation programs can consist of single or multiple interventions. A common single modality prehabilitation protocol is a preoperative exercise training program aimed to improve muscle strength and endurance, with the goal of reducing postoperative functional decline. Multimodal physical therapy programs include exercise and/or physical therapy, nutritional supplementation, anxiety reduction, medication reconciliation, and optimization of comorbid conditions.

13. **How can the postoperative course differ in geriatric patients?**
Evidence-based pathways exist that improve inpatient care of geriatric patients. Functional preservation with early physical therapy, delirium prevention with environmental supportive protocols, and care transition planning represent three distinct care pathways that can improve the inpatient care of geriatric patients.

14. **What is delirium?**
Delirium was historically defined by fluctuating level of consciousness. The DSM-5 definition includes disturbance in attention and orientation to the environment. This disturbance must follow a physiologic stress, develop over a short period of time, and represent an acute change from baseline.

15. **What is the differential diagnosis for delirium?**
Dementia, metabolic or infectious encephalopathy, cerebrovascular accident, alcohol or substance withdrawal, and depression.

16. **How can you diagnose delirium?**
The Confusion Assessment Method (CAM) involves verbal screening for acute onset and fluctuating course, inattention, and either disorganized thinking or alteration in consciousness.

17. **What is the incidence of delirium?**
Incidence ranges from 15% to 53% and is recognized as the most common postoperative complication in the elderly. Rates are highest in patients who undergo major operations requiring intensive care unit care (rates up to 80%). Initial onset of delirium typically occurs in the first 2 days postoperatively.

18. **What are the motor subtypes of delirium?**
Delirium can present in three distinct motor subtypes: hyperactive, hypoactive, or mixed. The Richmond Agitation and Sedation Scale (RASS) describes sedation level: positive is agitated (hyperactive), negative is sedate (hypoactive), and fluctuating is between agitated and sedated (mixed). The hypoactive motor subtype of delirium most commonly goes unrecognized. The hypoactive motor subtype of delirium is associated with poor long-term outcomes including 30% 6-month mortality.

19. **What is the proposed pathophysiology of delirium?**
Neurotransmitter alterations in the central nervous system play an important primary role, with fluctuations in serum serotonin, melatonin, and acetylcholine. Decreased acetylcholine synthesis or increased anticholinergic activity correlate directly with the confusional state. Delirium is a disturbance of global cortical and subcortical function, EEG changes include slowing of the dominant posterior alpha rhythm and abnormal slow-wave activity.

20. **What are preoperative, intraoperative, and postoperative risk factors for delirium?**
Preoperative: Advanced age, cognitive impairment, functional impairment, depression, psychotropic drug use, visual or hearing impairment, alcohol use, prior delirium, hypoalbuminemia

Intraoperative: Hypotension, increased blood transfusion, major surgical procedures, prolonged anesthesia time

Postoperative: Infection, hypoxia, substance withdrawal, narcotic use, medication side effects, anemia, electrolyte disturbances, inadequate pain control, lack of restorative sleep.

21. **What medications are known to cause delirium?**

    All anticholinergic drugs, tricyclic antidepressants, benzodiazepines, corticosteroids, H2-receptor antagonists, meperidine, and sedative hypnotics.

22. **What are nonpharmacologic interventions to prevent and treat delirium?**

    Nonpharmacologic delirium prevention involves early mobilization, reorientation, improving sleep-wake cycle, family presence, and availability of sensory aids including hearing aids and glasses. Sensory masking, such as eye masks and earplugs, can decrease delirium risk by up to 45%.

23. **Can pain cause delirium?**

    Both preoperative pain and inadequate pain control in the postoperative period are associated with development of delirium. However, high-dose opioids are also associated with an increased risk of postoperative delirium. This highlights the importance of nonnarcotic adjuncts and multimodal anesthesia.

24. **What are pharmacologic interventions to manage delirium?**

    Nonpharmacologic measures should be instituted first, along with pain assessment. Hyperactive delirium can progress to agitation and combative behavior; haloperidol and second-generation antipsychotics are frequently used as well as non-benzodiazepine–based sedation (dexmedetomidine or propofol).

25. **What are the sequelae of delirium?**

    The development of postoperative delirium is closely associated with increased complications, extended hospitalization, general decline in health, longer term neurocognitive decline, institutionalization, and death.

26. **How is delirium different from dementia (major neurocognitive disorder)?**

    Dementia is a long-term decline from a previous level of mental functioning. Previous definitions included memory impairment as a hallmark, although it may not be the first domain affected. Neurocognitive disorders can be divided into major and minor classifications based on degree of cognitive decline (substantial versus modest) and if the cognitive deficits are sufficient to interfere with independence.

27. **How can you screen for dementia?**

    The Mini-Cog test involves three-word registration, clock drawing, and three-word recall. This test is commonly used to screen for preoperative cognitive impairment.

28. **What are causes of dementia?**

    Alzheimer's disease represents >60% of dementia. Other progressive disorders include vascular dementia, Lewy body dementia, and frontotemporal dementia. Reversible causes such as drug toxicity, metabolic changes, thyroid disease, intracranial hemorrhage, or normal-pressure hydrocephalus represent <5% of etiologies.

29. **What is specific about geriatric depression?**

    Late-life depression is frequently underdiagnosed. Older adults frequently display fatigue and malaise in the setting of multimorbidity, making major depressive disorder difficult to diagnose. Consider testing with the Patient Health Questionnaire 2 (PHQ-2), which inquires for frequency of depressed mood and anhedonia over the past 2 weeks.

30. **What is the Beers list of medications?**

    The Beers list of medications outlines medications that have a high probability of adverse events when prescribed to older adults. This list of potentially inappropriate medications for use in older adults is widely recognized and should be considered when prescribing medications to the elderly. Medications on the Beers list that are commonly prescribed in the perioperative care that should be avoided include meperidine (Demerol), propoxyphene (Darvon), indomethacin (Indocin), pentazocine (Talwin), ketorolac (Toradol), cimetidine (Tagamet), ranitidine (Zantac), scopolamine, promethazine (Phenergan), cyclobenzaprine (Flexeril), and the benzodiazepines.

31. **What is the risk of falling in geriatric patients?**
    Falls have multiple contributors, such as intrinsic patient deficits (incontinence, poor balance, weakness, sensory impairment), medications, and environmental (slick socks, SCD tube or IV entanglement). Fall risk assessments include history, altered elimination, immobility, and cognitive impairment.

32. **What are forms of mistreatment of older adults?**
    Elder abuse and neglect is unfortunately common, with 500,000 reports to authorities and many more unreported. Types of elder abuse include abandonment, physical abuse, financial exploitation, neglect, and psychologic abuse. Diagnosis hinges on a high degree of suspicion and monitoring interaction between a senior and their caregiver.

KEY POINTS: FRAILTY

1. The geriatric population is physiologically different than adults, and additional preoperative assessment for frailty should be performed.
2. *Frailty* is a term used to describe physiologic vulnerability in older adults. Quantifying frailty assists with optimizing perioperative outcomes.
3. Delirium is the most common postoperative complication in the elderly population. Delirium prevention protocols are essential for older adults in the postoperative setting.

WEBSITES

- http://www.americangeriatrics.org/
- http://www.facs.org/~/media/files/quality%20programs/geriatric/acs%20nsqip%20geriatric%202016%20guidelines.ashx
- https://www.facs.org/quality-programs/acs-nsqip/geriatric-periop-guideline

BIBLIOGRAPHY

1. Robinson TN, Eiseman B, Wallace JI, et al. Redefining geriatric preoperative assessment using frailty, disability and co-morbidity. *Ann Surg.* 2009;250(3):449–455.
2. American Geriatrics Society Expert Panel on Postoperative Delirium in Older Adults. American Geriatrics Society abstracted clinical practice guideline for postoperative delirium in older adults. *J Am Geriatr Soc.* 2015;63(1):142–150.
3. Robinson TN, Walston JD, Brummel NE, et al. Frailty for Surgeons: review of a National Institute on Aging Conference on Frailty for Specialists. *J Am Coll Surg.* 2015;221(6):1083–1092.
4. Chow WB, Rosenthal RA, Merkow RP, et al. Optimal preoperative assessment of the geriatric surgical patient: a best practices guideline from the American College of Surgeons National Surgical Quality Improvement Program and the American Geriatrics Society. *J Am Coll Surg.* 2012;215(4):453–466.
5. Leung JM, Dzankic S. Relative importance of preoperative health status versus intraoperative factors in predicting postoperative adverse outcomes in geriatric surgical patients. *J Am Geriatr Soc.* 2001;49(8):1080–1085.
6. Mohanty S, Rosenthal RA, Russell MM, et al. Optimal perioperative management of the geriatric patient: a best practices guideline from the American College of Surgeons NSQIP and the American Geriatrics Society. *J Am Coll Surg.* 2016;222(5):930–947.
7. AGS/NIA Delirium Conference Writing Group. Planning Committee and Faculty. The American Geriatrics Society/National Institute on Aging Bedside-to-Bench Conference: Research Agenda on Delirium in Older Adults. *J Am Geriatr Soc.* 2015;63(5):843–852.
8. Fick DM, Semla TP. 2012 American Geriatrics Society Beers Criteria: new year, new criteria, new perspective. *J Am Geriatr Soc.* 2012;60(4):614–615.

II

TRAUMA

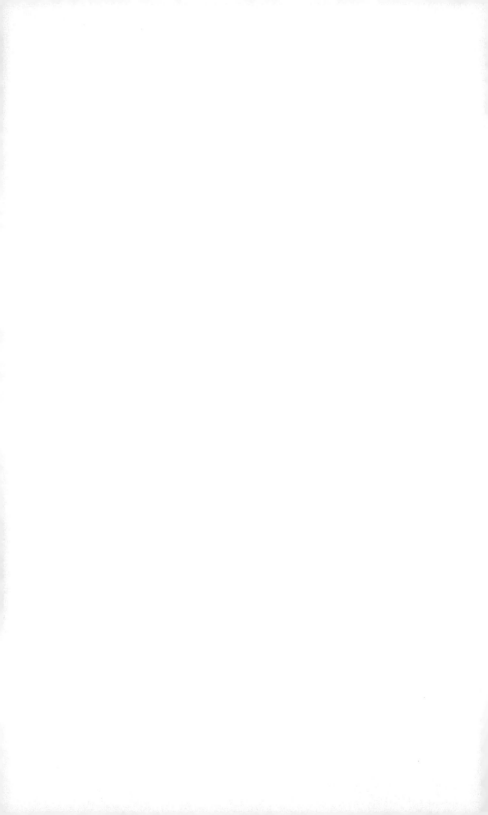

CHAPTER 17

INITIAL ASSESSMENT

David J. Skarupa, MD, FACS, Marie Crandall, MD, MPH, FACS

1. **What are the major components of the initial assessment of the trauma patient?**
   The major components of the initial assessment of the trauma patient are primary survey and resuscitation, primary survey adjuncts, secondary survey, reevaluation as needed, and transfer to definitive care center (if necessary).

2. **What is the purpose of the primary survey?**
   The purpose of the primary survey is to identify and treat life-threatening injuries, using a standard, reproducible approach, such as Advanced Trauma Life Support (ATLS).

3. **What are the components of the primary survey?**
   The primary survey follows A, B, C, D, Es. A—airway: Management with inline cervical spine immobilization; B—breathing: Evaluate and treat oxygenation and ventilation; C—circulation: Evaluate core pulses (femoral, carotid), large caliber (14 g or 16 g) upper extremity peripheral IV access (two), hemorrhage control; D—disability: Brief evaluation of neurologic status—Glasgow Coma Scale (GCS), pupillary exam, lateralizing signs; and E—exposure and environmental control: Fully expose, keep warm.

4. **What is the quickest way to assess the airway?**
   The fastest way to assess the airway is to ask the patient their name, or what happened. A clear accurate response in a normal voice tells you that the airway is patent, at least for now.

5. **What are causes of upper airway obstruction in the trauma patient?**
   The main causes of upper airway obstruction in the trauma patient are the tongue (from direct injury or obtundation), blood, loose teeth or dentures, vomit, and soft tissue edema.

6. **What are the initial maneuvers performed to manage an obstructed airway?**
   The initial maneuvers used to open an obstructed airway include positioning, such as a chin lift or jaw thrust, suctioning and removal of debris, and airway opening with oropharyngeal and nasopharyngeal tubes.

7. **What are the indications for a definitive airway?**
   Indications for a definitive airway include apnea, inability to protect airway (traumatic brain injury or intoxication), hypoxia, hypo- or hyperventilation, shock, need for deep sedation (surgeries or reduction of dislocations), and to facilitate safe workup and treatment of a dangerous or extremely agitated patient.

8. **What is a definitive airway?**
   A definitive airway is a tube in the airway with cuff inflated below the vocal cords. It must be connected to oxygen and secured in place.

9. **What are examples of definitive airways?**
   Examples of definitive airways include endotracheal intubation and a surgical airway.

10. **What are the types of definitive airways? List them in order of priority**
    Two types of definitive airways exist: Orotracheal intubation and surgical airway (cricothyroidotomy).

11. **What are some indications for a surgical airway?**
    Indications for a surgical airway are when an orotracheal intubation is unsuccessful, extensive maxillofacial trauma, and high-risk anterior neck trauma.

12. **What are some contraindications for a surgical airway?**
    Contraindications for a surgical airway are direct laryngeal trauma, tracheal disruption, and children <12 years old (consider needle cricothyroidotomy or tracheostomy).

13. **What are breathing problems that pose an immediate threat to the trauma patient?**

Tension pneumothorax is a breathing problem that can pose an immediate threat to the trauma patient. It is a form of obstructive shock. Physical exam findings of tension pneumothorax are absent breath sounds, hyperresonance to percussion of the chest, distended neck veins, and tracheal deviation away from the affected side. Prehospital treatment is often performed with needle decompression with an 8 cm needle in either the midaxillary line fifth interspace or the midclavicular line second interspace. If the patient is in the hospital, one may perform a finger thoracostomy followed by a tube thoracostomy at approximately the fifth interspace, or inframammary crease.

An **open pneumothorax** (a.k.a. sucking chest wound) is another breathing problem. This is when the chest wound communicating with the pleural space is more than two-thirds the tracheal diameter. Air follows via the path of least resistance, and if the wound is more than two-thirds the tracheal diameter, air will pass through the chest wall wound more readily than through the trachea with each respiration. Prehospital treatment is with a three-sided occlusive dressing. When the patient is in the trauma center the treatment is a chest tube and occlusive dressing over the wound (if possible), and transfer to the operating room for definitive management.

Flail chest is a breathing problem and defined by fractures of three or more ribs in two or more places. This causes paradoxical chest wall movement with respirations and is often associated with an underlying pulmonary contusion. Treatment starts with tube thoracostomy, pain control, and muscle relaxants. These patients may need to be intubated.

Simple pneumothorax on examination will likely have decreased breath sounds on the affected side and associated hypoxia. The treatment is a tube thoracostomy.

Massive hemothorax is often associated with physiologic changes (e.g., hypotension or shock) from hemorrhage and is defined by >1500 mL of blood in the pleural space. This space occupying volume prevents full lung expansion and results in decreased oxygenation and ventilation. On examination, the patient's chest will be dull to percussion and have decreased breath sounds on auscultation. Diagnosis usually occurs after placement of a tube thoracostomy. It is prudent to connect the tube to an underwater sealed collection chamber device for auto-transfusion. Definitive treatment is exploration of the pleural space (thoracotomy versus VATS) for hemorrhage control and evacuation of the pleural space. Blood transfusions often are required as well.

14. **What are some common simple ways to assess circulatory status of the trauma patient?**

The following are four simple ways to assess the circulatory status of the trauma patient:
a. Mental status (alert, verbal, pain, or unresponsive)
b. Skin perfusion (pink/warm versus pale/cool)
c. Hemodynamic parameters (BP, pulse, respiratory rate)
d. Gross estimate of systolic blood pressure:
    i. Radial pulse approximately 80 mm Hg
    ii. Femoral pulse approximately 70 mm Hg
    iii. Carotid pulse approximately 60 mm Hg

15. **What are some initial ways to stop hemorrhage?**

Initial ways to stop hemorrhage vary depending on the location. Extremity hemorrhage can be controlled with direct pressure or a tourniquet on the affected extremity proximal to the injury. Noncompressible areas (e.g., neck or axilla) may be controlled by a large Foley catheter (inflated with saline). If the pelvis is the source, a sheet or commercially available pelvic binder should be applied. Reduction and skeletal stabilization of long bone fractures will also help reduce bleeding.

16. **What are the preferred sites and types of IV access in an adult and pediatric trauma patient?**

The preferred type of IV access in an adult is two large-bore (14 g or 16 g) peripheral IV in the upper extremity (forearm or antecubital fossa). If peripheral IV access is not easily obtainable, intraosseous catheters should be inserted, preferably in the humeral heads or alternatively in the anteromedial tibia just inferior to the tibial tuberosity. A third option is placement of a central venous catheter (e.g., 8F cordis). The preferred access points are subclavian, femoral, and lastly the internal jugular vein. A cut down is the last resort.

Access preferences are similar in the pediatric (<6 years old) patient. Peripheral IV access with large-bore catheters is ideal, and should be placed in the antecubital fossa or saphenous vein at the ankle. A second choice is intraosseous access in the anteromedial tibia just inferior to the tibial tuberosity or in the distal femur. An 18 g should be used for an infant and 15 g for a child. Central venous access in the femoral vein and a cut down are the last resorts.

17. **What fluids should be used for initial resuscitation?**

Initial fluid resuscitation starts with lactated ringer's (LR). For an adult it is approximately 1 L and for pediatric patient (<40 kg) start with 20 mL/kg. Concepts such as "controlled resuscitation," "balanced resuscitation," "hypovolemic resuscitation," and "permissive hypotension" involve limiting crystalloid infusion in a patient who is mentating until bleeding has been controlled. In addition, crystalloids are nearly eliminated in someone who is in hemorrhagic shock. Blood and blood products are administered early.

18. **What is pericardial tamponade physiology?**

Tamponade physiology is classified under obstructive shock. It is most common after penetrating trauma. Pericardial fluid (blood) compresses the myocardium and inhibits diastolic filling. Patients may develop cardiogenic shock as the myocardium is stressed against the obstruction. Clinical signs of tamponade physiology include distended neck veins, muffled heart tones, and hypotension. This constellation of findings is called Beck's triad. One may also identify an abnormal peripheral pulse called pulsus paradoxus. This is when the systolic blood pressure decreases >10 mm Hg during inspiration. As a result, the radial, brachial, or femoral pulse is weakened or disappears momentarily. Distended jugular veins from a rise in venous pressure with inspiration is called Kussmaul's sign. An exaggerated drop in diastolic central venous pressure is known as Friedreich's sign. Definitive treatment is evacuation of the pericardial blood and repair of the myocardium via a sternotomy or anterolateral thoracotomy. Temporizing measures include pericardiocentesis with aspiration of blood. Leaving a flexible catheter with a three-way stopcock can be useful to frequently aspirate blood based on physiologic demands while transferring to definitive care.

19. **What is the Glasgow Coma Scale and what does it measure?**

The Glasgow Coma Scale (GCS) is a common way to score the level of consciousness of a person after a traumatic brain injury (TBI). It is composed of the following variables:
- Eyes: 1–4
- Motor: 1–6
- Verbal: 1–5

The lowest score is 3. The highest score is 15. The highest score if intubated is 11T (T = intubated). If the patient is paralyzed add P (e.g., GCS 3TP).

The GCS helps classify the severity of brain injury into the following:
- Mild TBI: 13–15
- Moderate TBI: 9–12
- Severe TBI: 3–8

20. **What are the adjuncts to the primary survey?**

The adjuncts to the primary survey are:
- EKG
- Catheters—urinary and gastric
- ABG
- Vital signs—respiratory/ventilator rate, pulse oximetry, pulse, blood pressure (place cuff on extremity opposite pulse oximeter)
- CXR
- Pelvic x-ray
- FAST or eFAST

These may be woven into the primary survey with a large team and multiple resources. Alternatively, when one does not have multiple personnel, it is done in a linear fashion after the primary survey.

21. **What does FAST mean, and what is its purpose?**

FAST stands for Focused Assessment Sonography in Trauma. Four views are obtained in the assessment: cardiac (sub-xiphoid four chamber view or parasternal long-axis view); right upper quadrant (RUQ), which visualizes Morrison's pouch (this is the space between the liver and kidney and is the most likely intraabdominal view to be positive); the left upper quadrant view (LUQ); and the pelvic view. In females, it visualizes the pouch of Douglas (posterior to the uterus/rectouterine pouch).

The extended FAST (eFAST) evaluates the pleural space for pneumothorax or hemothorax, the peritoneal cavity and the pericardial space for blood. The purpose of the exam is to detect free fluid. While it cannot differentiate the type of fluid, in trauma, it is presumed to be blood until proven otherwise. Combined with physiologic variables it helps with decision making to the operating room versus additional imaging.

22. **How much fluid can the FAST exam detect?**
The FAST exam can detect approximately 200 mL of intraperitoneal fluid.

23. **What is DPA or DPL?**
DPA stands for diagnostic peritoneal aspirate versus DPL, which stands for diagnostic peritoneal lavage. The FAST exam has largely replaced these more invasive tests. DPA and DPL have a more limited role in the modern era.

24. **What is the golden hour?**
The term *golden hour* is credited to Dr. R Adams Cowley and his extensive work on shock. The first 60 minutes are critical to reversing shock and getting out of the lethal triad. Injury is a disease of time— be prepared and work efficiently.

25. **What is the lethal triad?**
The components of the lethal triad are hypothermia (temperature $<34°C$), acidosis (pH <7.35), and coagulopathy. Coagulopathy can be determined either by clinical evidence of distorted clotting, PT/INR, or more en vogue methods such as thromboelastography (TEG) or rapid TEG (rTEG).

26. **How can I become proficient at initial assessment?**
The first step in becoming proficient in the initial assessment of the trauma patient is to take the ATLS course offered by the American College of Surgeons Committee on Trauma. Then practice the course in each injured patient interaction. Further proficiency can be obtained by taking the ATLS instructor course.

KEY POINTS: INITIAL ASSESSMENT

1. Follow the A, B, C, D, Es of the ATLS system when evaluating a trauma patient, and return to the same sequential order when reevaluating the patient.
2. Assume every trauma patient has a cervical spine injury until proven otherwise, and carefully assess methods to evaluate or clear the cervical spine.
3. Establish a secure airway based on the injury pattern present, or the neurological status of the patient (GCS).
4. Evaluate for presence of shock and initiate fluid, blood, or plasma resuscitation based on the level of shock and associated signs of coagulopathy, hypothermia, and acidosis via large-bore peripheral IV infusions.
5. Establish central venous catheterization to help assess hemodynamic stability.
6. Use FAST, DPL, and CT scan to evaluate the extent of injuries and triage the patient appropriately.

BIBLIOGRAPHY

1. American College of Surgeons Committee on Trauma. *Advanced Trauma Life Support Course.* 9th ed. Chicago: American College of Surgeons; 2012.
2. Kirkpatrick AW, Sirois M, Laupland KB, et al. Hand-held thoracic sonography for detecting post-traumatic pneumothoraces: the Extended Focused Assessment with Sonography for Trauma (EFAST). *J Trauma* 2004;57(2):288–295.
3. Cothren CC, Moore EE. Emergency department thoracotomy. In: *Trauma.* 6th ed. New York: McGraw Hill; 2008.
4. Inaba K, Byerly S, Bush LD, et al. Cervical spine clearance: a Western Association for the Surgery of Trauma multi-institutional trial. *J Trauma Acute Care Surg.* 2016;81(6):1122–1130.
5. Sperry J, Ochoa J, Gunn S, et al. An FFP:PRBC transfusion ratio of 1:1.5 is associated with a lower risk of mortality after massive transfusion. *J Trauma* 2008;65(5):986–993.

CHAPTER 18

POSTTRAUMATIC HEMORRHAGIC SHOCK

Hunter B. Moore, MD, Ernest E. Moore, MD, FACS

1. **What is hemorrhagic shock?**
   Shock exists when the cardiovascular system is no longer able to meet the body's metabolic and oxygen needs, resulting in cellular injury. In other words, the tissues are not adequately perfused to meet their oxygen and nutrient requirements. Hemorrhagic is a subtype of shock directly related to blood loss, which decreases oxygen delivery as a result of loss of circulating volume and oxygen-carrying red blood cells. The majority of deaths from bleeding occur within 2 hours of injury.

2. **What is the initial management of hemorrhagic or hypovolemic shock?**
   Depletion of the blood volume results in a decreased driving pressure returning blood to the heart, a decreased end-diastolic ventricular volume, and a decreased stroke volume, resulting in a decreased cardiac output (CO). Therefore, the priorities are to (1) control blood loss and (2) restore circulating blood volume. ATLS guidelines reinforce circulation (C in ABC) in the initial management of an injured patient. Circulation management requires vascular access, either through an IV catheter or intraosseous device. Hemorrhage control includes direct pressure, extremity tourniquets, pelvic binding, resuscitative endovascular aortic occlusion (REBOA), or aortic clamping via thoracotomy.

3. **Describe the cellular manifestations of hemorrhagic shock.**
   Inadequate tissue perfusion results in decreased cellular oxygen tension and disruption of normal oxidative phosphorylation with a decrease in the generation of adenosine triphosphate (ATP). The Na+ K+ ATPase slows, and the cell can no longer maintain membrane polarization integrity, impairing a number of important cellular processes. Anaerobic metabolism ensues, resulting in the production of lactic acid, creating a "gap" metabolic acidosis. The first evidence of this dysfunction is swelling of the endoplasmic reticulum, followed by mitochondrial damage, lysozyme rupture, and entry of interstitial water into the cell as intracellular sodium (Na+) accumulates. This loss of extracellular water exacerbates the intravascular volume deficit.

4. **What are the clinical manifestations of hemorrhagic shock?**
   - Heart rate (HR) >110 beats per minute, but can be paradoxically low in profound shock, patients taking cardiac medication may not manifest changes in HR.
   - Blood pressure (BP) <90 mm Hg is generally considered shock in adults, but requires age adjustment for pediatric and geriatric populations.
   - Altered mental status with lethargy and confusion.
   - Decrease in urine output <0.5 mL/kg per hour and low central venous pressure (CVP).
   - The skin becomes cool, clammy, and pale. The subcutaneous veins collapse (making it hard to start an IV line). Capillary refill is delayed 2–3 seconds.

5. **What is the formula for estimating total blood volume in adult and pediatric patients?**
   In adults and children, the average blood volume represents 7% and 9% of ideal body weight, respectively. Therefore, in adults, multiply the ideal weight in kg × 7% (70 mL/kg). In children, multiply ideal weight in kg × 9% (90 mL/kg).

6. **What are the potential sources of occult blood loss when trying to ascertain a patient's hemodynamic status?**
   The pleural spaces, abdominal cavity, retroperitoneal or pelvic space (pelvic fractures), major long bone fractures, and at the scene externally ("on the sidewalk"). Femur fractures can hide >1 L of blood, whereas each rib fracture can account for 150 mL.

7. **What is the first physiologic response to hypovolemia?**
   The patient tries to compensate for the decrease in stroke volume by increasing HR (tachycardia).

8. **Is the hematocrit a reliable guide for estimating acute blood loss?**
   No. A decrease in the hematocrit occurs with refill of the intravascular space from the interstitial space or during administration of exogenous crystalloid resuscitation fluid. However, this process is not immediate, and serial hematocrits are more helpful to assess blood loss.

9. **What is trauma-induced coagulopathy (TIC)?**
   One in four severely injured patients who present to the hospital will have an elevated INR (>1.3). This increase in INR is associated with a fourfold increase in mortality. The mechanisms driving TIC are complex and multifactorial related to hypocoagulation from autoheparinization from shedding of the glycocalyx and activated protein C with additional clotting impairment from platelet dysfunction due to post shock metabolites, and excessive clot degradation (hyperfibrinolysis) from endothelial release of tissue plasminogen activator.

10. **Should all trauma patients receive tranexamic acid?**
    No, despite the zealous use of tranexamic acid (TXA) in Europe, its efficacy in reducing mortality has been challenged. TXA is an antifibrinolytic medication that is proposed to inhibit fibrinolysis and reduce bleeding related mortality. The most cited paper for the use of TXA is the CRASH II trial, in which this medication reduced mortality by <2%. More recent retrospective studies in the United States have found no benefit, and one found a twofold increase in mortality with this medication. The mechanism to explain why TXA has limited efficacy after trauma may be because the majority of trauma patients present to the hospital with inhibition of fibrinolysis before any resuscitation efforts. A moderate amount of fibrinolysis following trauma is associated with improved survival. Thus, TXA should be used selectively and optimally guided by viscoelastic assays.

11. **What is the appropriate choice for IV solution during resuscitation?**
    Crystalloid (normal saline or lactated Ringer's) should be used for the initial resuscitation of most injured patients. However, patients who present to the hospital in overt hemorrhagic shock should undergo plasma-first resuscitation. Plasma is a physiologic colloid that is a metabolic buffer and contains coagulation proteins that attenuate TIC. The benefits of early plasma resuscitation have been validated in numerous retrospective studies and most recently in the PROPPR trial. Do not add artificial colloids or hypertonic saline to the initial fluids; this exacerbates underlying coagulopathy and, in animal models and human clinical trials, decreases survival.

12. **What is base deficit, and how is it useful during resuscitation?**
    The base deficit reflects the degree of metabolic acidosis in blood and is used in hemorrhagic shock as a surrogate marker of tissue hypoxia. The worse the base deficit the worse the patient's perfusion. Base deficit depends on the hematocrit, acid-base balance (pH), and partial pressure of carbon dioxide (pCO_2); if you correct the pCO_2 back to 40 mm Hg, the pH should be 7.40. If your patient is still acidotic, they have a base deficit, unless excessive normal saline is used during resuscitation. This creates an artificial base deficit from hyperchloremia. Additional laboratory assays such as lactate may aid in determining if the patient remains underresuscitated when excessive chloride has been used during resuscitation. Ideally, the strong ion gap should be used.

13. **What are the clinical classifications of shock and the associated clinical manifestations?**
    See Table 18.1. These are estimates and not nearly as accurate or valuable as determining your patient's response to therapy or resuscitation.

Table 18.1 Clinical Classifications of Shock

CLASS	DESCRIPTION	CLINICAL MANIFESTATIONS
Class 1	Blood volume loss = 15% Can compare this with a blood donor	Mild tachycardia, headache, and postural dizziness
Class 2	Blood volume loss = 30%	Moderate tachycardia, tachypnea, and decreased pulse pressure
Class 3	Blood volume loss = 40%	Marked tachycardia, tachypnea, decreased mental status, hypotension, and decreased urine output
Class 4	Blood volume loss >40%	Marked tachycardia, marked tachypnea, decreased systolic blood pressure, obtundation to unconscious mental status, and no urine output

14. **What are the other types of shock, and how do they differ from hemorrhagic shock?**

In addition to hemorrhagic or hypovolemic shock, there are neurogenic, cardiogenic, and septic types of shock. **Neurogenic shock** is caused by sudden loss of autonomic vascular tone from spinal cord injury (midthoracic or higher), resulting in vasodilation. The systolic BP is low, the pulse pressure is low, HR is low, but the skin remains warm. **Cardiogenic shock** results from pump failure secondary to intrinsic heart muscle damage (myocardial infarction) or mechanical compression (cardiac tamponade). In this setting, CO is low; however, intravascular volume is adequate reflected by increased CVP. **Septic shock** (more common in the surgical intensive care unit patients) is characterized by hypotension and low systemic vascular resistance (SVR). It is important to remember these categories of shock do not always exist in isolation. For example, a trauma patient may have cardiac tamponade and also be hemorrhaging into his pelvis.

15. **What is permissive hypotension?**

Permissive hypotension is a strategy to underresuscitate a patient until definitive hemorrhage control can be obtained. A systolic BP of <100 has previously been demonstrated to have a survival advantage in penetrating trauma. Its role in blunt trauma remains less clear and in patients with traumatic brain injury is contraindicated. This resuscitation strategy is utilized in the prehospital and emergency department setting, and should not be utilized once mechanical bleeding is controlled in the operating room. While it is inappropriate to wait until the trauma patient fits a precise physiologic classification of shock before starting volume restoration, overzealous use of crystalloid can be dangerous. Excessive crystalloid has several iatrogenic effects including dilution coagulopathy, "popping the clot" from rapid increase in systolic BP, increased edema leading to abdominal compartment syndrome, and organ failure.

16. **When are blood products indicated during initial resuscitation?**

Plasma and red blood cells (RBCs) should be available for immediate transfusion for all trauma patients at level I trauma centers. Hospitals with fewer resources may be dependent on an initial crystalloid resuscitation prior to blood products to temporize the patient's hemodynamic status until these products are available. While traditional ATLS guidelines suggest 2 L of crystalloid should be the threshold for initiating blood product use in trauma patients, the more modern approach is 1 L of crystalloid, and, if the patient remains hypotensive, plasma and RBCs transfusions should be initiated; AB plasma and O-negative RBCs can be transfused without cross matching the patient's blood. Do not wait for type-specific blood if immediate infusion is required; the blood bank is not generally using the same clock (they are not as frightened because they cannot see the patient). Platelets should be included after the patient has received >6 units of blood product or indicated by laboratory assessment (platelet count <100 or thromboelastography maximum amplitude [MA] <55).

17. **When should blood products stop being transfused?**

Once hemostasis is achieved. During active bleeding, the optimal hemoglobin of a patient is suggested to be 10 g as this adds to hemostasis through a process called margination. Transfusions beyond this level fail to improve oxygen delivery or any additional benefit. However, once bleeding is controlled, hemoglobin of 7 g is acceptable and should be the transfusion trigger for the patient while recovering in the intensive care unit. Goal-directed resuscitation with laboratory assays for blood products beyond RBCs is superior to guessing a patient's coagulation status. To date, viscoelastic assays (rotational thromboelstometry [ROTEM] or thromboelastometry [TEG]) can more accurately predict a patient's need for plasma, platelets, and cryoprecipitate.

18. **How does hemorrhagic shock lead to multiple organ failure?**

Multiple organ failure (MOF) is a syndrome that represents a complicated and dynamic pathophysiologic pathway leading to organ functional derangement and eventual death. Severe hemorrhagic shock begins an inflammatory cascade that cannot be reversed in some patients despite adequate resuscitation. This pathway is thought to begin within hours of injury. Patients with ARDS can be mechanically ventilated but later die from a combination of renal, liver, cardiac, and bone marrow failure. MOF is the leading cause of late postinjury mortality. In addition to the cellular derangement in ATP synthesis, shock causes the release of platelet-activating factor, interleukin-8, and arachidonic acid metabolites that prime neutrophils to adhere to endothelial cells and release cytotoxic mediators, which produce defects in the endovasculature, flooding the interstitial space and causing organ damage. The mesenteric circulation is a hotbed of proinflammatory mediator synthesis (the gut is the "motor for MOF") and appears to release agents (probably arachidonate and other toxic lipids) into the mesenteric lymph that causes systemic neutrophil priming and ultimately acute lung injury. The fibrinolysis system is also inhibited following injury and causes microvascular thrombosis causing organ

KEY POINTS: CLASSIFICATIONS OF SHOCK

1. Hemorrhagic (acute blood loss) is the most common cause of posttraumatic shock; low filling pressures and CO, low mixed venous oxygen saturation (SVO_2), high SVR.
2. Initial management of shock should focus on (1) controlling bleeding, (2) vascular access, and (3) restoration of blood volume.
3. One out of four patients in hemorrhagic shock present with evidence of TIC.
4. Plasma-first resuscitation is optimal in patients who present to the hospital in overt hemorrhagic shock.
5. Patients in neurogenic shock have a low blood pressure and low heart rate.

failure. This fibrinolysis shutdown is present in over 50% of severely injured patients on presentation to the hospital, and its incidence exceeds 80% of trauma patients within the first 24 hours of injury.

BIBLIOGRAPHY

1. Tisherman SA, Schmicker RH, Brasel KJ, et al. Detailed description of all deaths in both the shock and traumatic brain injury hypertonic saline trials of the Resuscitation Outcomes Consortium. *Ann Surg.* 2015;261(3):586–590.
2. Sauaia A, Moore EE, Johnson JL, et al. Temporal trends of postinjury multiple-organ failure: still resource intensive, morbid, and lethal. *J Trauma Acute Care Surg.* 2014;76(3):582–592; discussion 592–593.
3. Brohi K, Cohen MJ, Ganter MT, et al. Acute traumatic coagulopathy: initiated by hypoperfusion: modulated through the protein C pathway? *Ann Surg.* 2007;245(5):812–818.
4. Holcomb JB, Tilley BC, Baraniuk S, et al. Transfusion of plasma, platelets, and red blood cells in a 1:1:1 vs a 1:1:2 ratio and mortality in patients with severe trauma: the PROPPR randomized clinical trial. *JAMA.* 2015;313(5):471–482.
5. CRASH-2 trial collaborators, Shakur H, Roberts I, et al. Effects of tranexamic acid on death, vascular occlusive events, and blood transfusion in trauma patients with significant haemorrhage (CRASH-2): a randomised, placebo-controlled trial. *Lancet.* 2010;376(9734):23–32.
6. Valle EJ, Allen CJ, Van Haren RM, et al. Do all trauma patients benefit from tranexamic acid? *J Trauma Acute Care Surg.* 2014;76(6):1373–1378.
7. Moore HB, Moore EE, Gonzalez E, et al. Hyperfibrinolysis, physiologic fibrinolysis, and fibrinolysis shutdown: the spectrum of postinjury fibrinolysis and relevance to antifibrinolytic therapy. *J Trauma Acute Care Surg.* 2014;77(6):811–817. discussion 817.
8. Bickell WH, Wall MJ Jr, Pepe PE, et al. Immediate versus delayed fluid resuscitation for hypotensive patients with penetrating torso injuries. *N Engl J Med.* 1994;331(17):1105–1109.
9. Brown JB, Cohen MJ, Minei JP, et al. Goal-directed resuscitation in the prehospital setting: a propensity-adjusted analysis. *J Trauma Acute Care Surg.* 2013;74(5):1207–1212; discussion 1212–1214.
10. Gonzalez E, Moore EE, Moore HB, et al. Goal-directed hemostatic resuscitation of trauma-induced coagulopathy: a pragmatic randomized clinical trial comparing a viscoelastic assay to conventional coagulation assays. *Ann Surg.* 2016;263(6):1051–1059.

CHAPTER 19

TRAUMATIC BRAIN INJURY

Ramesh M. Kumar, MD, Kathryn Beauchamp, MD

1. **Is traumatic brain injury (TBI) a common problem?**
   Yes. In the United States, 1 in 12 deaths are due to injury. About 30% of traumatic deaths are associated with TBI. Of deaths resulting from motor vehicle accidents, 60% are a result of brain injury. Even more common is mild TBI, which accounts for 75% of admissions for head trauma. There are over 200,000 patients hospitalized with TBI in the United States per year and over 1.7 million mild TBIs that require a physician's attention. In 2010 TBI contributed to the death of more than 50,000 people in the United States. It is estimated that 2 million to 6 million people in the United States are living with TBI-associated disabilities.

2. **What is a concussion?**
   The definition of concussion or mild TBI per the Centers for Disease Control and Prevention is a complex pathophysiologic process secondary to trauma that results in a constellation of physical, cognitive, emotional, or sleep-related symptoms that may or may not involve loss of consciousness. The symptoms may include headache, dizziness, amnesia, and vomiting. There are about 128/100,000 population concussions in the United States per year. In pediatric patients, sports is the most common cause, whereas falls and motor vehicle accidents are the most common cause in adults.

3. **How is the Glasgow Coma Scale (GCS) score derived?**
   The GCS is a means of identifying changes in neurologic status. Its principal strengths are ease of use and reproducibility among observers. It is a 15-point scale, with 15 as the best score and 3 as the worst. TBIs are categorized according to severity based on the following ranges: mild, 13–14; moderate, 9–12; and severe, 3–8. The score is derived from the addition of the three individual components: best eye-opening response (1–4 points), best verbal response (1–5 points), and best motor response (1–6 points). The GCS is insensitive to pupillary response and focality.

4. **When should a neurosurgeon be consulted?**
   A neurosurgeon should be consulted for any trauma patient with an abnormal computed tomography (CT) scan of the head or with a normal head CT, but with a focal neurological deficit.

5. **How do you initially assess the patient with a brain injury?**
   Just like any trauma patient. The first steps are assessment of the ABCs (airway, breathing, and circulation) and rapid physiologic resuscitation. The neurologic examination is crucial. The initial examination includes (1) GCS assessment; (2) assessment of brainstem reflexes, including pupil size and reactivity, oculocephalic reflex (doll's eyes), corneal reflex, and cough and gag reflex; and (3) motor examination. Repetition of the neurologic examination is also crucial and may require monitoring in an intensive care unit. Finally, evaluate for concurrent cervical spine injury.

6. **What takes priority in a patient who is hypotensive also with a TBI?**
   Hypotension in patients with head injury may be a sign of other injuries. Do not assume that hypotension is a result of the brain injury alone. A single episode of hypotension is a poor prognostic factor in severe TBI as it doubles the mortality rate. Also, hypoxemia, as defined as a PaO_2 <60 or O_2 saturation <90%, significantly increases mortality in TBI.

7. **What is the significance of anisocoria in a patient with a decreased level of consciousness?**
   Anisocoria (unequal pupils) is a true neurologic emergency in a patient with TBI. It may be a sign of a mass lesion (e.g., subdural or epidural hematoma, contusion, or diffuse swelling of one hemisphere) causing uncal herniation and compression of the ipsilateral third nerve. Time is crucial. Give mannitol, get a CT scan, and proceed with surgical decompression (if deemed necessary). Anisocoria can also result from direct orbital injury, and if no neurological cause is found, an ophthalmologic consultation should be sought.

8. **What if the larger pupil is reactive?**

   Consider two separate possibilities. If the larger pupil is reactive to consensual and not direct light, it may be an afferent pupillary defect due to orbital or optic nerve injury, and ophthalmology should be consulted. If the larger pupil is reactive to direct and consensual light, the optic and third cranial nerve are functioning. Think of Horner's syndrome (miosis, ptosis, and anhidrosis) on the other side. This syndrome may be a result of injury to the sympathetic nerves traveling with the carotid artery in the neck. Consider evaluation (CT angiography) for a carotid dissection.

9. **Is the term *semicomatose* inaccurate?**

   Yes. Patients are either alert, lethargic (arousal is maintained by verbal interaction), obtunded (constant mechanical stimulation to maintain arousal), or comatose (neither verbal nor mechanical stimulation elicits arousal). GCS is a much better way to communicate a patient's level of consciousness. Change in level of consciousness is often the first sign of increasing intracranial pressure (ICP); it is also the most poorly documented part of the neurologic examination. Document all findings!

10. **How is motor response tested?**

    Ascertain the ability to follow commands by asking the patient to hold up fingers and move his or her arms and legs. If the patient does not follow commands, test response to painful central stimulus. Localization of painful stimulus is confirmed by the patient's hand reaching toward a sternal rub. The patient may be more severely injured if in response to pain he or she exhibits flexor posturing (decorticate), extensor posturing (decerebrate), or no response. Flexor posturing is concerning for a high brainstem injury, and extensor posturing is associated with lower brainstem dysfunction.

11. **What is the significance of periorbital ecchymosis (raccoon eyes) and ecchymosis over the mastoid (Battle's sign)?**

    In the absence of direct trauma to the eyes or mastoid regions, periorbital ecchymosis and ecchymosis over the mastoid are reliable signs of basilar skull fractures. Of patients with basilar skull fractures, 10% have cerebrospinal fluid (CSF) leaks, including rhinorrhea or otorrhea. Persistent CSF leaks are associated with an increased risk of meningitis; however, prophylactic antibiotics do not decrease the risk of meningitis.

12. **Should scalp lacerations be explored in the emergency department (ED)?**

    Usually not. A CT scan should be performed first to look for intracranial pathology or skull fracture. If surgical pathology is seen on the CT, the laceration will be closed in the operating room (OR). If not, the laceration can be washed and closed in the ED. If bleeding cannot be controlled before CT, then the laceration should be temporarily closed with staples to stop the blood loss.

13. **Which patients need CT scans of the head?**

    The CT scan is used partly as a triage tool with mild brain injuries and can be cost effective compared with admission to the intensive care unit for observation. Conversely, patients with a focal neurologic deficit do not proceed to the OR without a CT scan. Patients who definitely need a CT scan after mild TBI are those <16 years or >65 years, who are intoxicated, not dependable, on anticoagulants, have persistent amnesia or other neurological symptoms, signs of a basilar skull fracture, or abnormal neurological exam.

14. **What are the common traumatic surgical lesions?**

    Epidural hematomas (from arterial bleeding), subdural hematomas (from venous bleeding), and intra-parenchymal hematomas are common traumatic lesions that should be surgically treated if they have significant mass effect on the brain. If the ventricles are large (ventriculomegaly), a ventriculostomy can drain excessive CSF if ICP is elevated. A depressed skull fracture or foreign body (e.g., a bullet) may require a trip to the OR in certain clinical situations.

15. **When is ICP monitoring indicated?**

    ICP should be monitored in all salvageable patients with a severe TBI (GCS 3–8 after resuscitation) and an abnormal CT (defined as hemorrhage, contusions, swelling, herniation, or compressed cisterns). ICP monitoring is also indicated in patients with GCS <8 and normal CT if two or more of the following are noted: age >40, flexor or extensor posturing, or systolic blood pressure (SBP) <90 mm Hg. ICP monitoring serves as a very useful tool in treating patients with severe TBI; however, it has not been shown to significantly improve outcomes.

16. **Describe the initial treatment of patients with a suspected increase in ICP**
The brain, similar to every other organ, must have adequate blood flow and oxygen delivery. The ABCs come first. Airway should be established, and the patient should be intubated if necessary. Keep the SBP >90 mm Hg and avoid hypoxia. The head of the bed should be elevated to facilitate venous drainage, and cervical spine precautions followed. Mannitol should be given if patient has signs of impending herniation, such as anisocoria, or focal neurologic signs on examination such as posturing.

17. **Should all patients with elevated ICP be hyperventilated?**
Decreasing the partial pressure of carbon dioxide (pCO_2) is the most rapidly effective treatment for elevated ICP. Hyperventilation decreases ICP by causing cerebral vasoconstriction, thus decreasing cerebral blood volume. The goal is usually a pCO_2 of 30–35 mm Hg. Any patient with a depressed level of consciousness and inability to protect the airway should be intubated. Before a CT scan is obtained, patients with a neurologic examination concerning for uncal herniation (anisocoria with or without posturing) may be mildly hyperventilated until definitive treatment is achieved. Do not perform chronic hyperventilation as this can cause ischemic brain injury as a result of a decrease of cerebral blood flow (CBF). Because of this effect on CBF, hyperventilation should only be used as a temporizing measure.

18. **In hemodynamically stable patients, how do you decrease ICP?**
Start with the simple things first. Make sure the patient's head of the bed is elevated, and if the patient is wearing a cervical collar, ensure that it is not obstructing jugular venous outflow. If the patient is on continuous intravenous (IV) sedation, consider a bolus of sedative medication. If the patient has an external ventricular catheter, drain off 5 mL. For emergent treatment of refractory elevated ICP give mannitol, 0.25–1 g/kg, as an IV bolus, but remain alert for signs of resulting hypotension. More recent evidence also suggests that hypertonic saline may decrease ICP and maintain hemodynamic stability. Hypertonic saline may be given as a continuous infusion with a goal serum sodium or as bolus injections for bumps in ICP.
    Hypertonic saline can be given in varying concentrations ranging from 3% to 23.4% normal saline. Secondary causes of elevated ICP such as fever, hypercapnia or elevated intrathoracic pressures should be investigated and treated accordingly.

19. **What is the role for decompressive craniectomy in patients with severe TBI?**
Decompressive craniectomy involves removal of a large portion of the cranium and opening of the dura mater to relieve elevated ICP. Indications for this procedure remain unclear and controversial. Although it is effective at reducing elevated ICP, a large randomized control trial found that decompressive craniectomy leads to more unfavorable outcomes in patients with severe TBI than standard medical management.

20. **What is the end point of treatment with diuretics?**
There is no universally accepted end point; however, a serum sodium of 155 mEq/L and serum osmolality of 320 mOsm are usually the upper limits of diuresis. Anticipate intravascular hypovolemia and treat accordingly. The recent SAFE (Saline versus Albumin Fluid Evaluation) trial comparing albumin versus saline in resuscitation of patients with TBI has shown that resuscitating with albumin increases mortality and is more expensive than crystalloids. Thus, crystalloids should be used to replace the lost volume secondary to diuresis in TBI.

21. **What is the significance of cerebral perfusion pressure (CPP)?**
CPP is the difference between mean arterial pressure (MAP) and ICP:

$$CPP = MAP - ICP$$

CPP is important. Neurologic outcome is best in patients with CPPs in the 60s, and CPP <50 should be avoided. Some patients require treatment with pressors and fluids to maintain the CPP; however, aggressively maintaining CPP >70 should be avoided because of the increased risk of adult respiratory distress syndrome (ARDS).

22. **Why should all children with TBI be undressed and examined thoroughly?**
Half of children suffering nonaccidental trauma have TBI. A thorough examination may reveal additional injuries.

23. **Should posttraumatic seizures be treated prophylactically?**
Patients with brain parenchymal abnormalities on CT scan after head injury may benefit from 1 week of antiseizure prophylaxis. Early posttraumatic seizures (seizures occurring within 7 days of injury) can increase the metabolic demand of the injured brain and adversely affect ICP. Phenytoin and carbamazepine have been shown to decrease the incidence of early seizures, but not late seizures. Of patients who have seizures within the first 7 days of injury, 10% also have late seizures. Patients at increased risk of seizures are those with GCS <10, contusions, depressed skull fractures, brain hematomas, or penetrating injuries.

24. **Which coagulopathy is associated with severe brain injury?**
Disseminated intravascular coagulation. The presumed mechanism is massive release of thromboplastin from the injured brain into the circulation. The serum levels of fibrin degradation products roughly correlate with the extent of brain parenchymal injury. All patients who are severely brain injured should be evaluated with prothrombin time, partial thromboplastin time, platelet counts, and fibrinogen levels.

25. **What other medical complications may result from severe head injury?**
Diabetes insipidus (DI) secondary to the inadequate secretion of antidiuretic hormone is caused by injury to the posterior pituitary or hypothalamic tracts. The kidney is unable to reabsorb free water. Usually the urine output is >200 mL/h, and the urine specific gravity is <1.003. The serum sodium may rise precipitously and the patient may become hemodynamically unstable due to hypovolemia if DI is not treated promptly. The treatment of choice in trauma is 1-deamino-8-D-arginine vasopressin (DDAVP). Serum sodium levels must be watched closely after DDAVP administration as it can cause hyponatremia.

26. **If a patient is awake with significant neurologic symptoms but no abnormality on CT scan, what are the likely explanations?**
A spinal cord injury, or carotid or vertebral artery dissection resulting in a stroke.

27. **Are gunshot wounds that cross the midline of the brain uniformly fatal?**
No. The tract that the bullet takes is important, but so is the energy that it imparts to the brain. Prognosis and surgical treatment of gunshot wounds to the head must be considered on a case-by-case basis.

28. **What is the significance of concussion?**
In most studies of mild TBI, >50% of patients have complaints of headache, fatigue, balance problems, dizziness, irritability, depression, anxiety, and alterations of cognition and short-term memory. This constellation of symptoms has been called the postconcussive syndrome. It is important to alert the patient to the likelihood of developing these symptoms. The neurobehavioral problems significantly affect patients' lives. The symptoms generally only last a few days to a few weeks, but in rarer cases may take 3–6 months to resolve.

29. **Can patients with mild TBIs be discharged from the ED?**
Patients whose examination (including short-term memory) returns to normal and who have a normal head CT scan can be discharged to home if they are accompanied by a responsible person and given written instructions to return to the hospital if headache continues to worsen, if they experience increasing vomiting, weakness, drowsiness, or CSF leak appears.

30. **Is brain injury permanent? Is the outcome always poor?**
No and no. Brain injury occurs in two phases. The primary injury occurs at the moment of impact. Secondary injury is preventable and treatable. Conditions that can lead to secondary injury include hypoxia, hypotension, elevated ICP, and decreased perfusion to the brain secondary to ischemia, brain swelling, and expanding mass lesions. Rapid surgical management and avoidance of secondary injury improve outcome.

31. **What is the threshold for treating elevated ICP?**
Most studies agree that the threshold for treating ICP should be 20–25 mm Hg.

32. **Should high-dose steroids be given to TBI patients to treat increased ICP?**
No. There is evidence (CRASH [Corticosteroid Randomization After Significant Head Injury] study) that shows that high-dose steroids in TBI are associated with increased morbidity and mortality.

33. **Are patients with TBI at risk for deep venous thrombosis and pulmonary embolus?**

Yes. The risk of deep venous thrombosis (DVT) and pulmonary embolus (PE) in patients with TBIs can be as high as 30%. Sequential compression devices have been shown to reduce the rate of DVT/PE and should be used in all patients with TBIs unless a lower extremity injury prevents their use. Low-molecular-weight heparin (LMWH) has also been shown to decrease the risk of clot formation, but can also increase the risk of worsening intracranial hemorrhage.

KEY POINTS: TRAUMATIC BRAIN INJURY

1. Hypotension and hypoxia must be avoided in TBI.
2. Think of carotid or vertebral artery dissection in trauma patients with neurologic symptoms but a normal CT scan.
3. CPP = MAP − ICP. Try to maintain CPP between 50 and 60 mm Hg in severe TBI, especially in patients with ongoing ICP problems. Do not overtreat (CPP >70), as this increases the risk of ARDS.
4. Do not use high-dose steroids in TBI.

WEBSITES

- www.emedicine.com/pmr/topic212.htm
- www.cdc.gov/ncipc/tbi/mtbi/report.htm
- http://www.cdc.gov/traumaticbraininjury/get_the_facts.html

BIBLIOGRAPHY

1. Brain Trauma Foundation, American Association of Neurological Surgeons, Congress of Neurological Surgeons, et al. Guidelines for the management of severe traumatic brain injury. *J Neurotrauma.* 2007;24(suppl 1):S1–S106.
2. Brain Trauma Foundation. *Guidelines for the management of severe traumatic brain injury.* 4th ed. https://braintrauma.org/uploads/03/12/Guidelines_for_Management_of_Severe_TBI_4th_Edition.pdf. September 2016. Accessed March 15, 2017.
3. Carson J, Tator C. New guidelines for concussion management. *Can Fam Physician.* 2006;52:756–757.
4. Marion DW. Evidenced-based guidelines for traumatic brain injuries. *Prog Neurol Surg.* 2006;19:171–196.
5. Mazzola CA, Adelman PD. Critical care management of head trauma in children. *Crit Care Med.* 2002;0(suppl 11): S393–S401.
6. Narayan RK, Michel ME, Ansell B, et al. Clinical trials in head injury. *J Neurotrauma.* 2002;19:503–557.
7. Ogden AT, Mayer SA, Connolly Jr ES. Hyperosmolar agents in neurosurgical practice: the evolving role of hypertonic saline. *Neurosurgery.* 2005;57(2):207–215.
8. Ropper AH, Gorson KC. Clinical practice. Concussion. *N Engl J Med.* 2007;356(2):166–172.
9. SAFE Study Investigators, Australian and New Zealand Intensive Care Society Clinical Trials Group, Australian Red Cross Blood Service, et al. Saline or albumin for fluid resuscitation in patients with traumatic brain injury. *N Engl J Med.* 2007;357(9):874–884.
10. Shaw NA. The neurophysiology of concussion. *Prog Neurobiol.* 2002;67:281–344.
11. Chestnut RM, Temkin N, Carney N, et al. A trial of intracranial-pressure monitoring in traumatic brain injury. *N Engl J Med.* 2012;367(26):2471–2481.
12. Cooper DJ, Rosenfeld JV, Murray L, et al. Decompressive craniectomy in diffuse traumatic brain injury. *N Engl J Med.* 2011;364(16):1493–1502.
13. Thompson K, Pohlmann-Eden B. Pharmacological treatments for preventing epilepsy following traumatic head injury. *Cochrane Database Syst Rev.* 2015;(8):1–56.
14. Cancelliere C, Hincapie C, Keightley M, et al. Systematic review of prognosis and return to play after sport concussion: results of the International Collaboration on Mild Traumatic Brain Injury Prognosis. *Arch Phys Med Rehabil.* 2014;95(3 suppl 2):S210–S229.

CHAPTER 20

SPINAL CORD INJURIES

Todd F. VanderHeiden, MD, Philip F. Stahel, MD, FACS

1. **What is the difference between a spinal column injury and a spinal cord injury?**
Injuries to the spinal column can include damage to bone, disks, and/or ligaments. These injuries may induce spinal instability. Instability results when the spine can no longer maintain its alignment, protect the neural elements, or prevent incapacitating pain under physiologic loads. Injuries to the spinal column may also be associated with spinal cord injury, which is damage to the neural tissue within the spinal canal. This is often accompanied by a clinically detectable neurologic deficit. When evaluating trauma patients, it is crucial to determine the presence of a spinal column injury, a spinal cord injury, and/or the presence of spinal instability. Unstable spinal injuries often require surgical intervention to reestablish the "Holy Trinity of Spine." Upholding this triad (alignment, stability, neurology) mandates that treatment restore appropriate spinal alignment, proper decompression and protection of the neural elements, and provision of rock-solid stability.

2. **Describe the evaluation of a patient with a suspected spinal injury.**
Assume that all trauma patients have a spinal injury until proven otherwise. Start by ensuring that the patient is adequately immobilized while maintaining strict log-roll precautions. Initially, all trauma patients should be placed in a rigid cervical immobilizer. These cervical collars should be kept in place until the cervical spine is "cleared." Clearance is the process by which the treatment team confirms that a spinal injury is absent. Once this is done, the brace can be removed. On the contrary, if a spinal injury is identified, then a spinal surgery consult should be placed to determine the proper course of treatment. The care team should also work as a unit to remove patients from the backboard as soon as possible. This involves log-rolling the patient with a sufficient number of care team members so that it can be done safely. Simultaneously, the care provider should inspect the entire spine for external trauma while also palpating for irregularities and areas of step-off. A complete and thorough neurologic examination must then occur. Strength must be assessed in all myotomes of the four extremities. Sensory exam should include assessment of light-touch, proprioception, pain, and temperature in all dermatomes. Reflex examination should evaluate the upper and lower extremities, while also evaluating pathologic reflexes like Hoffman's and clonus. A complete sphincter exam must also be performed. This includes inspection of the anus, evaluation of perianal sensation with dull and sharp probes, detection of resting rectal tone with digital insertion, evaluation of voluntary anal sphincter contraction, and determining the presence or absence of the bulbocavernosus reflex. The examiner should also check for priapism. All examination results should be completely and thoroughly documented.

3. **How do you minimize the risk of additional spinal injury in the hospital?**
The best way to prevent further spinal injury in the hospital setting is to assume that a spinal injury exists until proven otherwise. This includes immobilization of the neck in a rigid cervical brace while also maintaining log-roll precautions. It is also important that the care team works together quickly and thoroughly to evaluate the entire spine. If it can be determined that no spinal injury is present, then the patient can be removed safely from braces and mobility precautions. If spinal injuries are detected, then a spinal surgery consultation must be obtained to determine the proper treatment course. Once this is accomplished, the care team must ensure that the appropriate precautions are obeyed and that the proper bracing is utilized effectively. Some patients may require acute internal fixation to provide rock-solid spinal stability. This will allow early mobilization of the patient. Spine boards should be removed very early in the course of the evaluation while the patient is still in the trauma bay. When in doubt, the care team should treat patients as if an unstable spinal injury exists. Only after completion of the spinal clearance pathway should providers be confident that spinal injuries are confirmed absent. If evaluation leads to detection of an injury then collar immobilization and log-roll precautions should be maintained until spinal surgery recommendations provide further guidance. A definitive treatment plan should be finalized and executed as soon as possible.

4. **How is the level of the spinal cord injury defined?**
   The spinal cord injury level does not refer to the level of the injury to the spinal column (vertebrae, disks, and/or ligaments). Rather, it refers to the most caudal level of normal spinal cord function. For example, if a patient has normal function of the deltoid musculature (C5) but little or no function of the musculature of the biceps (C6) or below, then the patient is said to have a "C5 motor-level" injury. Right and left sides should be documented separately.

5. **Which type of injury is commonly associated with cervical spinal injury?**
   Head injury. Forces associated with significant head and brain injury may be transmitted to the cervical spine. Of patients with spinal cord injuries, 50% have associated head injuries. Approximately 15% of patients with one spinal injury also have a noncontiguous second spinal injury. This highlights the importance of a complete and total spinal evaluation in all trauma patients.

6. **How can the spinal cord be evaluated in patients with associated head injury?**
   Trauma patients with head injuries can be very difficult to examine. In addition to significant cranial trauma, which limits the neurologic evaluation, these patients are also frequently intubated, sedated, and can even be pharmaceutically paralyzed. It is important for the examiner to be aware of these confounding variables. Despite these challenges, it is still possible to obtain important information concerning the neurologic examination and spinal cord function. Flaccid motor tone and absent reflexes should raise suspicion of spinal cord injury. These findings are extremely unusual with isolated brain injury. When patients cannot be assessed for motor and sensory function, it is important to examine reflexes and also to perform a complete and thorough sphincter examination. Spinal cord injured patients typically have flaccid paralysis with associated areflexia. It is important to compare the reflexes of the upper and lower extremities. The examiner should check for priapism. Priapism is common with spinal cord injury but not caused by head injury. The examiner should also perform a thorough anorectal examination as described above in Question 2. This detailed examination can be a "window" to the spinal cord. Examiners should have knowledge of spinal cord injury, conus medullaris syndrome, and cauda equina syndrome. Radiographic imaging should also be used liberally when a neurologic deficit is suspected.

7. **At presentation, which other significant injury may mimic a high thoracic cord injury?**
   Thoracic aortic dissection. Also known as the "great masquerader," presenting symptoms of aortic dissection can mimic pathology from any organ system including a high thoracic spinal cord injury. Diagnosis can be very challenging. Symptoms can include tearing, stabbing pain in the chest and/or back, and lower extremity ischemia and paraplegia. A thoracic aortic dissection may present as a T4-level spinal cord injury. T4 is typically a vascular watershed zone in the spinal cord between the vertebral arterial distribution and the aortic radicular arteries. Given the diagnostic dilemma associated with this condition, careful history and physical examination should be combined with liberal use of advanced diagnostic imaging.

8. **What is spinal shock?**
   Spinal shock is a clinical syndrome caused by trauma marked by the absence of all spinal cord function below the level of the injury. This condition results in flaccid motor paralysis, complete loss of sensation, and areflexia. As spinal shock evolves, return of reflex activity begins to occur. This happens in phases and begins with the bulbocavernosus reflex around 48–72 hours. Deep tendon reflexes may take days to weeks to return. The term *shock* in spinal shock does not involve end-organ hypoperfusion. Spinal shock, however, can lead to neurogenic shock. These two entities should not be confused. Neurogenic shock refers to diminished end-organ perfusion caused by hypotension that can result from cervical or upper-thoracic spinal cord injuries. This hypotension results from a lack of sympathetic vasomotor outflow innervation below the neurologic lesion. It is characterized by bradycardia from unbalanced vagal input to the heart. Fluid resuscitation should be utilized judiciously, and vasopressors should be used to keep the systolic blood pressure (SBP) >90 mm Hg. Atropine may be necessary to treat bradycardia.

9. **Describe an adequate radiologic evaluation.**
   Awake, alert, examinable, and reliable patients without neck pain or tenderness to palpation do not require imagining studies so long as there is no distracting injury and the patient is neurologically intact. In contrast, a three-view x-ray series (anteroposterior, lateral, and odontoid view) is recommended for radiographic evaluation of the cervical spine in symptomatic or unexaminable patients

following traumatic injury. The relationship between C7 and the top of the T1 vertebral body must be visualized on the lateral x-ray to be considered adequate. Plain films should be supplemented with computed tomography (CT) to further define areas that are suspicious or not well visualized on the plain cervical x-rays.

Patients with adequate cervical spine x-rays that are determined to be normal may still require brace treatment. Rigid cervical spine brace immobilization in awake and neurologically intact patients with the presence of neck pain and/or tenderness should be utilized for 10–14 days following the injury to adequately treat the cervical sprain/strain. Following this period of bracing, flexion and extension lateral cervical x-ray views should be obtained to confirm spinal stability. At that point, patients can be weaned from the cervical-collar and begin physical therapy targeted at improving strength and range-of-motion.

All obtunded and unexaminable patients with normal cervical spine x-rays should remain in a rigid cervical brace while they undergo high-quality CT imaging with coronal and sagittal reconstructions. If the results of this advanced study are normal, then the rigid cervical immobilizer can be safely removed. Although this is controversial, a normal CT of the cervical spine confers an extremely low risk of significant spinal injury. Furthermore, risks of ongoing rigid immobilization of an obtunded patient's neck are less important than the benefits of improved intensive care in this setting. Among other benefits, patients have lower risk of pressure sores, airway problems, and positioning difficulties once their cervical collars are removed. If questions remain following the CT, however, then magnetic resonance imaging (MRI) can be utilized to further supplement the diagnostic search. At this point, a spinal surgery consultation should be requested.

For the thoracic and lumbosacral spine, anteroposterior and lateral views are obtained based on mechanistic criteria or suspicion for injury. Patients with evidence of possible fractures on plain films should have CT scans to define the injury in greater detail. MRI is also useful to look for herniated disks and ligamentous injury. Currently, these spinal areas can be satisfactorily evaluated by images reconstructed from the body CT data done during the initial trauma workup (the "Pan-Man" Scan: CT scans of the chest, abdomen, and pelvis).

10. **Describe the proper way to read a lateral cervical spine film.**
It is important for the provider to make a habit of doing a thorough systematic review of the x-ray in the same way every time after it is determined to be an adequate film. First, look at the prevertebral soft tissue space. An enlarged space may be the only radiographic abnormality in up to 40% of C1 and C2 fractures. The space anterior to C3 should not exceed one-third of the vertebral body width of C3. At the C6 level, the entire body of C6 generally fits into the prevertebral soft tissue space. Second, sequentially check the alignment of the anterior and posterior edges of the vertebral bodies. There should be a smooth contour of these anterior and posterior cortical lines. Next, check the contour of the spinolaminar line. This should also have a smooth transition between levels. Pay close attention to the relationship between the cranium and the upper cervical spine. The occipital condyles, the ring of C1, and the odontoid should all maintain their intimate connections. Then, be sure to evaluate the intervertebral disk spaces and confirm that they are of relatively equal height. Further evaluation should include assessment of each facet joint confirming that there is no subluxation. Also check the spinous processes for alignment, congruity, and normal splaying. An abnormal relationship here may signify a ligamentous injury. Finally, evaluate each vertebral bone for fracture.

11. **What about the anteroposterior film?**
Check regional alignment of the cervical spine, being sure to note the presence of traumatic scoliosis or lateral listhesis. Carefully inspect the alignment of the midline spinous processes as well. Abrupt angulations can suggest unilateral facet dislocation. More subtle changes may indicate facet instability or fracture. Vertebral body fractures may be more obvious in the anteroposterior view. The anteroposterior view should always be inspected in tandem with the lateral view so that the provider can start to formulate a three-dimensional picture of these two-dimensional images.

12. **Can a patient have a spinal cord injury and normal plain radiographs?**
Yes. Spinal cord injury without radiographic abnormality (SCIWORA) is defined as neurologic signs and symptoms consistent with traumatic myelopathy despite normal x-rays. SCIWORA is rare, and is most common in children. Most series quote about 15% of spinal cord injuries (SCIs) in this age group, but the rate can be as high as 40% in children <9 years old. SCIWORA is less common in adults (about 5% of SCIs).

13. **Is magnetic resonance imaging useful in the evaluation of acute spine trauma?**
    Yes. If plain radiographs and CT scans do not adequately explain the extent of injury noted on the neurologic examination, an MRI should be used to further evaluate the spine. MRI scans are useful to investigate herniated disks, ligamentous injury, and evidence of damage to the neural tissue. Ongoing neurologic compression can also be identified. This may signify the need for surgical decompression. In addition, MRI is used routinely to further clarify injuries identified on CT imaging as well as for preoperative planning. Furthermore, MRI is an invaluable tool for spinal surgeons to select treatment. When examining the mechanism and morphology of the injury, it is important to not only evaluate the neurologic status of the patient but to also investigate the integrity of the posterior ligamentous complex of the spine. This analysis can guide the surgeon in choosing the proper approach for spinal fixation and stabilization when necessary.

14. **Fractures of C1 and C2 are visualized best with which view?**
    Odontoid view. When evaluating plain radiographs, it is best to scrutinize the open-mouth antero-posterior view to visualize the atlas and axis bones. However, assessment of this view should not preclude close analysis of the coronal and sagittal reconstructed CT images. Providers should look for overhang of the lateral masses of C1 compared to the lateral masses of C2 in the coronal plane. This occurs in C1 ring disruptions caused by burst injuries called Jefferson fractures. Axial CT images can add great detail to evaluation of these injuries. On the plain x-ray odontoid view, the sum total over-hang of both C1 lateral masses on C2 of >7 mm may be associated with disruption of the transverse atlantal ligament. This indicates possible atlantoaxial instability that may need internal fixation. The morphology of the axis bone should also be carefully analyzed on this view. Fractures of the odontoid are commonly encountered, and upon discovery should be assessed in all planes utilizing advanced imaging techniques. Odontoid fractures are grouped into three categories by type:
    • Type I: Avulsion fracture at the tip of the dens indicating injury to the alar ligament(s). Suspicion must be raised for occipitocervical dissociation (OCD) when this fracture is identified. If OCD is confirmed absent, then this dens fracture is well treated in a neck brace. If OCD is found, then craniocervical stabilization is necessary.
    • Type II: Fracture through the waist of the dens. This watershed area is a common site of fracture and can herald significant instability. Treatment is based on age and bone quality, and can employ braces, halo fixators, and/or surgery from anterior or posterior approaches. Sub-types A, B, and C can further be defined based on direction of fracture obliquity. This can further guide treatment and surgical approach.
    • Type III: Fracture at the base of the dens extending into the body of the axis. Fracture lines enter the C1-2 facet joints on the coronal views. These fractures occur in areas of plentiful cancel-lous bone with good healing potential and can be treated nonoperatively in a rigid cervical immobilizer.

15. **What is a Hangman's fracture?**
    A Hangman's fracture is the name typically given to the injury involving bilateral fractures through the pars interarticularis of C2. This injury is also referred to as traumatic spondylolisthesis of the axis when subluxation of C2 relative to C3 occurs. These injuries typically result from a hyperextension mechanism followed by a hyperflexion moment and are usually secondary to high-speed motor vehicle crashes. In judicial hangings, the fatal spinal injury can occur by spinal cord stretching combined with the C2 fracture. However, death by this technique is more commonly associated with compression or rupture of the vertebral and/or carotid arteries, which produce cerebral ischemia. Most patients with Hangman's fractures present neurologically intact because of the large diameter of the spinal canal at this level. There is also an autodecompression phenomenon that occurs due to the bilateral posterior element fractures, which results in widening of the spinal canal. Many cases of Hangman's fracture can be treated with external immobilization whether braces or halo fixators are utilized. More severe types of Hangman's fractures can be associated with C2–3 facet-joint and disk injuries, and also involve significant angulation. These injuries usually require open reduction and internal fixation.

16. **Define deficits found in complete spinal cord injury and compare them to deficits found in incomplete spinal cord syndromes, including anterior cord syndrome, central cord syndrome, and Brown-Séquard syndrome.**
    • **Complete spinal cord injury** may result from transection, stretch, or contusion of the spinal cord. All function—motor, sensory, and reflexive—below the level of the lesion is lost. This injury portends the worst prognosis.

- **Anterior cord syndrome** results from an injury of the anterior two-thirds of the spinal cord (the distribution of the anterior spinal artery), which carries motor, pain, and temperature tracts. Vibration sense and proprioception are left intact because the posterior columns are typically preserved. This injury usually stems from a vascular insult. Prognosis is poor.
- **Central cord syndrome** results from injury to the central area of the spinal cord. This entity is often found in patients with preexisting cervical stenosis resulting from spondylotic changes. Characteristic deficits are more severe in the upper extremities than in the lower extremities owing to the axial arrangement of the neuronal tracts. Distal deficits are more profound than proximal deficits within the limbs. Injury is thought to be a result of buckling of a thickened posterior ligamentum flavum into the spinal cord with an extension moment of the neck. Histologic analysis shows there is hemorrhage in the center of the spinal cord. Motor function is typically affected more than sensory function. Prognosis is variable, but there tends to be some clinically detectable recovery. Patients are often left with clumsiness of the hands.
- **Brown-Séquard syndrome** is usually seen in penetrating injuries that affect one side of the spinal cord through unilateral hemisection. This entity may also be seen in blunt injury, especially with unilateral traumatically herniated disks. The syndrome results from injury to half of the spinal cord, where clinical manifestations result in motor, position, and vibration deficits on the ipsilateral side of the injury, whereas the contralateral side shows deficits in pain and temperature sensation. This pattern of deficits occurs as a result of the decussation level of the neuronal tracts within the spinal cord. Prognosis is typically good.

17. **What is the role of methylprednisolone in the treatment of acute spinal cord injury?**
Patients that sustain acute traumatic spinal cord injury should not receive high-dose corticosteroid treatment. Although a highly debated topic for decades, it appears that the risks of such an intervention likely outweigh the benefits. Risks include pulmonary complications, gastrointestinal ulcers and bleeding, as well as infections. Historically, the results of the Second National Acute Spinal Cord Injury Study (NASCIS II) suggested that high-dose methylprednisolone resulted in a statistically significant neurologic improvement. Investigators used a dose of 30 mg/kg load, followed by 5.4 mg/kg per hour for 23 hours. The NASCIS III trial reported that patients dosed 3–8 hours after injury had improved neurologic outcomes when treated for 48 hours rather than 24 hours. In patients dosed within 3 hours of injury, no further gains were documented by treating beyond 24 hours. More recent analysis of the available data coupled with newer trials has put the value of these steroids in doubt. It is certain, however, that methylprednisolone is contraindicated in the management of penetrating spinal cord injury.

18. **Do patients with spinal cord injuries ever undergo acute surgery?**
Yes. Spinal cord injured patients will often require urgent surgery to reestablish the Holy Trinity of Spine. Spinal surgeons employ whatever techniques necessary to restore anatomic alignment, decompression of impinged neurologic structures, and provision of rock-solid stability. These goals should be accomplished as soon as patients are physiologically stable for surgery. Although there is currently no gold standard for the timing of surgery, the general guideline is to stabilize, align, and decompress the spine as soon as safely possible. This enables early mobilization, intensive care, and activation of spinal cord injury protocols. A higher level of urgency accompanies patients with incomplete injuries, deteriorating neurologic status, and patients that have a plateau in their improvement. Patients with complete spinal cord injuries have a less urgent status due to limited potential for neurologic recovery. However, these patients can still greatly benefit from early stabilization and proper alignment that will facilitate early therapeutic interventions. Neurologic deterioration may be encountered as a result of herniated disk material, bony impingement, epidural hemorrhage, or cord swelling within a narrowed canal that causes spinal cord compression and worsening symptoms. Early decompression can benefit these patients.

19. **How is the bony injury treated?**
The bony injury to the spinal column is treated in a variety of ways. The first step is for the spinal surgeon to determine if instability is present. Unstable fractures typically require surgery to openly reduce the spinal malalignment and internally fixate the spine to provide stability. Anterior, posterior, lateral, and combined techniques can be utilized. Spinal surgeons may use screws, rods, plates, struts, or a combination of implants to provide absolute stability to the spine, which will enable

immediate mobilization of the patient. One of the goals of spinal surgery in trauma patients is to provide rock-solid stability, thereby eliminating the need for any restrictions or precautions. In contrast, spinal fractures that are deemed stable may be treated in external orthoses that allow maintenance of alignment and support of the spine through nonsurgical means.

20. **What is the outcome in patients with spinal cord injury?**
    Variable. With complete spinal cord injury, chances of recovery are extremely poor. By definition, if detectable recovery does occur, then the injury was not complete in the first place. It is important to determine the presence of sacral sparing during the early evaluations of patients with spinal cord injury. The presence of sacral sparing defines the spinal cord injury as incomplete, even in the absence of detectable motor or sensory function below the lesion. Patients with incomplete injuries have a chance for recovery. In fact, patients with incomplete lesions have approximately a 75% chance of experiencing meaningful recovery. Early and appropriate treatment of the spinal column injuries helps to prevent pain and late neurologic deterioration.

21. **Are cervical spinal injuries associated with injuries to the carotid or vertebral arteries?**
    Yes. There are several spinal injury risk factors correlated to blunt vertebral artery injury. They are cervical fractures involving the foramen transversarium, fractures involving the C1-C2-C3 bones, and any injury involving subluxation of the cervical vertebrae. Screening of patients with these types of injuries utilizing computed tomographic angiography (CTA) can identify these vascular injuries. This enables timely classification and grading of the arterial insults and can enable employment of anticoagulation strategies that can help prevent cerebrovascular accident. Anticoagulation should be timed appropriately and should consider any needed spinal surgical intervention.

22. **Should all patients with spinal cord injuries have inferior vena cava filters placed to prevent pulmonary embolus?**
    No. Not all spinal cord injured patients require placement of an inferior vena cava filter. Indications for placement of such filters include patients with a contraindication to anticoagulation, patients that incur pulmonary emboli while receiving proper anticoagulation, and patients identified as having thrombi despite anticoagulation.

KEY POINTS: SPINAL CORD INJURY

1. Treat all trauma patients as if they have a significant spinal injury until proven otherwise.
2. Understand the proper clinical and radiographic evaluation of trauma patients with spinal injury.
3. Acknowledge and respect the Holy Trinity of Spine—alignment, stability, and neurology.
4. Understand the concept of spinal stability where, under physiologic loads, the spine maintains its alignment, protects its neurologic elements, and enables a tolerable amount of pain.
5. Evaluate spinal cord injured patients for concomitant vascular insults.
6. Investigate the vertebral and carotid arteries in patients with cervical spinal injuries.
7. Understand the difference between complete and incomplete spinal cord injuries.
8. Know the difference between spinal shock and neurogenic shock.
9. Understand that the concept of spinal clearance is proving that spinal injury is absent.
10. Early surgery in spinal cord injury works to restore alignment and provide rock-solid stability to enable early mobilization and proper nursing care.

WEBSITE

www.asia-spinalinjury.org

BIBLIOGRAPHY

1. Biffl WL, Egglin T. Sixteen-slice computed tomographic angiography is a reliable noninvasive screening test for clinically significant blunt cerebrovascular injuries. *J Trauma.* 2006;60(4):745–751.
2. Mahajan P, Jaffe DM, Olsen CS, et al. Spinal cord injury without radiologic abnormality in children imaged with magnetic resonance imaging. *J Trauma Acute Care Surg.* 2013;75(5):843–847.
3. Bracken MB, Shepard MJ, Holford TR, et al. Administration of methylprednisolone for 24 or 48 hours or tirilazad mesylate for 48 hours in the treatment of acute spinal cord injury: results of the Third National Acute Spinal Cord Injury randomized controlled trial. *JAMA.* 1997;277(20):1597–1604.
4. Cothren CC, Moore EE, Biffl WL, et al. Cervical spine fracture patterns predictive of blunt vertebral artery injury. *J Trauma.* 2003;55(5):811–813.
5. Cortez R, Levi AD. Acute spinal cord injury. *Curr Treat Options Neurol.* 2007;9(2):115–125.
6. Fehlings MG, Perrin RG. The timing of surgical intervention in the treatment of spinal cord injury: a systematic review of recent clinical evidence. *Spine.* 2007;31(suppl 11):S28–S35.
7. Hadley MN, Walters BC, Grabb PA, et al. Radiographic assessment of the cervical spine in symptomatic trauma patients. *Neurosurgery.* 2002;50(suppl 3):S36–S43.
8. Harris MB, Sethi RK. The initial assessment and management of the multiple-trauma patient with an associated spine injury. *Spine.* 2006;31(suppl 11):S9–S15.
9. Holmes JF, Akkinepalli R. Computed tomography versus plain radiography to screen for cervical spine injury: a meta-analysis. *J Trauma.* 2005;58(5):902–905.
10. Sliker CW, Mirvis SE, Shanmuganathan K. Assessing cervical spine stability in obtunded blunt trauma patients: review of medical literature. *Radiology.* 2005;234(3):733–739.
11. Teasell RW, Hsieh TJ, Aubut JA, et al. Venous thromboembolism following spinal cord injury. *Arch Phys Med Rehabil.* 2009;90(2):232–245.
12. Pearson AM, Martin BI, Lindsey M, et al. C2 vertebral fractures in the Medicare population: incidence, outcomes, and costs. *J Bone Joint Surg Am.* 2016;98(6):449–456.
13. Li XF, Dai LY, Lu H, et al. A systematic review of the management of Hangman's fractures. *Eur Spine J.* 2006;15(3):257–269.
14. Furlan JC, Noonan V, Cadotte DW, et al. Timing of decompressive surgery of the spinal cord after traumatic spinal cord injury: an evidence-based examination of pre-clinical and clinical studies. *J Neurotrauma.* 2001;28(8):1371–1399.
15. Evaniew N, Noonan VK, Fallah N, et al. Methylprednisolone for the treatment of patients with acute spinal cord injuries: a propensity score-matched cohort study from a Canadian multi-center spinal cord injury registry. *J Neurotrauma.* 2015;32(21):1674–1683.
16. Patel MB, Humble SS, Cullinane DC, et al. Cervical spine collar clearance in the obtunded adult blunt trauma patient. *J Trauma.* 2015;78(2):430–441.
17. Stahel PF, Vanderheiden T, Finn MA. Management strategies for acute spinal cord injury: current options and future perspectives. *Curr Opin Crit Care.* 2012;18(6):651–660.

CHAPTER 21

PENETRATING NECK TRAUMA

Stephanie N. Davis, MD, Clay Cothren Burlew, MD, FACS,
Ernest E. Moore, MD, FACS

1. **Why are penetrating neck wounds unique?**
   Although comprising only a small percentage of body surface area, the neck contains a heavy concentration of vital structures:
   - Vascular (common, internal, and external carotid arteries, vertebral arteries, internal and external jugular veins)
   - Respiratory (larynx, trachea)
   - Gastrointestinal (oropharynx, esophagus)
   - Lymphatic (thoracic duct)
   - Endocrine (thyroid and parathyroid glands)
   - Nervous (spinal cord, cranial nerves IX, X, XI, XII)
   - Skeletal (cervical vertebra, hyoid bone)

2. **What constitutes a penetrating neck wound?**
   Violation of the platysma muscle defines a penetrating neck wound. This investing fascial layer of the neck is superficial to vital structures. If the platysma is not penetrated, the wound is managed as a simple laceration and the patient is discharged from the emergency department (ED).

3. **Which side of the neck is more likely to be injured?**
   The left side because assailants are more commonly right handed.

4. **Do gunshot wounds and knife wounds cause the same relative injuries?**
   Gunshot wounds generally tend to inflict more tissue damage and typically penetrate deeper (see Table 21.1).

Table 21.1 Gunshot Versus Stab Wounds

STRUCTURE	GUNSHOT WOUNDS (%)	STAB WOUNDS (%)
Artery	20	5
Vein	15	10
Airway	10	5
Digestive	20	<5

5. **What are the three zones of the neck?**
   - Zone I: Is inferior to the clavicles and manubrium
   - Zone II: Extends from the clavicles to the angle of the mandible
   - Zone III: Comprises the area cephalad to the angle of the mandible (see Fig. 21.1)

6. **How do patients with penetrating neck wounds present?**
   - Hard signs: External hemorrhage, expanding hematoma, hemoptysis
   - Soft signs: Hoarseness, dysphagia, odynophagia, palpable crepitus, stable hematoma, stridor
   - Asymptomatic: No signs or symptoms of injury

7. **How often do patients with cervical crepitus have a significant injury?**
   One-third of patients with crepitus have an injury of the pharynx, esophagus, larynx, or trachea. In two-thirds of these patients, however, the air has been introduced through the wound entrance site, and there is no significant underlying injury.

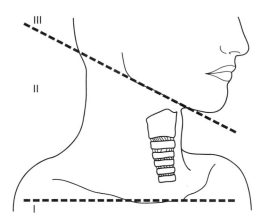

Fig. 21.1 The three zones of the neck.

8. **What are the priorities in the management of penetrating neck trauma?**
   The ABCs (airway, breathing, and circulation) are the priorities in every trauma patient. But digital control of active arterial bleeding is the top priority for neck wounds. If indicated, patients should be intubated orally, although cricothyrotomy may be necessary with an extensive neck hematoma or ongoing bleeding into the oropharynx. Although the patient may present with a patent airway, early elective airway control should be performed in patients with expanding hematomas. Based on the trajectory of injury, pneumothoraces, hemothoraces, or great vessel injury should be suspected.

9. **How should bleeding be controlled at the accident scene and in the ED?**
   Direct digital pressure is almost always successful, even for major arterial injuries. Blindly placing clamps inside a wound risks injury to other vital, uninjured structures, particularly nerves.

10. **Should you explore the neck wound in the trauma bay?**
    Not usually. Although careful visual inspection is warranted, probing the wound (digitally, with a Q-tip, or with a surgical instrument) may dislodge a blood clot, causing active hemorrhage.

11. **Why are penetrating injuries divided into zones?**
    Each zone has management implications. Because of the technical difficulties of injury exposure and varying operative approaches, a precise preoperative diagnosis is desirable for symptomatic Zone I and III injuries. Zone II injuries are more easily evaluated with physical examination (see Fig. 21.2).

12. **What are the indications for immediate operative exploration?**
    Hemodynamic instability or hard signs of injury.

13. **What is selective management of penetrating neck trauma?**
    Historically, all Zone II injuries violating the platysma were explored operatively. However, as a result of a prohibitive number of negative explorations, this approach lost support. Patients with soft signs of injury who are hemodynamically stable should undergo appropriate diagnostic imaging based on their symptoms. Asymptomatic patients with Zone II or III injuries may be observed. The exception is the patient with a transcervical gunshot wound; these patients should undergo computed tomographic angiography (CTA) to determine the tract of the missile and need for further diagnostic imaging.

14. **Should arteriography be performed on all patients?**
    CTA is performed in symptomatic, hemodynamically stable patients with Zone I or III injuries. In patients with Zone I trauma, CTA identifies great vessel injuries in the thoracic outlet that may require a thoracic operative approach. Diagnosis of Zone III injuries may be best managed with angioembolization or endovascular intervention.

15. **What is the value of other diagnostic studies, such as esophagography, esophagoscopy, laryngoscopy, and bronchoscopy?**
    CTA imaging is helpful because trajectory permits selective use of esophagography, bronchoscopy, and laryngoscopy to further evaluate patients with penetrating neck injuries. Esophagoscopy or

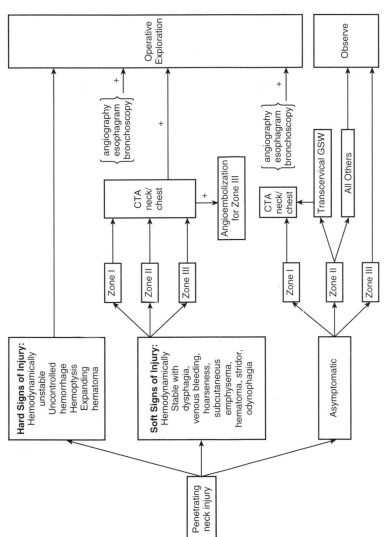

Fig. 21.2 Management of penetrating neck trauma.

esophagography may be utilized if an esophageal injury is suspected. For esophagography, water-soluble contrast material is used first; if this imaging does not show a leak, barium is used. Missed esophageal injuries can be deadly, with a 20% mortality rate if diagnosis is delayed only 12 hours. Intraoperative endoscopy with insufflation may be used provocatively to show an air leak and associated esophageal injury.

16. **Should an asymptomatic patient with a penetrating neck wound be sent home from the ED?**
No. Life-threatening penetrating neck wounds initially may be difficult to sort out; the safest policy is to observe all patients in the hospital for at least 24 hours.

KEY POINTS: PENETRATING NECK TRAUMA

1. Penetrating injury implies violation of the platysma.
2. Selective management is based on hemodynamic status, symptoms, and anatomic zones of injury.
3. Immediate operative intervention is indicated in patients with hemodynamic instability or hard signs of injury.
4. CTA is warranted for penetrating injuries in asymptomatic patients with Zone I or III wounds.

BIBLIOGRAPHY

1. Albuquerque FC, Javedan SP. Endovascular management of penetrating vertebral artery injuries. *J Trauma.* 2002;53(3):574–580.
2. Atteberry LR, Dennis JW. Physical examination alone is safe and accurate for evaluation of vascular injuries in penetrating zone II neck trauma. *J Am Coll Surg.* 1994;179(6):657–662.
3. Biffl WL, Moore EE. Selective management of penetrating neck trauma based on cervical level of injury. *Am J Surg.* 1997;174(6):678–682.
4. Demetriades D, Velmahos G. Cervical pharyngoesophageal and laryngotracheal injuries. *World J Surg.* 2001;25(8):1044–1048.
5. Ferguson E, Dennis JW. Redefining the role of arterial imaging in the management of penetrating zone 3 neck injuries. *Vascular.* 2005;13(3):158–163.
6. Gracias VH, Reilly PM, Philpott J, et al. Computed tomography in the evaluation of penetrating neck trauma. *Arch Surg.* 2001;136(11):1231–1235.
7. Hirshberg A, Wall MJ. Transcervical gunshot injuries. *Am J Surg.* 1994;167(3):309–312.
8. Inaba K, Munera F, McKenney M, et al. Prospective evaluation of screening multislice helical computed tomographic angiography in the initial evaluation of penetrating neck injuries. *J Trauma.* 2006;61(1):144–149.
9. Mazolewski PJ, Curry JD. Computed tomographic scan can be used for surgical decision making in zone II penetrating neck injuries. *J Trauma.* 2001;51(2):315–319.
10. Woo K, Magner DP. CT angiography in penetrating neck trauma reduces the need for operative neck exploration. *Am Surg.* 2005;71(9):754–748.

CHAPTER 22

BLUNT THORACIC TRAUMA

Erin L. Vanzant, MD, Martin D. Rosenthal, MD, Chasen A. Croft, MD, FACS

1. **How often do patients with isolated blunt chest trauma need an emergent operation?**
   Rarely. The majority of injuries can be managed with aggressive pain control, mechanical ventilation, tube thoracotomy, and other simple supportive care. Only 5% of patients with isolated blunt injury to the chest require thoracotomy, as operative injuries to pulmonary, vascular, and mediastinal structures are surprisingly rare.

2. **In a patient with a hemothorax after blunt chest injury, what is the most important guide for the decision to operate?**
   The hemodynamic status of the patient. Hemothorax after blunt injury is most often the result of nonoperative lesions of the lung and chest wall. In a stable patient, therefore, evacuation of the hemothorax, reexpansion of the lung, and correction of coagulopathy, hypothermia, and acidosis should be the initial focus. Chest tube output should be noted, as initial output >1500 mL is an indication for operative management, but is not the principle consideration.

3. **What is a tension pneumothorax?**
   Trapped air in the pleural space as a result of a one-way valve mechanism. In contrast to simple pneumothorax, tension pneumothorax causes hemodynamic compromise. This is a life-threatening condition because marked elevations in intrapleural pressure leading to impaired ventilation capacity, central venous return, and right ventricular filling produces circulatory collapse if left undiagnosed and untreated.

4. **What are the clinical signs of tension pneumothorax?**
   Hypotension, hyperresonance with absent breath sounds on the involved side, tachypnea, and distended neck veins.

5. **How is tension pneumothorax treated?**
   Immediate decompression through a hole in the chest. Tension pneumothorax should be treated on clinical suspicion and without delay for radiographic confirmation. For prehospital care, needle decompression via the second intercostal space in the midclavicular line. In the hospital setting, however, an experienced physician can completely decompress the pleural space just as rapidly with a tube thoracostomy.

6. **Does it matter how many ribs are broken?**
   Yes. Some studies indicate that the presence of three or more fractures is associated with significantly higher risk of mortality and six or more fractures indicate a higher risk of pneumonia and adult respiratory distress syndrome (ARDS), particularly in elderly patients.

7. **What is a flail chest?**
   A flail chest occurs when at least three consecutive ribs are fractured in two or more places resulting in loss of bony continuity with the rest of the chest. This results in the chest wall moving paradoxically ("flails") with respiration.

8. **How does flail chest impact ventilation?**
   In spontaneously breathing patients, the portion of the thoracic cage that has lost bony continuity retracts inward during inspiration and, conversely, outward during exhalation. This paradoxical motion can result in decreased tidal volumes and ultimately impaired ventilation.

9. **Do all patients with a flail segment then need to be put on a ventilator?**
   No. The impact of a flail segment on ventilation is not usually profound, and with good analgesia, many patients can maintain their own work of breathing. The elderly and those with decreased pulmonary reserve appear to be the most vulnerable, but no studies have shown prophylactic intubation to improve outcomes, and therefore standard indications for intubation should be used.

10. **Does flail chest affect oxygenation?**
    Flail chest, per se, has little direct impact on oxygenation. However, virtually all patients with flail chest have an underlying bruise on the lung—pulmonary contusion. The severity of the pulmonary contusion is a more important determinant of outcome and need for intubation than the impaired mechanics of the chest wall, as it has been shown that a large majority of patients with a pulmonary contusion of 20% or more develop ARDS. In general, pathophysiology of blunt injury to the chest with severe bony injury should be thought of as a single process (i.e., flail chest or pulmonary contusion).

11. **What is the natural history of pulmonary contusion?**
    It's like a bruise of the lung. Initially, the lung undergoes shearing of parenchyma and rupture of small blood vessels; this tissue injury is followed by edema and inflammation. The initial chest radiograph may appear deceptively benign and it can take up to 48 hours for the radiograph to depict the extent of injury as the contusion "blooms." Thus, patients with pulmonary contusion usually develop clinical deterioration within this time frame.

12. **What is the most common initial presentation of blunt injury to the thoracic aorta?**
    Death. Eighty-five percent of patients with a torn thoracic aorta die of exsanguination before they reach the hospital. Disruption of the heart and great vessels is second only to head injury as a cause of death as a result of blunt trauma.

13. **Of patients surviving to reach the hospital, where is the most common injury to the thoracic aorta?**
    A tear across the intima and media just distal to the takeoff of the left subclavian artery where the proximal thoracic aorta is tethered at the ligamentum arteriosum. Most who survive sustain partial tears or partial thickness tears of the wall with pseudoaneurysm; because the adventitia is intact, the patient does not immediately exsanguinate. With prompt diagnosis and treatment, the survival rate is 85%.

14. **What are the clinical signs of torn thoracic aorta?**
    There are no definitive signs. Suspicion must be based on mechanism of injury (rapid deceleration with lateral and frontal impact and fall from great heights). The physical signs associated with aortic disruption are not commonly observed; they include upper extremity hypertension, unequal upper extremity pressures, loss of lower extremity pulses, and expanding hematoma in the root of the neck.

15. **What findings on chest radiograph are associated with rupture of the descending thoracic aorta?**
    Like physical signs, no initial radiographic signs are definitive. The signs that have been associated with torn thoracic aorta include indistinct aortic knob, widened mediastinum (>8 cm at the level of the aortic knob), apical cap, left pleural effusion, depression of the left mainstem bronchus, rightward displacement of the esophagus (look for the nasogastric tube), first and second rib fractures, displacement of the trachea, and loss of the aortopulmonary window. Approximately 15% of patients with torn aorta have a normal mediastinum, and 7% have a completely normal chest radiograph.

16. **In the stable patient with a major mechanism of injury or chest radiographs consistent with aortic injury, how is the diagnosis made?**
    Dynamic helical computed tomography (CT) of the chest approaches 100% sensitivity for detecting aortic injury; it is widely available and applicable to all stable patients. Aortography can more precisely identify the site and extent of injury, but has largely been supplanted by CT angiography.

17. **Junior O'Flaherty was hit in the chest with a baseball bat. How can I tell if he has a bruise on his heart (myocardial contusion)?**
    You can't unless you are doing his autopsy.

18. **Okay, then how do I tell if something bad is going to happen to Junior's heart?**
    From a practical standpoint, only two things happen to the bruised heart: arrhythmia and pump failure. By far the most common manifestation of blunt cardiac injury is arrhythmia. Patients with an initial electrocardiogram (ECG) that is normal have an exceedingly small chance of developing clinically significant arrhythmias during their hospital course. Indications of acute injury include new elevated ST segments in leads I, aVL, and V2-V4, atrial fibrillation, and bundle branch blocks, though any ECG abnormality is an indication for admission and 24 hours of cardiac monitoring. Hemodynamic compromise from blunt cardiac injury is unusual and not subtle; echocardiography should be employed in patients with evidence of impaired contractility. Cardiac enzymes are poor predictors of arrhythmia or pump failure and are not recommended. Treatment is mainly supportive.

19. **Where do blunt injuries to the bronchus usually occur? How do they present?**

    Within a few centimeters of the carina. With deceleration, shearing force, and severe anteroposterior compression of the chest, the mainstem bronchi are splayed apart as the lungs are displaced laterally, the mainstem bronchi may tear near the site where they are fixed at the carina. The typical presentation is dyspnea, cyanosis, cervical subcutaneous air, massive air leak, or failure of lung reexpansion ("dropped lung") after a properly placed tube thoracostomy.

20. **What are the indications for emergency department thoracotomy after blunt chest injury?**

    Blunt trauma with witnessed arrest, cardiac activity on cardiac ultrasound, and <10 minutes of prehospital cardiopulmonary resuscitation. The outcome, however, is typically dismal; <1% of patients survive neurologically intact.

21. **What is traumatic asphyxia?**

    Traumatic asphyxia is the result of a protracted crush injury to the upper torso or epigastrium. In such an injury, venous hypertension is transmitted to the valveless veins of the upper body. Patients present with altered sensorium, petechial hemorrhages, cyanosis, and edema of the upper body. Although its initial presentation can be dramatic, with supportive care the outcome is usually good.

KEY POINTS: BLUNT THORACIC TRAUMA

1. Most blunt chest injuries—even significant ones—can be treated without operation. A chest tube, pain control, and supportive care is usually the most that is needed.
2. Tension pneumothorax is a preterminal event and should be treated immediately with a hole in the chest.
3. Do not bankrupt the hospital searching for a bruise on a patient's heart. Check his ECG and make sure it is pumping.
4. Patients leaking lots of air out of their lungs might have a tear in a major bronchus.
5. Rapid deceleration can result in a tear in the descending thoracic aorta. Despite a normal chest radiograph, patients with this mechanism deserve a CT scan.
6. ED thoracotomy after blunt chest is rarely indicated and carries a dismal outcome.

BIBLIOGRAPHY

1. Allen GS, Coates NE. Pulmonary contusion: a collective review. *Am Surg.* 1996;62(11):895–900.
2. Branney SW, Moore EE. Critical analysis of two decades of experience with postinjury emergency department thoracotomy in a regional trauma center. *J Trauma.* 1998;45(1):87–94.
3. Bulger EM, Arneson MA. Rib fractures in the elderly. *J Trauma.* 2000;48(6):1040–1046.
4. Demetriades D, Velmahos GC, Scalea TM, et al. Operative repair or endovascular stent graft in blunt traumatic thoracic aortic injuries: the AAST multicenter study. *J Trauma.* 2008;64(3):561–570.
5. Dyer DS, Moore EE, Ilke DN, et al. Thoracic aortic injury: how predictive is mechanism and is chest computed tomography a reliable screening tool? A prospective study of 1,561 patients. *J Trauma.* 2000;48(4):673–682.
6. Flagel BT, Luchette FA, Reed L, et al. Half-a-dozen ribs: the breakpoint for mortality. *Surgery.* 2005;138(4):717–723.
7. Gomez-Caro A, Ausin P, Moradiliellos FJ, et al. Role of conservative management of tracheobronchial injuries. *J Trauma.* 2006;61(6):1426–1434.
8. Karmy-Jones R, Jurkovich GJ, Nathens AB, et al. Timing of urgent thoracotomy for hemorrhage after trauma: a multicenter study. *Arch Surg.* 2001;136(5):513–518.
9. Kiser AC, O'Brien SM, Detterbeck FC. 2001 Blunt tracheobronchial injuries: treatment and outcome. *Ann Thorac Surg.* 2001;71(6):2059–2065.
10. Moore EE, Knudson MM, Burlew CC, et al. Defining the limits of resuscitative emergency department thoracotomy: a contemporary Western trauma association prospective. *J Trauma.* 2011;70(2):334–339.
11. Yeong EK, Chen MT. Traumatic asphyxia. *Plast Reconstr Surg.* 1994;93(4):739–744.
12. Mowery NT, Gunter OL, Collier BR, et al. Practice management guidelines for hemothorax and occult pneumothorax. *J Trauma.* 2011;70(2):510–518.

CHAPTER 23

PENETRATING THORACIC TRAUMA

Hunter B. Moore, MD, Ernest E. Moore, MD, FACS

1. **How often do patients with penetrating chest wounds need an operation?**
   Most penetrating injuries seen in civilian practice are from knives and low-energy handguns. Consequently, although injuries to the chest wall and lung are common, the vast majority can be treated with tube thoracostomy alone. Formal thoracotomy or median sternotomy is required in <15% of isolated penetrating chest injuries.

2. **What are the indications for emergency department thoracotomy after penetrating chest wounds?**
   Patients who arrive within 15 minutes of circulatory collapse (or arrest after arrival) can benefit from an emergency department thoracotomy (EDT). Unlike blunt injury, a treatable cause is more commonly found after penetrating injury (e.g., pericardial tamponade). EDT results in a survival of 25% in this setting. If the patient arrests in the emergency department with an isolated stab wound to the chest, survival exceeds 50%.

3. **When should resuscitative endovascular balloon occlusion of the aorta (REBOA) be used in chest trauma?**
   Never. REBOA can only occlude the aorta. EDT can accomplish this task, while also addressing interventions to improve perfusion including (1) relief of cardiac tamponade, (2) internal cardiac massage, (3) direct hemorrhage control of vital structures in the chest, and (4) control of acute air embolism with hilar clamp and selective air aspiration of the heart.

4. **What is the "6-hour rule" for chest injuries?**
   An upright chest radiograph with no evidence of pneumothorax after 6 hours makes a delayed pneumothorax or occult injury to an intrathoracic organ very unlikely. The 6-hour rule identifies patients who can be safely discharged.

5. **How much blood in the pleural space can be reliably detected by chest radiograph?**
   250 mL or more.

6. **If a stable patient with a penetrating chest wound has continued bleeding from a chest tube, when should a thoracotomy be done?**
   A good rule of thumb is that immediate return of over 1500 mL of blood or ongoing bleeding in excess of 250 mL/h for 3 consecutive hours should prompt operation. All unstable patients warrant an immediate operation.

7. **What is a "clam shell" thoracotomy?**
   Bilateral anterolateral thoracotomies with extension across the sternum. This procedure allows rapid access to pleural spaces, pulmonary hila, and the mediastinum.

8. **What is an open pneumothorax?**
   A defect in the chest wall that is open to the pleural space. In penetrating chest injuries, it most often is the result of a close-range shotgun blast.

9. **How is an open pneumothorax treated?**
   The defect in the chest wall should be covered with a dressing that is fixed on only three sides. This temporary fix prevents entry of air into the pleural space while allowing egress of air under pressure. A chest tube is then inserted. Formal repair of the chest wall can wait until more significant injuries are excluded.

10. **Where is "the box," and why is it important?**
    The box describes an area on the anterior chest where a wound should prompt concern about an underlying cardiac injury. Its borders are the midclavicular lines from clavicle to costal margin.

Although the typical patient with a penetrating cardiac injury has a wound in the box, the heart also can be reached from the root of the neck, axilla, and epigastrium.

11. **What is Beck's triad? Is it useful in penetrating chest injuries?**
Beck's triad consists of hypotension, distended neck veins, and muffled heart tones. These signs are difficult to appreciate in the trauma patient (particularly muffled heart sounds in a busy resuscitation room), and are present in a minority of patients with tamponade from penetrating injuries (<40%). The absence of distended neck veins might be expected because most patients have concomitant hypovolemia.

12. **In a stable patient with suspected penetrating cardiac injury, what is the most important initial study?**
After completion of the primary survey (airway, breathing, circulation [ABCs]), bedside ultrasonography should be performed. This rapid, sensitive method for detecting pericardial fluid will identify occult cardiac injury. Although the initial study may be negative with a small effusion, serial examinations detect virtually all cases.

13. **Junior O'Flaherty just got stabbed in the heart. What is he likely to die of?**
Cardiac tamponade. Knife wounds usually make a slitlike opening in the pericardium, which seals off with clot after the heart bleeds into the pericardial sac. Exsanguination is uncommon from stab wounds; tamponade is the most common threat to life.

14. **What is the initial therapeutic maneuver in the patient with a penetrating cardiac wound who is not yet hypotensive?**
Percutaneous pericardial drainage. One of the early effects of tamponade is subendocardial ischemia, which puts the patient at risk for refractory arrhythmias. Immediate decompression of the pericardium ensures safer transport to the operating room for definitive repair. Subxiphoid pericardial window is also an option (and popular on television), but ultrasound-guided decompression is the best choice.

15. **What is the eFAST?**
The extended focused assessment with sonography for trauma. This is an augmentation of the classic FAST exam when a probe is placed on the chest to detect a pneumothorax or hemothorax. The absence of "lung sliding" is indicative of air between the chest wall and lung pleura. This exam is operator dependent, but when performed with an experienced physician can have a sensitivity of >80% and can have a specificity >95%. It is important to make sure that the person conducting the exam does not turn the eFAST into a SLOW diagnostic assessment of the chest. Bilateral chest examination should take less than a minute, and if the operator is floundering, the chest x-ray should be taken without delay. The eFAST does not treat a pneumothorax, and a patient in extremis with high clinical suspicion should receive tube thoracostomy over ultrasonography.

16. **In a penetrating chest wound, how do I tell if the diaphragm is also injured?**
At end expiration, the dome of the diaphragm reaches the level of the nipples. In principle, then, any patient with penetrating injury below the level of the nipples may have an injury to the diaphragm. Computed tomography (CT) scanning is not reliable unless it shows obvious herniation of abdominal viscera into the chest. Diagnostic peritoneal lavage (DPL) is the preferred initial procedure. If the DPL fluid comes out a chest tube, there is a hole in the diaphragm. Absent this finding, the red blood cell count can also be used as a guide. Red blood cell counts <1000/mm^3 are negative. Counts >10,000 are positive; for counts of 1000–10,000, thoracoscopy or laparoscopy is often used to visualize the hemidiaphragm at risk.

17. **Why is it important to detect a small diaphragmatic laceration?**
Abdominal viscera can herniate from the positive-pressure abdominal cavity into the negative-pressure pleural space in a delayed fashion. The morbidity of a strangulated diaphragmatic hernia is not trivial, often because of delay in diagnosis. It is best to identify the hole at the time of the initial injury! However, vigilance for identification of left-sided injuries is much more important than on the right. Because of the bulky liver, most right-sided injuries do not require repair as the risk of abdominal herniation is low.

18. **Junior O'Flaherty was shot all the way through his mediastinum. He seems stable: does he need an operation?**
Probably not. Surprisingly, most wounds that appear to pass completely across the chest do not injure a critical structure. In fact, only about 35% of stable patients require exploration. Junior should be evaluated with history (odynophagia? hoarseness?), physical examination (deep cervical emphysema? expanding hematoma? pulseless extremity?), and CT scan to assess trajectory and evaluate for injury.

If the bullet tract indicates critical structures are at risk, follow-up angiography, bronchoscopy, and esophagoscopy may be necessary.

19. **Are prophylactic antibiotics warranted to prevent empyema after tube thoracostomy?**
Metaanalysis of currently published randomized studies on prophylactic antibiotics for tube thoracostomy suggests a benefit. The number of doses required is unclear; further, the use in patients with blunt multisystem injuries may be questioned because of the risk of emergence of resistance.

20. **What is the most important risk factor for posttraumatic empyema?**
Persistent hemothorax with a tube thoracostomy. Blood is an excellent incubation medium for bacteria; therefore, expedient evacuation of blood from the pleural space via video-assisted thoracoscopic surgery is central in the management of traumatic hemothorax.

21. **What is the indication for video-assisted thoracoscopic surgery in the subacute setting of chest trauma?**
Persistent air leak or hemothorax for greater than 48 hours from injury.

22. **What is a bronchovenous air embolism?**
An air embolism occurs when gas under pressure leaks from a lacerated bronchus into an adjacent lacerated pulmonary vein. Air then travels to the left side of the heart and into the coronary arteries. The classic presentation is a patient with a penetrating chest injury who arrests after intubation and application of positive-pressure ventilation.

23. **How is bronchovenous air embolism diagnosed and treated?**
Diagnosis is based only on the typical history (see question 22). Therapy is directed toward removal of air from the left ventricle and coronary arteries: Trendelenburg (head down) position with right side down, immediate thoracotomy and aspiration of the apex of the left ventricle, the aortic root, and occasionally the coronary arteries.

24. **In a penetrating esophageal injury, where may air be evident on physical examination?**
The deep subcutaneous tissues of the neck. In the upright position, air in the mediastinum dissects into a plane continuous with the deep cervical fascia.

25. **How do penetrating tracheobronchial injuries present?**
Laceration of the trachea and major bronchi presents with subcutaneous emphysema, hemoptysis, and dyspnea. Chest radiographs reveal a pneumothorax or pneumomediastinum. After tube thoracostomy, continuous air leak and failure of the lung to reexpand should prompt suspicion of a major bronchial injury.

26. **What does a blurry bullet on a chest radiograph indicate?**
A bullet lodged in the myocardium. Movement of the heart causes the image to be blurry on the radiograph. Beware the blurry bullet.

KEY POINTS: PENETRATING THORACIC TRAUMA

1. Most patients with a penetrating chest wound do not need an operation. A chest tube is usually the only definitive treatment necessary.
2. If there is not a pneumothorax after 6 hours, the patient is unlikely to have a significant chest injury.
3. If a weapon penetrates the anterior chest in the box, use an ultrasound to look for pericardial blood.
4. Cardiac tamponade is what is likely to kill you after a stab wound to the heart.
5. Diaphragm injuries are important to identify, particularly on the left side.

BIBLIOGRAPHY

1. Moore HB, Moore EE, Burlew CC, et al. Establishing benchmarks for resuscitation of traumatic circulatory arrest: success-to-rescue and survival among 1,708 patients. *J Am Coll Surg.* 2016;223(1):42–50.
2. Ibirogba S, Nicol AJ, Navsaria PH. Screening helical computed tomographic scanning in haemodynamic stable patients with transmediastinal gunshot wounds. *Injury.* 2007;38(1):48–52.

3. Rhee PM, Foy H, Kaufmann C, et al. Penetrating cardiac injuries: a population-based study. *J Trauma.* 1998;45(2):366–370.
4. Cothren C, Moore EE. Lung-sparing techniques are associated with improved outcome compared with anatomic resection for severe lung injuries. *J Trauma.* 2002;53(3):483–487.
5. Stassen NA, Lukan JK, Spain DA, et al. Reevaluation of diagnostic procedures for transmediastinal gunshot wounds. *J Trauma.* 2002;53(4):635–638. discussion 638.
6. Nagy KK, Lohmann C, Kim DO, et al. Role of echocardiography in the diagnosis of occult penetrating cardiac injury. *J Trauma.* 1995;38(6):859–862.
7. Mandal AK, Sanusi M. Penetrating chest wounds: 24 years experience. *World J Surg.* 2001;25(9):1145–1149.
8. Montoya J, Stawicki SP, Evans DC, et al. From FAST to E-FAST: an overview of the evolution of ultrasound-based traumatic injury assessment. *Eur J Trauma Emerg Surg.* 2016;42(2):119–126.
9. Ties JS, Peschman JR, Moreno A, et al. Evolution in the management of traumatic diaphragmatic injuries: a multicenter review. *J Trauma Acute Care Surg.* 2014;76(4):1024–1028.

CHAPTER 24

BLUNT ABDOMINAL TRAUMA

Angela R. LaFace, MD, David J. Ciesla, MD, MS

1. **What are the key components of the history and physical exam when evaluating a patient with blunt abdominal trauma?**
   The tenets of the initial assessment and resuscitation of patients with blunt abdominal trauma remain the same as with all trauma patients. Evaluation is divided into the primary and secondary surveys, with resuscitation, intervention, and reevaluation as needed. The primary survey aims to identify and treat immediately life-threatening conditions and evaluates the airway, breathing, and circulation, with attention to disability/deformity and complete patient exposure. The focused assessment with sonography for trauma (FAST) exam is then performed, followed by the secondary survey, which is a full history and physical examination. A key history element is the injury mechanism (e.g., motor vehicle collision, automobile-pedestrian accident, fall from height) as injury patterns vary with mechanism. In motor vehicle crashes, note the position of the victim in the car, velocity of impact, type of crash (head-on, side impact, rollover), and type of occupant restraint. Information about damage to the vehicle, such as a broken windshield or bent steering wheel, may raise suspicion of cervical or thoracic injuries. Serial vital signs and mental status assessments are critical. Physical exam alone is unreliable for the diagnosis of intraabdominal injury and additional screening and diagnostic measures are often necessary.

2. **How does the evaluation and management of blunt abdominal trauma differ from penetrating abdominal trauma?**
   Minimal diagnostic imaging is typically indicated before laparotomy in penetrating abdominal trauma that violate the peritoneal cavity(especially in gunshot wounds) as up to 90% may have injuries that require operative intervention. In blunt abdominal trauma, however, injury patterns are less predictable, and many stable patients with solid organ injuries may be managed nonoperatively.

3. **Which organs are most frequently injured in blunt abdominal trauma?**

Solid	Hollow	Miscellaneous
Liver 50%	Small bowel 10%	Mesentery 10%
Spleen 40%	Colon 5%	Urologic 10%
Pancreas 10%	Duodenum 5%	Vascular 4%
	Stomach 2%	
	Gallbladder 2%	

4. **What accounts for the difference in abdominal injury patterns in penetrating versus blunt abdominal trauma?**
   The pattern of injury conferred by penetrating trauma is a reflection of the volume an organ takes up within the abdominal cavity. In blunt trauma, the ability of the organ to absorb transferred energy determines its risk for injury. Solid organs have nondistendable capsules that respond to mechanical stress by fracture. Hollow organs are compliant, muscular, and generally absorb energy well. Potential for closed loops puts hollow viscus at risk of rupture (i.e., duodenum, sigmoid colon).

5. **What imaging modalities are useful in blunt abdominal trauma?**
   - **Ultrasound (US):** Reliably identifies peritoncal fluid (blood) >200 cc and pericardial fluid, but may miss up to 25% of isolated solid organ injuries.
   - **X-Ray:** Chest and pelvis films performed as part of the early secondary survey identify rib and pelvic fractures raising suspicion for associated intraabdominal injuries (splenic laceration, bladder injury, etc.). Traumatic diaphragmatic hernia may be identified.

- **Computed tomography (CT) scan:** Identifies the presence and severity of solid organ injury, detects intraabdominal air and fluid, and aids in evaluation of pelvic fractures. CT scanning can also identify retroperitoneal and mesenteric hematomas and vascular injuries. It is least useful in diagnosing hollow organ injuries especially in the absence of oral contrast. Mesenteric injuries that raise the suspicion of associated hollow viscus injuries may often be demonstrated, however. It is an excellent modality, with a 99.97% negative predictive value for blunt abdominal trauma that continues to improve as multidetector technology advances.

6. **How is US used in the evaluation of blunt abdominal trauma?**
The FAST exam, performed during the early secondary survey, has become the initial screening modality for intraabdominal injury. Since blood tends to pool in the peritoneal recesses, Morrison's pouch (hepatorenal), left upper quadrant (splenorenal), and pelvis special attention is given to these areas. Free fluid, noted as a black "stripe" on US, denotes a positive FAST. While the sensitivity for detecting >250 mL of fluid is excellent, the source of the bleeding or severity of injury is not reliably determined. Its most useful application is to identify intraabdominal hemorrhage in unstable patients, especially in the presence of other bleeding sources (i.e., pelvic fracture). A positive FAST is an indication for abdominal exploration in hemodynamically unstable patients and a CT scan in stable patients.

7. **What is diagnostic peritoneal lavage?**
Diagnostic peritoneal lavage (DPL) is a modality for diagnosing intraabdominal injury (bleeding, injury to hollow viscus or hepatobiliary system) in abdominal trauma. An infraumbilical incision is made and a soft catheter is placed into the peritoneal cavity. Aspiration of peritoneal contents is performed with a grossly positive result obtained if >10 mL blood is returned suggesting significant hemoperitoneum. If grossly negative, a liter of normal saline is instilled into the abdomen via the catheter. The effluent is siphoned and sent to the laboratory for evaluation of red blood cell (RBC) and white blood cell (WBC) count, amylase, bilirubin and alkaline phosphatase levels. The DPL is considered positive if RBC >100,000/mL, WBC >500/mL, 19 amylase >IU/L, bilirubin >0.01 mg/dL, or alkaline phosphatase >2 IU/L. Effluent exiting through a chest tube or urinary catheter indicates diaphragmatic or bladder injury. Today, the DPL has largely been replaced by newer, noninvasive imaging measures.

8. **What are the indications for abdominal exploration in blunt abdominal trauma?**
The major consideration for operation is hypotension due to suspected intra-abdominal hemorrhage, physical exam suggesting perforation (peritonitis, pneumoperitoneum), or traumatic abdominal wall or diaphragmatic hernia.

9. **What are the goals of exploratory laparotomy in abdominal trauma?**
The major goals in abdominal exploration for trauma are control of hemorrhage and contamination, restoration of perfusion and gastrointestinal continuity (function), and wound closure. The steps in an operation are (1) incision, (2) rapid assessment and control of bleeding (direct pressure, evacuation of hemoperitoneum with resection or surgical repair as able), (3) systematic exploration to identify all injuries, (4) resection/repair/reconstruction of nonviable tissue, and (5) wound closure.

10. **What is the lethal triad?**
Acidosis, coagulopathy, and hypothermia comprise the lethal triad: a vicious cycle in which progression of each element exacerbates the others. Severely injured and critically ill patients are subject to this pathology with a resultant high risk of mortality. The second stage of the damage control operation (resuscitation) is aimed at halting this cycle.

11. **What is a damage control operation or abbreviated laparotomy?**
True damage control is a strategy where the definitive operation is suspended to restore normal physiology and reverse the lethal triad. The first phase (initial operation) has a limited scope, such that only lifesaving interventions are performed and definitive repairs are delayed. Resuscitation occurs in phase two (rewarming, correction of coagulopathy and acidosis). In phase three, surgical reconstruction and wound closure is performed if possible. Most often, this occurs 24–48 hours after initial operation, but may require multiple procedures. Other indications for abbreviated laparotomy include a planned second look to assess the viability of the viscera and the inability to close the abdomen safely at the index operation due to excessive visceral swelling. While these techniques are often necessary, their use has decreased with contemporary resuscitation strategies.

12. Do all patients with abdominal bleeding require operation for hemorrhage control?

No. Many patients with mild solid organ bleeding will stop spontaneously with resuscitation and correction of coagulopathy. Select patients with moderate abdominal bleeding can be managed with angioembolization of the liver, spleen, or pelvis. Such patients generally have evidence of ongoing hemorrhage (transfusion requirement) but are not in shock or in immediate danger of exsanguination. Angioembolization increases the success of nonoperative management of solid organ injuries.

KEY POINTS: BLUNT ABDOMINAL TRAUMA

1. Physical exam is often unreliable in the diagnosis of blunt abdominal injuries necessitating liberal screening and diagnostic imaging.
2. Abdominal free fluid in the absence of solid organ injury raises special concern for mesenteric and hollow organ injuries.
3. Angioembolization is an effective means of intraabdominal hemorrhage control in select patients.
4. Peritonitis and intraabdominal hemorrhage with refractory shock are strong indications for abdominal exploration.

BIBLIOGRAPHY

1. Cirocchi R, Abraha I. Damage control surgery for abdominal trauma. *Cochrane Database Syst Rev.* 2010;(1):CD007438.
2. Cotton BA, Reddy N, Hatch QM, et al. Damage control resuscitation is associated with a reduction in resuscitation volumes and improvement in survival in 390 damage control laparotomy patients. *Ann Surg.* 2011;254(4):598–605.
3. Higa G, Friese R, O'Keeffe T, et al. Damage control laparotomy: a vital tool once overused. *J Trauma.* 2010;69(1):53–59.
4. Hoff MG, Holevar M, Nagy K, et al. Practice management guidelines for the evaluation of blunt abdominal trauma: the EAST practice management guidelines work group. *J Trauma.* 2002;53(3):602–615.
5. Ochsner MG, Knudson MM, Pachter HL, et al. Significance of minimal or no intraperitoneal fluid visible on CT scan associated with blunt liver and splenic injuries: a multicenter analysis. *J Trauma.* 2000;49(3):505–510.
6. Smith CB, Barrett TW. Prediction of blunt traumatic injury in high acuity patients: bedside examination vs computed tomography. *Am J Emerg Med.* 2011;29(1):1–10.
7. Stengal D, Bauwens K, Sehouli J, et al. Emergency ultrasound based algorithms for diagnosing blunt abdominal trauma. *Cochrane Database Syst Rev.* 2005;(2):CD004446.
8. Capecci LM, Jeremitsky E. Trauma centers with higher rates of angiography have a lesser incidence of splenectomy in the management of blunt splenic injury. *Surgery.* 2015;158(4):1020–1024. discussion 1024–1026.

CHAPTER 25

PENETRATING ABDOMINAL TRAUMA

Aidan D. Hamm, MD, Clay Cothren Burlew, MD, FACS,
Ernest E. Moore, MD, FACS

1. **Why is the evaluation different for patients with stab wounds (SWs) versus gunshot wounds (GSWs)?**
   Although one-third of SWs to the anterior abdomen do not penetrate the peritoneum, 80% of GSWs violate the peritoneum. Additionally, of those wounds that penetrate the peritoneum, 95% of GSWs have associated visceral or vascular injuries, while only one-third of SWs do (Fig. 25.1).

2. **What are the indications for emergent laparotomy in patients with SWs?**
   Hypotension, peritonitis, other signs of abdominal visceral injury (hematemesis, proctorrhagia, palpation of diaphragmatic defect on chest tube insertion, and radiologic evidence of injury to the gastrointestinal [GI] tract) mandate immediate exploration. Most authorities also advocated prompt exploration for omental or intestinal evisceration because of the high risk of visceral injury.

3. **What are the indications for immediate laparotomy in patients with GSWs?**
   Because of the high incidence of visceral injury, early exploration is indicated for virtually all GSWs that violate the peritoneum. The exception is penetrating trauma isolated to the right upper quadrant; in hemodynamically stable patients with bullet trajectory confined to the liver by computed tomography (CT) scan, nonoperative observation may be considered. Similarly, in obese patients, if the GSW is thought to be tangential through the subcutaneous tissues, CT scan can delineate the tract and exclude peritoneal violation. Laparoscopy is another option to assess peritoneal penetration.

4. **When is emergency department (ED) thoracotomy indicated for a penetrating abdominal wound?**
   Resuscitative thoracotomy should be considered when a patient presents in cardiac arrest (cardiopulmonary resuscitation <15 minutes) or with profound hypotension (systolic blood pressure [SBP] <60 mm Hg) that is refractory to initial resuscitation. Although external wounds may point to penetrating abdominal injury, intrathoracic structures may be injured as well. Therefore, following anterolateral thoracotomy, the heart should be assessed for injury; if cardiac tamponade is present, the pericardium is opened vertically in a plane anterior to the phrenic nerve. If an injury is identified, hemorrhage from the injury is controlled. Once the cardiac injury is controlled, or if no injury is identified, the descending aorta is cross-clamped to decrease subdiaphragmatic hemorrhage and improve coronary and cerebral perfusion. Open cardiac massage is performed if necessary. If these measures restore circulatory perfusion to a SBP >70 mm Hg, the patient is transferred to the operating room for definitive repair.

5. **What are the key elements of the secondary survey?**
   Examine the patient systematically; it is easy to overlook synchronous injuries. The examination includes looking for additional sites of penetrating wounds; be sure to look thoroughly in the axilla and perineum as wounds can be hidden in folds of skin. Evaluation for blood in the GI, genitourinary, and gynecologic systems should be done, and associated blunt mechanisms of injury should be considered; some patients are assaulted with both knives and fists (Fig. 25.2). A neurologic exam is important to document any deficits prior to operative intervention as well as to determine the etiology.

6. **What are the appropriate initial studies?**
   A chest radiograph ensures that the bullet did not traverse the diaphragm causing a hemothorax or pneumothorax; the chest film also determines the position of any new tubes or lines (e.g., central venous catheters endotracheal tubes, nasogastric tubes, and thoracostomy tubes). Biplanar abdominal radiographs are helpful in locating retained foreign bodies (i.e., bullets) and may reveal

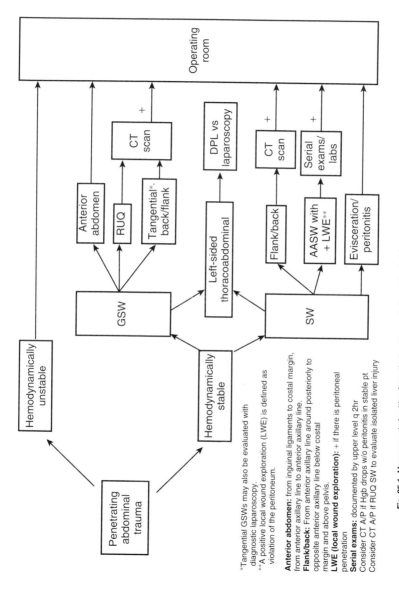

*Tangential GSWs may also be evaluated with diagnostic laparoscopy.
**A positive local wound exploration (LWE) is defined as violation of the peritoneum.

Anterior abdomen: from inguinal ligaments to costal margin, from anterior axillary line to anterior axillary line.
Flank/back: From anterior axillary line around posteriorly to opposite anterior axillary line below costal margin and above pelvis.
LWE (local wound exploration): + if there is peritoneal penetration
Serial exams: documented by upper level q 2hr
Consider CT A/P if Hgb drops w/o peritonitis in stable pt
Consider CT A/P if RUQ SW to evaluate isolated liver injury

Fig. 25.1 Management algorithm for patients with penetrating abdominal trauma.

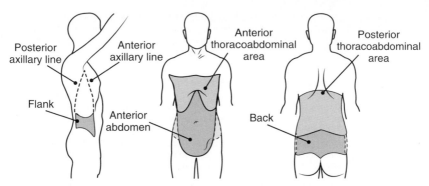

Fig. 25.2 An example of how the path of a bullet through a contorted body can produce confusion when the patient is examined in the ED. An entrance wound will be found at the left upper arm and an exit wound at the medial aspect of the right knee. The bullet could have damaged any structure between these two wounds when the patient's body was contorted. *(From Legome E, Shockley LW, eds.* Trauma: a comprehensive emergency medicine approach. *Cambridge: Cambridge University Press; 2011:215.)*

pneumoperitoneum. In penetrating abdominal trauma from GSWs, it is important to obtain a plain radiograph of the abdomen plus films one space above and below the site of injury; this helps locate retained missiles and gain information regarding the trajectory of the bullet. A general idea of trajectory is helpful to direct abdominal exploration at the time of laparotomy. For example, a single wound at the umbilicus with an abdominal film demonstrating a bullet in the pelvis would heighten one's concern for an iliac or rectal injury versus identifying a bullet in the right upper quadrant. Determining trajectory utilizing plain films to identify retained bullets is especially important when only one wound is evident. Radiopaque markers applied to the skin at the site of evident wounds are also helpful in determining the trajectory of missiles. Injuries in proximity to the rectum obligate sigmoidoscopy (see Chapter 29), and those with proximity to the urinary tract should be evaluated with CT scanning (see Chapters 31 and 32).

Focused abdominal sonography for trauma (FAST) exams are performed to assess for hemoperitoneum and may be an adjunct in the initial evaluation of the patient sustaining penetrating trauma. FAST includes examining four locations: the right supra-renal recess (Morrison's pouch), the pelvis around the bladder, the splenorenal fossa, and the pericardium. The extended FAST (eFAST) includes examining the pleura for normal lung slide, which if absent indicates a pneumothorax. All of this imaging is performed in the ED resuscitation bay. Only hemodynamically stable patients should undergo CT scanning. Of note, FAST may be unreliable in anterior abdominal SWs. FAST may not reveal fluid if less 250 cc is not present. Initial labs should include a spun hemoglobin, complete blood count, basic metabolic panel, lactate, arterial blood gases, and coagulation studies (ideally thromboelastography or rotational thromboelastography). These studies guide transfusion and resuscitation.

7. **What is the difference between a penetrating wound to the anterior abdomen versus the flank or back?**
   Because the incidence of injury is higher for anterior wounds, and injuries are within the peritoneal cavity, diagnostic evaluation differs.

8. **How is an anterior abdominal SW evaluated in asymptomatic patients?**
   The first step in asymptomatic patients is local exploration of the wound to determine peritoneal penetration. If the tract clearly terminates superficially, above the fascia, no further evaluation is required and the patient is discharged from the ED. If the fascia is penetrated or the peritoneum violated, further evaluation is warranted with serial examinations and labs over 24-hour observation as up to 50% may require laparotomy. The majority of patients with visceral injury will manifest signs or symptoms of their injury (fever, tachycardia, increasing abdominal tenderness, peritoneal signs, or increasing white blood cell count) within 8–12 hours. The optimal diagnostic approach remains debated in hemodynamically stable patients with thoracoabdominal SWs, defined as adjacent to the

costal margin. Options for evaluation include diagnostic peritoneal lavage (DPL) or diagnostic laparoscopy. Diagnostic laparoscopy is preferred if there are findings suggestive of diaphragmatic violation such as a hemothorax or pneumothorax, particularly on the left side, which has a much higher risk of delayed diaphragmatic visceral herniation. DPL may be technically challenging in combative as well as obese patients.

9. **How is a local wound exploration (LWE) performed?**
   This is performed in the ED. Local anesthesia is infiltrated around the wound and the wound is explored under direct vision to follow the tract through the tissue layers. The skin incision can be extended if needed for exposure. Handheld retractors facilitate visual inspection of the fascia to determine if there is violation.
   Penetration of the posterior fascia is considered a positive LWE. Penetration of the peritoneum is difficult to identify. Penetration of the anterior fascia with identification of the posterior fascia is considered an equivocal study and mandates observation.

10. **What constitutes a positive diagnostic peritoneal lavage result after penetrating trauma?**
    A grossly positive tap (aspiration of >10 mL of blood or aspiration of GI or biliary contents) mandates immediate exploration. A negative initial aspirate result is followed by the instillation of 1000 mL of saline (15 mL/kg in children) into the abdomen through a dialysis catheter, followed by gravity drainage of the fluid back into the saline bag. The finding of >100,000/μL red blood cells (RBCs), >500 μL WBCs, amylase >20 IU/L, alkaline phosphatase >3 IU/L, or elevated bilirubin level are considered positive and thus are indications for operation.

11. **Is a positive diagnostic peritoneal lavage result after penetrating thoracoabdominal SW different than after an abdominal SW?**
    The role of a DPL is to identify hollow viscus injury (stomach, small bowel, colon) or a diaphragm injury. To identify all patients with a diaphragm injury following a thoracoabdominal SW, a lower cutoff for RBCs is used on the DPL count. A RBC count >10,000/μL is considered positive, and an indication for laparotomy; patients with a DPL RBC count between 1000/μL and 10,000/μL should undergo laparoscopy or thoracoscopy.

12. **How are SWs to the flank and back evaluated in asymptomatic patients?**
    The incidence of significant injuries is 10% for SWs to the back and 25% for SWs to the flank. SWs to the flank and back should undergo multislice CT to detect occult retroperitoneal injuries of the colon, duodenum, and urinary tract. The most valuable aspect of CT scanning is determining the wound trajectory. Evidence or concern of injury to the these structures may include intra or extraperitoneal fluid and air, wound track extending through the peritoneum, bowel wall defect, bowel wall thickening, extravasation of contrast (enteric, vesicular, or vascular), or a diaphragmatic injury.

13. **How is a lower chest SW evaluated?**
    SWs to the lower chest are associated with abdominal visceral injury in 15% of cases, whereas GSWs to the lower chest are associated with abdominal visceral injury in nearly 50% of cases. The lower chest is defined as the area between the nipple line (fourth intercostal space) anteriorly, the tip of the scapula (seventh intercostal space) posteriorly, and the costal margins inferiorly. Because the diaphragm reaches the fourth intercostal space during expiration, the abdominal organs are at risk of injury even after what appears to be an "isolated chest" wound. Thus, wounds to the lower chest should also be managed as thoracoabdominal wounds to rule out intraabdominal and diaphragmatic injury (see Chapter 23).

14. **Which patients with abdominal GSWs are candidates for nonoperative management?**
    Hemodynamically stable patients with tangential, subcutaneous missile tracts or those with isolated hepatic trauma (see Chapter 26). Selective management of GSWs to the back and flank are based on triple-contrast CT scan results.

15. **If abdominal operative exploration is indicated, what is the general approach?**
    A midline laparotomy provides rapid entry and wide exposure; it may be extended as a median sternotomy to access the chest. The aorta should be palpated just below the diaphragm to assess the patient's blood pressure. Liquid and clotted blood is evacuated with multiple laparotomy pads and suction to identify the major source(s) of active bleeding. After localizing the source of hemorrhage,

direct digital occlusion (vascular injury) or laparotomy pad packing (solid organ injury) are used to control bleeding. Hollow visceral injuries are temporarily isolated with noncrushing clamps, are rapidly oversewn, or segmentally excised using a GIA stapler. The entire abdomen is systematically explored before undertaking extensive repairs so that injuries can be prioritized for definitive treatment.

16. **How is the retroperitoneum anatomically divided?**
    The retroperitoneum is divided into three zones that correlate with the underlying structures and likelihood of injury to those structures. Management of trauma to the retroperitoneum differs based upon mechanism of injury and zone of injury.
    - Zone I: Midline retroperitoneal hematoma from diaphragmatic hiatus to distal to the aortic and IVC bifurcation. Concern for major vascular injury to the great vessels. These are always explored in penetrating trauma, usually via a left or right medial visceral rotation for supracolic injuries, and isolation of pelvic vasculature for distal IVC, aorta, or proximal iliac injuries.
    - Zone II: Lateral retroperitoneal hematoma. Concern for injury to the renal hilum and vessels or renal pelvis. In penetrating trauma, these are generally explored unless very small, nonpulsatile, and not expanding.
    - Zone III: Pelvic retroperitoneal hematoma. In penetrating injuries, this should be explored to rule out injury to major pelvic vessels.

KEY POINTS: PENETRATING ABDOMINAL TRAUMA

1. GSWs to the abdomen generally require operative exploration; an exception is the right upper quadrant wounds with isolated hepatic injury.
2. Following a SW, patients with hypotension, peritonitis, or evisceration should undergo operative exploration.
3. Anterior abdominal SWs in stable patients are initially evaluated with local wound exploration; penetration of the peritoneum requires further evaluation with serial examinations and labs.
4. Flank and back SWs in stable patients are evaluated with contrast CT scan.

CONTROVERSIES

17. **What is the role of laparoscopy and thoracoscopy after penetrating abdominal trauma?**
    Although an intriguing diagnostic modality with additional therapeutic capabilities, laparoscopy thus far has had limited application in the United States. With the exception of suspected diaphragmatic injury, an isolated solid organ injury, or evaluation for peritoneal penetration, laparoscopy has yet to demonstrate advantages over the algorithm delineated previously. The potential for missed injuries and poor evaluation of the retroperitoneum are major concerns. Therapeutic laparoscopy, however, has been used extensively in Latin American and some European countries.

18. **Nonoperative management of GSWs penetrating the peritoneum**
    Although most trauma centers in the United States follow the guidelines outlined above, there are several major trauma centers (e.g., LA County), that manage patients nonoperatively based on CT scanning.

BIBLIOGRAPHY

1. Biffl WL, Kaups KL, Cothren CC, et al. Management of patients with anterior abdominal stab wounds: a Western Trauma Association multicenter trial. *J Trauma*. 2009;66(5):1294–1301.
2. Boyle Jr EM, Maier RV, Salazar JD, et al. Diagnosis of injuries after stab wounds to the back and flank. *J Trauma*. 1997;42(2):260–265.
3. Chiu WC, Shanmuganathan K. Determining the need for laparotomy in penetrating torso trauma: a prospective study using triple-contrast enhanced abdominopelvic computed tomography. *J Trauma*. 2001;51(5):860–868.
4. Demetriades D, Hadjizacharia P, Constantinou C, et al. Selective nonoperative management of penetrating abdominal solid organ injuries. *Ann Surg*. 2006;244(4):620–628.
5. Freeman RK, Al-Dossari G, Hutcheson KA, et al. Indications for using video-assisted thoracoscopic surgery to diagnose diaphragmatic injuries after penetrating chest trauma. *Ann Thorac Surg*. 2001;72(2):342–347.
6. Henneman PL, Marx JA. Diagnostic peritoneal lavage: accuracy in predicting necessary laparotomy following blunt and penetrating trauma. *J Trauma*. 1990;30(11):1345–1355.

7. McAnena OJ, Marx JA. Peritoneal lavage enzyme determinations following blunt and penetrating abdominal trauma. *J Trauma*. 1991;31(8):1161–1164.
8. Moore EE, Marx JA. Penetrating abdominal wounds: a rationale for exploratory laparotomy. *JAMA*. 1985;253(18):2705–2708.
9. Reber PU, Schmied B. Missed diaphragmatic injuries and their long-term sequelae. *J Trauma*. 1998;44(1):183–188.
10. Simon RJ, Rabin J. Impact of increased use of laparoscopy on negative laparotomy rates after penetrating trauma. *J Trauma*. 2002;53(2):297–302.
11. Berg RJ, Karamanos E. The persistent diagnostic challenge of thoracoabdominal stab wounds. *J Trauma Acute Care Surg*. 2014;76(2):418–423.

HEPATIC AND BILIARY TRAUMA

Hunter B. Moore, MD, Trevor L. Nydam, MD,
Ernest E. Moore, MD, FACS

CHAPTER 26

1. **How often is the liver injured in trauma?**
   The liver is both large and central, so it is vulnerable to blunt trauma and an easy target for penetrating wounds. It is the most frequently injured intraabdominal organ in trauma.

2. **What are the determinants of mortality after acute liver injury?**
   The mechanism of injury, grade of injury, and the associated abdominal organs injured determine mortality. The mortality for stab wounds to the liver is 2%; for gunshot wounds, 8%; and for blunt injuries, 15%. The mortality rate for isolated grade III hepatic injuries is 2%; for grade IV, 20%; and for grade V, 65%. Retrohepatic vena cava injuries carry mortality rates of 80% for penetrating trauma and 95% for blunt trauma.

3. **What history and physical signs suggest acute liver injury?**
   Any patient sustaining blunt abdominal trauma (BAT) with hypotension must be assumed to have a liver injury until proven otherwise. Specific signs that increase the likelihood of hepatic injury are contusion over the right lower chest, fracture of the right lower ribs (especially posterior fractures of ribs 9–12), and penetrating injuries to the right lower chest (below the fourth intercostal space, flank, and upper abdomen). Physical signs of hemoperitoneum may be absent in as many as one-third of patients with significant hepatic injury.

4. **What diagnostic tests are helpful in confirming acute liver injury?**
   Diagnostic peritoneal lavage is sensitive for hemoperitoneum (99%), but not specific for liver injury. Ultrasound (US) is highly sensitive in identifying >200 mL of intraperitoneal fluid. It is noninvasive and may be repeated at frequent intervals, but it is relatively poor for staging liver injuries. Contrast-enhanced US is in development at the moment. Abdominal computed tomography (CT) scan is used in patients who are hemodynamically stable who are candidates for nonoperative management. Grading of liver injuries by CT scan is useful in determining the success rate of nonoperative management because higher-grade injuries are more likely to require intervention.

5. **What is the role of hepatic angiography?**
   Selective hepatic artery embolization is effective therapy for hepatic arterial bleeding, both for avoidance of surgery and for recurrent postoperative bleeding. Embolization should be considered for patients with active contrast extravasation into the peritoneum seen on CT scan because they are less likely to tamponade.

SURGICAL ANATOMY OF THE LIVER

6. **How many anatomic lobes are present in the liver? What is their topographic boundary?**
   The Brisbane nomenclature has been developed to standardize the way liver anatomy is defined, based on three orders of divisions. The first order of division is the right and left hemiliver. The boundary between the hemilivers lies in an oblique plane extending from the gallbladder fossa anteriorly to the inferior vena cava (IVC) posteriorly. The next order of division is based on the watershed areas between the hepatic artery and bile duct branches. While there are no visible landmarks to identify the right segments of the liver, the left hemiliver is divided into two segments via the umbilical fissure. These sections are further divided into segments that have no distinct topical anatomic markers aside from segment one (caudate segment), which is wrapped around the vena cava. These segments are numbered I–VIII, based on the portal vein.

7. **What is the blood supply to the liver and the relative contribution of each structure to hepatic oxygenation?**
The hepatic artery supplies approximately 30% of the blood flow to the liver and 50% of its oxygen supply. The portal vein provides 70% of the liver's blood flow and 50% of its oxygen. The relative significance of arterial flow in cirrhotic patients is greater; therefore, hepatic artery ligation is not recommended in patients with cirrhosis.

8. **What are the most common variations in hepatic arterial supply to the right and left lobes of the liver?**
In most people, the common hepatic artery originates from the celiac axis and divides into right and left hepatic arterial branches within the porta hepatis. Approximately 15% of people have a replaced right hepatic artery (sole arterial supply to the right lobe) that originates from the superior mesenteric artery (SMA). A replaced right hepatic artery always supplies a cystic artery; thus, ligation should be followed by cholecystectomy. A replaced left hepatic artery (approximately 15% of people) arises from the left gastric artery; it may be the sole blood supply to the left lobe or may contribute to blood supply in conjunction with a normal left hepatic artery. In 5% of people, the hepatic arterial supply does not arise from the celiac axis. In these people, either the right and left hepatic arteries are replaced or a single main hepatic trunk derives from the SMA.

9. **What is the venous drainage of the liver?**
The right, middle, and left hepatic veins are the major venous tributaries and enter the IVC below the right hemidiaphragm.

OPERATIVE MANAGEMENT OF LIVER INJURY

10. **How are acute liver injuries classified?**
Liver wounds are generally graded on a scale of I–VI according the depth of parenchymal laceration and involvement of the hepatic veins or retrohepatic portion of the IVC. Optimal methods of obtaining hemostasis vary with the severity of the injury (see Table 26.1).

Table 26.1 Liver Injury Scale

		Description of Injury		
GRADE	SUBCAPSULAR HEMATOMA	LACERATION	PARENCHYMAL HEMATOMA	VASCULAR
I	<10% surface area	<1 cm deep	—	—
II	10%–50% surface area	1–3 cm deep	≤10 cm long	—
III	>50% surface area	>3 cm deep	>10 cm long	—
IV	—	25%–75% of lobe or 1–3 Couinaud segments	—	—
V	—	>75% of the lobe or >3 Couinaud segments	—	Retrohepatic inferior vena cava or major hepatic veins

Data from Moore EE, Cogbill TH. Organ injury scaling: spleen and liver (1994 revision), *J Trauma.* 1995;38(3):323–324.

11. **Do all patients with a traumatic liver injury require surgery?**
No. Nonoperative treatment is the standard for victims of blunt trauma who remain hemodynamically stable. One-third of such patients require blood transfusions, but if the volume exceeds 6 units in the first 24 hours, angiography should be done. Complications, including perihepatic infection, biloma, bilhemia, and hemobilia, have been reported in 10% of nonoperative patients.

12. **Which patients are more likely to fail nonoperative management?**
    Although not all studies consistently agree on the following parameters, several large retrospective studies suggest a low systolic blood pressure at admission, number of blood transfusions, peritoneal signs, high injury severity score, and evidence of other intraabdominal injury are risk factors for failure of Nonoperative management (NOM) of blunt hepatic trauma. There is no single predictor for which patients will eventually fail NOM, which in a recent analysis suggested around 10%. Therefore, any patients with a liver injury greater than grade II should be observed closely in the intensive care unit.

13. **Do all penetrating liver injuries require the operating room?**
    No, penetrating anterior abdominal injuries to the right upper quadrant are one of the exceptions to the classic thought that all penetrating trauma to the abdomen requires an operation. Patients who are hemodynamically stable and have no signs of peritonitis can be successfully managed nonoperatively when CT imaging is suggestive of an isolated liver injury. The success rate is not as high as blunt trauma, but, overall, penetrating abdominal liver trauma nonoperative management is successful in the majority of patients.

14. **What are the options for temporary control of significant hemorrhage in victims of hepatic trauma?**
    Ongoing hemorrhage leads to the vicious cycle of acidosis, hypothermia, and coagulopathy. Manual compression, perihepatic packing, angioembolization, and the Pringle maneuver are the effective temporary strategies.

15. **What is the Pringle maneuver?**
    The Pringle maneuver is a manual or vascular clamp occlusion of the hepatoduodenal ligament to interrupt blood flow into the liver. Included in the hepatoduodenal ligament are the hepatic artery, portal vein, and common bile duct. Failure of the Pringle maneuver to control liver hemorrhage suggests either (1) injury to the retrohepatic vena cava or hepatic vein, or (2) arterial supply from an aberrant right or left hepatic artery (see question 9).

16. **What is the finger fracture technique?**
    Finger fracture hepatotomy or tractotomy is the method of exposing bleeding points deep within liver lacerations by blunt dissection. Separating the liver parenchyma enables bleeding points to be identified and ligated.

17. **What is the role of selective hepatic artery ligation in securing hemostasis in patients with a major liver injury?**
    Deep lacerations of the right or left hepatic lobe may result in bleeding that cannot be completely controlled by suture ligation of specific bleeding points within the liver parenchyma. In this situation, either the right or left artery can be ligated for control of the bleeding with little risk of ischemic liver necrosis.

18. **Why is retrohepatic vena caval laceration lethal?**
    Exposure requires either extensive hepatotomy, extensive mobilization of the right lobe, right lobectomy, or transection of the vena cava. The large caliber and high flow of the IVC results in massive hemorrhage during surgical exposure, whereas clamping of the IVC often results in hypotension attributable to an abrupt decrease in venous return to the heart.

19. **What is the physiologic rationale for use of a shunt in attempted repair of retrohepatic vena caval injuries?**
    Hemorrhage control requires maintenance of venous return to the heart while both antegrade and retrograde bleeding through the laceration is stopped. These requirements are met by shunting blood through a tube spanning the laceration between the right atrium and lower IVC.

20. **What is the intrahepatic balloon tamponading device?**
    For transhepatic penetrating injuries, a 1-inch Penrose drain is sutured around a red rubber catheter. This forms a long balloon that is threaded through the bleeding liver injury and inflated with contrast media through a stopcock in the red rubber catheter. The balloon tamponades liver hemorrhage. The catheter is brought out through the abdominal wall, deflated, and removed 24–48 hours later.

21. **What are the indications for perihepatic packing?**
    Liver packing with planned reoperation for definitive treatment of injuries in patients who have hypothermia, acidosis, and coagulopathies is a life-saving maneuver (damage control laparotomy). Laparotomy pads (>10) are packed around the liver to compress and control hemorrhage. A temporary dressing is then placed over the open abdomen (damage control laparotomy), and the patient's metabolic abnormalities and coagulopathy are corrected with planned reoperation within 24 hours.

22. **What is the abdominal compartment syndrome?**

    The abdominal compartment syndrome is a potentially lethal complication of perihepatic packing or large volume resuscitation. It may occur when intraabdominal pressure exceeds 20 cm H_2O. Intraabdominal pressure increases because of bowel and liver edema secondary to ischemia and reperfusion injury or continued hemorrhage into the abdominal cavity. As pressure increases beyond 20 cm H_2O, venous return, cardiac output, and urine output decrease, but ventilatory pressures increase. Patients must return promptly to the operating room for decompression of the abdomen. A manometer attached to the Foley catheter is useful in following intraabdominal pressure.

23. **What are the common complications related to liver injury?**

    After blunt injury to the liver, overall, 13% develop hepatic complications. Complications include bleeding, biliary leaks or fistulae, abdominal compartment syndrome, and infection. Complications occur more frequently in higher grades of injury: 5% in grade III, 22% in grade IV, and 52% in grade V.

BILIARY TRACT INJURY

24. **Why are complications associated with bile duct leaks?**

    Bilomas (i.e., collections of bile) frequently become infected and may result in lethal peritonitis. Biliopleural fistula, a communication between the biliary system and pleural cavity, persists because of the relative negative pressure in the thorax and may result in a bile empyema. Bilhemia results from an intrahepatic fistula between the bile ducts and hepatic veins, resulting in severely elevated bilirubinemia. Hemobilia occurs from the rupture of an arterial pseudoaneurysm into the biliary system, resulting in upper gastrointestinal hemorrhage.

25. **What is the incidence of bile duct leak?**

    For patients managed nonoperatively, the leak rate is 3%, and they are rarely seen for grade I, II, or III injuries. Leak rates are higher for those who undergo operations or angioembolization. Perihepatic fluid collections identified by US suggest a leak; however, they are more accurately identified by hepatobiliary iminodiacetic acid scan or endoscopic retrograde cholangiopancreatography (ERCP).

26. **What is the initial management of a bile leak?**

    ERCP is usually quite useful in diagnosing and treating leaks. Biliary stenting with or without sphincterotomy and percutaneous drainage of bilomas frequently allows spontaneous resolution of bile duct injuries. Extensive injuries require hepaticojejunostomy or reconstruction.

KEY POINTS: HEPATOBILIARY TRAUMA

1. Liver injuries are common following BAT and should be considered in all patients who are hypotensive.
2. Ninety percent of patients with blunt liver injuries can be treated nonoperatively. Angioembolization is an important adjunct.
3. Penetrating liver injuries can also be managed nonoperatively in the setting of hemodynamic stability and lack of peritonitis.
4. Damage control laparotomy should be considered for severe hepatic injuries.
5. The hepatic artery delivers 30% of blood flow, and the portal vein delivers 70% of blood flow.
6. Biliary injuries can occur with severe hepatic injury, but most are treated by minimally invasive techniques.

WEBSITE

www.facs.org

BIBLIOGRAPHY

1. Croce MA, Fabian TC, Menke PG, et al. Nonoperative management of blunt hepatic trauma is the treatment of choice for hemodynamically stable patients. *Ann Surg.* 1995;221(6):744–753.
2. Hiatt JR, Gabbay J. Surgical anatomy of the hepatic arteries in 1000 cases. *Ann Surg.* 1994;220(1):50–52.
3. Hurtuk M, Reed RL. Trauma surgeons practice what they preach: the NTDB story on solid organ injury management. *J Trauma.* 2006;61(2):243–255.
4. Strasberg S. Nomenclature of hepatic anatomy and resections: a review of the Brisbane 2000 system. *J Hepatobiliary Pancreat Surg.* 2005;12(5):351–355.
5. Meredith JW, Young JR. Nonoperative management of adult blunt hepatic trauma: the exception or the rule. *J Trauma.* 1994;36(4):529–534.
6. Moore EE. Staged laparotomy for the hypothermia, acidosis, and coagulopathy syndrome. *Am J Surg.* 1996;172(5):405–410.
7. Moore EE, Cogbill TH, Malangoni MA, et al. Organ injury scaling. *Surg Clin North Am.* 1995;75(2):293–303.
8. Boese CK, Hackl M. Nonoperative management of blunt hepatic trauma: a systematic review. *J Trauma Acute Care Surg.* 2015;79(4):654–660.
9. Demetriades D, Hadjizacharia P, Constantinou C, et al. Selective nonoperative management of penetrating abdominal solid organ injuries. *Ann Surg.* 2006;244(4):620–628.
10. Poggetti RS, Moore EE. Balloon tamponade for bilobar transfixing hepatic gunshot wounds. *J Trauma.* 1992;33(5):694–697.
11. Tai NR, Boffard KD. A 10-year experience of complex liver trauma. *Br J Surg.* 2002;89(12):1532–1537.
12. Velmahos GC, Toutouzas K, Radin F, et al. High success with nonoperative management of blunt hepatic trauma: the liver is a sturdy organ. *Arch Surg.* 2003;138(5):475–481.
13. Verous M, Cillo U, Brolese A, et al. Blunt liver injury: from non-operative management to liver transplantation. *Injury.* 2003;34(3):181–186.
14. Wahl WL, Brandt MM. Diagnosis and management of bile leaks after blunt liver injury. *Surgery.* 2005;138(4):742–748.

CHAPTER 27

SPLENIC TRAUMA

Chadrick R. Evans, MD, Eric M. Campion, MD, Ernest E. Moore, MD, FACS

1. **What is the physiologic role of the spleen?**
   In fetal development, the spleen serves as a major site of hematopoiesis. Later in life the spleen produces immunoglobulin M (IgM), properdin, and tuftsin, important factors in immunologic function. The spleen also acts as a filter, allowing resident macrophages to remove abnormal red blood cells, cellular debris, and encapsulated and poorly opsonized bacteria.

2. **What injury patterns are associated with splenic trauma?**
   Mechanisms associated with splenic injury include direct blunt force, deceleration, and compression to the left torso. Splenic injuries should be considered after any significant motor vehicle accident or fall—lower rib fractures, left-side-only rib fractures, and high-energy transfer increase the probability of splenic injury.

3. **What are the signs and symptoms of splenic injury?**
   The most common sign is pain in the left upper quadrant produced by stretching of the splenic capsule. Peritoneal irritation (rebound tenderness) is caused by extravasated blood. Vital signs vary depending on the associated blood loss and are not specific for injuries to the spleen. On the other hand, patients with a significant splenic injury may exhibit no signs or symptoms at all.

4. **What is Kehr's sign?**
   Kehr's sign is pain from blood irritation of the left diaphragm that is referred to the posterior left shoulder. A common scenario is to have a shoulder radiograph performed after a fall when the pain is actually from a ruptured spleen.

5. **What studies can help in the diagnosis of splenic trauma?**
   Focused assessment with sonography for trauma (FAST) is routinely performed in the emergency department and can rapidly identify as little as 200 mL of fluid or blood, although this finding is nonspecific for splenic injury. When FAST is equivocal, diagnostic peritoneal lavage is an accurate and sensitive measure of intraabdominal bleeding but is also nonspecific. Computed tomography (CT) scanning is the gold standard diagnostic test because of its ability to identify splenic injuries with a high sensitivity, define the magnitude of injury, and identify concomitant injuries.

6. **How are splenic injuries classified, and why is that important?**
   Splenic injuries are classified based on the American Association for the Surgery of Trauma splenic injury scale (Table 27.1). Operative versus nonoperative management (NOM) is governed by the hemodynamic status of the patient and concomitant injures. NOM is influenced by the CT grade of splenic injury. NOM is usually successful in grades I–III, whereas further intervention including splenic angioembolization (SAE) is often recommended for grade IV–V injuries because of their high rate of failure of nonoperative management (FNOM).

7. **Do splenic injuries require laparotomy?**
   Hemodynamically unstable patients should undergo operative management of splenic injuries. However, in hemodynamically stable patients, NOM should be considered in approximately 75%–85% of all blunt splenic injuries in adults, with an overall success rate >90%. The overall NOM success in children <6 years old is >95%. SAE has increased the rate of successful NOM and should be considered in high-risk patients, including grade IV–V injuries as well as all splenic injuries with contrast extravasation on CT scan.

8. **What are the contraindications to NOM of splenic injury?**
   - Hemodynamic instability
   - Peritonitis
   - Abdominal injury requiring operative intervention
   - Lack of facility capabilities; for example, ready availability of operating room, monitored bed, and blood products

Table 27.1 Grades of Splenic Injury

GRADE	DESCRIPTION
I	Hematoma: Nonexpanding subcapsular <10% surface area Laceration: Nonbleeding capsular <1 cm parenchymal depth
II	Hematoma: Nonexpanding, subcapsular <50% surface area, Nonexpanding intraparenchymal <5 cm diameter Laceration: Bleeding, capsular <3 cm parenchymal depth
III	Hematoma: Subcapsular >50% surface area, expanding, ruptured with active bleeding, Intraparenchymal >5 cm diameter or expanding Laceration: Capsular >3 cm parenchymal depth, involving trabecular vessel
IV	Hematoma: Ruptured, intraparenchymal, with active bleeding Laceration: Involves segmental or hilar vessels with >25% splenic devascularization
V	Laceration: Shattered spleen Vascular: Hilar avulsion or complete splenic devascularization

9. **What are the benefits of NOM of splenic injury?**
   NOM has been associated with preserved splenic function, avoidance of nontherapeutic laparotomies and their associated intraabdominal complications, reduced transfusion rates, decreased length of stay, and lower hospital costs.

10. **What defines FNOM, and how often does it occur?**
    No standard definition for FNOM exists. Hemodynamic instability, persistent bleeding/continued need for blood products, and peritonitis should be considered FNOMs. FNOM occurs in less than 10% of cases.

11. **What are indications for SAE?**
    Current data suggests severe splenic injuries (grade IV–V) and any splenic injury with contrast extravasation or pseudoaneurysm benefits from angioembolization because of the high risk of FNOM. FNOM ranges from 26% to 60% in these high-risk patients, but can be reduced to <10% with the addition of SAE.

12. **What are the complications of SAE?**
    The SAE complication rate ranges from approximately 3% to 10%. Complications include splenic infarction, splenic abscess, visceral vessel injury, complications related to vascular access, and contrast induced nephropathy.

13. **How long should patients remain on bedrest during NOM of splenic injuries?**
    No consensus exists on the optimal timing of mobilization. However, current data suggest early mobilization is not associated with an increased incidence of delayed splenic rupture.

14. **When should patients managed nonoperatively receive venous thromboembolism prophylaxis?**
    Optimal timing of venous thromboembolism (VTE) prophylaxis remains controversial. Recent data suggest early initiation of VTE prophylaxis (<48 hours after injury) does not increase the rate of FNOM or blood transfusion needs. Up to a fourfold increase in VTE events have been noted in patients who do not receive VTE prophylaxis until after 72 hours postinjury.

15. **What is delayed rupture of the spleen?**
    This is an uncommon event, but delayed splenic rupture should be distinguished from a delayed diagnosis of splenic injury. True delayed splenic rupture occurs >48 hours in a patient with a history of abdominal trauma and no overt clinical evidence of intraabdominal injury on initial presentation.

16. **Should a follow-up CT scan be performed, and when can patients managed nonoperatively return to full activity?**
    Routine follow-up imaging in splenic injuries undergoing NOM is controversial. FNOM occurs by 72 hours in 85%–95% of FNOM cases and are often recognized without the need for repeat imaging. Consideration for postdischarge repeat imaging should be given to patients desiring significant physical activity, such as contact sports. Timing of return to activity also remains a debated topic. Eighty

percent of grade I–II injuries heal by 50 days, whereas 80% of grade III–V injuries heal by 75 days. Some advocate restricting activity until CT documented healing for grade II–V injuries. Many trauma surgeons advocate activity restrictions of 4–8 weeks for grade I–II injuries and at least 8 weeks or until image documented healing for grade III–V injuries.

17. **What are the general principles of operative management of the injured spleen?**
The first priority is to control bleeding. When there is complete disruption of the spleen, a vascular clamp should be applied to the hilum. In most cases, bleeding can be temporarily controlled by gauze packing and manual compression of the spleen. If successful, the abdomen is then thoroughly explored for other injuries. Mobilization of the spleen to the midline by division of the splenocolic, splenorenal, phrenosplenic, and gastrosplenic ligaments is required for complete assessment of the spleen. The short gastric vessels can be ligated with division of the gastrosplenic ligament. Repair of the spleen can be accomplished by application of hemostatic agents, direct pledgeted suture repair of the splenic parenchyma, partial splenectomy, and construction of a "splenic wrap" using absorbable mesh. Splenic preservation should only be considered in the hemodynamically stable patient. If splenectomy is required, the splenic artery and vein should be ligated individually before removing the spleen.

18. **What is splenic autotransplantation and does it preserve splenic function?**
Splenic autotransplantation is the implantation of splenic parenchyma into the gastrocolic omentum. Autotransplantation after splenectomy is controversial. After autotransplantation, immunoglobulin G (IgG) and IgM levels are increased in response to pneumococcal vaccine compared with patients after splenectomy alone but the clinical significance is unknown.

19. **What early complications arise after splenectomy?**
Recurrent bleeding, acute gastric dilatation, gastric perforation, pancreatitis, pancreatic tail injury with pancreatic fistula formation, and subphrenic abscess.

20. **Does postsplenectomy leukocytosis predict infection?**
Elevations in white blood cell (WBC) count and platelet count (PC) after splenectomy are a common physiologic event. After the fourth postoperative day, however, a WBC >15 × 10^3 and a PC/WBC <20 have been associated with sepsis and should not be confused with the physiologic response to splenectomy. A PC that fails to rise to >200 × 10^3 by the seventh postoperative day has also been associated with a higher likelihood of infection.

21. **What is overwhelming postsplenectomy infection (OPSI)?**
OPSI is a highly lethal bacteremia (typically encapsulated bacteria) that occurs in 0.5%–2% of patients after splenectomy. The risk of OPSI is greatest when splenectomy is performed during infancy or for hematologic disorders. The most common organisms are pneumococcus, meningococcus, *Escherichia coli*, *Haemophilus influenzae*, staphylococcus, and streptococcus. Although rare, OPSI carries a mortality rate of 50%–75% if not treated immediately.

22. **How is overwhelming postsplenectomy infection prevented?**
Vaccinations against pneumococcus, meningococcus, and haemophilus, as well as yearly influenza vaccinations, should be administered to all postsplenectomy patients. The optimal timing in the emergency splenectomy patient is controversial. Evidence suggests increased antibody production if vaccinations are given after 14 days postsplenectomy. But some advocate vaccination prior to discharge because of the high rate of loss of follow-up in the trauma population. Pneumococcal revaccination should be guided by antibody titers where available. If titers are unavailable revaccination should occur every 5 years. High-risk patients (age <2 years, inadequate vaccination response, history of invasive pneumococcal disease, and immunosuppression) should receive antibiotic prophylaxis with oral penicillin (oral macrolide in penicillin allergy).

KEY POINTS: EXPECTANT MANAGEMENT OF SPLENIC INJURIES

1. NOM can be considered in 75%–85% of blunt splenic injury patients.
2. NOM has a success rate >90% in appropriately selected patients.
3. Contraindications to NOM include hemodynamic instability, peritonitis, additional intraabdominal injury requiring operative intervention, and lack of facility capabilities.
4. SAE should be considered in grade IV–V splenic injuries and any injuries with contrast extravasation or pseudoaneurysm.

BIBLIOGRAPHY

1. Banerjee A, Kelly KB, Zhou HY, et al. Diagnosis of infection after splenectomy for trauma should be based on lack of platelets rather than white blood cell count. *Surg Infect.* 2014;15(3):221–226.
2. Bhullar IS, Frykberg ER. At first blush: absence of computed tomography contrast extravasation in grade IV and V adult blunt splenic trauma should not preclude angioembolization. *J Trauma Acute Care Surg.* 2013;74(1):105–112.
3. Davies JM, Lewis MPN, Wimperis J, et al. Review of the guidelines for the prevention and treatment of infection in patients with an absent of dysfunctional spleen: prepared on behalf of the British Committee for Standards in Haematology by a working party of the Haemato-Oncology Task force. *Br J Haematol.* 2011;155(3):308–317.
4. Ekeh AP, McCarthy MC. Complications arising from splenic embolization after blunt splenic trauma. *Am J Surg.* 2005;189(3):335–339.
5. Fata P, Robinson L. A survey of EAST member practices in blunt splenic injury: a description of current trends and opportunities for improvement. *J Trauma.* 2005;59(4):836–841.
6. Haan JM, Biffl W, Knudson MM, et al. Splenic embolization revisited: a multicenter review. *J Trauma.* 2004;56(3):542–547.
7. Harbrecht BG, Ko SH. Angiography for blunt splenic trauma does not improve the success rate of nonoperative management. *J Trauma.* 2007;63(1):44–49.
8. Leemans R, Harms G. Spleen autotransplantation provides restoration of functional splenic lymphoid compartments and improves the humoral immune response to pneumococcal polysaccharide vaccine. *Clin Exp Immunol.* 1999;117(3):596–604.
9. London JA, Parry L. Safety of early mobilization of patients with blunt solid organ injuries. *Arch Surg.* 2008;143(10):972–976.
10. McCray VW, Davis JW. Observation for nonoperative management of the spleen: how long is long enough? *J Trauma.* 2008;65(6):1354–1358.
11. Miller PR, Chang MC. Prospective trial of angiography and embolization for all grade III to V blunt splenic injuries: nonoperative management success rate is significantly improved. *J Am Coll Surg.* 2014;218(4):644–648.
12. Moore EE, Cogbill TH. Organ injury scaling: spleen and liver (1994 revision). *J Trauma.* 1995;38(3):323–324.
13. Requarth JA, D'Agostino RB, Miller PR. Nonoperative management of adult blunt splenic injury with and without splenic artery embolotherapy: a meta-analysis. *J Trauma.* 2011;71(4):898–903.
14. Rostas JW, Manley J, Gonzalez RP, et al. The safety of low molecular-weight heparin after blunt liver and spleen injuries. *AM J Surg.* 2015;210(1):31–34.
15. Sartorelli KH, Frumiento C. Nonoperative management of hepatic, splenic, and renal injuries in adults with multiple injuries. *J Trauma.* 2000;49(1):56–61.
16. Savage SA, Zarzaur BL, Magnotti LJ, et al. The evolution of blunt splenic injury: resolution and progression. *J Trauma.* 2008;64(4):1085–1092.
17. Shatz DV, Schinsky MF. Antibody responses in postsplenectomy trauma patients receiving the 23-valent pneumococcal polysaccharide vaccine at 1 versus 7 versus 14 days after splenectomy. *J Trauma.* 1998;44(5):760–766.
18. Skattum J, Naess PA. Refining the role of splenic angiographic embolization in high-grade splenic injuries. *J Trauma Acute Care Surg.* 2013;74(1):100–104.
19. Stassen NA, Bhullar I, Cheng JD, et al. Selective nonoperative management of blunt splenic injury: an Eastern Association for the Surgery of Trauma practice management guideline. *J Trauma Acute Care Surg.* 2012;73(5 suppl 4):S294–S300.
20. Velmahos GC, Zacharias N, Emhoff TA, et al. Management of the most severely injured spleen: a multicenter study of the Research Consortium of New England Centers for Trauma (ReCONECT). *Arch Surg.* 2010;145(5):456–460.
21. Weng J, Brown CVR, Rhee P, et al. White blood cell and platelet counts can be used to differentiate between infection and normal response after splenectomy for trauma: prospective validation. *J Trauma.* 2005;59(5):1076–1080.

CHAPTER 28

PANCREATIC AND DUODENAL INJURY

Ryan A. Lawless, MD, Ernest E. Moore, MD, FACS

1. **How common are pancreatic and duodenal injuries?**
   Injury to the pancreas and duodenum remain uncommon, likely because of the intimate association with other vital structures within the retroperitoneum. The recently documented incidence of duodenal injury is 0.2%–0.3%, followed by 0.004%–0.6% for pancreas injury. In patients undergoing laparotomy for trauma the incidence is 3%–6%. Traditionally, the incidence of pancreatic injury is higher in penetrating trauma; however, recent experience has suggested a reversal of this with the majority of pancreatic injuries resulting from a blunt mechanism.

2. **What other injuries are typically associated with penetrating pancreatic trauma?**
   Isolated injuries to the pancreas and duodenum are the exception rather than the rule, with more than 90% being associated with a concomitant injury. Liver injury is the most frequent concomitant injury, with a reported incidence of 50%. Other commonly associated injuries include the stomach (40%), large abdominal vessels such as the aorta and vena cava (40%), spleen (25%), kidney (2%), and duodenum (20%).

3. **How are pancreatic injuries diagnosed preoperatively?**
   Penetrating trauma to the pancreas is usually discovered during exploration for associated injuries. Such patients may present with hemodynamic instability from bleeding, positive focused abdominal sonography in trauma examination, or peritonitis. Patients with blunt injury who are hemodynamically stable should undergo abdominal computed tomography (CT) scan, and possible endoscopic retrograde cholangiopancreatography (ERCP) if proximal ductal disruption is suspected. The sensitivity for detecting pancreatic injury and pancreaticoduodenal injury is low for both 16- and 64-multidetector CT scan; however, the specificity is >90%. ERCP is the most accurate method of identifying an injury to the pancreatic duct. Magnetic resonance cholangiopancreatography (MRCP) is a useful modality to identify pancreatic injury with ductal involvement, and has an added advantage of evaluating the duct distal to a transection; however, therapeutic maneuvers are not possible with MRCP. Elevated serum amylase concentrations are nonspecific for pancreatic injury and can be normal initially in a high proportion of patients.

4. **What are some of the commonly used surgical options for the treatment of pancreatic injuries?**
   The majority of pancreatic injuries can be treated with the placement of closed suction drains at the time of initial laparotomy. In situations of more severe trauma, the integrity of the pancreatic duct must be investigated through direct inspection or pancreatography. Injuries involving the duct portion of the pancreatic duct are managed with a distal pancreatectomy and drain placement. If the patient is in extremis, a splenectomy should be performed during the distal pancreatectomy. However, if a patient is hemodynamically stable, a spleen preserving distal pancreatectomy is preferred. Injuries involving the pancreatic duct proximal to the mesenteric vessels may require a significant resection such as a pancreaticoduodenectomy. Extensive resections such as these are generally performed following a damage control situation at the follow-up operation.

5. **What are the common complications of pancreatic trauma?**
   Exsanguination, as with most traumatic injuries, is the most common cause of early death, prompting the use of damage control. For patients who survive their initial operation, the two most common complications are pancreatic fistulas and intraabdominal abscesses. Other late problems include pancreatitis, pancreatic pseudocyst, and pancreatic hemorrhage. Pancreatic insufficiency is a concern when resecting >80% of the pancreas. Careful attention to the injury pattern and location of injury in relation to the mesenteric vessel should lead to the correct surgical operation. Resection of the pancreas distal to the mesenteric vessels should allow enough pancreas to remain for sufficient exocrine and endocrine function. Most patients who die after sustaining injuries to the pancreas do so as a result of late complications and not from the pancreatic injury itself.

KEY POINTS: SURGICAL OPTIONS FOR PANCREATIC INJURIES

1. Low-grade injuries are treated with simple closed suction drainage at the time of initial operation.
2. Concomitant injuries are common and should be investigated early.
3. In a hemodynamically unstable patient, debridement of devascularized tissue, hemostasis, and drainage should be performed with reconstruction delayed until the patient is stable.
4. If a proximal ductal injury is suspected in a stable patient, visualize with ERCP, MRCP, or cholangiogram.
5. Consider establishing enteral nutritional access by placing a jejunal feeding tube in patients with more than minor injuries.

DUODENUM

6. **What is the role of CT scanning in diagnosing blunt duodenal injuries?**
CT evaluation of a hemodynamically stable patient sustaining blunt trauma is the diagnostic modality of choice. Specific direct signs of bowel injury, pneumoperitoneum, or oral contrast extravasation indicate injury to the hollow viscus and mandate operative exploration. Indirect evidence of a duodenal injury includes periduodenal fluid or hematoma, focal pneumatosis, adjacent vascular or organ injury, and fatty stranding in the retroperitoneum, which are nonspecific findings. A recent analysis identified 11% of patients with nonspecific CT findings suggestive of duodenal injury required operative repair. Eighteen percent of patients failed nonoperative management as defined by worsening findings on interval CT scan or physical examination; however, upon operative exploration, only 5% of the nonoperative failure was secondary to a duodenal injury.
    Isolated periduodenal fluid or hematoma does not mandate an operative exploration. A safe management algorithm should include observation with serial examinations and an interval CT scan at 24 hours.

7. **What is the importance of the Kocher maneuver?**
In 1903, E. Theodor Kocher described a maneuver to visualize and repair injuries to the duodenum, distal common bile duct, and pancreatic head during exploratory surgery. The avascular lateral peritoneal attachments to the duodenum are incised sharply, and the duodenum is elevated and reflected medially from the retroperitoneum to the border of the inferior vena cava. This allows for inspection and palpation of the posterior surface of the duodenum and head of the pancreas.

8. **What are the four portions of the duodenum and their surgical relationships?**
The **first portion** of the duodenum begins at the pylorus, making it an intraperitoneal structure. It then migrates into the retroperitoneum as it passes by the gallbladder. The **second portion** descends 7–8 cm through the retroperitoneum anterior to the vena cava. The medial border of the duodenum is adherent to the head of the pancreas where the common bile and pancreatic ducts enter; it shares a common blood supply with the head of the pancreas through the pancreaticoduodenal arcades. The **third portion** of the duodenum turns horizontally through the retroperitoneum contacting the uncinate process along its superior border and passing behind the root of the mesentery. The **fourth portion** continues horizontally, ascending slightly and crossing the spine anterior to the aorta, where it is fixed to the suspensory ligament of Treitz at the duodenojejunal flexure, medial to the inferior mesenteric vein.

9. **How are duodenal injuries classified?**
An organ injury scale has been adopted that allows for standardized descriptions of duodenal injuries, which extend from grade I (less severe) to grade V (most severe). The grading of duodenal injuries assists surgeons in selecting the appropriate surgical procedure for the repair or reconstruction of these frequently complex injuries (see Table 28.1).

10. **What are the main surgical options for penetrating duodenal injuries?**
The majority of simple lacerations involving <50% of the duodenal circumference can be repaired primarily. Complex lacerations with devitalized tissue or lacerations that involve >50% of the duodenal circumference require debridement of the margins and reanastomosis of the divided ends. If tension on the suture line is anticipated following resection of devitalized tissue, adjunctive techniques such as Roux-en-Y duodenojejunostomy or pyloric exclusion in conjunction with a gastric drainage procedure are more appropriate. Injuries involving the distal common bile duct and pancreatic head may warrant a pancreaticoduodenectomy after damage control procedure. Consideration should be given to establishing enteral access, especially in all complex repairs.

Table 28.1 Grades of Pancreatic and Duodenal Injury: Grade Injury Description

		Pancreas Injury Scale
GRADE	**TYPE OF INJURY**	**DESCRIPTION OF INJURY**
I	Hematoma	Minor contusion without duct injury
	Laceration	Superficial laceration without duct injury
II	Hematoma	Major contusion without duct injury or tissue loss
	Laceration	Major laceration without duct injury or tissue loss
III	Laceration	Distal transection/parenchymal injury with duct injury
IV	Laceration	Proximal transection/parenchymal injury involving ampulla
V	Laceration	Massive pancreatic head disruption
		Duodenum Injury Scale
GRADE	**TYPE OF INJURY**	**DESCRIPTION OF INJURY**
I	Hematoma	Involving single portion of duodenum
	Laceration	Partial thickness
II	Hematoma	Involving >1 portion of duodenum
	Laceration	<50% circumference involved
III	Laceration	50%–75% circumference of D2
		50%–100% circumference of D1, D3, D4
IV	Laceration	>75% circumference D2
		Involves ampulla or distal common bile duct
V	Laceration	Massive disruption of duodenopancreatic complex
	Vascular	Devascularization of duodenum

KEY POINTS: SURGICAL OPTIONS FOR DUODENAL INJURIES

1. Concomitant injuries are common, particularly to the pancreas, and they should be searched for and addressed.
2. Blunt duodenal injuries are difficult to diagnose and the decision to operate should include subtle clinical signs and indirect imaging evidence.
3. Appropriate duodenal evaluation upon abdominal exploration requires a Kocher maneuver.
4. Operative repair is determined by injury grade and extent of devitalized tissue. Most injuries can be managed with simple primary repair. Extensive resections should be delayed in hemodynamically unstable patients via damage control procedures.
5. Enteral access should be considered in all but the simplest injuries.

BIBLIOGRAPHY

1. Huerta S, Bui T. Predictors of morbidity and mortality in patients with duodenal injuries. *Am Surg.* 2005;71(9):763–767.
2. Kao LS, Bulger EM. Predictors of morbidity after traumatic pancreatic injury. *J Trauma.* 2003;55(5):898–905.
3. Lopez PP, Benjamin R, Cockburn M, et al. Recent trends in the management of combined pancreatoduodenal injuries. *Am Surg.* 2005;71(10):847–852.
4. Moore EE, Cogbill T, Malangoni M, et al. Organ injury scaling II: pancreas, duodenum, small bowel, colon, and rectum. *J Trauma.* 1990;30(11):1427–1429.
5. Patel SV, Spencer JA. Imaging of pancreatic trauma. *Br J Radiol.* 1998;71(849):985–990.

6. Subramanian A, Dente CJ, Feliciano DY. The managing of pancreatic trauma in the modern era. *Surg Clin North Am.* 2007;87(6):1515–1532.
7. Takishima T, Sugimoto K. Serum amylase level on admission in the diagnosis of blunt injury to the pancreas: its significance and limitations. *Ann Surg.* 1997;226(1):70–76.
8. Timaran CH, Daley BJ. Role of duodenography in the diagnosis of blunt duodenal injuries. *J Trauma.* 2001;51(4): 648–651.
9. Vassiliu P, Toutouzas KG. A prospective study of post-traumatic biliary and pancreatic fistuli. The role of expectant management. *Injury.* 2004;35(3):223–227.
10. Velmahos GC, Constantinou C. Safety of repair for severe duodenal injuries. *World J Surg.* 2008;32(1):7–12.
11. Wales PW, Shuckett B. Long-term outcome after nonoperative management of complete traumatic pancreatic transection in children. *J Pediatr Surg.* 2001;36(5):823–827.
12. Girard E, Abba J, Cristiano N, et al. Management of splenic and pancreatic trauma. *J Visc Surg.* 2016;153(4 suppl):45–60.
13. Velmahos GC, Tabbara M, Gross R, et al. Blunt pancreatoduodenal injury: a multicenter study of the research consortium of New England Centers for Trauma (ReCONECT). *Arch Surg.* 2009;144(5):413–419.
14. Cogbill TH, Moore EE, Morris Jr JA, et al. Distal pancreatectomy for trauma: a multicenter experience. *J Trauma.* 1991;31(12):1600–1606.
15. Krige JE, Kotze UK. Morbidity and mortality after distal pancreatectomy for trauma: a critical appraisal of 107 consecutive patients undergoing resection at a Level 1 Trauma Centre. *Injury.* 2014;45(9):1401–1408.
16. Bradley M, Bonds B, Dreizin D, et al. Indirect signs of blunt duodenal injury on computed tomography: is non-operative management safe? *Injury.* 2016;47(1):53–58.
17. Siboni S, Benjamin E. Isolated blunt duodenal trauma: simple repair, low mortality. *Am Surg.* 2015;81(10):961–964.
18. Melamud K, LeBedis CA. Imaging of pancreatic and duodenal trauma. *Rad Clin Nor Am.* 2015;53(4):757–771.

CHAPTER 29

TRAUMA TO THE COLON AND RECTUM

Emily Miraflor, MD, Jahanara Graf, MD

COLON TRAUMA

1. **How do most colon injuries occur?**
   Nearly all (>95%) colon injuries are caused by penetrating trauma from a gunshot, a stab wound, an iatrogenic injury, or a sexual injury. Blunt colonic trauma is rare and usually results from seat belts during motor vehicle crashes.

2. **How are colon injuries diagnosed?**
   They are usually diagnosed during laparotomy for penetrating trauma. For patients in whom the need for laparotomy has not been established, a rectal examination may show blood in the stool, which suggests a left-sided or rectal injury. Elevated white blood cell counts or enzyme levels (amylase, alkaline phosphatase) may reflect a bowel injury. While no longer commonly performed, fecal material in diagnostic peritoneal lavage is highly suggestive of a bowel injury. Imaging findings that are concerning for a colonic injury include free air, extravasation of contrast, retroperitoneal gas, or fluid adjacent to the colon. All significant injuries are generally clinically manifest within 18 hours of injury.

3. **How are colon injuries graded?**
   - Grade I: Contusion or hematoma without devascularization or partial-thickness laceration
   - Grade II: Laceration <50% circumference
   - Grade III: Laceration >50% circumference
   - Grade IV: Transection of the colon
   - Grade V: Transection with segmental tissue loss or devascularization

4. **What are three primary surgical options for managing a colon injury?**
   a. Primary repair: Nondestructive colon wounds without devascularization and involving <50% of the bowel wall can be primarily repaired with suture.
   b. Resection with primary anastomosis: Destructive wounds that feature devascularization or involve more than 50% of the bowel wall should be resected. In these cases, it is safe to perform a primary reanastomosis in patients with good hemodynamic status, minimal contamination, and minimal comorbidities.
   c. Resection with colostomy formation: Some patients are too sick to undergo primary anastomosis. These are the patients that are in persistent shock, coagulopathic, multiply injured, or affected by other comorbidities. In this situation, it is appropriate to perform a resection with a colostomy.

5. **What are the advantages and disadvantages of each of these options?**
   a. Primary repair and resection with primary anastomosis provides definitive treatment at the initial operation. The patient is spared the morbidity of a colostomy and its reversal. The disadvantage is that suture lines are created in suboptimal conditions giving rise to the concern for anastomotic breakdown. A randomized trial of primary repair versus diversion failed to show a benefit for diversion.
   b. A proximal colostomy avoids an unprotected suture line in the abdomen but it does require a second operation to close the colostomy. Additionally, stomas carry a morbidity of their own, such as necrosis, stenosis, obstruction, and prolapse. A significant portion of patients who undergo stoma creation never have their stoma closed, those who undergo stoma closure experience a 15%–25% complication rate.

6. **How are most patients with colon injuries surgically managed?**
   Primary repair is safe and effective in most patients with colon trauma. Hand sewn and stapled anastomoses have equivalent complication rates. Prophylactic antibiotics are administered for no longer than 24 hours postoperatively.

7. **How should the surgical incision and penetrating wound be managed?**
Wounds should be left open to heal by secondary intention to decrease the incidence of wound infection and fascial dehiscence. Negative pressure wound therapy can be used to simplify management of the open midline wound.

8. **What complications are associated with colonic injury and its treatment?**
   - Wound infection (65% if the skin incision is closed primarily; do not be tempted to close a dirty incision)
   - Intraabdominal abscess (20%)
   - Fascial dehiscence (10%)
   - Stoma complications (5%)
   - Anastomotic leak (5%)
   - Mortality (<1%)

RECTAL TRAUMA

9. **How do rectal injuries occur?**
Similar to colon injuries, most rectal injuries result from penetrating trauma as a result of gunshot, stab, iatrogenic, or sexual injury. Patients with blunt pelvic fractures should be assessed for rectal and urethral injuries.

10. **How are rectal injuries diagnosed?**
The diagnosis is suggested by the course of the projectile and the presence of blood on digital rectal examination. A computed tomography scan may help delineate the trajectory of the bullet or stab wound. If rectal trauma is suspected, the patient should undergo proctoscopy to look for hematoma, contusion, laceration, or gross blood. If the diagnosis is in question, radiographs with soluble-contrast enemas should be performed.

11. **How are patients with intraperitoneal rectal injuries treated differently from those with extraperitoneal injuries?**
The portion of the rectum proximal to the peritoneal reflection is called the intraperitoneal segment. Injuries of this portion are treated similar to colonic injuries. The portion of the rectum below the peritoneal reflection is the extraperitoneal segment.
  Extraperitoneal rectal injuries can be difficult to diagnose because peritonitis does not occur. A high level of suspicion for rectal injury must be maintained for any patient with penetrating trauma to the lower abdomen, the buttocks, or in patients with a significant pelvic fracture.

12. **What are the four basic principles for managing simple extraperitoneal rectal injuries?**
Historically, treatment of extraperitoneal rectal injury consisted of four components:
 a. Diversion: Either a loop or an end sigmoid colostomy
 b. Drainage: Placement of a presacral drain into the retrorectal space via a perineal incision
 c. Repair: Transanal repair when possible
 d. Washout: Irrigation of the distal rectum with isotonic solution until the effluent is clear
  The most recent guidelines recommend proximal diversion for management of extraperitoneal rectal injuries; however, they recommend avoidance of routine presacral drains and distal rectal washout.

13. **How are complex extraperitoneal rectal injuries managed?**
In patients with massive pelvic trauma and an associated rectal injury, an abdominoperineal resection may be required for adequate debridement and hemostasis. An abdominoperineal resection is also required in rare instances in which anal sphincters have been destroyed. This type of injury is extremely rare.

14. **What complications are associated with rectal trauma and its treatment?**
The complications are similar to those in colonic injuries, such as intraabdominal abscess and wound infection. In addition, pelvic osteomyelitis may occur. In this case, debridement and long-term culture-specific intravenous (IV) antibiotics may be necessary.

15. **What is the role of antibiotics in colorectal trauma?**
Antibiotics are given prophylactically preoperatively to prevent postoperative infections. They should be initiated preoperatively (you need a good blood level at the time you make your incision) and ended quickly (24 hours postoperatively).

Broad-spectrum combination therapy is superior to single-agent therapy. Whenever the possibility of colorectal injury is entertained, broad-spectrum IV prophylactic antibiotics should be started immediately.

KEY POINTS: COLORECTAL TRAUMA

1. Primary repair of colon injuries is safe.
2. Hand sewn and stapled anastomoses have equal complication rates.
3. A preoperative dose of antibiotic therapy, to be continued for 24 hours or less, is advantageous.
4. The management of extraperitoneal rectal injuries is evolving. Diversion is the most conservative strategy.

BIBLIOGRAPHY

1. Beck DE, Roberts PL, eds. *The ASCRS Textbook of Colon and Rectal Surgery*. 2nd ed. Springer Science; 2011.
2. Bosarge PL, Como JJ, Fox N, et al. Management of penetrating extraperitoneal rectal injuries: an Eastern Association for the Surgery of Trauma practice management guideline. *J Trauma Acute Care Surg*. 2016;80(3):546–551.
3. Cayten CG, Fabian TC. Patient management guidelines for penetrating intraperitoneal colon injuries. Eastern Association for the Surgery of Trauma. https://www.east.org/education/practice-management-guidelines/penetrating-colon-injuries-management-of-. 1998. Accessed 14.02.17.
4. Curran TJ, Borzotta AP. Complications of primary repair of colon injury: literature review of 2,964 cases. *Am J Surg*. 1999;177(1):42–47.
5. Demetriades D, Murray J, Chan LS, et al. Handsewn versus stapled anastomosis in penetrating colon injuries requiring resection: a multicenter study. *J Trauma*. 2002;52(1):117–121.
6. Demetriades D, Murray J, Chan L, et al. Penetrating colon injuries requiring resection: diversion or primary anastomosis? An AAST prospective multicenter study. *J Trauma*. 2001;50(5):765–775.
7. Gonzalez RP, Phelan 3rd H. Is fecal diversion necessary for nondestructive penetrating extraperitoneal rectal injuries? *J Trauma*. 2006;61(4):815–819.
8. Miller PR, Fabian TC, Croce MA, et al. Improving outcomes following penetrating colon wounds. *Ann Surg*. 2002;235(6):775–781.
9. Mulholland MW, Lillemoe KD, eds. *Greenfield's Surgery: Scientific Principles and Practice*. 5th ed. Lippincott Williams & Wilkins; 2011:402–403.

PELVIC FRACTURES

Philip F. Stahel, MD, FACS, David J. Hak, MD, MBA, FACS

1. **What are the first steps in the evaluation and treatment of a patient with pelvic ring injuries?**
   Severely injured patients with high-energy acute pelvic ring disruptions are at high risk of mortality from associated exsanguinating hemorrhage. Diagnostic workup strategies in the emergency room must be standardized to avoid an unnecessary delay to definitive surgical bleeding control, as the time elapsed between injury and operating room has been shown to inversely correlate with survival.

2. **What are the sources and potential volume of bleeding in the displaced pelvic fracture?**
   The main source of acute retroperitoneal hemorrhage in patients with hemodynamically unstable pelvic ring disruptions is attributed to venous bleeding in 80%–90%, originating from presacral and paravesical venous plexus and from bleeding cancellous bone surfaces from sacral and iliac fractures and sacroiliac joint disruptions. Only 10%–20% of all retroperitoneal pelvic bleeding sources are of arterial origin.

3. **What is the most common source of arterial bleeding associated with a pelvic fracture?**
   The superior gluteal artery.

4. **Should a Foley catheter be placed in trauma patients with displaced pelvic fractures?**
   Contraindications to Foley placement include urethral injuries, which should be suspected when blood is observed at the penile meatus or presence of a high-riding prostate on digital rectal exam. A retrograde urethrogram may be used to diagnose a urethral injury. If a urethral injury is suspected or confirmed, a suprapubic catheter should be placed instead of a Foley. In all other cases, a Foley should be placed.

5. **What is the incidence of urologic injury associated with pelvic fractures?**
   Overall, in unstable pelvic fractures (B and C types), 10%–20%, with a high prevalence in APC-3 or LC-3 equivalent pelvic ring disruptions and "vertical shear" injury mechanisms.

6. **Which gender and what portion of the urethra is most commonly injured in patients with a displaced pelvic fracture?**
   The male urethra is more commonly injured. The urethra passes through the urogenital diaphragm or pelvic floor, transitioning in an abrupt fashion from the membranous to the bulbous urethra. The urethra at this point is attenuated and relatively fixed above, accounting for the large number of injuries at the membranous bulbous junction. The female urethra is much shorter, and the most common site of urethral injury in women is at the bladder neck.

7. **Describe the mechanism that results in a bladder rupture.**
   The bladder is both an intraperitoneal and extraperitoneal structure. Compression of a distended bladder results in an intraperitoneal rupture along the bladder dome. Extraperitoneal rupture, a more common injury, results from the laceration of the bladder by displaced pubic rami fracture fragments, mainly in lateral compression type mechanisms equivalent to LC-2 and LC-3 injuries.

8. **What are the commonly used radiographic classification schemes for pelvic fractures?**
   The mechanistic classification by Young and Burgess describes pelvic fractures as antero-posterior compression (APC), lateral compression (LC), vertical shear (VS), or combined mechanism (CM). The alphanumeric AO/OTA classification, which is equivalent to the Tile classification, categorizes fractures by ascending severity into three groups (A, B, C) with numbered subgroups (1, 2, 3) based on increasing severity of ligamentous and bony disruption.

9. **What is an open pelvic fracture?**
An open pelvic fracture is defined by a breach through the skin envelope or the mucosa (rectum, vagina) leading to exposed and contaminated pelvic bone elements. Open pelvic fractures are associated with a significantly increased postinjury mortality due to exsanguinating hemorrhage, infections, and sepsis. The initial clinical assessment of patients with pelvic fractures therefore mandates a rectal and vaginal examination as well as a rectoproctoscopy. Open pelvic fractures in the rectal or perineal region require a temporary diverting colostomy for decontamination and infection control.

10. **When is acute mechanical stabilization of a pelvic fracture indicated?**
The application of noninvasive external pelvic compression devices (pelvic binders or sheets) represents an established measure for acute resuscitation of bleeding pelvic fractures with the intent of reducing intrapelvic volume and mitigating the extent of acute retroperitoneal blood loss. Placement of pelvic binders at the level of the greater trochanter has been shown to improve temporary pelvic ring stability.

11. **What is pelvic packing and when is it used?**
The concept of pelvic packing was first described in Europe as a transabdominal open pelvic packing technique through an explorative midline laparotomy. More recently, the concept of "direct" preperitoneal pelvic packing (PPP) was adapted in the United States by a suprapubic midline incision that allows a direct retroperitoneal approach to the retroperitoneal space. The modified PPP technique allows for more effective packing within the concealed preperitoneal space, without the necessity of opening the retroperitoneal space through a laparotomy. As the main source of pelvic bleeding is of venous origin, pelvic packing in conjunction with external pelvic fixation has been show to provide an effective "tamponade" for acute hemorrhage control during the early resuscitation phase of patients with hemodynamically unstable pelvic ring disruptions. Pelvic packings have to be removed in a subsequent "second look" procedure within 24–48 hours, to decrease the risk of infection.

12. **What is the role of angiography in an acute pelvic fracture?**
Most current clinical guidelines recommend the use of early angiography and percutaneous transcatheter angioembolization as one of the main therapeutic options for acute bleeding control in patients with hemodynamically unstable pelvic fractures. The apparent shortcoming of angioembolization is related to the inability of controlling venous bleeding, which represents the main source of hemorrhage in 80%–90% of all patients with unstable pelvic ring injuries.

13. **Why do patients die from pelvic fractures?**
The main cause of death in patients with unstable pelvic ring disruptions is from acute exsanguination from uncontrolled retroperitoneal hemorrhage. Delayed causes of mortality include infections, sepsis, and multiple organ failure.

14. **What is the rationale for pelvic external fixation?**
Pelvic ring disruptions in hemodynamically unstable patients should be temporarily stabilized to prevent further hemorrhage and to support measures of hemorrhage control, including angiography and pelvic packing. The rationale for acute external pelvic fixation consists of reducing the intrapelvic volume in "open book" equivalent (APC-2/-3) and "vertical shear" injuries by decreasing the retroperitoneal bleeding space, and to provide a stable counter-pressure to the packed lap sponges for effective pelvic packing. The external fixation devices must be placed in a manner that permits abdominal access for laparotomy, diagnostic imaging, and the definitive operative approach for open reduction and internal fixation of pelvic fractures.

15. **Is there a role for pneumatic antishock garments in the treatment of pelvic fractures?**
Pneumatic antishock garments (PASGs) are falling out of favor in the treatment of pelvic fractures. Their potential role is limited to emergency transportation and initial stabilization of patients "in extremis" with unresponsive traumatic-hemorrhagic shock. The application of PASGs is associated with increased risk of lower extremity and gluteal compartment syndromes.

16. **When can patients with a pelvic fracture ambulate?**
The pelvic fracture classification and modality of definitive pelvic ring fixation dictates the patients' mobility and ambulation status. For example, stable A-type injuries per AO/OTA (Tile) classification can be mobilized immediately without restrictions. Similarly, APC-1 and LC-1 fractures per Young and Burgess classification are amenable to immediate full weight bearing. Most pelvic ring disruptions

with unstable posterior pelvic elements at the level of the iliosacral joint, or complete (vertically unstable) sacral fractures, require partial protective weight bearing for 10–12 weeks post injury, to avoid a secondary displacement.

17. **What are the three radiographic views required to evaluate patients with pelvic fractures?**
    a. Anteroposterior pelvis view.
    b. Pelvic "inlet" view, in which the x-ray beam is angled caudad by 45 degrees providing a view down the pelvic ring.
    c. Pelvic "outlet" view, in which the x-ray beam is angled cephalad by 45 degrees providing optimal assessment of the sacrum and any associated displacement in the superior-inferior plane.

18. **What percent of patients with an unstable pelvic fracture will suffer an associated neurologic injury?**
    Associated injuries of the lumbosacral plexus, sacral foramina, and sacral canal are rare (<5%) in most pelvic ring injuries, yet the rates of associated neurologic injuries are significantly increased in complete pelvic ring disruptions (e.g., "vertical shear" mechanisms) and in displaced zone 2 and zone 3 sacral fractures.

19. **What is the significance of an L5 transverse process fracture in a patient with a pelvis fracture?**
    A transverse process fracture at the level of L5 is a surrogate marker of vertical instability of the pelvic fracture due to the attachment of the iliolumbar ligaments. Most "vertical shear" injuries have an associated L5 transverse process fracture.

KEY POINTS: BLOOD LOSS FROM PELVIC RING DISRUPTIONS

1. Severe pelvic ring disruptions are associated with massive exsanguinating hemorrhage into the retroperitoneal space, which can hold as much as the entire intravascular blood volume (4–6 L). Around 80%–90% percent of deaths related to pelvic bleeding result from venous and cancellous bone bleeding in the retroperitoneal space.
2. Noninvasive external pelvic compression devices (pelvic binders, sheets) are effective "first-line" pelvic ring reduction and stabilization tools to mitigate ongoing intrapelvic hemorrhage. Only 10%–20% of pelvic bleeding sources are of arterial origin, most commonly from the superior gluteal artery. Angioembolization is effective in controlling pelvic arterial bleeding sources.
3. Direct preperitoneal pelvic packing in conjunction with external pelvic fixation represents a "damage control" measure that has been shown to successfully reduce hemorrhage and mortality in patients with hemodynamically unstable pelvic ring injuries, from 40% to 60% historic mortality, to 15% to 20% reported in the current literature.

VIDEO RESOURCE

Technique of direct preperitoneal pelvic packing: https://www.youtube.com/watch?v=RYHbEPE-Tno

BIBLIOGRAPHY

1. Smith W, Williams A, Agudelo J, et al. Early predictors of mortality in hemodynamically unstable pelvis fractures. *J Orthop Trauma.* 2007;21(1):31–37.
2. Sathy AK, Starr AJ, Smith WR, et al. The effect of pelvic fracture on mortality after trauma: an analysis of 63,000 trauma patients. *J Bone Joint Surg Am.* 2009;91(12):2803–2810.
3. Costantini TW, Coimbra R, Holcomb JB, et al. Current management of hemorrhage from severe pelvic fractures: results of an American Association for the Surgery of Trauma multi-institutional trial. *J Trauma Acute Care Surg.* 2016;80(5):717–725.
4. Stahel PF, Smith WR. Current trends in resuscitation strategy for the multiply injured patient. *Injury.* 2009;40(suppl 4): S27–S35.
5. Mauffrey C, Cuellar 3rd DO, Pieracci F, et al. Strategies for the management of haemorrhage following pelvic fractures and associated trauma-induced coagulopathy. *Bone Joint J.* 2014;96-B(9):1143–1154.

6. Gansslen A, Hildebrand F. Management of hemodynamic unstable patients "in extremis" with pelvic ring fractures. *Acta Chir Orthop Traumatol Cech.* 2012;79(3):193–202.

7. Hou Z, Smith WR, Strohecker KA, et al. Hemodynamically unstable pelvic fracture management by advanced trauma life support guidelines results in high mortality. *Orthopedics.* 2012;35(3):e319–e324.

8. Magnone S, Coccolini F, Manfredi R, et al. Management of hemodynamically unstable pelvic trauma: results of the first Italian consensus conference (cooperative guidelines of the Italian Society of Surgery, the Italian Association of Hospital Surgeons, the Multi-specialist Italian Society of Young Surgeons, the Italian Society of Emergency Surgery and Trauma, the Italian Society of Anesthesia, Analgesia, Resuscitation and Intensive Care, the Italian Society of Orthopaedics and Traumatology, the Italian Society of Emergency Medicine, the Italian Society of Medical Radiology -Section of Vascular and Interventional Radiology- and the World Society of Emergency Surgery). *World J Emerg Surg.* 2014;9(1):18.

9. Ertel W, Keel M. Control of severe hemorrhage using C-clamp and pelvic packing in multiply injured patients with pelvic ring disruption. *J Orthop Trauma.* 2001;15(7):468–474.

10. Heetveld MJ, Harris I. Guidelines for the management of haemodynamically unstable pelvic fracture patients. *ANZ J Surg.* 2004;74(7):520–529.

11. Ertel W, Eid K. Therapeutical strategies and outcome of polytraumatized patients with pelvic injuries. *Eur J Trauma.* 2000;26:278–286.

12. Giannoudis PV, Pape HC. Damage control orthopaedics in unstable pelvic ring injuries. *Injury.* 2004;35(7):671–677.

13. Lustenberger T, Meier C. C-clamp and pelvic packing for control of hemorrhage in patients with pelvic ring disruption. *J Emerg Trauma Shock.* 2011;4(4):477–482.

14. Burlew CC, Moore EE, Smith WR, et al. Preperitoneal pelvic packing/external fixation with secondary angioembolization: optimal care for life-threatening hemorrhage from unstable pelvic fractures. *J Am Coll Surg.* 2011;212(4):628–635. discussion 635–627.

15. Osborn PM, Smith WR, Moore EE, et al. Direct retroperitoneal pelvic packing versus pelvic angiography: a comparison of two management protocols for haemodynamically unstable pelvic fractures. *Injury.* 2009;40(1):54–60.

16. Perkins ZB, Maytham GD. Impact on outcome of a targeted performance improvement programme in haemodynamically unstable patients with a pelvic fracture. *Bone Joint J.* 2014;96-B(8):1090–1097.

17. Li Q, Dong J, Yang Y, et al. Retroperitoneal packing or angioembolization for haemorrhage control of pelvic fractures– Quasi-randomized clinical trial of 56 haemodynamically unstable patients with Injury Severity Score ≥33. *Injury.* 2016;47(2):395–401.

18. Jang JY, Shim H. Preperitoneal pelvic packing in patients with hemodynamic instability due to severe pelvic fracture: early experience in a Korean trauma center. *Scand J Trauma Resusc Emerg Med.* 2016;24:3.

19. Chiara O, di Fratta E, Mariani A, et al. Efficacy of extra-peritoneal pelvic packing in hemodynamically unstable pelvic fractures, a Propensity Score Analysis. *World J Emerg Surg.* 2016;11:22.

20. Suzuki T, Smith WR. Pelvic packing or angiography: competitive or complementary? *Injury.* 2009;40(4):343–353.

21. Tai DK, Li WH, Lee KY, et al. Retroperitoneal pelvic packing in the management of hemodynamically unstable pelvic fractures: a level I trauma center experience. *J Trauma.* 2011;71(4):E79–E86.

22. Rossaint R, Duranteau J. Non-surgical treatment of major bleeding. *Anesthesiol Clin N Am.* 2007;25:35–48.

23. Metsemakers WJ, Vanderschot P. Transcatheter embolotherapy after external surgical stabilization is a valuable treatment algorithm for patients with persistent haemorrhage from unstable pelvic fractures: outcomes of a single centre experience. *Injury.* 2013;44(7):964–968.

24. Abrassart S, Stern R. Unstable pelvic ring injury with hemodynamic instability: what seems the best procedure choice and sequence in the initial management? *Orthop Traumatol Surg Res.* 2013;99(2):175–182.

25. Hagiwara A, Minakawa K. Predictors of death in patients with life-threatening pelvic hemorrhage after successful transcatheter arterial embolization. *J Trauma.* 2003;55(4):696–703.

26. Shapiro M, McDonald AA. The role of repeat angiography in the management of pelvic fractures. *J Trauma.* 2005;58(2):227–231.

27. Thorson CM, Ryan ML, Otero CA, et al. Operating room or angiography suite for hemodynamically unstable pelvic fractures? *J Trauma Acute Care Surg.* 2012;72(2):364–370. discussion 371–362.

28. Chu CH, Tennakoon L. Trends in the management of pelvic fractures, 2008-2010. *J Surg Res.* 2016;202(2):335–340.

29. Marzi I, Lustenberger T. Management of bleeding pelvic fractures. *Scand J Surg.* 2014;103(2):104–111.

30. Lustenberger T, Wutzler S. The role of angio-embolization in the acute treatment concept of severe pelvic ring injuries. *Injury.* 2015;46(suppl 4):S33–S38.

31. Bakhshayesh P, Boutefnouchet T. Effectiveness of non invasive external pelvic compression: a systematic review of the literature. *Scand J Trauma Resusc Emerg Med.* 2016;24(1). 73.

32. Pizanis A, Pohlemann T. Emergency stabilization of the pelvic ring: clinical comparison between three different techniques. *Injury.* 2013;44(12):1760–1764.

33. Prasarn ML, Small J. Does application position of the T-POD affect stability of pelvic fractures? *J Orthop Trauma.* 2013;27(5):262–266.

34. Stahel PF, Mauffrey C, Smith WR, et al. External fixation for acute pelvic ring injuries: decision making and technical options. *J Trauma Acute Care Surg.* 2013;75(5):882–887.

35. Halawi MJ. Pelvic ring injuries: Emergency assessment and management. *J Clin Orthop Trauma.* 2015;6(4):252–258.

36. Poenaru DV, Popescu M. Emergency pelvic stabilization in patients with pelvic posttraumatic instability. *Int Orthop.* 2015;39(5):961–965.

37. Rommens PM, Hofmann A. Management of acute hemorrhage in pelvic trauma: an overview. *Eur J Trauma Emerg Surg.* 2010;36(2):91–99.

38. Burgess A. Invited commentary: Young-Burgess classification of pelvic ring fractures: does it predict mortality, transfusion requirements, and non-orthopaedic injuries? *J Orthop Trauma.* 2010;24(10):609.
39. Koller H, Keil P. Individual and team training with first time users of the Pelvic C-Clamp: do they remember or will we need refresher trainings? *Arch Orthop Trauma Surg.* 2013;133(3):343–349.
40. Kim FJ, Pompeo A, Sehrt D, et al. Early effectiveness of endoscopic posterior urethra primary alignment. *J Trauma Acute Care Surg.* 2013;75:189–194.
41. Hak DJ, Baran S. Sacral fractures: current strategies in diagnosis and management. *Orthopedics.* 2009;32:752–757.

CHAPTER 31

UPPER URINARY TRACT INJURIES

Rodrigo Donalisio da Silva, MD, Fernando J. Kim, MD, MBA, FACS

1. **What is the most common type of renal trauma in the United States, blunt or penetrating?**
   Approximately 90% of renal injuries are caused by blunt mechanism in the United States.

2. **Why are pediatric patients more susceptible to major renal injuries?**
   Pediatric patients have weaker abdominal muscle, less ossified thoracic cage, decreased perirenal fat, and increased renal size in relation to the rest of the body.

3. **When should a patient be investigated for renal trauma?**
   All blunt trauma patients with gross hematuria or those with shock and microscopic hematuria should be investigated for renal injuries. For penetrating trauma, all patients with hematuria (gross or microscopic) should be investigated.

4. **When does one suspect renal trauma?**
   The mechanism of injury and physical examination will raise the suspicion for renal trauma. Flank ecchymosis, location of penetrating wounds, associated injuries (e.g., rib fracture), gross hematuria, and hypovolemic shock are things associated with renal injuries. Patients with anatomic renal abnormalities (e.g., hydronephrosis, ureteropelvic junction obstruction, ectopic kidney) can have hematuria out of proportion to the history of renal trauma. Injury to the renal hilum can cause little or no hematuria despite a severe injury.

5. **What imaging study is the best to evaluate renal trauma?**
   Computerized axial tomography (CAT) scan of the abdomen and pelvis with intravenous (IV) contrast is the best image modality to investigate renal trauma. Delayed images (excretory phase) should be performed to delineate the collecting system and ureters.

6. **When do you perform a single-shot intravenous pyelogram (IVP)?**
   The single-shot IVP can be used in patients when a CAT scan could not be performed before surgical exploration (e.g., shock). This image study is not adequate to diagnose and classify renal and ureteral injuries; however, it can help to determine the presence of contralateral kidney. A single film is taken 10 minutes after the administration of 2 mg/kg of contrast (max 150 mg).

7. **How do you classify renal trauma?**
   - Grade I: Subcapsular hematoma and/or contusion
   - Grade II: Laceration <1 cm in depth and into cortex, small hematoma contained in the Gerota's fascia. Nonexpanding perirenal hematoma
   - Grade III: Laceration >1 cm in depth and into cortex, small hematoma contained in the Gerota's fascia. Nonexpanding perirenal hematoma
   - Grade IV: Laceration extends to renal pelvis or urinary extravasation, vascular injury to main renal artery or vein with contained hemorrhage, segmental infarctions without associated lacerations, expanding subcapsular hematomas compressing the kidney
   - Grade V: Shattered kidney or avulsion of renal hilum

8. **What are the different types of renal hilum trauma?**
   The main renal vessels can be interrupted by thrombosis or avulsion. In both instances, there will be no contrast enhancing the injured kidney in the CAT scan with IV contrast. Hematuria may not be present in these cases. The renal artery injury is often stretched with blunt trauma and an intimal flap may cause obstruction and ischemia. Main renal artery trauma with intimal flap can be successfully managed with arterial endovascular stent placement by interventional radiology.

9. **How long can a nonperfused kidney tolerate warm ischemia?**
   If the injured kidney had normal function, irreversible damage to the kidney can happen after 30 minutes. After 8 hours of ischemia, renal salvage is minimal.

10. **How is renal trauma managed?**
    Hemodynamically stable patients with blunt renal injury can be managed nonoperatively in 98% of cases. Unstable patients with high-grade renal trauma (grade IV and V) and patients with severe urine leakage or lack of clinical progression (severe abdominal distension with severe pain due to ileus, hematoma, and/or urine leakage) are more prone to renal exploration. Arterial stent placement and segmental embolization of the kidney can be performed successfully by interventional radiologists and a moderate urine leak may be treated with ureteral stents.

11. **Is surgery recommended for most traumatic renal injuries?**
    No. Conservative treatment is the most common treatment for renal trauma. Surgical exploration is necessary in only 2% of patients.

12. **What is the significance of delayed gross hematuria?**
    Hematuria that occurs 3–4 weeks after the trauma may be due to arteriovenous fistula formation. When conservative treatments fail, arterial embolization is the appropriate next step. Rarely, partial or total nephrectomy is required in these cases.

13. **How do you manage unexpected retroperitoneal bleeding during exploratory laparotomy?**
    Pulsatile or expanding retroperitoneal hematomas suggest a major vascular injury. The surgeon may gain vascular control (both proximal and distal) prior to the exploration of the retroperitoneum or attain manual renal parenchymal compression while the assistant evacuates the hematoma and dissection of vasculature is possible. Often, acute arterial bleeding is followed by arterial spasm and contraction, while venous bleeding can be continuous. Stable hematomas may be left unexplored if preoperative images are not concerning. It is recommended to involve the urological team prior to the surgical exploration of hematomas to increase the chance of renal salvage and reconstruction.

14. **What are the treatment options for urinary leakage after renal trauma?**
    Urinary extravasation usually does not require surgical intervention. Initially these patients should be managed with bladder drainage to decompress the upper urinary tract. In cases of penetrating injury and gunshot trauma, the ureter can suffer a blast effect that can result in delayed urine extravasation in 48–72 hours, with urinoma formation. In these cases, ureteral stents with or without percutaneous drainage of the urine collection can effectively manage this injury. Surgical repair should be reserved for patients who failed minimally invasive treatments.

15. **What is conservative treatment of traumatic renal injuries?**
    Bedrest until gross hematuria is improved. Drainage of the bladder in cases of urinary extravasation. Monitoring of vital signs, hemoglobin, hematocrit, and urinary output. After hospital discharge, microscopic hematuria can take months to resolve. Blood pressure should be monitored, and urine analysis. Follow-up imaging should be considered for symptomatic patients and/or high-grade renal injury.

16. **What is the likelihood of subsequent hypertension in patients with renal trauma?**
    Posttraumatic hypertension can occur in <2% of renal trauma patients. The onset usually occurs in the first several months of the trauma. The mechanism of posttraumatic hypertension is renin mediated and can be a result of renal artery stenosis or occlusion, renal parenchyma compression, and posttraumatic arteriovenous fistula. Acute hypertension may occur in cases of "Page kidney" due to large retroperitoneal hematoma with or without urine leak that compresses the kidney.

17. **What are the most common causes of ureteral injuries?**
    The ureter is injured in <2.5% of traumas caused by external violence. The most common cause of ureteral injury is iatrogenic and external violence. The ureter can be compromised in around 3% of gunshot wounds to the abdomen. Iatrogenic injuries to the ureters can occur due to ligation with suture, hemostatic clamp, thermal injury, and/or endoscopic injuries (ureteroscopies).

18. **How do I evaluate and identify ureteral injuries?**
    In external violence patients with penetrating injuries, gross hematuria can be present. In stable patients, CAT-IVP can identify the injury showing contrast extravasation. In unstable patients that need exploratory laparotomy, a suspicion for ureteral injury should indicate exploration of the ureter. Indigo

carmine (1 vial IV in bolus) can be used to check for urinary extravasation. Retrograde pyelogram can be performed in the operating room to identify ureteral injuries.

19. **What are the complications of a missed ureteral injury?**
Urinary leakage and the formation of urinoma can lead to fever, leukocytosis, azotemia, pain, ileus, or urinary extravasation through the laparotomy incision.

20. **What is the treatment of ureteral injuries?**
The management of ureteral injuries will depend on the location (proximal, mid, or distal ureter), trauma mechanism (iatrogenic, high energy, stab, avulsion), and complete or partial tear of the ureter. Surgical options will be endoscopic ureteral stent placement, primary excision and anastomosis, ureteral reimplantation (distal ureter) with or without psoas hitch and/or Boari flap, or autotransplant. The surgical technique will be determined by the ureteral lesion and location, surgeon's preference, and patient's clinical stability.

KEY POINTS: UPPER URINARY TRACT INJURIES

1. The vast majority of renal injuries are caused by blunt trauma.
2. Hematuria workup should be performed for all patients with gross hematuria or those with microscopic hematuria and cystolic blood pressure <90 mmHg.
3. CAT scan of the abdomen and pelvis with IV contrast and delayed image is the best image modality to investigate renal trauma.
4. Conservative management can be performed in up to 80% of patients with renal trauma.
5. Urine extravastion can initially be managed conservatively.

BIBLIOGRAPHY

1. Baker LA, Silver RI, Docimo SG. Cryptorchidism. In: Gearhart JP, Rink RC, eds. *Pediatric Urology.* Philadelphia: WB Saunders; 2001:738–753.
2. Siomos VJ, Sehrt D. Surgical treatment of kidney and urinary tract trauma. In: Di Saverio S, Tugnoli Gregorio, eds. *Trauma Surgery: Volume 2: Thoracic and Abdominal Trauma.* Milano: Springer-Verlag; 2014.
3. Kim FJ. Genito-urinary trauma. In: Moore EE, Feliciano DV, eds. *Trauma.* 8th ed. (in press).
4. Morey A, Brandes S, Dugi III D, et al. Urotrauma: AUA Guideline. *J Urol.* 2014;192(2). 327–335.
5. Pompeo A, Molina WR, Sehrt D, et al. Laparoscopic ureteroneocystostomy for ureteral injuries after hysterectomy. *JSLS.* 2013;17(1):121–125.
6. Serafetinides E, Kitrey ND, Djakovic N, et al. Review of the current management of upper urinary tract injuries by the EAU Trauma Guidelines Panel. *Eur Urol.* 2015;67(5):930–936.
7. Shariat SF, Trinh QD, Morey AF, et al. Development of a highly accurate nomogram for prediction of the need for exploration in patients with renal trauma. *J Trauma.* 2008;64(6):1451–1458.

CHAPTER 32

LOWER URINARY TRACT INJURY AND PELVIC TRAUMA

Rodrigo Donalisio da Silva, MD, Fernando J. Kim, MD, MBA, FACS

1. **What are the causes of bladder injury?**
   Bladder injury can be caused by trauma or iatrogenic manipulation. Traumatic bladder injuries can be classified as intraperitoneal or extraperitoneal, blunt or penetrating. The most common sign of bladder injury is gross hematuria. Other signs of bladder injury are pelvic pain, inability to void, or incomplete recovery of catheter irrigation.

2. **What types of bladder injury may occur with blunt trauma?**
   Blunt trauma to the bladder can cause bladder contusion or intraperitoneal or extraperitoneal bladder rupture. Gross hematuria with normal cystography in the absence of upper tract injuries defines bladder contusion. Extraperitoneal injury is the most common bladder injury. Usually it is located at the bladder base. Extraperitoneal injuries can be managed conservatively with bladder drainage with a Foley catheter for 7–10 days. Intraperitoneal bladder ruptures usually occur at the bladder dome, caused by a blunt trauma in a distended bladder. These lesions should be repaired surgically using a two-layer closure with absorbable suture and bladder drainage with a Foley catheter for 7–10 days. Before removing the Foley catheter, a computerized axial tomography (CAT) cystogram should be performed to confirm proper bladder healing.

3. **What is the likelihood of a bladder injury in patients with a fractured pelvis?**
   Extraperitoneal bladder injury occurs in 10% of all pelvic fractures. Conversely, approximately 85% of blunt bladder injury is associated with pelvic fracture. Bladder injuries occur more often with parasymphyseal pubic arch fractures and more often with bilateral than unilateral fractures. Isolated ramus fractures produce bladder laceration in 10% of cases.

4. **How is bladder injury evaluated?**
   CAT cystography provides diagnostic accuracy when performed with the bladder filled with 300–400 mL of 50% diluted contrast agent using the Foley catheter under gravity. If CAT scan is not available, voiding cystogram should be performed with postvoid images.

5. **What are the retrograde cystourethrographic patterns of bladder injury?**
   Bladder contusion has a normal cystography in the presence of gross hematuria and absence of upper urinary tract injury. In the extraperitoneal bladder rupture, contrast is seen adjacent and confined to the bladder base. In intraperitoneal bladder rupture, the contrast extravasation is seen at the dome of the bladder, usually delineating bowel loops, or collected in the gutters.

6. **How is bladder rupture managed?**
   Bladder contusion requires drainage until gross hematuria is resolved. Extraperitoneal rupture can be managed conservatively with indwelling catheter for 7–10 days. If laparotomy is performed, bladder injury can be repaired. Intraperitoneal bladder injuries should be managed surgically. In selected cases, laparoscopic repair can be performed. Cystography should be performed to confirm resolution of extravasation before removing the catheter (approximately 14 days after injury and drainage).

7. **When should you suspect urethral injury?**
   The presence of blood in the urethral meatus associated with trauma mechanism (straddle injury, trauma to the genitals, pelvic fracture). Penile, scrotal swelling and ecchymosis, inability to void, and inability to pass a urethral catheter should be investigated for urethral injury. In males, digital rectal exam can reveal total disruption of the urethra when the prostate is not palpable. In females, urethral disruption results from severe mechanism of injury, and it is associated with high mortality.

8. **When patients present with pelvic fracture, is concomitant urethral injury a major concern?**

Yes. Concomitant urethral injury occurs in approximately 10% of patients with pelvic fracture. It is more common in anterior disruption of the pelvic ring. Unilateral fracture is associated with 20% of urethral injury and bilateral fractures, 50%.

9. **How are urethral injuries diagnosed?**

Retrograde urethrography (RUG) must be performed in all cases that a urethral injury is suspected. Incomplete urethral disruption will demonstrate contrast extravasation in the urethra with bladder opacification. Total disruption of the urethra will show extensive contrast extravasation, and the bladder will not receive much or any contrast.

10. **How is urethral injury managed?**

Incomplete urethral transection can be managed by catheter stenting across the injury. This should be performed by a urologist who will use cystoscopy to pass a guide wire up to the bladder. A council tip Foley catheter will be passed using the guide wire. Complete transection of the urethra can be managed with early endoscopic urethral realignment when possible. Diversion by suprapubic cystostomy should be used when primary realignment fails or when the patient is too unstable to proceed with primary realignment. Patients often require some type of surgical reconstruction or dilatation of the urethra.

11. **What are the complications of urethral injury?**

The most common long-term complication of urethral injury is urethral stricture. Erectile dysfunction can occur in posterior total urethral disruption associated with pelvic fracture.

12. **What is the differential diagnosis of blunt scrotal trauma?**

Testicular rupture, hematocele, scrotal hematoma, intratesticular hematoma, and testicular torsion. Ultrasonography is a helpful diagnostic tool to differentiate among the possible diagnoses.

13. **What is the sonographic sign of testicular rupture?**

The loss of the normal homogeneous echo texture of the testicle, with areas of hyperechogenicity or hypoechogenicity.

14. **How is testicular rupture managed?**

When suspicious for testicular rupture in the ultrasonography, surgical exploration should be performed. Debridement of the extruded, nonviable testicular tissue should be performed, followed by tunica albuginea repair. Evacuation of the hematoma and careful hemostasis should be performed. Some cases will require orchiectomy because of the lack of viable remaining testicular tissue.

15. **What is the most common cause of penile fracture?**

Sexual intercourse or aggressive masturbation is associated with penile fracture. Rupture of the corpus cavernosum occurs when abnormally forced bending of the erect penis. A popping sound followed by immediate penis detumescence is frequently reported by patients.

16. **What are the physical examination findings in a patient with penile fracture?**

Hematoma and penile deviation of the penile shaft to the opposite side of the rupture. The hematoma will be confined to the penis (eggplant deformity) if the Buck's fascia is intact. Rupture of the Buck's fascia will cause hematoma in the perineum and abdominal wall because the blood will spread under the Colle's and Scarpa's fascia.

17. **How do you treat a penile fracture?**

Treatment of penile fracture is surgical repair. The penile shaft should be exposed by degloving the penis to identify the defect(s). Concomitant urethral injury can occur in up to 20% of the cases. RUG should be performed if urethral injury is suspected.

18. **In penile amputation injuries, how should the amputated portion of the penis be preserved for transport?**

The amputated portion of the penis should be wrapped in saline-soaked gauze and placed in a sealed sterile bag, and then the bag containing the protected penis is placed in an ice-slush bath (double-bag procedure). The ice should not be in direct contact with the penis. Penile reimplantation should be performed within the first 24 hours.

19. **How do you manage a major scrotal loss?**
    If primary repair is not possible, meshed split-thickness grafts may be used to cover the testis. When delayed repair is necessary, thigh pouches can be created until permanent reconstruction is feasible.

20. **What are the most common causes of vesicovaginal fistulas?**
    Obstetric (prolonged childbirth), trauma, and iatrogenic. Vesicovaginal fistula presents clinically as urinary leakage through the vagina.

21. **What is the best time to repair a vesicovaginal fistula secondary to an uncomplicated hysterectomy?**
    Although 3–6 months after injury has been recommended in the past, early repair can be successful if there is minimal inflammation and there is no complicating factors. Repair can be done with open surgery, laparoscopy, or vaginal approach.

KEY POINTS: LOWER URINARY TRACT INJURY AND PELVIC TRAUMA

1. Extraperitoneal bladder rupture can be managed with urinary Foley catheter only.
2. Intraperitoneal bladder rupture should be managed with surgical repair.
3. Urethral injuries should be diagnosed with RUG and managed with urinary catheter acutely.
4. Penile fracture should be managed surgically.
5. Testicular injuries should be managed surgically.

BIBLIOGRAPHY

1. Kim FJ, Chammas Jr MF. Laparoscopic management of intraperitoneal bladder rupture secondary to blunt abdominal trauma using intracorporeal single layer suturing technique. *J Trauma.* 2008;65(1):234–236.
2. Kim FJ, Pompeo A, Sehrt D, et al. Early effectiveness of endoscopic posterior urethra primary alignment. *J Trauma Acute Care Surg.* 2013;75(2):189–194.
3. Lumen N, Kuehhas FE, Djakovic N, et al. Review of the current management of lower urinary tract injuries by the EAU Trauma Guidelines Panel. *Eur Urol.* 2015;67(5):925 929.
4. Kim FJ. Genito-urinary Trauma. In: Moore EE, Feliciano DV, eds. *Trauma*, 8th ed. McGraw Hill. (in press).
5. Morey AF, Brandes S, Dugi DD, et al. Urotrauma: AUA guideline. *J Urol.* 2014;192(2):327–335.

CHAPTER 33

EXTREMITY VASCULAR INJURIES

Steven R. Shackford, MD, FACS

1. **What is the pathophysiology of extremity vascular injury?**
   Peripheral arteries are composed of three layers: outer adventitia, central muscular, and inner endothelial, or intima. Trauma, either blunt or penetrating, can produce hemorrhage (from laceration or puncture), thrombosis (from intimal disruption and exposure of the subendothelial matrix), or spasm—either alone or in combination. The intima is the least compliant of the vascular layers, and it fractures when the more flexible layers bend when deformed by an adjacent broken bone or joint dislocation. The injured intima may form a flap that can prolapse into the arterial lumen as a result of the forward blood flow dissecting under it. Penetrating injuries produce focal injury, while blunt injuries tend to be diffuse and injure not only the vascular structures but also the adjacent bone, muscle, and nerves. This adjacent tissue contains small, unnamed vessels or collaterals that are often injured in diffuse blunt trauma, thus exaggerating any existing ischemia. Transection of a vessel causes it to retract in spasm, which usually stops or reduces bleeding, but results in a hematoma, sometimes of large proportions. Puncture of an artery produces hemorrhage and a large hematoma, eventually tamponaded by surrounding tissue, but producing a pseudoaneurysm. Intimal prolapse may produce dissection and eventual thrombosis. Finally, injury to an artery and a vein in close proximity produces a local hematoma and eventually a pathologic connection between them—an arteriovenous fistula. These pathologies (hemorrhage, ischemia, thrombosis, pseudoaneurysm, and arteriovenous fistula) and their consequences should be considered in the diagnosis as one approaches a patient with extremity vascular injury.

2. **Which are the most commonly injured arteries in the upper and lower extremity?**
   In the upper extremity, the brachial artery is most frequently injured, primarily because of its length and relative exposure to harm. The forearm arteries (radial and ulnar) are next most common, followed by the axillary and the subclavian. In the lower extremity, the most frequently injured artery is the superficial femoral, followed by the popliteal. The leg arteries (tibials and peroneal) and the common femoral are infrequently injured.

3. **What orthopedic injuries commonly have associated vascular injuries?**
   There are several orthopedic injuries that mandate an arterial assessment because they are associated with arterial injuries, which, not infrequently, are missed. These are a supracondylar fracture of the humerus, an anterior or posterior dislocation of the knee and midshaft, or a supracondylar fracture of the femur.

4. **How does one proceed with the evaluation of a patient with suspected vascular injury of the extremity? What are the physical findings or signs of vascular injury?**
   As with every trauma patient, the sequence follows that prescribed by the Advanced Trauma Life Support program. If the patient is in shock or extremis, treatment precedes evaluation. It is imperative that patients in shock are resuscitated to the endpoint of a palpable peripheral pulse in an uninjured extremity. If possible, the following information (obtained from the patient and/or prehospital providers) is helpful in managing a patients with a potential vascular injury: time of injury, amount of blood loss visible at the scene, mechanism of injury, initial vital signs, and trends in vital signs. After the primary survey is completed, the secondary survey for extremity arterial injury must include the following (for both the injured and uninjured extremity for comparison): neurologic exam (including motor and sensory), proximal and distal pulse examination, and assessment of capillary refill. The "hard" signs (in this context "hard" does not mean difficult to ascertain, but firm or solid) of vascular injury are pulsatile bleeding, expanding hematoma, palpable thrill, audible bruit (assessed distal to the injury), and evidence of regional ischemia (the six Ps: pain, pallor, poikilothermia, paralysis, paresthesia, and pulselessness). One might think of the acronym "hard" as *hardly a reasonable doubt* that

a vascular injury is present. "Soft" signs are less firm and *suggest* the presence of a vascular injury: diminished but present pulse (diminished compared to the uninjured extremity), large but stable hematoma, injury to a peripheral nerve that is anatomically adjacent to a major artery, penetrating wound in the proximity of a major extremity artery, and history of moderate blood loss. The presence of "hard" signs reliably indicates the need for surgical therapy. The presence of "soft" signs indicates the need for additional diagnostics.

5. **What diagnostic measures should be pursued when "soft" signs are present?**
In addition to a well-done repeat secondary survey (see above), in the presence of a reduced or diminished pulse (compared to the uninjured limb in a resuscitated patient), one must perform an arterial pressure (systolic) index (API) comparing the injured limb to the uninjured limb. This is done using an appropriately sized sphygmomanometer cuff and a continuous wave (handheld Doppler device). The cuff should be placed just above the site of the injury. An artery distal to the injury is interrogated with the Doppler transducer, and the cuff **slowly** inflated until the Doppler signal can no longer be heard. The pressure at which the signal disappears as the cuff is slowly inflated is recorded and compared to the uninjured extremity with the cuff in a similar position. Using the systolic pressure in the injured limb as the numerator and the systolic pressure in the uninjured limb as the denominator, the API is calculated. An API of >0.9 can reliably rule out an arterial injury (API of <0.9 has a sensitivity of 95% and specificity of 97% for major arterial injury; an API >0.9 has a negative predictive value of 99%). However, repeated follow-up is strongly advised. For the other "soft" signs, imaging is necessary and is best done with a computed tomography (CT) arteriogram, which, for several reasons, has replaced catheter-based arteriography. Catheter-based arteriography can itself produce an arterial injury. Arteriography, at best, can provide biplanar or oblique images that are certainly helpful, but they may still miss occult injuries and definitely increase the dye load. CT angiograms require only a single venous dye injection and can provide not only coronal, sagittal, and axial views but also three-dimensional reconstructions that can be rotated and magnified to better view an area of interest. CT angiograms are less costly and can be performed much more quickly than catheter-based arteriography. The only potential limitation of CT angiography is the diffraction produced by metallic fragments that can overlie a possible injury.

6. **What abnormalities on CT angiography determine a positive test result?**
The following are considered to be "positive" findings: obstruction of flow, extravasation of contrast, early venous filling (suggesting arteriovenous fistula), contrast in a contained hematoma (pseudoaneurysm), intimal defect, and focal narrowing (spasm). It is absolutely imperative that the surgeon caring for the patient carefully review the images because what the radiologist reports may not have clinical significance. For example, obstruction of flow in a branch of a major nutrient artery (such as the profunda femoris) will not be symptomatic nor should it be treated. Other examples include the intimal defect, which can heal without producing symptoms, and spasm, which will usually resolve with simple observation.

7. **What is the most effective way to control arterial bleeding in an injured extremity?**
In the prehospital arena and in the emergency room, hemorrhage is best controlled with a **correctly applied** tourniquet. If not correctly applied, it will not control hemorrhage. If loosely applied, arterial flow continues, but the loose tourniquet obstructs venous outflow, thereby increasing hemorrhage. Attempts at controlling bleeding in the emergency room by the direct application of clamps is discouraged as a misplaced clamp can further damage the artery or an adjacent nerve.

8. **How should a patient with an extremity vascular injury be prepared and draped in the operating room?**
The entire involved extremity should be circumferentially prepped and draped into the sterile field. An uninjured lower extremity should also be circumferentially prepped and draped for the possible harvesting of greater or lesser saphenous vein for conduit. Injuries involving the proximal thigh or the shoulder must have the ipsilateral upper chest or lower abdomen prepped for proximal control, if needed.

9. **What are the operative principles for the repair of vascular injuries?**
The **first step** is obtaining proximal control. This must be done utilizing the incisions that are used for elective cases. It is inadvisable to directly approach the injury without proximal vascular control as it increases blood loss and does not save any time. Occasionally, if obtaining proximal control is hindered by anatomic structures such as the inguinal ligament or the angle of the mandible, a Fogarty

balloon catheter with a three-way stopcock can be inserted and the balloon inflated. This will allow the time necessary to dissect the proximal artery to provide sufficient area to apply a clamp or vessel loop and repair the artery in question. Once proximal control is obtained and there is no evidence of cavitary hemorrhage or brain injury, systemic heparinization should be considered. The **second step** is to obtain distal control—again staying away from the area of injury, if possible. The **third step** is to assess the injuries and plan accordingly. The primary considerations are the time since injury, the nature of the arterial injury, and the nature of the associated injuries to bone and soft tissue. If there is complete occlusion of the artery and signs of ischemia were present on arrival, reperfusion of the distal extremity becomes the priority. This can be done with insertion of a temporary vascular shunt (see below). The **fourth step** is debridement of the artery back to uninjured tissue. If possible, leave the injured back wall of the artery intact as dividing it will cause both ends of the vessel to retract. After debridement and appropriate preparation, temporarily unclamp proximally first and then distally to assure there is antegrade and retrograde bleeding. Then pass a Fogarty catheter both proximally and distally to assure there is no residual thrombus either proximally or distally. After passing the catheter, inject heparinized saline into both the proximal and distal ends. The **fifth step** is repair, which can be done with a primary arteriography, patch angioplasty, end-to-end anastomosis (without tension), or interposition grafting. The **sixth step** is assessment of the repair by checking for the presence of a distal pulse, interrogating both inflow and outflow with a continuous wave Doppler, or intraoperative arteriography. One or all may be chosen and the result(s) documented. The **final step** is coverage of the repair with vascularized tissue.

10. What is the best conduit to use for extremity vascular injuries if primary repair is not possible?
    Greater or lesser saphenous should be the primary choice. Cephalic vein from the uninjured extremity is also feasible; however, it lacks the muscular coat of the lower extremity veins and can become aneurysmal with time. In the absence of the primary venous choices, prosthetic grafts (polytetrafluoroethylene [PTFE, heparin bonded] is recommended) have been used in the larger major peripheral arteries (i.e., common femoral, superficial femoral, and subclavian).

11. Should injuries to major veins of the extremities be repaired?
    If the patient is stable, repair of major veins should be undertaken because repair of the vein enhances the success of a concomitant arterial repair by improving outflow. This is most applicable to popliteal venous injuries. The types of procedures used in repairing arterial injuries are also applicable to venous repairs—venorrhaphy, end-to-end anastomosis, and interposition grafting. The choice of conduit is dependent on the size of the vein. For the popliteal artery greater saphenous vein is the conduit of choice. For larger veins, such as the common femoral, heparin bonded, externally supported PTFE is recommended. Late thrombosis often occurs after venous repair, but this initial patency allows collateral circulation to develop. This may also reduce the incidence of postoperative venous insufficiency.

12. When should injured major veins be ligated?
    Major veins should be ligated rather than repaired when the patient is hemodynamically unstable.

13. What complications can develop after ligation of major extremity veins?
    Possible complications include rapid increase in muscle compartment pressure, leading to compromised venous or arterial flow and compartment syndrome (see question 14). Postoperative venous stasis may also occur, which can be attenuated with intermittent pneumatic calf compression and leg elevation.

14. What is compartment syndrome?
    Compartment syndrome is characterized by increased tissue pressure as a result of swelling (edema combined with vascular congestion) within a compartment. The increase in tissue pressure initially impairs substrate diffusion from the capillary into the interstitium, reduces venous return and, eventually, arterial inflow. In the extremity, the muscular fascial envelopes combine with bone to form nondistensible compartments.

15. What is the most common cause of an extremity compartment syndrome?
    An extremity compartment syndrome most commonly occurs following reperfusion of a previously ischemic limb. Ischemia depletes intracellular energy stores, and reperfusion leads to the generation of toxic free radicals, causing cellular swelling and interstitial fluid accumulation. Compartment syndrome of the leg can occur with a fibular or tibial fracture and associated swelling.

16. **What is the earliest sign of compartment syndrome after vascular repair of an extremity? How is the objective diagnosis of compartment syndrome made? What is the treatment?**
    The initial sign is loss of light touch sensation (sensory nerves appear to be the most sensitive to anoxia as the compartment becomes more swollen). This is followed by weakness and considerable pain on active or passive movement of the limb. On exam, the compartment is firm to the touch. Distal pulses are usually normal. The diagnosis is made by measuring compartment pressures with a percutaneous needle and pressure transducer. A tissue pressure of >25–30 torr confirms the diagnosis and mandates fasciotomy. The treatment is emergency fasciotomy with complete decompression of the compartment.

17. **What is the result of untreated compartment syndrome?**
    Untreated compartment syndrome results in myonecrosis within the compartment and the subsequent release of myoglobin into the circulation. Myoglobin is cleared by the kidney and can precipitate in the acid milieu of the nephron leading to acute renal failure.

18. **In an injured extremity with concomitant fracture and vascular injury, which repair should be performed first?**
    This does present a dilemma, but it is easily resolved with the use of a temporary silastic shunt that can be easily and quickly inserted to reestablish blood flow in the ischemic extremity. Such shunts are commercially available or can be constructed from sterile intravenous tubing for smaller diameter vessels (i.e., superficial femoral artery) or pediatric chest tubes for larger vessels (i.e., common femoral or iliac). After obtaining proximal and distal control, the shunt is carefully inserted into the appropriately prepared proximal vessel (proximal and distal control should be obtained using vessel loops rather than a clamp so that the shunt can easily pass). Once inserted proximally, the vessel is allowed to "bleed," assuring that the shunt is in the lumen and there are no obstructions to flow. It is then carefully inserted into the distal vessel. After insertion, flow is assessed with the continuous wave Doppler proximally and distally and then tied in place proximally and distally. The orthopedist can now proceed with fracture fixation, but must be mindful of the presence of the shunt. If possible, the trauma surgeon can harvest conduit from an uninjured lower extremity while the orthopedic procedure is ongoing. Shunt patency should be intermittently assessed. When the orthopedic repair is completed the vascular repair can be performed. Shunts have a low complication rate and can have extended dwell times with or without heparinization.

19. **After reducing or fixing an extremity fracture, what must you always do?**
    Evaluate the distal pulses to ensure adequate vascular inflow (especially if fixation or any manipulation follows a vascular repair).

20. **What is damage control vascular surgery and when is it indicated?**
    Damage control is reserved for a patient with a vascular injury who is hemodynamically unstable, hypothermic, acidotic, and coagulopathic. In this case, a temporary vascular shunt (see question 18) is inserted to reestablish flow to the distal extremity. Wounds are expeditiously packed and the patient is taken to the intensive care unit for physiologic resuscitation and rewarming. The shunt is left in place until the metabolic problems are corrected and the patient stabilized. After that occurs, definitive vascular repair can be undertaken.

21. **What is the likely diagnosis in a patient with repetitive palmar trauma and finger ischemia or necrosis?**
    The most likely diagnosis is hypothenar hammer syndrome, which is produced by repetitively using the palm of the hand as a blunt instrument. It occasionally coexists with palmar artery fibrodysplasia. (The arteriogram shows digital artery occlusions with segmental ulnar artery occlusion or "corkscrew" elongation.) (See Fig. 33.1.)

22. **What are the complications of a percutaneous closure device?**
    Percutaneous closure devices are used following catheter-based diagnostic and therapeutic procedures. Complications include thrombosis of the access artery (due to the device "catching" the posterior wall of the artery), distal emboli from the access site, and pseudoaneurysm formation due to incomplete closure.

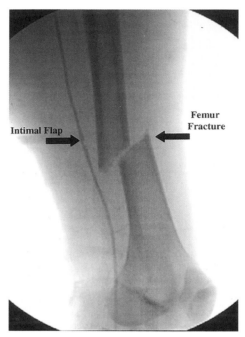

Fig. 33.1 Angiography demonstrating intimal flap in superficial femoral artery associated with femur fracture.

KEY POINTS: DIAGNOSIS AND MANAGEMENT OF PERIPHERAL VASCULAR INJURY

1. Assessment of a patient with a potential vascular injury must include a physical examination of the injured and uninjured extremity following resuscitation.
2. Hard signs indicate the presence of a vascular injury; soft signs suggest the presence of a vascular injury and the need for additional testing.
3. Arterial vascular imaging is best done with CT angiography, except when metal fragments overlie the area of injury.
4. The optimal conduit for interposition grafting is autogenous greater saphenous vein.
5. Extremity compartment syndrome following a vascular injury is the result of ischemia followed by reperfusion; it can also occur in the leg following blunt injury without vascular compromise.
6. Complications of compartment syndrome include amputation and acute renal failure.
7. The treatment of compartment syndrome is emergency complete fasciotomy.
8. Temporary vascular shunts are useful in combined vascular and orthopedic injuries and for reestablishing perfusion when damage control is necessary.

WEBSITES

- www.east.org/tpg/lepene.pdf
- https://westerntrauma.org/algorithms/algorithms.html

BIBLIOGRAPHY

1. Sise MJ, Shackford SR. Peripheral vascular injury. In: Moore EE, Feliciano DV, eds. *Trauma*. 7th ed. New York, NY: McGraw Hill Medical; 2013:816–849.
2. Ode G, Studnek J. Emergency tourniquets for civilians: can military lessons in extremity hemorrhage be translated? *J Trauma Acute Care Surg*. 2015;79(4):586–591.
3. Inaba K, Siboni S, Resnick S, et al. Tourniquet use for civilian extremity trauma. *J Trauma Acute Care Surg*. 2015;79(2):232–237.
4. Inaba K, Hand A, Seamon MJ, et al. Multicenter evaluation of temporary vascular shunts in vascular injury. *J Trauma Acute Care Surg*. 2016;80(3):359–365.
5. Sise MJ, Shackford SR. Extremity vascular trauma. In: Rich NM, Mattox K, eds. *Vascular Trauma*. 2nd ed. Philadelphia, PA: Elsevier Saunders; 2004:353–389.
6. Palacios FS, Rathbun SW. Medical treatment of postthrombotic syndrome. *Semin Intervent Radiol*. 2017;34:61–67.
7. Mathew S, Smith BP, Cannon JW, et al. Temporary arterial shunts in damage control: experience and outcomes. *J Trauma Acute Care Surg*. 2017;82:512–517.

CHAPTER 34

FACIAL LACERATIONS

Karen K. Lo, MD, David W. Mathes, MD, FACS

1. **What distinguishes facial lacerations from other?**

   After facial trauma, restoration of the appearance of the face is of the utmost concern. Successful primary closure of a facial laceration can be best achieved with irrigation, minimal debridement, gentle handling of the tissue, and eversion of the skin edges. Adherence to these principles gives the best chance for the least noticeable scar.

   The face has abundant blood supply, when compared to the rest of the body. Thus, lacerations on the face should be closed even after more than 6 hours from injury. Furthermore, as the face has laxity of skin, most wounds may be primarily repaired. In the majority of cases, the use of local flaps should be avoided immediately after injury and once the wound is stable used in a secondary procedure.

2. **How do you anesthetize a wound for repair?**

   If the wound is small, lidocaine with epinephrine may be injected into the wound directly. However, the infusion may distort the anatomy.

   For larger wounds, the following nerve blocks may be performed. The advantage of this technique is that it allows adequate analgesia without the confounding distortion/edema of a local infusion. One must be careful to not inject the nerves directly, and remember to withdraw while inserting. The following are the nerve blocks for the face:

   - **Mental nerve block (for ipsilateral lower lip and the chin):** The mental nerve is a branch of the inferior alveolar nerve, which is a branch of cranial nerve (CN) V3. The mental nerve exits the mental foramen, which is usually located at the second premolar, about 2 cm inferior to the alveolar ridge.
   - Studies have found that an intraoral injection is less painful than a percutaneous injection, but care must be taken to not directly inject the nerve or inject into the foramen. This may be done by retracting the cheek and inserting the needle along the lower gum line where there is a buccal mucosal fold around the premolar teeth, this is a shallow injection about 5 mm deep. One to 2 mL of local anesthetic is slowly injected. If a percutaneous approach is taken, insert the needle midway between the oral commissure and the inferior mandible.
   - **Infraorbital nerve (for ipsilateral upper lip, lateral nose, cheek, and lower eyelid):** The infraorbital nerve is a branch of the second division of CNV, the maxillary nerve. The maxillary nerve exits the foramen rotundum and branches prior to exiting the infraorbital canal where it becomes the infraorbital nerve.
   - An infraorbital nerve block can be done with 1–3 mL of anesthetic agent. The infraorbital foramen is best located by having the patient look straight ahead and imagine a line extending from the pupil down to the inferior border of the infraorbital ridge (midpupillary line). Retract the lip, and insert the needle near the second bicuspid, keeping the needle parallel with the tooth. Protect the foramen by placing a finger on the inferior orbital rim, and slowly inject 2–3 mL of local anesthetic.
   - Alternatively, a percutaneous injection can be done by sterilely inserting the needle approximately 1 cm below the infraorbital rim at the midpupillary line at a perpendicular angle. Again, one should take care not to enter the foramen.
   - **Supraorbital nerve and supratrochlear nerves (ipsilateral forehead):** The supraorbital and supratrochlear nerve is located at the superior medial orbital rim and 1.5 cm medial respectively. To block the forehead, identify the supraorbital foramen where you can feel the notch at the superior orbital rim and inject just lateral to that. Inject 2 mL of lidocaine.
   - Furthermore, for children, eutectic mixture of local anaesthetics (EMLA) cream may be applied, but the cream takes 60 minutes for optimal analgesia.

3. **How do you clean a wound?**

   Irrigate wound with normal saline after local anesthesia, taking care to remove all foreign bodies and devitalized tissue.

4. **What sutures should one use?**
For clean lacerations, the deep dermal layer should be reapproximated with interrupted buried 4-0 Vicryl or PDS. For skin, 5-0 or 6-0 interrupted nylon or another type of monofilament suture such as Prolene should be used to close a wound on the face. For mucosal lacerations, Chromic or Vicryl should be used.
   N-Butyl-2-cyanoacylate (Dermabond) or fast absorbing gut (absorbable suture) may be used on a child who would not tolerate suture removal, or a patient who will likely not return for suture removal. Skin adhesive, like N-Butyl-2-cyanoacylate should only be used if it is a low-tension laceration without concern for infections.

5. **How do you place sutures?**
Sutures on the face should be placed a little closer together than usually recommended because of cosmetic concerns. The sutures should be placed 1–2 mm from the skin edge and 3 mm apart to achieve better tissue approximation.

6. **How long do sutures stay in place?**
Sutures should be removed after 3–5 days to minimize scarring and "railroad tracks." After removal of the sutures, consider placement of Steri-Strips over the wound for 1–2 weeks.

7. **What parts of the face require special attention?**
The Lip: The **vermilion border** is the edge of the lip where the red part of the lip meets with the skin edge. It is essential to realign the vermilion border meticulously as any break in the vermilion border is very noticeable.
   The lip can be divided into two parts. The part of the lip that is visible when the mouth is at rest is called the **dry mucosa.** This is the part of the lip to which we apply chap-stick. Continuing past the dry mucosa, into the mouth, is the **wet mucosa.** This is the surface that lies against the teeth and is moist at baseline. These distinctions are important. Try to align the border between dry and wet mucosa to prevent a subtle but noticeable irregularity. In order to ease the visualization of these discrete borders, it is often times easier to use a nerve block, as this will not distort the anatomy, while a local infusion will. These landmarks can also be marked with methylene blue before injecting local anesthesia into the lip.

8. **How do you care for lip mucosal lacerations?**
   • The most important aspect of mucosal laceration is to realign the wet-dry mucosal border.
   • Place the first stitch at the border between the wet and dry surfaces.
   • Use absorbable 4-0 sutures to sew the wet mucosa to wet mucosa and the dry mucosa to dry mucosa.

9. **How do you repair partial-thickness lip lacerations that cross the vermilion border?**
   • Realign the vermilion border first by placing an interrupted suture in the skin above the vermilion border. Use 5-0 or 6-0 suture monofilament.
   • Realign the lip mucosa using absorbable sutures (4-0 or 5-0). Be sure to evert the skin edges.

10. **How do you repair full-thickness lip lacerations?**
The skin, lip muscle, and mucosa have all been cut in full-thickness lip lacerations. These lacerations often appear to be missing tissue due to the muscle retraction but generally there is little missing tissue.
   • **Irrigate the wound:** Use normal saline.
   • **Repair the muscle:** Repair the muscle by using an interrupted or a figure of eight suture in the muscle only. Use an absorbable suture, 3-0 or 4-0. Do not get any mucosa in this muscle bite.
   • **Repair the innermost mucosa:** Repair the inner aspect of the lip first. Use an absorbable 4-0 suture, and place minimal sutures.
   • **Repair the skin:** Realign the vermilion border, then repair the wet and dry border.

11. **How do you repair a full-thickness cheek laceration?**
A full-thickness cheek laceration goes from the skin through the subcutaneous tissues and the intraoral mucosa. These wounds should be repaired in layers. One must examine the parotid gland to ensure that there is no injury to the parotid gland. A proper facial nerve exam should also be performed.

If there is no suspicion of parotid or facial nerve injury:
- Irrigate the wound.
- Repair the intraoral mucosa first. Use absorbable 4-0 suture.
- Irrigate the wound again, as the oral mucosa is now separated from the subcutaneous tissue.
- Reapproximate the subcutaneous tissue if needed with the minimal absorbable 4-0 sutures.
- Repair the skin using interrupted 5-0 nonabsorbable monofilament.

12. **How do you identify a parotid gland injury?**
A high level of suspicion for a parotid gland injury should be raised if there is a facial injury that is inferior to an imaginary line from the tragus to the upper lip. Furthermore, a facial nerve injury should be ruled out too. One way of identifying a parotid gland injury is by palpating and "milking" the parotid gland to see if saliva pools in the wound. One may also use a lacrimal probe or inject methylene blue into the duct from its oral opening. Parotid duct injuries and facial nerve injuries should be taken to the operating room by specialized surgeons for operative repair.

13. **Should eyebrows be shaved for laceration repair?**
No, the eyebrows should not be shaved! They provide good landmarks and they may not grow back normally.
- Eyebrow lacerations are repaired using the natural curve of the eyebrow as well as possible.
- Use 5-0 or 6-0 monofilament that are a different color from the eyebrow, and leave the suture ends long so that you can easily find them for removal.
- Do not place sutures excessively tight as that may damage underlying hair follicles and lead to brow alopecia.

14. **When are antibiotics indicated in facial lacerations?**
Generally, copious irrigation and minimal debridement of facial lacerations should be enough to prevent infection. If antibiotics are given, a first-generation cephalosporin is given. If allergic to penicillin, clindamycin is given. Systemic antibiotic coverage should be used in bite wounds and in patients with underlying cardiac conditions associated with high risk of adverse outcomes from infective endocarditis. Furthermore, systemic antibiotics should be considered in patients at high risk for infections, such as the elderly, immunocompromised patients, and patients with wounds involving the oral cavity.

15. **How should a facial laceration be cared for after repair?**
Postoperative antibiotic ointment may be applied during the first 48 hours after repair. Patients should be instructed to avoid the sun and to use sunscreen on the scar for the first year. The scar will tan differently than the surrounding skin; thus, sun exposure will make a scar become hyperpigmented and more noticeable.

16. **When should scars be revised?**
Scars usually appear their worst during the first couple of months. Scar revision should await until the scar is mature, which may take 4–24 months. Generally, no revision should be undertaken for at least 6–12 months.

KEY POINTS: FACIAL LACERATIONS

1. Appearance and function are of paramount importance in facial repairs.
2. Most clean lacerations can be treated with placement of deep dermal sutures and fine monofilament interrupted sutures that are removed in 3–5 days.
3. The vermilion border should be carefully reapproximated.
4. Eversion of wound edges is important to the favorable outcome of a scar.
5. Good anesthesia in the form of local infiltration, nerve block, or topical applications is essential for an optimal repair.
6. Look for a parotid gland injury if there is a facial injury that is inferior to a line from the tragus to the upper lip.

BIBLIOGRAPHY

1. Goldwyn RM, Rueckert F. The value of healing by secondary intention for sizable defects of the face. *Arch Surg.* 1977;112(3):285–292.
2. Gordin EA, Daniero JJ. Parotid gland trauma. *Facial Plast Surg.* 2010;26(6):504–510.
3. Gurunluonglu R. Facial lacerations. In: Harken AH, Moore EE, eds. *Abernathy's Surgical Secrets.* 6th ed. Philadelphia, PA: Elsevier; 2008:165–168.
4. Lazaridou M, Iliopoulos C. Salivary gland trauma: a review of diagnosis and treatment. *Craniomaxillofac Trauma Reconstr.* 2012;5(4):189–196.
5. Neligan PC. Facial injuries. In: Neligan PC, Buck DW, eds. *Core Procedures in Plastics Surgery.* Philadelphia, PA: Elsevier; 2013:91–109.
6. Medel N, Panchal N. Postoperative care of facial laceration. *Craniomaxillofac Trauma Reconstr.* 2010;3(4):189–200.
7. Syverud SA, Jenkins JM. A comparative study of the percutaneous versus intraoral technique for mental nerve block. *Acad Emerg Med.* 1994;1(6):509–513.
8. Wu PS, Beres A. Primary repair of facial dog bite injuries in children. *Pediatric Emerg Care.* 2011;27(9):801–803.

CHAPTER 35

MAXILLOFACIAL TRAUMA

Chan M. Park, MD, DDS, FACS, Erica Shook, DDS,
A. Thomas Indresano, DMD, FACS

1. **What is the overall treatment goal in repairing facial fractures?**
   Restoration of form and function to premorbid condition is the primary goal in treatment of facial fractures. In regards to midface and mandibular fractures, restoration of dental occlusion restores function and restoration of facial width and projection restores form. With orbital fractures, restoration of orbital volume and freeing of any incarcerated orbital fat and/or muscles restores both form and function.

2. **A patient presents with ecchymosis in bilateral mastoid process and periorbital ecchymosis. What is the clinical significance?**
   Bilateral mastoid process ecchymosis is also known as Battle's sign, and bilateral periorbital ecchymosis is also known as raccoon eyes. Both of these should lead one to suspect basilar skull fracture.

3. **A patient has limited superior gaze in one of the eyes on examination. What is the clinical significance?**
   In the presence of an injury to the orbit or periorbital region, entrapment must be suspected. Entrapment is incarceration of inferior rectus muscle. Other disturbances must be ruled out, including cranial nerve injury, periorbital fat herniation, hematoma, and edema.

4. **What is a normal intraocular pressure (IOP), and when is lateral canthotomy indicated?**
   Normal IOP is 10–21 mm Hg. An elevated IOP >40 mm Hg and clinical evidence of visual disturbance, pain, and proptosis warrants emergent lateral canthotomy and urgent ophthalmologic consultation.

5. **What is the main difference between superior orbital fissure syndrome and orbital apex syndrome?**
   The two share many of the same clinical symptoms, including, but not limited to, ophthalmoplegia, lid ptosis, proptosis, fixated and dilated pupil, and anesthesia of the upper eyelid and forehead. Superior orbital fissure syndrome results from compression of contents within the superior orbital fissure, whereas in orbital apex syndrome, symptoms result from compression of contents within the superior orbital fissure and optic canal. Therefore, orbital apex syndrome will result in visual disturbances, including blindness, whereas superior orbital fissure syndrome will not result in visual disturbances.

6. **A vertical laceration to which region of the face is concerning for injury to the facial nerve?**
   An injury proximal to an imaginary vertical line down from the lateral canthus should be concerning for facial nerve injuries.

7. **With injuries to lips, what percent of a lip can be avulsed and still closed primarily?**
   With lip injuries, up to 25%–30% of the lips can be avulsed and closed primarily. In general, anything greater than this will have a more favorable outcome if reconstructed with local flaps.

8. **What are some general principles in repairing tongue lacerations?**
   The tongue has rich blood supply and abundance of muscle. Attention must be made to close the tongue laceration in multiple layers to avoid opening of wounds and excess hemorrhage. The deep structures should be reapproximated with 3-0 Vicryl and the mucosal layer with 3-0 chromic gut or 3-0 Vicryl.

9. **What is traumatic telecanthus?**
   It is widening of the intercanthal distance due to trauma, usually naso-orbital-ethmoid (NOE) fractures. The average intercanthal distance is 28–35 mm for Caucasians (varies per ethnicity). Intercanthal distances >35 mm are suggestive of injury, whereas distances >40 mm are diagnostic for injury involving the medial canthal attachment.

10. **How do you manage a septal hematoma?**
A septal hematoma will appear as a fluctuant and tender enlargement of the septum and should be drained immediately via a small incision or by needle aspiration. To prevent reformation, placement of packing materials such as Silastic stents or a running suture through and through the septum should be performed. Untreated septal hematoma may lead to abscess, necrosis of the cartilage, subperichondrial fibrosis, and/or saddle nose deformity.

11. **In a patient with NOE fractures who has a clear substance draining from his or her nose, what do you suspect and how will you verify?**
This could be cerebrospinal fluid (CSF) rhinorrhea (disruption in dura leading to CSF leak into nasal cavity). This is verified with a bedside halo test (CSF will form an outer ring around the blood on a piece of filter paper). The most accurate verification is via testing the fluid for β_2 transferrin; however, this test can take up to 4 days to process in the laboratory.

12. **In what patients should nasal tubes (i.e., nasoendotracheal tubes, nasogastric tubes) be used cautiously and possibly avoided?**
In patients with midface fractures such as LeFort and NOE fractures because of risk of intracranial placement.

13. **What are the different types of LeFort fractures and how do you assess for them?**
There are three types of LeFort fractures, which are fracture patterns of the midface. LeFort I fractures are transverse fractures of the maxilla with a characteristic presentation of anterior open bite malocclusion, ecchymosis of the maxillary buccal vestibule and palate, and mobility of the maxilla. LeFort II fractures extend superiomedially to include the medial aspect of the inferior orbital rims and nasal bones and present with mobility of the maxilla and nose as a combined segment as well as bilateral periorbital edema and ecchymosis (raccoon eyes), epistaxis, anterior open bite malocclusion, ecchymosis of the maxillary buccal vestibule and palate, and possible CSF rhinorrhea. LeFort III fractures cause craniofacial disjunction with a fracture pattern that causes a mobilized segment to include the maxilla, nose, and zygomas. Other possible clinical findings in LeFort III patients include bilateral periorbital edema and ecchymosis (raccoon eyes), ecchymosis of the maxillary buccal vestibule and palate, lengthening of facial height, orbital hooding, enophthalmos, ecchymosis over the mastoid region (Battle's sign), CSF rhinorrhea, CSF otorrhea, and hemotympanum.
   When assessing for LeFort fractures, grasp and attempt to mobilize the anterior maxilla with your dominant hand while stabilizing the head with your nondominant hand at the nasofrontal region. By doing this, one is able to have a stable point of reference with one hand while assessing for mobility of the maxilla with the other hand. The type of LeFort fracture can determined by which regions are mobile.

14. **How are maxillary sinus fractures managed?**
Patients should be put on sinus precautions to include no nose blowing, sneezing with mouth open, and no drinking through straws. This is to minimize soft tissue emphysema. Depending upon the patient's health and wound healing capabilities, antibiotics may be considered. Isolated maxillary sinus fractures are rarely operative, although injuries of adjacent/related structures (i.e., zygomaticomaxillary complex [ZMC] or NOE fractures) may be.

15. **What is a tripod fracture?**
The term *tripod* is a misnomer and an antiquated term given the four articulations. It refers to a fracture of the ZMC, which has four sutures: zygomaticomaxillary, zygomaticotemporal, zygomaticofrontal, and zygomaticosphenoid. The determination of whether a given ZMC fracture is operative depends on the degree of displacement, deformity, stability, and functional impairment (i.e., limited mouth opening due to impingement of the mandibular coronoid process on the collapsed zygomatic arch).

16. **What are signs of dentoalveolar fractures and/or mandible fractures?**
Clinical signs of dentoalveolar fractures and/or mandible fractures may include malocclusion, steps in occlusion, mobility of segments, sublingual or vestibular ecchymosis, and gingival lacerations.

17. **When should antibiotics be prescribed for mandibular fractures?**
Fractures that communicate with the oral cavity have a high risk of infection; thus, antibiotic coverage is indicated. This includes any fracture with a laceration of the mucosa/gingiva overlying it or any fracture involving a tooth as the periodontal ligament surrounding that tooth serves as a connection with the oral cavity.

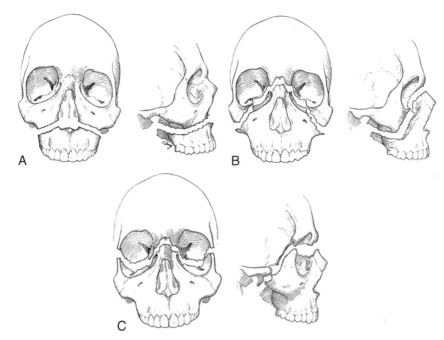

Fig. 35.1 The LeFort classification of midface fractures: (A) LeFort I, (B) LeFort II, and (C) LeFort III. *(From Salin MB, Smith BM. Diagnosis and treatment of midface fractures. In: Fonseca RJ, ed. Oral and Maxillofacial Trauma. Vol. 2. St. Louis: Elsevier; 2005:645–646; with permission.)*

18. **What type of mandible fractures can cause acute airway distress?**
    Bilateral mandibular body fractures can allow posterior collapse of the anterior mandible and tongue, thus causing airway obstruction. Any mandible fracture with active bleeding in a patient unable to protect his or her airway can also cause airway compromise, as can swelling or a hematoma.

19. **When is a neurosurgical consultation indicated for a frontal sinus fracture?**
    Frontal sinus fractures in which there is a suspicion of intracranial injury, such as fractures involving the posterior table, warrant neurosurgical consultation.

KEY POINTS: MAXILLOFACIAL TRAUMA

1. A thorough clinical examination should not be underrated in its importance in identifying facial traumatic injuries.
2. The goal of treatment of facial fractures is restoration of form and function.
3. It is paramount to identify urgent conditions including retrobulbar hematoma, septal hematoma, CSF leak, orbital entrapment, and airway distress.

BIBLIOGRAPHY

1. Fonseca RJ, Walker RV, eds. *Oral and Maxillofacial Trauma*. 3rd ed. St. Louis: Elsevier Saunders; 2005.
2. Freihofer HP. Inner intercanthal and interorbital distances. *J Maxillofac Surg*. 1980;8(4):324–326.
3. Gentile MA, Tellington AJ. Management of midface maxillofacial trauma. *Atlas Oral Maxillofac Surg Clin North Am*. 2013;21(1):69–95.
4. Paskert JP, Manson PN. Nasoethmoidal and orbital fractures. *Clin Plast Surg*. 1988;15(2):209–223.
5. Spinnato G, Alberto PL. Teeth in the line of mandibular fractures. *Atlas Oral Maxillofac Surg Clin North Am*. 2009;17(1):15–18.
6. Zweig BE. Complications of mandibular fractures. *Atlas Oral Maxillofac Surg Clin North Am*. 2009;17(1):93–101.

CHAPTER 36

HAND INJURIES

Krister Freese, MD, Stephanie D. Malliaris, MD, Kyros Ipaktchi, MD, FACS

1. **How are hand fractures and hand injuries splinted?**
   Immobilization should include splinting the joint above and below the injury. For example, a splint for a metacarpal fracture includes the wrist and metacarpal phalangeal (MCP) joints.

2. **Name commonly used splints**
   - **Volar wrist splint:** Ideal resting splint for the hand after burn and soft tissue injuries.
   - **Thumb spica splint:** Ideal for injuries located on the radial side of the hand including tendinitis of the first dorsal compartment (de Quervain's Tenosynovitis) and thumb fractures.
   - **Ulnar gutter splint:** Commonly used for fractures of the fourth and fifth metacarpals (Boxer's fracture).
   - **Stack splint:** Immobilizes the distal interphalangeal joint (DIP) joint and is used for mallet finger injuries and nailbed trauma. It allows proximal interphalangeal joint (PIP) flexion, thereby decreasing risk of joint contractures.
   - **Moldable aluminum splint:** Used for phalangeal fractures and PIP dislocations. Dorsal placement facilitates hand use.
   - **Dorsal blocking splint:** Used for flexor tendon lacerations. The splint is placed over the dorsal hand and wrist, with wrist in slight flexion and MCP joints in 90 degrees of flexion. The interphalangeal (IP) joints are in full extension.

3. **What are the signs of flexor tenosynovitis?**
   The four Kanavel's signs are (1) flexed posture of the digit, (2) circumferential swelling, (3) tenderness along the flexor tendon sheath, (4) and pain with passive extension of the digit.

4. **How is flexor tenosynovitis treated?**
   Urgent decompression of the tendon sheath in the operating room (OR), culture specific antibiotics, and wound care.

5. **How and where should hand injuries be explored?**
   Hand wounds should be explored under tourniquet control with adequate analgesia using delicate instruments in a well-lit surgery suite. Visual magnification is usually mandatory. As a general rule, dorsal wounds can be explored in the emergency department (ED), and simple, clean extensor tendons can be repaired there. Volar wounds with concomitant tendon or nerve injuries generally require exploration in the OR.

6. **How is emergency hemostasis of injured hands achieved?**
   In the acute setting (outside the operating suite), hemostasis may be achieved by elevating the extremity and applying constant direct compression of the wound. For persisting bleeding, a tourniquet above the level of injury may be applied. Application time must be documented and should not exceed 2 hours to prevent ischemic damage to muscle and nerves. Avoid blind clamping and/or suture tying of any deep structure in order to prevent iatrogenic neurovascular damage.

7. **How are fingertip injuries treated?**
   Wounds with minimal pulp disruption will heal spontaneously with daily cleansing and dressing changes with nonadherent, moist gauze. Larger defects may require a skin graft, which can be obtained from the defatted amputated piece. Locally exposed bone can often be successfully treated with occlusive dressings, which are changed twice per week until epithelialized tissue covers the defect. In cases of protruding exposed bone, flap coverage may be necessary if digital length is to be maintained as in thumb defects. In distal phalangeal defects of a digit, bony shortening can be an option. If shortening for coverage needs to exceed proximally beyond the flexor digitorum profundus insertion, then a flap is indicated. Digital nerves cannot be repaired distal to the DIP joint.

8. **What is the classification system for fingertip amputations?**
Fingertip amputations are classified based on the amount of remaining sensate volar skin. Favorably angulated amputations commonly involve loss of dorsal structures: nail and bone. In these injuries, the volar glabrous skin is still available for easy coverage. This amputation type can be treated by dressings only, allowing wound repair by contraction and epithelialization. Volarly angulated amputation angles are deemed "unfavorable" for conservative management and usually require reconstructive procedures (see Fig. 36.1).

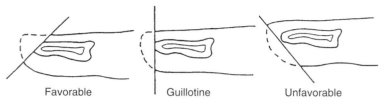

| Favorable | Guillotine | Unfavorable |

Fig. 36.1 Fingertip amputations. *From Ditmars Jr, DM. Fingertip and nail bed injuries. In Kasdan ML, ed.* Occupational Hand and Upper Extremity Injuries and Disease. *Philadelphia: Hanley & Belfus; 1991; with permission.*

9. **How are nailbed injuries repaired?**
Repair of disrupted germinal matrix must be meticulously approximated under magnification and the nailbed splinted, preferably with the avulsed part. Nailbed injuries are repaired with 5-0 fast absorbing chromic sutures. Alternatively, a cyanoacrylate tissue adhesive can be used. This does not obviate the need for meticulous reapproximation of the nailbed. Subungual hematomas can be evacuated by a hot-tipped paperclip or battery-powered electric cautery. The eponychial fold should be stented with either the original nail plate or some other inert material. Often, nailbed disruptions cannot be diagnosed without removal of the nail. The nail plate should be removed if a subungual hematoma extends to >50% of the nail surface area.

10. **What is the initial management of flexor tendon laceration?**
Flexor tendon lacerations are not an emergency, and should therefore not be repaired in the ED. If a hand surgeon is unavailable, the wound is copiously irrigated and skin sutured closed. Prophylactic antibiotics need to be administered and the hand splinted in a metacarpophalangeal (MP) and IP joint flexing dorsal splint. This injury should be treated within the first 10 days. Delays in treatment can preclude the ability to perform primary tendon repairs.

11. **What is the proper management of an open fracture?**
Open fractures proximal to the MCP joint should be cleaned and dressed in the ED, but not probed or cultured. A first-generation cephalosporin, such as Ancef, is administered and tetanus immunization updated. Open fractures meeting the criteria of the Gustilo and Anderson classification should receive additional penicillin and an aminoglycoside, such as Gentamicin.

 A saline-soaked dressing is applied over the wound, and the hand is splinted in a functional position using a bulky dressing. Urgent irrigation and debridement in the OR is indicated followed by fracture stabilization and wound closure. Open fractures distal to the MCP joint can be washed out in the ED and treated nonemergently.

12. **What is the proper treatment for hand infections?**
The extremity should be immobilized and elevated, and antibiotics should be administered. Serial examinations should be used to assess for improvement. The patient should be referred for possible surgical drainage especially if concern for abscess or deeper infection exists.

13. **What is the proper management of human and animal bites?**
After wound cleansing, radiographs are obtained to rule out foreign bodies (e.g., broken teeth). Wounds are left open and antibiotics are started. Keep a high level of suspicion for infection in all puncture bites that inoculate deep structures and have no drainage (e.g., cat bites). All wounds are rechecked at 24 and 48 hours. If evidence of infection is present, parenteral antibiotics should be instituted and the patient referred for possible surgical drainage. In human bites, the most common microorganisms are *Staphylococcus aureus*, alpha hemolytic *Streptococcus*, and *Eikenella corrodens*. They are best treated with penicillinase resistant penicillin, such as amoxicillin/clavulanate. In animal

bites, *Pasteurella multocida*, *Staphylococcus aureus*, and alpha hemolytic *Streptococci* prevail and are treated with amoxicillin/clavulanate. So-called "fight bites" occur over the MCP or PIP joint when a clenched fist is impaled on the incisors of an adversary. This often inoculates the MCP joint with anaerobic Streptococci. The resulting traumatic arthrotomy can be difficult to identify, especially when examining the hand flat on the examination table and not in the initial clenched position. These injuries require irrigation and debridement in the OR.

14. Name common hand infections
    - **Paronychia:** Infection of the dorsal soft tissue surrounding the nail plate. Early infections can be treated with antibiotics and soaks. More established infections require drainage under digital block.
    - **Felon:** Infection of the fingertip pulp. Drainage through a longitudinal incision is the recommended treatment. Other incisions may destabilize the fingertip pulp from the underlying distal phalanx.
    - **Collar button abscess:** Infection of the web space that involves both the palmar and dorsal sides.
    - **Deep space infections:** Three deep fascial spaces in the hand are known as sites for deep infections: The thenar space, midpalmar space, and hypothenar space. Infections in these locations can be missed.

15. How are injection injuries treated?
    Despite their innocuous appearance, injection injuries may cause profound destruction of hand structures. Any such injury requires immediate hospitalization with emergent irrigation and debridement. Multiple, second look debridements may be required. The prognosis is guarded when oil-based paint or industrial solvents are involved. Latex and water-based paints cause less tissue damage.

16. What are the most preventable causes of secondary functional disability in hand injuries?
    Edema and infection lead to increased scarring and restricted function. Prolonged immobilization in a poor position also impairs function. Failure to obtain radiographs may lead to a missed or delayed diagnosis of an injury.

17. What is the proper ED treatment of the patient with an amputated part?
    Patients need to be treated according to the advanced trauma life support protocol. In addition to cardiopulmonary stabilization, tetanus immunization and prophylactic antibiotics are administered. Broad-spectrum antibiotics should be given in heavily contaminated wounds or in diabetic or immunocompromised patients. Radiographs of the injured extremity and the amputated part are ordered as are laboratory studies such as hemoglobin/hematocrit content, blood type and screening, and other tests as indicated (blood glucose for diabetics, etc.). Photo documentation of soft tissue injuries is helpful. While tests are pending, a replantation center is contacted for transfer. Prolonged ischemia of the amputated part risks the possible success of replantation attempt. Once the patient is accepted, expedited transfer is mandatory, which may include airlifting. Digital replantation is usually possible up to 24 hours. The larger the amputate size including the amount of severed muscle (forearm and arm level injuries) the shorter the ischemia tolerance. Major amputations (proximal to the palmar arch) are usually not replantable beyond 6 hours of cold ischemia time.

18. How should the amputated part be transported to the replantation center?
    The amputated part is wrapped in saline-soaked gauze and sealed in a plastic bag. This bag in turn is placed in a container with iced saline maintaining the temperature around 4°C. Direct contact with ice must be avoided to prevent freezing. Hypotonic and hypertonic solution should not be used to prevent osmotic damage to the part.

19. What is acute carpal tunnel syndrome?
    Acute compression of the median nerve in the carpal tunnel is a condition associated with trauma to the hand, wrist, or forearm. Examples are distal radius fractures or a perilunate dislocation. This clinical diagnosis presents with worsening wrist pain and sensory changes in the median nerve distribution, which typically include paresthesias in the volar thumb, index, middle, and half of the ring finger. The hallmark of acute carpal tunnel syndrome is progressive neurologic changes in the median nerve distribution.

20. How is acute carpal tunnel treated?
    Emergent decompression of median nerve by releasing the transverse carpal ligament.

KEY POINTS: EMERGENCY ROOM CARE OF HAND INJURIES

1. Do not explore volar sided lacerations in the ER. When concerned for possible neurovascular and/or tendinous injuries, examine and document in writing neurovascular status and motor function in a standardized hand examination format.
2. Never clamp or suture tie suspected upper extremity arterial bleeders in the field or the emergency room. Instead, use direct pressure/elevation, compression dressings or a tourniquet placed above injury level. Document tourniquet time, which cannot exceed >2 hours of tourniquet ischemia.
3. Always obtain x-rays for bite injuries or suspected foreign body intrusion. Consider ultrasound/MRI when dealing with possible radiolucent/organic foreign bodies (e.g., wood splinters/rose thorns).
4. Always leave puncture wounds and bite injuries open to drain. No suture closure of bite wounds in the ER.
5. Mandatory operative exploration and debridement in the OR of:
   a. All fight bite injuries to the MCP joint area
   b. Paint gun injuries
   c. Suspected flexor tendon sheath (FTS) (positive Kanavel's Signs)

BIBLIOGRAPHY

1. Hile D, Hile L. The emergent evaluation and treatment of hand injuries. *Emerg Med Clin North Am.* 2015;33(2): 397–408.
2. Higgens JP. Replantation. In: Wolfe S, Pederson WC, eds. *Green's Operative Hand Surgery.* 7th ed. Philadelphia: Elsevier; 2016.
3. Gustilo RB, Anderson JT. Prevention of infection in the treatment of one thousand and twenty-five open fractures of long bones: retrospective and prospective analyses. *J Bone Joint Surg Am.* 1976;58(4):453–458.
4. Hansen TB, Carstensen O. Hand injuries in agricultural accidents. *J Hand Surg Br.* 1999;24(2):190–192.
5. Amirtharajah M, Lattanza L. Open extensor tendon injuries. *J Hand Surg Am.* 2015;40(2):391–397.
6. Jebson PJL, Louis DS. Hand infections. *Hand Clin.* 1998;14(4):511–711.
7. Kennedy SA, Stoll LE. Human and other mammalian bite injuries of the hand: evaluation and management. *J Am Acad Orthop Surg.* 2015;23(1):47–57.
8. Tosti R, Ilyas AM. Acute carpal tunnel syndrome. *Orthop Clin North Am.* 2012;43(4):459–465.
9. Martin C, Gonzalez Del Pino J. Controversies in the treatment of fingertip amputations: conservative versus surgical reconstruction. *Clin Orthop Relat Res.* 1998;353:63–73.
10. Taras JS, Lamb MJ. Treatment of flexor tendon injuries: surgeons' perspective. *J Hand Ther.* 1999;12(2):141–148.
11. Van der Molen AB, Matloub HS. The hand injury severity scoring system and Workers' Compensation cases in Wisconsin, USA. *J Hand Surg Br.* 1999;24(2):184–186.
12. Strauss EJ, Weil WM. A prospective, randomized, controlled trial of 2-octylcyanoacrylate versus suture repair for nail bed injuries. *J Hand Surg Am.* 2008;33(2):250–253.

CHAPTER 37

BURNS

Karel D. Capek, MD, David N. Herndon, MD, FACS

1. Where do burn injuries occur?

Eighty percent of burn-related injuries occur in the home, mostly in low-income, multifamily dwellings.

2. Who is at risk of suffering burns?

The incidence of burn injuries and deaths in the United States is substantially higher than that of the rest of the industrialized world. The male-to-female ratio for burn injuries is roughly 2:1. Alcohol abuse and illicit drug activity increase the risk of burn injury.

3. What factors influence burn outcomes most profoundly?

The overall mortality risk of burns is 7.6%. Pediatric burn centers record mortalities between 2% and 3%, whereas mortality for those older than 50 years is more than three times higher than the national mean, and above 70 years of age, mortality exceeds 33%. In pediatric burns, we have seen 14 survivors of 25 patients with subtotal (97%–99% total body surface area [TBSA]) burn injury. Age in years + % body surface area burned + 17 if inhalation injury present = (modified) Baux score. Survivors currently reported to 140.

4. What happens to burned tissues?

- Extensive damage to the skin (considered the largest single organ in the body and consuming almost 20% of the cardiac output) sets the stage for bacterial invasion.
- The interior milieu is protected from the environment by a complex integumentary system; serious homeostatic derangements occur when the skin is destroyed.
- Heat-denatured integumentary proteins enter the circulation. Systemic infection or sepsis remains the dominant precipitant of organ failure and death; this points to a burn injury-related Immune dysfunction or failure.

5. What happens in burned tissues?

The injury site may be divided into three zones by standard light microscopy: An inner zone of necrosis, a middle zone of stasis, and an outer zone of hyperemia. In the zone of necrosis, proteins are denatured; all microvascular and macrovascular structure and function are destroyed. Surrounding this central zone is a zone of stasis. Here, cellular morphology is intact, but cells are swollen with microstructural changes with extravasation of leukocytes and red blood cells into the interstitial space, increased interstitial fluid, and capillary stasis. A third zone of hyperemia then transitions into the adjacent normal tissues where no abnormalities are seen.

6. Besides the skin injury, what other associated injuries may occur?

Inhalation injury is diagnosed in 10% of all hospitalized burn victims. Other physical trauma is frequently associated with explosions or merely the attempts to escape the fire. Awareness of associated trauma justifies the importance of a careful advanced trauma life support trauma evaluation. Depending on mechanism, eye injuries, tympanic membrane rupture (explosions), and pneumothorax may accompany burn injury.

7. How is inhalation injury diagnosed?

a. Obvious hoarseness or stridor.
b. Substantial head and neck or facial burns.
c. Entrapment in enclosed space or direct proximity to an explosion.
d. Event history of superheated steam.
e. Bronchoscopic evidence of carbonaceous material or mucosal hyperemia.

8. What changes occur systemically?

Systemic events become clinically significant beyond an injury size of 10% TBSA. Several abnormalities occur:

- A trend to fluid retention with generalized edema, caused by an increased systemic microvascular permeability of rapid onset (minutes to hours).

- A definite and reproducible decrease in cardiac output (and increased systemic vascular resistance) that shifts over 12–36 hours into a vasodilated, cardiovascularly hyperdynamic state by 36 hours postinjury. Thus, burn injury is accompanied by interrelated changes in volume status, vascular tone, and cardiac pump function.
- There is an increase in whole-body oxygen consumption and CO_2 production (metabolic rate) to as much as twice the Harris Benedict predicted resting energy expenditure. This increase in metabolic rate leads to rapid catabolic consumption of lean body mass, which is only partially ameliorated by the protein/calorie feeding at supranormal levels.
- There is a marked, prolonged elevation in circulating catecholamines.
- There is a marked, prolonged elevation of endogenous glucocorticoids.
- There is a marked impairment in cell-mediated and natural killer cell immunity, increasing susceptibility to fungal, viral, and opportunistic bacterial infections.
- Thermal (body heat) homeostasis becomes progressively deranged, with concurrent reset of the hypothalamic thermal set-point. This includes alterations in heat exchange via all four mechanisms of heat dissipation: radiant (body surface blood flow), convective (hair position), evaporative (sweating and wound exudate), and conductive (determined by the ambient temperature and temperature of objects in contact with the patient).

9. **What can first responders do when witnessing a burn injury?**
First, do no harm. No ice, butter, dry ice, or any other substance should be applied to the wound after extinguishing the fire. If the burn is minor (<10% TBSA), running tepid tap water over the burn with a handheld shower for 20 minutes is beneficial. Applying wet towels appears to provide no benefit and may provoke hypothermia. If stranded in a remote area, encourage oral fluid intake and cover the wound with clean towels. Aspirin or ibuprofen may benefit the patient and the wound. Elevate any burned extremities. Cover the victim if cold/shivering and protect from further environmental exposure.

10. **What actions are needed from prehospital providers (i.e., after the prehospital crew arrives, what are their priorities)?**
The American College of Surgeons' Committee on Trauma (ACS-COT) advises that all ambulance crews follow "scoop and run" procedure guidelines for all burn victims within 60 minutes of an appropriate hospital (level I or II trauma center or burn facility).

Maintain elevation of burned extremities. If facial burns or swelling are present, elevate the head above the level of the heart. If spinal precautions are necessary, this may be done via reverse Trendelenburg positioning. Attempt to place an intravenous (IV) line en route, but this is not essential if the travel time is <60 minutes. Lines may be placed through burned skin, preferably in antecubital veins. Intraosseous access is often faster and may be lifesaving in major burns when IV access cannot be rapidly obtained in the field.

Actively maintain body temperature around 36°C–38°C. Protect from environmental exposure; maintain ambient environmental temperature of 80°F–90°F (e.g., using ambulance heater) if possible. There is an exception to above: In the setting of hypoxic insult or possible cyanide/carbon monoxide intoxication, patients with frank neurologic abnormality (e.g., Glasgow Coma Scale <12) may be maintained between 35°C and 37°C body temperature, with a normal room temperature ambulance cabin (permissive hypothermia).

11. **How does the hospital-based emergency department contribute to the care of the patients with major burns?**
Urgency in caring for the victim, not the wound, is pivotal for the ultimate survival of the victim:
a. Airway. Look for soot in the pharynx and for extensive facial burns.
b. Breathing. Identify hoarseness or stridor. Listen for breath sounds on both sides.
c. Circulation. Place two peripheral IV lines; start fluids as lactated Ringer's solution; calculate the Parkland formula = 4 mL× kg body weight × % body burn [half of volume in first 8 hours; other half over 16 hours].
d. Neurologic deficit. Examine central nervous system and cranial nerves; assess the neurologic status all extremities.
e. Expose and examine the skin, log roll and meticulously determine burn size on the posterior body, and then cover and preserve body heat. The patient's environment should be heated to 90°F, and suitable protection from environmental exposure (e.g., cold hallways) provided.
f. Fluid therapy should be assessed and titrated hourly to maintain 1 mL urinary output per kilogram of body weight every hour. Urethral catheterization (preferably with temperature probe) is indicated for burn resuscitation.

g.   Pain management and psychologic emotional support are also important. Provide analgesia and anxiolytics with small, titrated doses of short- or medium-acting medications.

12. **How is burn size estimated?**
This determination is done clinically, with the aid of three important clinical tools:
a.   The volar surface of the victim's opened hand (including fingers) is about 1% of TBSA; most useful for the sizing of small scattered wound areas.
b.   Rule of nines: Most commonly used, easy to memorize, accuracy OK for adults:
      i.   Adult head 9%
      ii.   Total each upper extremity 9%
      iii.   Total each anterior lower extremity 9%
      iv.   Total each posterior lower extremity 9%
      v.   Anterior torso 18%
      vi.   Posterior torso including buttocks 18%
      vii.   Genitals 1%
      viii.   Note that adults and children differ significantly by the difference in the relative size of the head (9% in adults, 15% in infants). By contrast, a thigh in an infant is much smaller than in an adult (6% versus 10%).
c.   Lund and Browder chart: More accurate, necessary for pediatric patients.
d.   Three-dimensional burn size estimation is also possible via smartphone or tablet devices.

13. **How is inhalation injury defined?**
In contrast to the visible and somewhat quantifiable external burn injury to the skin, the inhalation of heat, carbon monoxide, cyanide, and other toxic or noxious vapors is less visible and less quantifiable, yet quite dangerous. Four separate mechanisms of injury are generally called inhalation injury:
a.   Carbon monoxide intoxication.
b.   Heat damage to upper airways.
c.   Inhalation of toxic smoke components that are produced by the combustion of modern synthetic materials used in the interior decoration of houses, buildings, and cars.
d.   Cyanide poisoning: The combustion of many synthetic materials also produces cyanide gas, which binds to the cytochrome enzyme system and inhibits mitochondrial function and cellular respiration. Blood cyanide levels should be assessed in all patients with carbon monoxide levels >10%.

14. **What treatments have most influenced the outcome of burn victims over the past 100 years?**
Adequate and timely fluid resuscitation, early and complete excision of the burn wound, aggressive nutritional support, early and comprehensive rehabilitation of functional deficits.

15. **How should fluid be resuscitated, and by what route?**
All patients with burns >10% TBSA should receive fluid. Formulaic or decision-support system guided fluid resuscitation should be initiated above 15%–20% TBSA. Enteral resuscitation via orogastric tube is useful in burns <30% and can be used in austere environments or mass casualty situations. By default, burn resuscitation is usually via IV route.

16. **How is fluid therapy managed?**
The fluid management plan has two components. First, determine the burn wound size and the patient's weight in kilograms; calculate the hourly fluid rate using one of the available formulas. Administer lactated Ringer's solution at the hourly rate calculated. In infants and small children, added 5% dextrose is needed to prevent hypoglycemia.
   The second component of the plan is just as important. Monitor (hourly) the effectiveness of your fluid therapy plan and adjust it promptly when indicated. The goal is a patient who is hemodynamically normalized, with a urine output of 0.5–1.0 mL of urine per kilogram body weight per hour. Pulmonary edema developing during the resuscitation phase indicates over-resuscitation, but can be difficult to diagnose in the setting of inhalation injury. Examination of the jugular veins (supine and head of bed elevated), central venous pressure, cardiac apical impulse, changes in heart size with serial chest x-ray, and/or focused intensive care unit cardiac sonography can be helpful in this difficult setting. By ultrasound, full ventricles and no (<15%) respiratory variation in inferior vena cava diameter indicates intravascular volume status is adequate. Supranormal (90%) ejection fraction can be seen in acute hypovolemia (burn shock).

17. **What should be done if this treatment algorithm fails to achieve clinical improvement and patient stabilization?**
Failure to respond to the resuscitation formula is indicative of a poor prognosis. However, some additional measures may be beneficial but are not currently considered as part of the standard care. These include the use of mannitol (hypertonic) solutions, use of colloid (albumin or plasma) in massive burns, and the early use of inotropes (dobutamine once volume replete).

18. **How are fluid requirements calculated when there has been a delay in the initiation of therapy?**
Current teaching is to proportionally increase the fluid volume in an attempt to get the desired total volume for 8 hours into the patient before the first 8-hour period elapses. This remedy does require some common sense, accounting for hemodynamics and urine output.

19. **What is the best way to care for burn wounds initially?**
Early on, these wounds need simple coverage with a surgically clean or, if available, sterile sheet or surgical drape. The ACS-COT burn and trauma guidelines state that definitive wound care need not occur up to 24 hours postinjury. No ointment or specific antibacterial treatment is initially required. The patient should be kept warm because exposure precipitates systemic hypothermia. For definitive wound care, the entire patient is washed or showered, and residual debris and damaged epidermis are removed. Then the extent of the injury is mapped, usually on a Lund and Browder chart, along with preliminary attempts to determine the depth of the injury. A burn wound is usually a mosaic of different areas injured to varying degrees (depths). All burn wounds deepen to some extent over the first 48–96 hours, so a better prediction of which areas require grafting will come with time.

20. **Why and how is the depth of a burn injury graded?**
This depends on the presence of skin appendages (hair follicle and sweat gland) that carry the germinal layer (skin stem cell niche) deep into the dermis, from which reepithelialization can occur. On the day of injury, the visual ability to differentiate a burn wound that will heal from that which will not is poor (50% accuracy). Over time (next 3–7 days), the accuracy of clinical prediction will improve somewhat (90%). Table 37.1 helps to elucidate these aspects.
   Fourth-degree burns involve damage to structures deeper than the dermis (e.g., fat, muscle, bone, tendon, nerve, joint capsule). Burns are designated as fifth degree when tissue is lost, blown off, or vaporized by the burn or blast.

Table 37.1 Depth of Injury With Clinical Signs and Probable Outcome

DEPTH OF INJURY	CLINICAL SIGNS AND SYMPTOMS	OUTCOME
First degree (superficial injury limited to epidermis)	Erythema of the skin with mild to moderate discomfort	Wounds heal spontaneously in 5–10 days; damaged epithelium peels off, leaving no residual effects
Second degree: Superficial (involves entirety of epidermis and superficial portion of dermis)	Wounds are blistered or weeping, erythematous, and painful. Skin is desiccated, blistered, white eschar often seen	Wounds heal spontaneously within 2–3 weeks without residual scarring and with good-quality skin; pigmentation may be altered
Deep (involves deeper dermis, but viable portions of epidermal appendages remain)	Wounds are occasionally moist and difficult to distinguish from third-degree burn	Wounds heal spontaneously beyond 3–4 weeks; hypertrophic scarring often occurs and, occasionally, unstable epithelium. For best results, remove eschar by tangential excision and cover with split-thickness skin graft
Third degree (all epidermal appendages destroyed)	Avascular, waxy, white, leathery brown or black, insensate eschar	Unless small in size (<2 cm in diameter), wounds require removal of eschar and coverage with skin graft for healing

21. **When should surgical excision of the burn wound begin?**
    It should start as soon as possible, but it should be blended with common sense and pragmatism. This can be as soon as 12–24 hours after injury if the patient is stable and resuscitated.

22. **How is the excised area managed?**
    A significant advance in burn management occurred in the early 1970s when Janzekovic demonstrated that excised wounds should be immediately grafted with skin. This remains the goal. If donor sites are insufficient, cadaver skin, pigskin, amniotic membrane, or biosynthetic products (e.g., Integra, Biobrane, or Transcyte) can be used for wound coverage. These areas require subsequent autografting. Cultured autologous keratinocytes are an attractive theoretical alternative, but they remain fragile and require meticulous care to prevent shearing and infection.

23. **How can we best supply fuel to the metabolic furnace of the body?**
    Place a (postpyloric) feeding tube on arrival. Nutritional support of the burn victim is paramount. Total enteral nutrition may have the added benefit of maintaining the intestinal barrier function, which may reduce septic events by preventing bacterial translocation.

24. **What is the role of antibiotics in burn care?**
    Antibiotics are never administered prophylactically for burn injuries. However, early and appropriate antibiotic therapy is a life-saving tool in the management of established infections in burn patients. Culture ill-appearing patients early and often to diagnose changes in microbial species or antibiotic resistance. When they were introduced, topical antimicrobial soaks (silver nitrate 0.5% or mafenide acetate 5%) drastically decreased invasive burn wound infections (ecthyma gangrenosum).

25. **How are chemical burn injuries approached?**
    Wear protective equipment if chemical agent is still present. Brush off all chemicals that remain in powdered form on the victim. Thereafter, immediate and prolonged irrigation (1–4 hours, or until pH is neutral) of the contaminated skin should be done with running tap water; in the case of alkali burns, irrigate longer. Some chemicals may be absorbed; therefore, immediate contact with a toxicology center is indicated. Be especially wary of systemic effects of hydrofluoric acid or phenol burns. If eye involvement is noted, irrigate immediately and copiously, urgent ophthalmology consultation is warranted.

26. **How are patients with electrical burns managed?**
    An injury caused by electricity may either be an electrical flash burn or contact or conduction injury. In electrical flash injury, the air or atmosphere is ionized by the electrical discharge, without conduction of current through the body. Thus, the injury is only cutaneous. A true electrical flash burn most frequently heals without much grafting. Airway compromise is rare. In electrical conduction injury, however, tissue is damaged through the actual transfer of electrical energy through the patient from entry point to exit. Thermal energy is generated within the tissues because of the relative resistance to the conduction of current, with resultant protein denaturation and cell death. Different structures (e.g., bone, skin, muscle, nerve, tendon, and lung) exhibit different electrical conductivity, resulting in unpredictable conduction pathways. Thus, the skin is often only minimally involved at the entry and exit sites, with extensive muscle, nerve, tendon, and even bone necrosis in erratic patterns. Neurologic injury, compartment syndrome, and myoglobinuria are frequent complications. Rapid and complete tissue decompression (i.e., fasciotomy) is essential with early and repeated reexploration to remove necrotic tissue. The goal of fluid therapy should be to achieve high urine volumes (>1.0–1.5 mL/kg per hour). Alkalization of the urine and mannitol can be beneficial.

27. **After burn injuries have healed, what important issues remain to be addressed in the rehabilitation period?**
    The rehabilitation of a burn victim must begin on the day of admission and is a total team effort that involves physiatrists, plastic surgeons, occupational therapists, physical therapists, nutritionists, psychologists, social workers, pulmonologists, microbiologists, pharmacists, speech therapists, and nurses. Rehabilitation of the mind and body must occur in concert.

KEY POINTS: SEVERITY OF THE BURN INJURY

Age in years + percent body surface area burned + 17 if inhalation injury present = (modified) Baux score. Survivors currently reported to 140.

BIBLIOGRAPHY

1. Herndon DN, ed. *Total Burn Care*. 5th ed. Philadelphia, PA: Elsevier. In press.
2. Blumetti J, Hunt JL. The Parkland formula under fire: is the criticism justified? *J Burn Care Res.* 2008;29(1):180–186.
3. Demling RL. Burn care in the immediate resuscitation period. In: *American College of Surgeons Surgery: Principles and Practice*. Chicago: American College of Surgeons; 2002.
4. Prevention Gibbons J. In: Gibbons J, ed. *Fire! 38 Lifesaving Tips for You and Your Family*. Seattle: Ballard Publishing; 1995.
5. Hart DW, Wolf SE, Gore DC, et al. Determinants of skeletal muscle catabolism after severe burn. *Ann Surg.* 2000;232(4):455–465.
6. Krzywiecki A, Ziora D. Late consequences of respiratory system burns. *J Physiol Pharmacol.* 2007;58(suppl 5):319–325.
7. McDonald-Smith GP, Saffle JR, Edelman L, et al. *National Burn Repository 2002 Report*. Chicago: American Burn Association; 2002.
8. McGill V, Kahn S. The impact of substance use on mortality and morbidity from thermal injury. *J Trauma.* 1995;38(6):931–934.
9. Mustonen KM, Vuola J. Acute renal failure in intensive care burn patients. *J Burn Care Res.* 2008;29(1):227–237.
10. Pruitt BA, Goodwin CW, Mason Jr AD. Epidemiological, demographic and outcome characteristics of burn injury. In: Herndon DN, ed. *Total Burn Care*. 2nd ed. Philadelphia: WB Saunders; 2002.

CHAPTER 38

PEDIATRIC TRAUMA

Shannon N. Acker, MD, Jonathan P. Roach, MD,
David A. Partrick, MD, FACS, FAAP

1. **What is the leading cause of death in children in the United States?**
   Traumatic injuries cause more death and disability in children from ages 1 to 18 years than all other causes combined. Unintentional injury accounts for 65% of all injury deaths in children under 19 years of age. Each year, approximately 20,000 children and teenagers die as a result of injury and 50,000 children suffer permanent disability. Each year, nearly one in four children receives medical treatment for an injury. The estimated annual cost is $15 billion.

2. **What age groups are at particular risk for traumatic death?**
   Infants younger than age 2 years have a consistently higher mortality rate for the same severity of injury compared to older children. During adolescence, however, injury takes the greatest toll, accounting for nearly 80% of deaths.

3. **What primary mechanisms account for pediatric traumatic injuries?**
   Blunt (90%), penetrating (9%), and crush injuries (<1%). Motor vehicle crashes are the most common cause of injury (40%–50%) and death in childhood followed by falls (36%).

4. **Do the rates of traumatic injury vary between male and female children?**
   Yes. Boys account for about two-thirds of all pediatric trauma patients. Boys and men are at a 4 times greater risk for "successful" suicide (although boys try it less often), 3 times greater risk for drowning, 2.5 times greater risk for homicide, and 2 times greater risk for motor vehicle-related trauma.

5. **How is a child's airway different from an adult's?**
   Children are at increased risk of airway obstruction because of their large tongue, floppy epiglottis, increased lymphoid tissue, and short, small-diameter trachea. Uncuffed endotracheal tubes are appropriate in children younger than age 8 years to minimize vocal cord trauma, subglottic edema, and ulceration. The narrowest part of a child's airway is the cricoid ring, which functions as a seal for the uncuffed endotracheal tube.

6. **What is the appropriate size of endotracheal tube to place in a child?**
   The internal diameter of the endotracheal tube should be the same size as the child's small finger. For newborns, use a 3-mm tube; children in first year of life, 4-mm tube; children older than 1 year, internal diameter of the endotracheal tube is equal to the child's age in years divided by 4, plus 4 (but in an urgent situation do not resort to extensive calculations, simply look at the child's fifth finger).

7. **What if oral endotracheal intubation cannot be accomplished?**
   A needle cricothyrotomy is preferable to surgical cricothyrotomy and can be performed with a 14-gauge catheter. Conceptually, this is the same as transtracheal jet ventilation in adults. Surgical cricothyrotomy is much more difficult in small children and has a high association with secondary subglottic stenosis.

8. **What is a child's total blood volume?**
   It is 80 mL/kg (8% of body weight).

9. **What is the first sign of significant blood loss in children?**
   Tachycardia. Young children are incredibly resilient and have a remarkable tolerance to blood loss. Hemorrhage of 30% of blood volume may result in no blood pressure (BP) change, but such blood loss does cause a rapid increase in heart rate (HR). A child's cardiac output depends largely on HR; unlike adults, children have a limited capacity to increase stroke volume. Elevated shock index, pediatric age adjusted (SIPA) (maximum normal HR/minimum normal systolic BP adjusted for age) may help identify the most severely injured children in the trauma bay. Children with elevated SIPA on presentation have higher injury severity scores, longer hospital length of stay, and higher overall mortality compared with children with a normal SIPA on presentation.

10. **What are signs of hypovolemic shock in children?**
Tachycardia (progressing to bradycardia), hypotension, altered mental status, respiratory compromise, delayed capillary refill (>2 s), and decreased or absent peripheral pulses.

11. **Is hypotension a reliable indicator of blood loss in children?**
No. Fewer than half of injured children with documented hypotension have an identifiable insult resulting in significant volume loss. Hypotension is often associated with an isolated closed head injury, especially in children younger than age 6 years.

12. **Why are children at increased risk for hypothermia during resuscitation?**
The child's body surface area is large relative to internal body mass; an unclothed child can lose heat fast. Cold intravenous (IV) fluids and inhaled gases can exacerbate hypothermia, leading to hypoxemia, which causes pulmonary hypertension and progressive metabolic acidosis. Infants <6 months of age are particularly vulnerable as they lack significant subcutaneous fat and an effective shivering mechanism.

13. **What sites are preferred for venous access in children?**
Two large-bore IV catheters should be inserted percutaneously in the upper extremities. The second choice is percutaneous access to the distal saphenous vein (or a cutdown).

14. **What if you cannot establish an IV line?**
The intraosseous (IO) route is safe and requires less time than a venous cutdown. The anteromedial surface of the proximal tibia is the preferred site for access, with the needle placed 3 cm distal to the tibial tuberosity. The proximal femur, distal femur, and distal tibia are other potential sites. In general, any medication that can be administered via an IV line can be administered via the IO route. Complications are rare and result primarily from infection or extravasation. IO volume resuscitation facilitates subsequent cannulation of the venous circulation.

15. **What are the appropriate crystalloid and blood resuscitation volumes in children?**
Initial resuscitation should include a bolus of 20 mL/kg of either lactated Ringer's solution or normal saline. Adequate response is evident with a decrease in HR and an increase in urinary output. The 20-mL/kg bolus should be repeated if assessment reveals inadequate tissue perfusion. If evidence of shock persists after two bolus infusions of crystalloid solution, 10 mL/kg of packed red blood cells (type specific if available or O-negative) should be administered.

16. **Why are head injuries more common in children than adults?**
Relative to body size, a child's head is larger than an adults until age 10. Central nervous system injury is the leading cause of death among injured children and thus is the principal determinant of outcome.

17. **What types of head injuries are more common in children?**
Concussion is the leading cause of head injury in children. Epidural hemorrhage is the most common type of intracranial bleed; subdural hemorrhage is relatively rare. However, mortality from subdural hemorrhage is 40% compared to only 4% for an epidural bleed. Pediatric patients also tend to sustain injuries that produce diffuse edema rather than focal, space-occupying lesions.

18. **Can children have significant chest trauma without rib fractures?**
Absolutely. The chest wall is much more compliant in children than in adults; thus, kinetic energy is transmitted more readily to structures within the thorax. A child with significant blunt chest trauma is at increased risk of life-threatening contusion to the lungs or heart even with no or relatively few rib fractures. When present, rib fractures in children may indicate nonaccidental trauma and should prompt further evaluation. Thoracic injury is the second leading cause of death (after head trauma) in children. However, children with clinically significant chest trauma have abnormalities identified on chest radiograph. Among pediatric trauma patients with normal chest radiograph, computed tomography (CT) of the chest is not indicated. CT should only be obtained in the setting of an abnormal chest x-ray.

19. **What types of thoracic injuries are common or uncommon in children?**
Pulmonary contusion, traumatic asphyxia, and tracheobronchial injuries are common in children. Traumatic aortic rupture, flail chest, diaphragmatic rupture, and open pneumothorax are unusual.

20. **What is the frequency of abdominal organ injury in blunt trauma?**
In decreasing order of frequency, they are spleen, liver, kidneys, intestine, pancreas, urinary bladder, and major blood vessels. Approximately one-third of children with major trauma have significant intraperitoneal injuries that must be recognized and treated expeditiously.

21. **What is the utility of clinical examination in blunt abdominal trauma?**
Thorough clinical examination can help determine which patients do not need CT scan of the abdomen to evaluate for intraabdominal injury. In a large series of injured children, Holmes et al. demonstrated that the absence of seven clinical signs (Glasgow Coma Scale >13, no evidence of abdominal wall trauma, no complaints of abdominal pain, no abdominal tenderness on exam, no vomiting, no thoracic wall trauma, and no decreased breath sounds) has a negative predictive value for intraabdominal injury of 99%.

22. **What are the advantages and disadvantages of CT in children?**
Abdominal CT scan is safe, noninvasive, and can assess retroperitoneal structures and identify specific organ injuries. It is the gold standard for diagnosis of blunt intraabdominal injury. However, CT scanning does not come without risk to children. The risk of radiation induced malignancy ranges from one new malignancy for every 500–6000 scans performed. Risk of radiation induced malignancy is higher in younger children as their tissues are still dividing and are more susceptible to radiation induced injury. Additionally, CT scan has a poor ability to detect hollow viscus injury, requires IV contrast with associated risks of renal injury and allergic reaction, and requires time and transport to radiology, which can be critical in an injured child.

23. **Is ultrasonography effective in the evaluation of children with abdominal trauma?**
Unfortunately, the focused abdominal sonography for trauma (FAST) exam does not have the same sensitivity and specificity in children as it does in adults. In the adult trauma population, the sensitivity and specificity of the FAST exam to detect intraabdominal injury exceed 95%. However, in the pediatric population, the FAST exam remains specific (>90% specificity) but lacks sensitivity (50%). This is secondary to the fact that children are more likely to have only intracapsular hematoma without associated hemoperitoneum following solid organ injury, whereas adults are more likely to have free hemoperitoneum.

24. **Is there a reliable method to diagnose hollow visceral injury in children?**
No. Serial physical examinations remain the gold standard. Repeat physical examination by the trauma surgical team is mandatory.

25. **What are the "soft signs" of pediatric intraabdominal injury?**
   - Seat-belt sign: Ecchymosis in the distribution of the child's seat belt correlates with a high incidence of solid organ injury, hollow viscus injury, and lumbar spine injury.
   - Gross hematuria has a 30% risk for significant intraabdominal injury, including injury outside of the genitourinary system.
   - Elevation of the liver enzymes aspartate aminotransferase (>250 U/L) or alanine aminotransferase (>450 U/L) corresponds to a 50% risk of blunt liver injury.
   - Children with documented pelvic fracture have at least a 20% risk for associated intraabdominal injury.
   - Children with severe neurologic impairment (Glasgow Coma Scale score <8) frequently suffer concurrent intraabdominal injury.

26. **What should be suspected in children with seat belt or handlebar injuries?**
The seat-belt complex consists of ecchymosis of the abdominal wall, a flexion-distraction injury to the lumbar spine (Chance fracture), and small bowel injury. Approximately 30% of children with the seat belt sign have an associated small bowel injury. A handlebar injury classically causes disruption of the pancreatic duct at the junction of the body and tail where the pancreas crosses the vertebral column and is vulnerable to anterior blunt compression.

27. **Does the presence of hemoperitoneum in children require laparotomy?**
No. Unlike in adults, <15% of children with hemoperitoneum require laparotomy for control of bleeding or repair of an injury.

28. **Do all children with solid organ injuries require operative repair?**
No. As with adult patients, selective nonoperative management of solid organ injuries is now the standard of care. Failure rates of nonoperative management of blunt liver and spleen injuries are now <5% in most pediatric trauma centers; this rate is significantly lower than in the adult trauma population.

29. **When is nonoperative management of solid organ injury in children appropriate?**
Children who can be safely monitored for ongoing bleeding following blunt solid organ injury include those children who remain hemodynamically stable without other injuries that mandate operative intervention. The need for initial packed red blood cell transfusion does not mandate operative intervention unless the child fails to achieve hemodynamic stability following transfusion. Children should be closely monitored for signs of ongoing bleeding, which include tachycardia, hypotension, altered mental status, decreased urine output, delayed capillary refill, or respiratory compromise.

30. **What are the long-term consequences of nonoperative management of a splenic injury in children?**
Vascular pseudoaneurysm may form following blunt splenic injury. However, in pediatric patients these complications are exceedingly rare (<1%). Up to 15% of children (depending on grade of injury) may experience prolonged pain >4 weeks after injury. In almost all cases, though, this pain is related to the healing process or is entirely unrelated to the spleen. Additionally, children are at risk for rebleeding from the injury during the healing process. The American Pediatric Surgical Association recommends that children undergo a period of activity restriction following hospital discharge to allow time for healing and decrease the risk of rebleeding.

31. **What are the indications for operative intervention for solid organ injuries?**
Hemodynamic instability, failure to stabilize with blood product transfusion, other intraabdominal injuries that mandate laparotomy.

32. **What is SCIWORA?**
SCIWORA stands for spinal cord injury without radiologic abnormalities and typically manifests as cervical spine injury with no bony or ligamentous abnormalities on complete plain radiographs or CT. Abnormalities are usually evident on MRI. SCIWORA is unique to children because a child's spine has increased elasticity, shallow and horizontally oriented facet joints, anterior wedging of the vertebral bodies, and poorly developed uncinate processes compared to adults. The spinal cord can be completely disrupted in young children without apparent disruption of the vertebral elements. Two-thirds of SCIWORA cases are seen in children under 8 years of age.

33. **What is the hallmark of SCIWORA?**
SCIWORA manifests as a documented neurologic deficit that may have changed or resolved by the time the child arrives in the emergency department. Danger lies in the fact that immediate re-injury of the same area may produce permanent disability. Many children with SCIWORA tend to develop neurologic deficits hours to days after the reported injury. Therefore, spinal immobilization should continue, and thorough neurosurgical evaluation is essential in any child with reliable evidence of even a transient neurologic deficit.

34. **What percentage of pediatric deaths attributed to injury are caused by intentional trauma?**
Twenty-five percent. More than 80% of deaths from head trauma in children younger than 2 years are caused by intentional abuse.

35. **What signs are suspicious for nonaccidental trauma (NAT)?**
- History of failure to thrive
- Delay in seeking medical care
- History of multiple previous injuries
- Absent or uninterested caregiver
- Fluctuating or conflicting histories
- History inconsistent with the injury or developmental level of the victim

Suspicious physical findings include bite, pinch, slap, or cord marks or bruises in various stages of healing; multiple or bilateral skull fractures; a skull fracture in a fall <4 feet; retinal hemorrhages (from shaking), rib fractures, and perineal burns or linear burn borders (from "dipping" the child into scalding liquid).

36. **List the characteristics of abusive head trauma**
- Diffuse axonal injury
- Subdural hemorrhage
- Age <2 years
- Little external evidence of trauma

37. **What fracture patterns are suspicious for NAT?**
    - Multiple rib fractures at various stages of healing
    - Extremity fractures including metaphyseal "chip" or "bucket-handle" fractures
    - Diaphyseal spiral fracture in children <9 months of age
    - Transverse midshaft long-bone fracture
    - Femur fracture in infants <2 years of age
    - Fracture of the acromion process of the scapula
    - Proximal humerus fracture

38. **What percentage of NAT cases involves burn injuries? What are their characteristics?**
    Twenty percent of cases of abuse involve burns. Scalding by hot water is the most common cause of burn. Specific patterns of injury may raise suspicion of abuse, including burns involving the buttocks and perineum (bathing trunk distribution), back, dorsum of the hand, and stocking-glove distribution. Cigarette burns look like circular punched-out ulcers of similar size and are also concerning for NAT.

39. **What are the necessary steps in evaluation of a child with suspected NAT?**
    Any child with suspected NAT should have a detailed physical examination with thorough documentation (drawings and photographs can be quite helpful) of all injuries, head CT scan, skeletal survey, and retinal fundoscopic examination. The appropriate child protective services should be contacted immediately.

40. **How common is postinjury multiple organ failure (MOF) in children?**
    It is rare. With equivalent injury severity, MOF in children is much lower than in adults and carries a much lower mortality.

41. **What is the role of glycemic control in the pediatric trauma population?**
    Euglycemia (glucose 90–130 mg/dL) is associated with decreased rate of infection, decreased hospital length of stay, and increased survival.

KEY POINTS: PEDIATRIC TRAUMA

1. Trauma is the leading cause of death and disability in the pediatric population.
2. The majority of pediatric trauma is due to blunt mechanisms.
3. Tachycardia, not hypotension, is the first sign of significant blood loss in children.
4. Serial physical examination remains key to the care of blunt injured children.
5. Among children under age 2 years, if the clinical history does not match the patient's presentation, the physician should maintain a high index of suspicion for NAT.

BIBLIOGRAPHY

1. Calkins CM, Bensard DD, Moore EE, et al. The injured child is resistant to multiple organ failure: a different inflammatory response? *J Trauma*. 2002;5(6)3:1058–1063.
2. Dare AO, Dias MS. Magnetic resonance imaging correlation in pediatric spinal cord injury without radiographic abnormality. *J Neurosurg*. 2002;97(1 suppl):33–39.
3. Kristoffersen KW, Mooney DP. Long-term outcome of nonoperative pediatric splenic injury management. *J Pediatr Surg*. 2007;42(6):1038–1041.
4. Holmes JF, Gladman A. Performance of abdominal ultrasonography in pediatric blunt trauma patients: a meta-analysis. *J Pediatr Surg*. 2007;42(9):1588–1594.
5. Mazzola CA, Adelson PD. Critical care management of head trauma in children. *Crit Care Med*. 2002;30(11 suppl):S393–S401.
6. Mehall JR, Ennis JS, Saltzman DA, et al. Prospective results of a standardized algorithm based on hemodynamic status for managing pediatric solid organ injury. *J Am Coll Surg*. 2001;193(4):347–353.
7. Partrick DA, Bensard DD. Is hypotension a reliable indicator of blood loss from traumatic injury in children? *Am J Surg*. 2002;184(6):555–559.
8. Roaten JB, Partrick DA, Nydam TL, et al. Nonaccidental trauma is a major cause of morbidity and mortality among patients at a regional level I pediatric trauma center. *J Pediatr Surg*. 2006;41(12):2013–2015.
9. St. Peter SD, Keckler SJ. Justification for an abbreviated protocol in the management of blunt spleen and liver injury in children. *J Pediatr Surg*. 2008;43(1):191–193.

10. Stafford PW, Blinman TA. Practical points in evaluation and resuscitation of the injured child. *Surg Clin North Am.* 2002;82(2):273–301.
11. Tuggle DW, Kuhn MA. Hyperglycemia and infections in pediatric trauma patients. *Am Surg.* 2008;74(3):195–198.
12. Acker SN, Roach JP. Beyond morbidity and mortality: the social and legal outcomes of non-accidental trauma. *J Pediatr Surg.* 2015;50(4):604–607.
13. Acker SN, Ross JT. Pediatric specific shock index accurately identifies severely injured children. *J Pediatr Surg.* 2015;50(2):331–334.
14. Roach JP, Acker SN. Head injury pattern in children can help differentiate accidental from non-accidental trauma. *Pediatr Surg Int.* 2014;30(11):1103–1106.
15. Holscher CM, Faulk LW, Moore EE, et al. Chest computed tomography imaging for blunt pediatric trauma: not worth the radiation risk. *J Surg Res.* 2013;184(1):352–357.
16. Holmes JF, Lillis K, Monroe D, et al. Identifying children at very low risk of clinically important blunt abdominal injuries. *Ann Emerg Med.* 2013;62(2):107–116.
17. Miglioretti DL, Johnson E, Williams A, et al. The use of computed tomography in pediatrics and the associated radiation exposure and estimated cancer risk. *JAMA Pediatr.* 2013;167(8):700–707.

III

ABDOMINAL SURGERY

CHAPTER 39

APPENDICITIS

Laurel R. Imhoff, MD, MPH, Alden H. Harken, MD, FACS

1. **What is the classic presentation of acute appendicitis?**
   Periumbilical pain that migrates to the right lower quadrant (RLQ) in a patient who is anorexic. Associated symptoms include nausea, vomiting, and bowel changes.

2. **What is the pathophysiology of appendicitis?**
   The appendix is susceptible to luminal obstruction via lymphoid hyperplasia, a retained fecalith, tumor, foreign body, or kink. Any of these processes may result in lymphatic and venous obstruction that increases intraluminal pressure and causes distention of the appendiceal lumen. Consequently, an acute inflammatory response develops that leads to ischemia, bacterial overgrowth, and eventually necrosis. Unless surgically removed, the gangrenous appendix will perforate, releasing the appendiceal contents into the peritoneal cavity. Subsequently, a phlegmon, intraperitoneal abscess, or local peritonitis develops.

3. **What is the mechanism of the periumbilical pain?**
   The intestines are insensitive to touch or inflammation unless the enclosing peritoneum is involved. Epigastric pain results from a distended section of intestine. This pain is referred along midline.

4. **Where is McBurney's point?**
   One-third the distance between the anterosuperior iliac spine and the umbilicus.

5. **What is McBurney's point?**
   The point of maximal tenderness in acute appendicitis. It results from local inflammation of the parietal peritoneum.

6. **Was McBurney a cop from Boston?**
   Probably. Another McBurney was a surgeon from New York who, in collaboration with a surgeon named Fitz, coined the term appendicitis In classic papers published in 1886 and 1889.

7. **What are the typical laboratory findings of a patient with appendicitis?**
   - White blood cell (WBC) count: 12,000–14,000
   - Negative urinalysis results (no WBCs)
   - Negative pregnancy test result

8. **What layers does the surgeon encounter on exposing the appendix through a Rockey-Davis incision?**
   Skin, subcutaneous fat, aponeurosis of the external oblique muscle, internal oblique muscle, transversalis abdominis muscle, transversalis fascia, and peritoneum.

9. **What are other possible signs in appendicitis?**
   - **Rovsing's sign:** Pain in the RLQ with palpation of the left lower quadrant.
   - **Dunphy's sign:** Increased pain with coughing (a cough jostles the inflamed peritoneum).
   - **Psoas sign:** Pain on passive extension of the right thigh. It is present when the inflamed appendix is retrocecal and overlying the right psoas muscle.
   - **Obturator sign:** Pain on passive internal rotation of the hip when the right knee is flexed. It is present when the inflamed appendix is in contact with the obturator internus muscle.

10. **Who was Rockey-Davis?**
    Rockey-Davis was a pair of surgeons—AE Rockey and GG Davis—who developed RLQ transverse, muscle-splitting incisions that extend into the rectus sheath.

11. **What is the blood supply to the appendix and right colon?**
    The ileocolic and right colic arteries, which come off the superior mesenteric artery.

12. **Does surgery for appendicitis involve a risk of mortality?**
    No, surgical procedure is devoid of risk.

    Mortality rate
    Nonperforated appendix   <0.1%
    Perforated appendix   <0.3%

13. **What patient groups are at higher risk of death from perforated appendicitis?**
    a. Very young patients (younger than 2 years)
    b. Elderly patients (older than 70 years) who exhibit diminished abdominal innervation and present late
    c. Diabetic patients, who present late because of diabetic visceral neuropathy
    d. Patients taking steroids; steroids mask everything

14. **What is a "white worm"?**
    A normal appendix.

15. **What is the differential diagnosis of RLQ pain?**
    - Meckel's diverticulum
    - Diverticulitis
    - Ectopic pregnancy
    - Crohn's disease
    - Ovarian torsion
    - Tubo-ovarian abscess (TOA)
    - Pelvic inflammatory disease (PID)
    - Carcinoid tumor
    - Cholecystitis
    - Ruptured ovarian cyst

16. **What is an acceptable negative appendectomy rate?**
    This is a controversial topic currently being debated in surgical literature. Traditionally, up to a 15% negative appendectomy rate was considered acceptable. Now with the adjunct of imaging (ultrasound [US] and computed tomography [CT]) lower negative rates are expected.

17. **What is the role of imaging in the diagnosis of acute appendicitis?**
    US and CT can be both negatively and positively helpful. They may eliminate alternative diagnoses such as ectopic pregnancy or TOA when a perfectly normal right fallopian tube and ovary is seen. They may establish the diagnosis when an inflamed, edematous appendix is visualized. CT is particularly useful in visualizing periappendiceal tissue and may reveal that the appendix has already perforated by showing a phlegmon or abscess.

18. **What sonographic and CT findings are suggestive of appendicitis?**
    a. An appendix of 7 mm or greater in anteroposterior diameter
    b. Thickened or enhancing appendiceal wall
    c. Periappendiceal inflammation, such as fat stranding, fluid, phlegmon, or abscess
    d. The presence of an appendicolith

19. **Has laparoscopic appendectomy replaced the traditional "open" approach?**
    Yes, "lap appy" is now the standard. Laparoscopic appendectomy takes a little longer in the operating room, a little shorter in the hospital, is a little more expensive, and is associated with more rapid return to work.

KEY POINTS: APPENDICEAL CARCINOID

1. Sixty percent of carcinoid tumors occur in the appendix; 0.03% of appendectomies reveal incidental carcinoid.
2. This malignant but slow tumor spreads to lymph nodes, liver, and right heart.
3. If tumor size is <2 cm and does not involve the base of the appendix, appendectomy alone may suffice; however, the bowel should be assessed because of a 30% chance of synchronous lesion.
4. If tumor size is >2 cm or involves the base of the appendix, right hemicolectomy is necessary.

20. **What is a Meckel's diverticulum?**
    Meckel's diverticulum is a congenital omphalomesenteric mucosa remnant that may contain ectopic gastric mucosa. It is found in 2% of the population, 2 feet upward from the ileocecal valve. It becomes inflamed in 2% of patients (i.e., the rule of 2s).

21. **Can chronic diverticulitis masquerade as appendicitis?**
    Yes. Fifty percent of patients aged 50 years and older have colonic diverticula. The appendix is just a big cecal diverticulum. Thus, it makes sense that appendicitis and diverticulitis should look, act, and smell alike.

22. **Can a woman with a negative pregnancy test present with an ectopic pregnancy?**
    Yes. The fallopian tube must be inspected for a walnut-sized lump. Appropriate surgical therapy is a longitudinal incision to "shell out" the fetus with subsequent repair of the tube. This approach (as opposed to salpingectomy) is designed to preserve fertility. Methotrexate also may precipitate spontaneous evacuation in early-term pregnancy.

23. **Can Crohn's disease initially present as appendicitis?**
    Yes. This presentation is typical. Crohn's disease is boggy, edematous, granulomatous inflammation of the distal ileum. Traditional surgical dictum suggests that it is appropriate to remove the appendix in patients with Crohn's disease unless the cecum at the appendiceal base is involved.

24. **Is it possible to confuse appendicitis with a TOA?**
    Of course. An ovarian abscess buried deep in an inflamed, edematous, matted right adnexa can be treated successfully with intravenous antibiotics alone. Do not drain pus into the free peritoneal cavity; this will only make the patient sicker.

25. **Can PID resemble appendicitis?**
    PID can look exactly like appendicitis except for a positive "chandelier sign." On pelvic examination, manual tug on the cervix moves the inflamed, painful adnexae, and the patient hits the chandelier. Patients with PID should be treated with antibiotics (either orally or intravenously, depending on how sick the patient is).

26. **How does one deal with an appendiceal carcinoid tumor?**
    Carcinoid tumors may present anywhere along the gastrointestinal tract; 60%, however, are in the appendix. An obstructing carcinoid tumor, much like a fecalith, can lead to appendicitis, and in 0.3% of appendectomies, carcinoid tumors are the culprit. Most carcinoid tumors are small (<1.5 cm) and benign; 70% are located in the distal appendix. They are effectively treated with appendectomy alone. A large carcinoid tumor (>2.0 cm) at the appendiceal base, especially with invasion into the mesoappendix, must be considered malignant and mandates a right hemicolectomy.

27. **Can appendicitis be mistaken for acute cholecystitis?**
    Occasionally, yes. Both entities reflect acute, localized, intraperitoneal inflammation. Laboratory studies may be identical: WBC count of 12,000–14,000, negative urinalysis result, and negative pregnancy test result. Thus, if one is thinking "appendicitis," the major difference may be only right upper quadrant pain versus RLQ pain. Laparoscopic cholecystectomy is possible for acute cholecystitis, but conversion to an open procedure should be more frequent.

WEBSITES

* http://www.websurg.com (Excellent lectures/videos/photos of surgery; registration required.)

BIBLIOGRAPHY

1. Silen W, ed. *Cope's Early Diagnosis of the Acute Abdomen.* 19th ed. Oxford University Press; 1996.
2. Fitz RH. Perforating inflammation of the vermiform appendix with special reference to its early diagnosis and treatment. *Trans Assoc Am Physicians.* 1886;1:107–144.
3. Rockey AE. Transverse incisions in abdominal operations. *Med Rec.* 1905;68:779–780.
4. Guss DA, Behling CA. Impact of abdominal helical computed tomography on the rate of negative appendicitis. *J Emerg Med.* 2008;34(1):7–11.
5. Huynh V, Lalezarzadeh F. Abdominal computed tomography in the evaluation of acute and perforated appendicitis in the community setting. *Am Surg.* 2007;73(10):1002–1005.
6. Pokala N, Sadhasivam S. Complicated appendicitis—is the laparoscopic approach appropriate? A comparative study with the open approach: outcome in a community hospital setting. *Am Surg.* 2007;73(8):737–741. discussion 741–742.

7. Samuel M. Pediatric appendicitis score. *J Pediatr Surg.* 2002;37(6):877–881.
8. Urbach DR, Cohen MM. Is perforation of the appendix a risk factor for tubal infertility and ectopic pregnancy? An appraisal of the evidence. *Can J Surg.* 1999;42(2):101–108.
9. van Rossem CC, Bolmers MD, Schreinemacher MH, et al. Diagnosing acute appendicitis: surgery or imaging? *Colorectal Dis.* 2016;18(12):1129–1132.
10. Hansen W, Mariam M, Paladin A, et al. Evolving practice patterns in imaging pregnant patients with acute abdominal and pelvic conditions. *Curr Probl Diagn Radiol.* 2016;46(1):10–16.

CHAPTER 40

GALLBLADDER DISEASE

Ning Lu, MD, Walter L. Biffl, MD, FACS

1. **What is the prevalence of gallstones in Western society for women and men 60 years of age?**
   Women, 50%; men, 15%, although there is formidable ethnic predilection with gallstones endemic in American Indians.

2. **What is the difference between cholelithiasis, cholecystitis, choledocholithiasis, and cholangitis?**
   Cholelithiasis refers to the presence of gallbladder stones. Symptomatic cholelithiasis is the most common indication for cholecystectomy. **Cholecystitis** is an inflammatory condition of the gallbladder, usually initiated by gallstone impaction in the gallbladder neck with obstruction of the cystic duct. **Choledocholithiasis** is the presence of stones in the common bile duct (CBD). **Cholangitis** is an infection of the biliary tree, generally as a result of obstruction, usually secondary to choledocholithiasis.

3. **What percentage of asymptomatic gallstones becomes symptomatic?**
   Ten percent at 5 years, 15% at 10 years, and 18% by 15 years.

4. **Should patients with asymptomatic gallstones undergo cholecystectomy?**
   No. The risk of observation of patients with asymptomatic gallstones is less than or equal to the risk of operation.

5. **In what groups of patients with asymptomatic gallstones is prophylactic cholecystectomy beneficial?**
   • Patients with congenital hemolytic anemia who have gallstones at the time of splenectomy
   • Patients undergoing small bowel resection for carcinoid tumor in whom somatostatin therapy or hepatic angioembolization is anticipated

6. **What is the optimal timing for laparoscopic cholecystectomy in acute cholecystitis?**
   "Cooling the gallbladder down" and delaying surgery for 6 weeks is associated with recurrent cholecystitis in 20% of patients. Prospective randomized studies have consistently found that early cholecystectomy allows shorter hospital stays, with no difference in morbidity or mortality, compared with delayed cholecystectomy. Procedures performed within the first 24 hours generally are easier because the area of dissection is not yet maximally inflamed, and fibrosis and increased blood vessel proliferation have not yet occurred. Moreover, this approach is cost-effective.

7. **What is the conversion rate from laparoscopy to the open approach in acute cholecystitis and in symptomatic cholelithiasis?**
   The overall conversion rate is 5%; it occurs in 10%–15% for acute cholecystitis but <5% for symptomatic cholelithiasis.

8. **What is the incidence of acalculous cholecystitis?**
   Ten percent of all cases of cholecystitis.

9. **What organisms require antibiotic coverage in biliary infections?**
   Escherichia coli, Klebsiella species, *Streptococcus faecalis, Clostridium welchii, Proteus* species, *Enterobacter* species, and anaerobic *Streptococcus* species.

10. **What is the incidence of CBD injury in open and laparoscopic cholecystectomy?**
    It is 0.2%–0.3% for open and 0.4%–0.6% for laparoscopic cholecystectomy.

11. **How does laparoscopic intraoperative ultrasound (LUS) compare with laparoscopic intraoperative cholangiography (LIOC)?**
    The sensitivity of LUS is high (90%) and comparable to that of LIOC. Potential advantages of LUS include less time and less dissection than LIOC.

12. **Does LUS or LIOC prevent CBD injuries during cholecystectomy?**
In population-based studies, there are fewer CBD injuries among patients undergoing LIOC; however, there is no level I evidence that the LIOC was preventive. LIOC does, however, identify injuries at the time they occur. Advocates of LUS argue that identifying the anatomy before a duct is transected (and LIOC catheter inserted) may prevent CBD injuries.

13. **What percentage of patients undergoing cholecystectomy have unsuspected choledocholithiasis?**
Although as many as 15% of patients with symptomatic gallstones have choledocholithiasis, only about 2% are clinically unsuspected. If the patient has no history of jaundice or biliary pancreatitis, and a CBD <6 mm in diameter, there is no role for routine laboratory screening. The vast majority of these stones will pass spontaneously.

14. **Should patients with suspected choledocholithiasis undergo surgery first, or CBD assessment?**
In a recent prospective randomized clinical trial, among patients at intermediate risk of a common duct stone, initial cholecystectomy compared with sequential common duct endoscopy assessment and subsequent surgery resulted in a shorter length of stay without increased morbidity.

15. **When, if ever, should laparoscopic cholecystectomy be performed during pregnancy?**
Most attacks of acute biliary colic during pregnancy resolve spontaneously. To avoid preterm labor, cholecystectomy should be performed after delivery. If surgery is necessary, however, the second trimester is preferred for any surgical intervention.

16. **What is the prevalence of gallbladder carcinoma found incidentally during cholecystectomy?**
Open, 1%; laparoscopic, 0.1%. This compares with an incidence in the general population of 0.01%.

17. **Why is cholecystectomy increasing in the pediatric population?**
Gallstone identification has increased because of the more liberal use of ultrasonography in patients with abdominal pain.

KEY POINTS: GALLBLADDER DISEASE

1. Overall incidence in United States: women >60 years old, 50%; men >60 years old, 15%.
2. Fifteen percent to 20% of patients with gallstones become symptomatic.
3. Patients with acute cholecystitis should have surgery as soon as possible after the onset of symptoms.
4. Routine LUS may identify CBD stones and may help avoid CBD injuries.
5. Patients with moderate risk of choledocholithiasis should proceed directly to cholecystectomy with intraoperative bile duct evaluation.

BIBLIOGRAPHY

1. Biffl WL, Moore EE, Offner PJ, et al. Routine intraoperative laparoscopic ultrasonography with selective cholangiography reduces bile duct complications during laparoscopic cholecystectomy. *J Am Coll Surg.* 2001;193(3):272–280.
2. Cabarrou P, Portier G, Chalret Du Rieu M. Prophylactic cholecystectomy during abdominal surgery. *J Visc Surg.* 2013;150(4):229–235.
3. de Mestral C, Rotstein OD. A population-based analysis of the clinical course of 10,304 patients with acute cholecystitis, discharged without cholecystectomy. *J Trauma Acute Care Surg.* 2013;74(1):26–31.
4. Ghumman E, Barry M. Management of gallstones in pregnancy. *Br J Surg.* 1997;84(12):1646–1650.
5. Iranmanesh P, Frossard JL, Mugnier-Konrad B, et al. Initial cholecystectomy vs sequential common duct endoscopic assessment and subsequent cholecystectomy for suspected gallstone migration: a randomized clinical trial. *JAMA.* 2014;312(2):137–144.
6. Koti RS, Davidson CJ. Surgical management of acute cholecystitis. *Langenbecks Arch Surg.* 2015;400(4):403–419.

CHAPTER 41

PANCREATIC CANCER

Martin D. McCarter, MD, FACS

1. **What is the magnitude of the problem?**
   For the year 2016, there were an estimated 53,000 new cases of pancreatic cancer in the United States, and more than 41,790 deaths, making this arguably one of the most lethal tumors. It is now the third most common cause of cancer death in the United States for both men and women, with an annual incidence of approximately 12.3 cases/100,000.

2. **What are the histologic types of pancreatic cancer?**
   Adenocarcinoma is far and away the most common (and lethal) type. Neuroendocrine tumors, making up approximately 1%–5% of cases, generally have a more indolent course. Other rare tumor types such as sarcoma, lymphoma, pseudopapillary, and intraductal papillary mucinous (IPMN) tumor can occur as well.

3. **What are the presenting signs of pancreatic cancer?**
   - Painless jaundice: 40% of patients
   - Pain (epigastric, right upper quadrant, back) with jaundice: 40%
   - Metastatic disease (e.g., hepatomegaly, ascites, lung nodules) with or without jaundice: 20%
   Most patients also have other nonspecific gastrointestinal symptoms such as bloating, food intolerance, or pancreatic insufficiency, and weight loss.

4. **What is the estimated survival for pancreatic cancer patients?**
   Overall 5-year survival for those undergoing a complete resection ranges from 5% to 25%.

Stage	At Diagnosis	Estimated Median Survival
Resectable	10%–20%	10–24 months
Locally Advanced	40%–45%	9–12 months
Metastatic	40%–45%	6–9 months

5. **Why is there such a high rate of advanced disease at diagnosis?**
   The pancreas is retroperitoneal, relatively insensate, and symptoms of disease do not manifest themselves until local obstruction of duodenum, pancreatic, or biliary duct forms. About 80% arise in the head of the gland, 10% arise in the body, and 10% in the tail.

6. **What is IPMN?**
   IPMN is a type of neoplasm, or precancerous tissue that grows within the pancreas ducts and is characterized by the production of a thick mucinous fluid. IPMNs are classified as main duct, side branch, or a mixed type based on their radiographic appearance. IPMNs are analogous to adenomatous colon polyps in that they have malignant potential, but not all IPMNs will transform into an invasive cancer.

7. **What are the indications to operate on IPMNs?**
   The concern for a current occult malignancy or the risk of developing a malignancy drives much of the decision making around when to operate. In general, the indications to operate on IPMNs are for those that are symptomatic (i.e., causing pancreatitis or digestive problems from pancreatic insufficiency), those that involve the main pancreatic duct with >10 mm dilation (higher risk), those associated with mural nodules or high-grade dysplasia, side branch IPMNs associated with cysts >3 cm, or those that rapidly change under surveillance.

8. **What is the significance of a "double-duct" sign?**
   This refers to the presence of a dilated pancreatic and biliary ductal system identified on computed tomography (CT) scan or endoscopic retrograde cholangiopancreatography (ERCP). In the absence of a biliary stone, this nearly always implies the presence of an underlying cancer as the etiology.

9. **What in the world is CA 19-9?**

CA 19-9 stands for carbohydrate antigen 19-9. It is a tumor marker associated with pancreatic and biliary tumors, which is measured in the patient's serum. It is nonspecific (may be elevated in inflammation and other benign conditions), but may be helpful in monitoring a patient's progress/response to therapy. Its sensitivity and specificity can be limited by certain conditions. For example, the blood test for CA 19-9 is dependent on the Lewis blood group antigen phenotype and is not detectable in patients with Lewis AB- phenotype (approximately 5%–10% of the population). In addition, inflammatory conditions and biliary obstruction cause artificial elevation and therefore limit its usefulness under these conditions.

10. **What do you do when the ultrasound (US), ERCP, and CT scan show dilated extrahepatic bile ducts, a mass in the head of the pancreas, and no obvious cause other than cancer? The tumor seems separate from the portal vein and mesenteric arteries, and there are no liver metastases. What should be done next?**

Make an assessment of operative risk. If the patient is a poor operative risk, one should consider percutaneous or endoscopic US-guided fine-needle aspiration (FNA) to document cancer, if possible, and endoscopic stenting of the bile duct; surgery probably is not a good option. If the patient is a good operative risk, the next step is surgery. The clinical picture is accurate in at least 90% of cases, and FNA adds no useful information at this time. If no malignant tissue is obtained, surgery is still indicated to relieve the jaundice and because a negative biopsy does not rule out a cancer.

11. **We are in the operating room, the abdomen is open, and the discussion revolves around taking out the tumor. What is a Whipple procedure?**

Pancreaticoduodenectomy involves the removal of the gallbladder, distal common duct, duodenum, gastric antrum, and the portion of pancreas to the right of the portal vein; in essence, a proximal pancreatectomy.

12. **What is distal pancreatectomy? A total pancreatectomy?**

Distal pancreatectomy removes the portion of gland to the left of the portal vein, along with the spleen. Total pancreatectomy combines both procedures, again, with antrectomy in some centers.

13. **Why remove the gallbladder, duodenum, and stomach if the problem is in the pancreas?**

After the ampulla of Vater is removed, the gallbladder does not function well and forms gallstones. The second and third portions of the duodenum share a blood supply with the head of the pancreas and are usually devascularized when the head is removed. Historically, the gastric antrum was removed to improve resection margins.

Removing the antrum adds little to the scope of the operation, however, and marginal ulceration can be prevented by placing the gastrojejunostomy downstream from where bile and pancreatic secretions enter the gut. Thus, many surgeons choose to perform a pylorus-preserving Whipple procedure when feasible.

14. **How does one determine whether to perform a Whipple procedure, distal pancreatectomy, or total pancreatectomy? What is the cure rate?**

Whipple procedures are used for mobile tumors in the head of the pancreas and periampullary region. Distal pancreatectomy is used for lesions of the body and tail unaccompanied by signs of spread. Total pancreatectomy is generally reserved for a few rare situations in which a diffuse cancer involves most of the gland but nowhere else. Median survival with each procedure is about 18–24 months, and 5-year survival is about 5%–25%. This procedure has about 1%–3% operative mortality and 25%–40% morbidity in centers with extensive experience; in other settings, the operative risk and complication rate can be much higher.

15. **What should be done if there is tumor extension or nodal metastases along the aorta or root of mesentery?**

The patient cannot be cured with surgery, so the goal is palliation. If obstructive jaundice is present, a biliary-enteric bypass or endoscopic stenting should be performed. If a tumor obstructs the duodenum, a gastroenterostomy should also be carried out. Some surgeons believe gastroenterostomy should be done routinely for cancers of the pancreatic head, regardless of whether duodenal compromise is present because up to 20% of patients without this problem at the time of surgery may require intervention for poor gastric emptying in the future.

16. **What are other signs of inoperability?**
General contraindications to resection include metastatic disease, invasion of the inferior vena cava, or major local arteries (celiac axis, hepatic artery, superior mesenteric artery). Relative contraindications to resection include invasion of the portal or superior mesenteric vein. Resection of the portal vein and reconstruction can be done with less morbidity than in the past, but it is debatable whether this technical exercise has led to improved survival or just better patient selection.

17. **What is a borderline resectable pancreatic cancer?**
Borderline resectable pancreas cancer refers to a locally advanced tumor (not overtly metastatic) that abuts or involves a short segment of the portal vein, superior mesenteric vein, or, in some cases, abuts the hepatic artery or superior mesenteric artery. The evolving concept is to assess the tumor biology by treating these patients with some combination of chemotherapy, then reassess for response, and then treat with local radiation therapy and reassess with imaging again. If the disease has not progressed and no new lesions are found, some patients seem to benefit from an aggressive operative approach with planned vascular reconstruction.

18. **A patient is found to have unsuspected spread to the celiac axis. You carry out a biliary and gastric bypass. What other palliative options can you consider?**
Some of these patients, if suffering from preoperative back pain, can be relieved of this by intraoperative alcohol celiac ganglion block. Alternatively, such treatment can be carried out postoperatively by gastroenterology or interventional radiology. Palliative chemotherapy and radiation therapy can also provide pain relief.

19. **Are there any other treatments (chemotherapy, radiation therapy, pet therapy) that improve outcomes in resected pancreatic cancer?**
Marginally. This is not as a result of a lack of interest or effort. There is some evidence that chemotherapy (gemcitabine) or a combination of chemotherapy and radiation therapy may add a few months to overall survival following resection. The vast majority of prospective adjuvant trials have failed to make a significant difference in overall survival, though retrospective studies suggest some benefit. Here is a genuine opportunity for bright students such as the present reader to make a difference!

20. **With high morbidity and low cure rates, why are surgeons so eager to do Whipple procedures?**
Resection represents the only chance for cure. In addition, pancreatic resection—when carried out safely—probably offers the best long-term palliation in those destined to die of their disease. Finally, future advances in adjuvant therapy may provide hope for improvement in overall survival.

KEY POINTS: DIAGNOSTIC WORK-UP OF A PATIENT WITH JAUNDICE

1. Liver function tests: Determine degree of jaundice (obstructive versus nonobstructive) and hepatic dysfunction.
2. US of right upper quadrant: Rules out gallstones, evaluates intrahepatic versus extrahepatic ductal dilatation.
3. If hepatic ducts are dilated: ERCP or percutaneous transhepatic cholangiography to delineate site of mechanical obstruction.
4. CT: Evaluates size of tumor if present, degree of regional spread, or liver metastases.

WEBSITES

- www.nccn.org
- www.cancer.org

BIBLIOGRAPHY

1. Christians KK, Heimler JW, George B, et al. Survival of patients with resectable pancreatic cancer who received neoadjuvant therapy. *Surgery.* 2016;159(3):893–900.
2. Tanaka M. International consensus on the management of intraductal papillary mucinous neoplasm of the pancreas. *Ann Transl Med.* 2015;3(19):286.
3. Helmink BA, Snyder RA. Advances in the surgical management of resectable and borderline resectable pancreas cancer. *Surg Oncol Clin N Am.* 2016;25(2):287–310.
4. Giuliani J, Bonetti A. The role of palliative surgery in the management of advanced pancreatic cancer in patients with biliary and duodenal obstruction. *Eur J Surg Oncol.* 2016;42(4):581–583.
5. Tsuchikawa T, Hirano S. Concomitant major vessel resection in pancreatic adenocarcinoma. *Postgrad Med.* 2015;127(3):273–276.
6. Hüttner FJ, Fitzmaurice C, Schwarzer G, et al. Pylorus-preserving pancreaticoduodenectomy (pp Whipple) versus pancreaticoduodenectomy (classic Whipple) for surgical treatment of periampullary and pancreatic carcinoma. *Cochrane Database Syst Rev.* 2016;16:2.
7. Sinha R, Gardner T. Double-duct sign in the clinical context. *Pancreas.* 2015;44(6):967–970.
8. Verbesey JE, Munson JL. Pancreatic cystic neoplasms. *Surg Clin North Am.* 2010;90(2):411–425.
9. Wargo JA, Warshaw AL. Surgical approach to pancreatic exocrine neoplasms. *Minerva Chir.* 2005;60(6):445–468.
10. Roeder F. Neoadjuvant radiotherapeutic strategies in pancreatic cancer. *World J Gastrointest Oncol.* 2016;8(2):186–197.

CHAPTER 42

ACUTE PANCREATITIS

Brooke C. Bredbeck, MD, Carlton C. Barnett, Jr., MD, FACS

1. **What are the common causes and incidence of acute pancreatitis?**
   Gallstones (40%–70%), alcohol (25%–35%), idiopathic (10%), and other (<5%). The incidence of acute pancreatitis is estimated 13–45 per 100,000 people, making it the second highest cause of total hospital stays in the United States.

2. **What are the uncommon causes?**
   Hyperlipidemia, hypercalcemia (hyperparathyroidism, multiple myeloma), iatrogenic factors (4% of patients undergoing endoscopic retrograde cholangiopancreatography [ERCP] may experience pancreatitis), drugs (didanosine, thiazide diuretics, H2 blockers, azathioprine, octreotide, estrogens, opiates, acetaminophen), infections (mumps, coxsackievirus), genetic factors (cystic fibrosis, hereditary pancreatitis, etc.), ischemia, pancreas divisum, malignancy, scorpion bites, and signs and autoimmune pancreatitis.

3. **What are the characteristic symptoms?**
   Acute onset of severe epigastric pain that is boring in nature and often radiates to the back. Pain is frequently accompanied by nausea and vomiting. Physical exam reveals diffuse abdominal tenderness, abdominal distention, "boardlike" abdominal guarding, and hypoactive bowel sounds. Patients may be febrile, tachycardic, and dehydrated. Evidence of jaundice or identification of gallstones on right upper quadrant ultrasound suggests a biliary cause of pancreatitis. Severe pancreatitis may result in retroperitoneal bleeding, leading to periumbilical or flank discoloration (called Cullen's sign and Grey Turner sign, respectively).

4. **What is the appropriate therapy for mild to moderate pancreatitis?**
   The critical component of supportive therapy is adequate fluid resuscitation to restore circulating volume. This can be measured by urine output, so place a Foley catheter. Appropriate treatment also includes pain medications, alcohol withdrawal prophylaxis, and nasogastric decompression for persistent emesis. Enteral nutrition maintains the gut mucosal barrier and prevents infection, so oral diet with on-demand nasoenteric tube feeding is recommended after 72 hours.

5. **Which is the better laboratory test, amylase or lipase?**
   Serum amylase levels tend to peak sooner than lipase levels, which may remain elevated for 4–5 days. Up to 30% of patients have normal amylase levels, particularly alcoholics with chronic "burned-out" pancreatitis. Serum lipase has a greater sensitivity and specificity than amylase levels. Three times the upper limit of normal serum lipase or amylase is diagnostic of pancreatitis.

6. **What other disease states cause hyperamylasemia?**
   Perforated peptic ulcers, small bowel obstruction, parotid gland inflammation or tumor, renal failure, and ovarian tumors are associated with elevated amylase levels.

7. **What is the significance of hypoxemia early in the course of pancreatitis?**
   Patients with necrotizing pancreatitis may develop respiratory failure requiring mechanical ventilation, which may progress to multiple organ failure. Hypoxemia is an ominous sign, as are infiltrates on admission chest radiograph.

8. **What is the revised Atlanta classification?**
   The classification system stratifies patients into mild, moderately severe, and severe forms of acute pancreatitis. Its purpose is to identify high-risk patients who may require specialist consultation or escalation in care.

Revised Atlanta classification of acute pancreatitis

Mild	No organ failure
	No local or systemic complications
Moderately severe	ANY of the following:
	Organ failure that resolves within 48 hr
	Local or system complications without organ failure
Severe	Persistent organ failure (POF) in one or more organs
	POF in the first week carries 33% mortality

9. What clinical scoring systems are used in acute pancreatitis, and what are their limitations?

   Clinical scoring systems use a defined set of clinical, radiologic, and laboratory measures to determine patient severity and predict outcomes. The calculations can be cumbersome because of the large number of criteria and the need to wait for follow-up labs. The **modified Marshall score** can define POF within the revised Atlanta classification if the value is over 2. The score examines three systems: respiratory, renal, and cardiovascular. The **Ranson score** measures 11 indices and a score of 3 or higher is considered severe disease. It cannot be calculated until after 48 hours of inpatient treatment. Other predictive indices include the acute physiology and chronic health evaluation II (APACHE II) scoring system and the Balthazar scoring system. The **APACHE II score** achieves positive and negative predictive values that are comparable to the Ranson's criteria. The **Balthazar score**, based on findings from computed tomography (CT) scanning (amount of inflammation, presence and extent of necrosis, and presence of fluid collections), is also acceptable for evaluation of expected morbidity and mortality.

10. What is necrotizing pancreatitis?

    The inflammation and edema of acute pancreatitis may progress with subsequent devitalization of pancreatic and/or peripancreatic tissue. Pancreatic necrosis occurs in approximately 20% of acute episodes.

11. Why is it important to differentiate acute pancreatitis from necrotizing pancreatitis?

    The presence and extent of necrosis are key determinants of the clinical course. Approximately 20% of patients with pancreatic necrosis develop infected pancreatic necrosis. Infection accounts for 80% of all deaths from pancreatitis. A step-up approach to treatment of infected necrotizing pancreatitis begins with antibiotics (culture-guided if possible). If conservative management fails, drainage and surgical debridement in later stages are the current standard of care.

12. What is the optimal method for diagnosing pancreatic necrosis with or without associated infection?

    Dynamic CT scans with intravenous contrast allow visualization and differentiation of healthy, perfused parenchyma from patchy, poorly perfused necrotic tissue. Sensitivity of CT imaging is not diagnostically useful for identification of necrosis until >4 days from onset. Therefore, a CT scan should be obtained in patients that do not clinically improve in response to fluid resuscitation and supportive treatment. CT-guided aspiration of the necrotic tissue may be performed to determine the presence of infection.

13. When is surgery indicated in patients with acute pancreatitis?

    Patients with persistent infected pancreatic necrosis after antibiotic therapy alone should receive step-up care beginning with percutaneous drainage. If this is not successful, open drainage and necrosectomy can be performed. Open drainage is best accomplished via a bilateral subcostal incision, placement of the greater omentum over the transverse colon to prevent enteric fistulas, and removal of necrotic material from the lesser sac. Alternately, drainage through the colonic mesentery can be accomplished with care taken to avoid the middle colic arterial pedicle. The patient may require multiple trips to the operating room for repeated debridement; typically, the abdomen is not formally closed until only viable tissue remains. Operative intervention for sterile pancreatic necrosis is controversial. The only absolute indications for surgery in sterile pancreatic necrosis are (1) abdominal compartment syndrome, (2) suspected enteric perforation, or (3) bleeding (splenic artery pseudoaneurysms, which can complicate the disease). Although there is a high incidence of infection in patients with >50% necrosis, "preemptive" debridement is not recommended because of high morbidity and mortality.

14. **Are there alternatives to open pancreatic necrosectomy?**
Although open surgical debridement is considered the gold standard for the treatment of infected pancreatic necrosis it is associated with significant morbidity. Continued improvement endoscopic and laparoscopic technology as well as interventional radiology techniques has led to interest in less invasive approaches, which may have lower morbidity. These include retroperitoneal pancreatic necrosectomy (video-assisted retroperitoneal debridement or minimally invasive retroperitoneal pancreatic necrosectomy), laparoscopic necrosectomy, endoscopic necrosectomy, and percutaneous approaches that can be combined with less invasive techniques.

15. **When should antibiotic therapy be added?**
There is no role for antibiotic prophylaxis to prevent infection. Therefore, patients with mild cases of pancreatitis should be treated with supportive measures. Patients with infected necrotizing pancreatitis should be treated with culture-guided antibiotic therapy. In patients with signs of sepsis, treatment with empiric antibiotics is reasonable while a source of infection is sought (i.e., CT-guided aspiration of pancreatic necrosis).

16. **What is the most common complication of acute pancreatitis?**
Pancreatic pseudocysts. Patients with pseudocysts typically present with persistent abdominal pain, nausea and vomiting, or an abdominal mass. CT scan imaging is diagnostic. Since one-third of pseudocysts spontaneously resolve, intervention is generally avoided unless patients are symptomatic. Operative (cyst-gastrostomy or cyst-jejunostomy) or endoscopic transmural drainage can be performed 6–12 weeks after presentation, once the pseudocyst is "mature," meaning it has a thick wall that can be sutured to the bowel. Further, pseudocysts smaller than 6 cm in diameter often spontaneously resolve.

17. **What is the natural history of cholelithiasis following gallstone pancreatitis?**
Cholecystectomy is curative and should be performed before patient discharge in the 80% of patients with uncomplicated, acute edematous pancreatitis. Cholecystectomy is performed when the patient's initial symptoms resolve. Cholecystectomy should be accompanied by an intraoperative cholangiogram or laparoscopic ultrasonography; if a retained stone is seen in the common bile duct, laparoscopic common duct exploration or ERCP should be performed before discharge.

18. **What is the natural history of alcoholic pancreatitis?**
Attacks recur. Abstinence from alcohol and tobacco, a common associated risk factor, should be encouraged because many patients develop chronic pancreatitis.

KEY POINTS: ACUTE PANCREATITIS

1. Causes: Gallstones (40%–70%), alcohol (25%–35%), idiopathic (10%), other (<5%).
2. Symptoms: Acute onset of epigastric pain that radiates to back with associated nausea or emesis.
3. Lab tests: Elevated amylase and/or lipase (more sensitive).
4. Imaging: CT scan diagnoses pancreatic necrosis, peripancreatic fluid collections, and pseudocysts.
5. Treatment: Crystalloid resuscitation, oral feeding as tolerated, and pain control; 20% of cases progress to necrotizing pancreatitis. If infection occurs, a step-up approach to treatment starts with antibiotics and may progress to percutaneous drainage and/or operative debridement.

BIBLIOGRAPHY

1. Bell D, Keane MG. Acute pancreatitis. *Medicine*. 2014;43(3):174–181.
2. Gimenez TR, Calvo AG. Etiology of acute pancreatitis. *Cent Eur J Med*. 2014;9(4):530–542.
3. Johnson CD, Besselink MG. Clinical review: acute pancreatitis. *BMJ*. 2014;349:4859.
4. Lankisch PG, Apte M. Seminar: acute pancreatitis. *Lancet*. 2015;386(9988):85–96.
5. Rosing DK, de Virgilio C, Yaghoubian A, et al. Early cholecystectomy for mild to moderate gallstone pancreatitis shortens hospital stay. *J Am Coll Surg*. 2007;205:762–766.
6. Stevenson K, Carter CR. Acute pancreatitis. *Surgery*. 2013;31(6):295–303.
7. Talukdar R, Vege SS. Acute pancreatitis. *Curr Opin Gastroenterol*. 2015;31(5):374–379.
8. Tenner S, Baillie J. American College of Gastroenterology guideline: management of acute pancreatitis. *Am J Gastroenterol*. 2013;108(9):1400–1415.
9. Thoeni R. Imaging of acute pancreatitis. *Radiol Clin N Am*. 2015;53(6):1189–1208.
10. Uhl W, Warshaw A, Imrie C, et al. IAP guidelines for the surgical management of acute pancreatitis. *Pancreatology*. 2002;2(6):565–573.
11. Dua MM, Worhunsky DJ. Surgical strategies for the management of necrotizing pancreatitis. *J Pancreas*. 2015;16(6):547–558.

CHAPTER 43

DIAGNOSIS AND MANAGEMENT OF CHRONIC PANCREATITIS

Brooke C. Bredbeck, MD, Carlton C. Barnett, Jr., MD, FACS

1. **What is chronic pancreatitis?**
   The classic description is a prodrome of smoldering abdominal pain and eventual pancreatic insufficiency. Histologically, chronic fibroinflammatory processes result in destruction of the functioning endocrine and exocrine pancreatic cells.

2. **What is the most common cause?**
   Alcohol abuse is a common cause in the developed world, accounting for 34%–60% of cases. Because only 3%–10% of those with alcohol use disorder develop pancreatitis, genetic risk factors and smoking are garnering more attention for their role in chronic pancreatitis. Other known causes include posttraumatic strictures, pancreas divisum, autoimmune disorders, and metabolic disorders (hypertriglyceridemia and hypercalcemia). The overall incidence is estimated to be 2–200 per 100,000 people.

3. **Is chronic pancreatitis the result of acute pancreatitis?**
   Acute and chronic pancreatitis are viewed as being opposite ends of the same disease spectrum. For example, alcohol may cause damage to acinar cells through reactive oxygen species, leading to pancreatic stasis. The stasis causes inflammation from release of pancreatic enzymes, which eventually leads to fibrosis and stricture. Severe fibrosis is a hallmark of end-stage chronic pancreatitis.

4. **How is chronic pancreatitis diagnosed?**
   A step-wise, image-guided approach starts with computed tomography (CT) to rule out masses and look for calcifications or pseudocysts. Magnetic resonance (MR)/magnetic resonance cholangiopancreatography (MRCP) and endoscopic ultrasound (EUS) better visualize the parenchyma and duct. Endoscopic retrograde cholangiopancreatography (ERCP) is less common because of higher procedure risks. Pancreatic function tests (PFTs) show promise but are not yet widely available.

5. **What are the signs of pancreatic insufficiency?**
   Insulin-dependent diabetes mellitus (found in up to 30% of patients) and steatorrhea (in 25%) at diagnosis. The form of diabetes associated with chronic pancreatitis is termed *IIIc*; it can be particularly difficult to manage because of the destruction of both the insulin and glucagon producing cells.

6. **How much of the pancreas must be destroyed before endocrine or exocrine insufficiency develops?**
   Approximately 90%.

7. **What is steatorrhea? How does one confirm the diagnosis?**
   Steatorrhea is soft, greasy, foul-smelling stools caused by exocrine insufficiency. A 72-hour fecal fat analysis confirms the diagnosis. The D-xylose test for small bowel function shows normal results. The Schilling test is for B_{12} absorption is not sensitive. Patients with steatorrhea are managed with a variable combination of low-fat diet, pancreatic enzyme replacement therapy (PERT), and proton pump inhibitors.

8. **Is serum amylase elevated in patients with chronic pancreatitis?**
   No. The serum amylase level is usually normal in cases of burned-out pancreatitis.

9. **What are the complications of chronic pancreatitis?**
   Pancreatic pseudocyst, abscess, fistula, or neoplasm may occur. Obstruction of the duodenum or biliary tree is possible. Malnutrition increases risk for osteoporosis and fracture.

10. **What is a possible source of upper gastrointestinal bleeding (UGIB) in a patient with chronic pancreatitis?**
    Although gastritis and peptic ulcer disease are more common causes of UGIB, splenic vein thrombosis with associated gastric varices and hypersplenism (known as sinistral hypertension) should also be considered. (Your attending will love this answer!)

11. **What is the "chain of lakes"?**
    During ERCP, contrast dye is injected into the pancreatic duct; sequential areas of narrowing followed by dilatation of the duct cause the appearance of a string of beads or chain of lakes.

12. **What are the treatment options for chronic pancreatitis?**
    Initially, medical therapy includes pain medications, abstinence from alcohol and tobacco, and PERT and/or insulin therapy as indicated. Patients with evidence of pancreatic insufficiency and persistent abdominal pain requiring repeated hospitalizations should consider more invasive therapeutic options. For patients with main duct obstruction and upstream ductal dilation, endoscopic treatment (sphincterotomy, stricture dilation, stone extraction or lithotripsy, stent placement) may be successful. The remainder of patients with refractory symptoms may undergo surgical intervention.

13. **What are the indications for surgery?**
    There are no steadfast rules. Relative indications include pain refractory to medical management, a dilated main pancreatic duct, biliary or gastric outlet obstruction, pancreas divisum, symptomatic or enlarging pseudocyst, and suspicion of malignancy. Recent studies indicate that surgery may be more beneficial in select patients who are early in the disease process.

14. **Which operative procedures are commonly performed?**
    A Roux-en-Y lateral pancreaticojejunostomy (Puestow procedure) provides pain relief through ductal drainage while preserving pancreatic parenchyma. The pancreatic duct is opened head-to-tail, and the Roux jejunal limb is sutured to the pancreatic capsule around the "filleted" duct to provide a drainage route. Pancreaticoduodenectomy (i.e., a Whipple procedure) or duodenum preserving pancreatic head resection (Beger and Frey procedures) may be performed for patients with an inflammatory mass in the head of the pancreas. The Frey procedure "cores out" the pancreatic head and drains both the pancreatic head ducts and the length of the pancreatic duct. Beger procedures may be better in patients who would be pancreatic auto islet transplant candidates for improved islet cell harvest. Distal pancreatectomy or retrograde drainage into a pancreaticojejunostomy may also be used for isolated distal disease.

15. **What is the result of operative intervention?**
    Pain relief occurs in approximately 70% of patients at the end of 1 year and in 50% of patients at the end of 5 years. Although associated morbidity ranges from 6% to 50% based on the type of operation, overall mortality from these procedures is 1%–3%.

KEY POINTS: CHRONIC PANCREATITIS

1. Causes: Alcohol (34%–60%), other/idiopathic.
2. Symptoms: Smoldering abdominal pain and pancreatic insufficiency (diabetes, steatorrhea).
3. Lab tests: PFTs are not widely available. Check for associated endocrine and exocrine insufficiency.
4. Imaging: CT scan diagnoses pancreatic masses, ductal dilation, calcifications, and pseudocysts; MR/MRCP, EUS, and ERCP evaluate the pancreatic duct; MR and EUS evaluate the parenchyma.
5. Treatment: Pain medications, abstinence from alcohol and tobacco, PERT and insulin therapy, antioxidants; corticosteroids for autoimmune type; if pain is refractory to medical management, may be treated with endoscopic or surgical intervention.

BIBLIOGRAPHY

1. Braganza J, Lee SH. Chronic pancreatitis. *Lancet.* 2011;377(9772):1184–1197.
2. Brock C, Nielsen LM. Pathophysiology of chronic pancreatitis. *World J Gastroenterol.* 2013;19(42):7231–7240.
3. Conwell DL, Bechien UW. Chronic pancreatitis: making the diagnosis. *Clin Gastroenterol Hepatol.* 2012;10(10):1088–1095.
4. DiMagno MJ, DiMagno EP. Chronic Pancreatitis. *Curr Opin Gastroenterol.* 2013;29(5):531–536.
5. Forsmark CE. Management of chronic pancreatitis. *Gastroenterology.* 2013;144(6):1282–1291.
6. Gupte AR, Forsmark CE. Chronic pancreatitis. *Curr Opin Gastroenterol.* 2014;30(5):500–505.
7. Issa Y, Bruno MJ, Bakker OJ, et al. Treatment options for chronic pancreatitis. *Nat Rev Gastroenterol Hepatol.* 2014;11:556–564.

CHAPTER 44

PORTAL HYPERTENSION AND ESOPHAGEAL VARICES

James Cushman, MD, MPH, FACS

1. **Describe the common causes of upper gastrointestinal bleeding (UGIB) in US populations.**
   Peptic ulcer disease is the number one cause of UGIB in the United States. The gram-negative bacteria *Helicobacter pylori* plays a significant role in the pathogenesis for many. Esophageal varices (EV) related to portal hypertension (PH) is another leading cause, followed by a number of disorders including Mallory-Weiss tears, and arteriovenous malformations.

2. **What is the definition of PH?**
   An hepatic venous pressure gradient (HVPG) >5 mm Hg defines PH. HVPG is measured between the portal vein and the inferior vena cava. In practice, the pressure is measured free and in a wedged fashion in the hepatic veins. PH becomes significant when the HVPG becomes >10 mm Hg. It should be noted that HVPG is not commonly tested or utilized in many US centers.

3. **What are the causes of PH?**
   Chronic injury to the liver from a variety of sources leads to increased resistance to portal blood flow. In the United States, this resistance is most commonly within the liver and the most common cause (>90%) is chronic alcohol abuse. Structural changes include distortion of liver microcirculation from fibrosis and vascular occlusion. The resistance can also be prehepatic (e.g., portal vein thrombosis) or posthepatic (e.g., Budd-Chiari syndrome). Worldwide causes of cirrhosis include schistosomiasis and other infectious sequelae.
   One way to stratify patients with cirrhosis is by characterizing them as either with compensated cirrhosis (i.e., those who do not have ascites, encephalopathy, jaundice, or variceal hemorrhage) versus decompensated.

4. **How is PH diagnosed?**
   PH is often asymptomatic until complications develop. Clinical signs may include abdominal wall collateral vessels, splenomegaly, and thrombocytopenia. Thus, the diagnosis of cirrhosis is a clinical one; however, imaging studies may reveal the characteristic nodular liver, ascites, and/or the existence of EV. Up to 60% of patients with newly diagnosed cirrhosis present with clinically significant PH. Additional diagnostic confirmation can be accomplished by obtaining an HVPG measurement if needed.

5. **Describe screening and prevention strategies for patients with known PH.**
   Among asymptomatic patients with cirrhosis, approximately 85% will have an elevated HVPG and 40% of these will have EV. Some literature suggests that gastroesophageal varices are present in almost half of patients with cirrhosis at the time of diagnosis. Given the 6-week mortality with each episode of variceal hemorrhage is approximately 15%–20%, it is prudent to offer screening and prevention strategies for such patients. The recommended screening method to determine the presence and size of gastroesophageal varices is esophagogastroduodenoscopy. The current consensus is that every known cirrhotic be endoscopically screened for varices at the time of diagnosis. The rationale behind screening is the existence of effective therapies that reduce the likelihood of first and subsequent bleeding episodes.

6. **Describe the Child-Turcotte-Pugh classification of cirrhosis.**
   Gastroesophageal varices occur with the highest rate in patients with Child's class B or C cirrhosis, and the mortality for any given episode of variceal hemorrhage is higher in class B or C cirrhotics. (The table below is available from multiple sources. Class A= 5–6 points, Class B= 7–9 points, and Class C = 10–15 points.)

Clinical Criteria	1 Point	2 Points	3 Points
Encephalopathy	None	Mild to moderate	Severe
Ascites	None	Mild to moderate	Large or refractory to diuretics
Bilirubin (mg/dL)	<2	2–3	>3
Albumin (g/dL)	>3.5	2.8–3.5	<2.8
Prothrombin time (seconds prolonged)	<4	4–6	>6
International normalized ratio	<1.7	1.7–2.3	>2.3

7. **What is the pathogenesis of PH leading to varices, variceal hemorrhage, and portosystemic collaterals?**

   Increased resistance to portal blood flow results from cirrhosis, and this leads to increases in portal venous pressure as stated. This results in decreased vasodilating factors (e.g., nitric oxide [NO]) and increased angiogenic factors (e.g., vascular endothelial growth factor) and the formation of new vessels. Splanchnic vasodilation occurs leading to increased portal blood flow, which completes a cycle by increasing portal venous pressure. Dilation of preexisting vessels leads to formation of varices and/or collaterals. Collaterals develop at watershed zones between the portal venous drainage (e.g., stomach, small bowel, large bowel, and spleen) and systemic venous drainage (e.g., esophagus, distal rectum). Collaterals can also develop from recanalization of embryonic connections (e.g., umbilical vein, persistent ductus venosus).

   Note: EV refers to esophageal varices, but it should be noted that gastric varices are present in 20% of patients with cirrhosis, either in isolation or in combination with EV. In this chapter, the term *EV* and gastroesophageal varices may be used interchangeably with this caveat.

8. **Describe how the HVPG and Child's classification help in both risk assessment and management of bleeding from EV in patients with cirrhosis and PH?**

   In cirrhotic patients with an HVPG >10 mm Hg, a higher risk of complications such as ascites and varices exist. In addition, these patients have double the risk of developing EV (50% at 5 years) when compared to patients with HVPG below this threshold (25% at 5 years). With an HVPG >12 mm Hg, there is an increased risk of EV rupture and bleeding. As stated previously, patients with decompensated cirrhosis, Child's class B and C, carry the highest rate of EV formation and a higher mortality for any given episode of variceal hemorrhage.

9. **What are the current methods used for the primary and secondary prophylaxis of esophageal variceal bleeding and are they effective?**

   Current evidence cannot recommend ß-adrenergic blockers for the primary prevention of the development of EV. However, once EV are present then criteria including varix size, characteristics, and patient's Child class are evaluated for determination if prophylaxis of bleeding is warranted. Nonselective ß-blockers and endoscopic variceal ligation (EVL) are both effective in preventing first bleeding episodes in existing EV, according to a 2008 metaanalysis of randomized clinical trials, and would be used for medium- and large-sized EV, or in small-sized EV with red wale signs and/or Child's class B or C cirrhosis. (Nonselective ß-blockers are effective by both ß1 and ß2 actions by reduction of cardiac output and splanchnic vasoconstriction respectively. The reader is referred to the references for further reading regarding the advantages and disadvantages between medical therapy and endoscopic therapy.)

10. **What is the recommended treatment approach for the patient who has experienced an acute variceal bleed?**

    Patients with Child class A or B disease or who have an HVPG <20 mm Hg have a low or intermediate risk. Standard therapy involves the combination of a safe vasoconstrictor (octreotide in the United States) administered from the time of admission for 2–5 days; endoscopic therapy (EVL) performed at <12 hours from admission on diagnostic endoscopy; and short-term prophylactic antibiotics (e.g., ciprofloxacin or ceftriaxone). Placement of a transjugular intrahepatic portosystemic shunt (TIPS) is currently considered salvage therapy for the 10%–20% of patients in whom standard medical therapy fails and will be discussed below.

11. **What is the general approach to the patient who has survived one episode of EV bleed in an effort to reduce a recurrent bleed?**

    A patient who survives an initial episode of bleeding secondary to EV has a 60% chance of recurrence. All such patients are thus recommended to have some form of treatment for the prevention of recurrent bleed prior to their discharge from the hospital, and treatment recommendations apply to all patients with variceal hemorrhage. Examples of such treatments include medical therapy, EVL, TIPS, and surgical shunts. A number of metaanalyses discuss matching specific therapies or combination of therapies for differing patient characteristics. Patients with Child class A disease have a good response to current therapies with a 0%–5% mortality. As previously noted, patients in whom their HVPG decreases to <12 mm Hg (or reduced by >20% from baseline) have the lowest rate of recurrent variceal bleeding.

12. **What are the specifics in current recommended therapy for patients who have survived one episode of EV bleed?**
    Current guidelines (see reference 1) recommend the combined use of EVL and nonselective ß-blockers for the prevention of recurrent variceal bleed. This is based on a randomized controlled trial showing a significantly lower rate of variceal rebleeding with combined modalities. However, the rate of bleeding from all sources was not significantly different because of the bleeding from esophageal ulcers induced by the EVL (a known complication of EVL). Patients who have rebleeding despite this combined therapy should undergo early placement of a TIPS or surgical shunt.

13. **A restrictive transfusion strategy, defined as a posttransfusion hemoglobin threshold of 7 g/dL, has been shown in various clinical settings to not increase, and perhaps decrease, mortality. Has such a strategy been shown to be similarly effective in cases of acute gastrointestinal (GI) bleeding?**
    Current international guidelines recommend decreasing the hemoglobin threshold for transfusion in a variety of critical care settings, including the condition of normovolemic anemia seen in patients who have had a GI bleed.
    A recent study (see reference 2) demonstrates that even in patients with an acute bleed, a restrictive transfusion strategy significantly reduced the rates of therapeutic failure factors such as further rebleeding, need for salvage or rescue therapy, and reduced length of hospital stay. Such a strategy should be used cautiously in the patient with active GI hemorrhage and shock.

14. **By what possible mechanisms is a restrictive strategy advantageous in acute GI bleeders, and those PH in particular?**
    Transfusion of red blood cells may lead to an impairment in hemostasis by dilution of coagulation factors and platelets. Splanchnic vasoconstriction in the setting of hypovolemia may be ameliorated by transfusion, leading to increase in splanchnic blood flow. Restoring blood volume may induce a rebound increase in portal venous pressure and precipitate bleeding. These concerns have been validated by experimental evidence that patients undergoing a liberal transfusion strategy had a significant increase in portal pressure not seen in the restrictive strategy group.

15. **Outpatient management of the patient with cirrhosis of the liver involves what major complications or sequelae in addition to variceal bleeding (name three)?**
    The three primary clinical issues that are caused by PH are ascites, variceal bleeding, and hepatic encephalopathy (HE). Hepatorenal syndrome (HRS) and spontaneous bacterial peritonitis are two less common but severe manifestations of decompensation.

16. **How common is ascites in the setting of cirrhosis and how is it managed?**
    Ascites is the most common manifestation of decompensated cirrhosis and affects 60% of previously compensated cirrhotics within 10 years of diagnosis. Rates of mortality once ascites is manifested varies depending on the study but are uniformly grave. First-year mortality is described at 15%, and by 3–5 years ranges between 44% and 50%. The mainstay of medical therapy is sodium restriction in the diet to prevent volume overload. A goal of <2000 mg/day is recommended. The use of oral diuretics such as spironolactone and furosemide is considered standard medical therapy, with typical starting dosages being 100 mg and 40 mg daily, respectively. Persistent ascites despite a low salt diet and maximal diuretic therapy is defined as refractory ascites and generally leads to a referral for orthotopic liver transplant, repeated paracentesis, placement of a TIPS, or peritovenous shunt. Use of peritovenous shunts have declined because of high complication rates with one remaining indication for it being in a patient with refractory ascites but ineligible for a TIPS or repeated paracentesis.

17. **How common is HE in the setting of cirrhosis and how is it managed?**
    HE is a manifestation of cirrhosis that if it occurs in the hospitalized patient carries a 3.9-fold increased mortality risk. Estimates are that 30%–40% of patients with cirrhosis will develop HE during the course of their disease, and relapse rates are high despite maximal suppressive therapy.

Pathophysiology is multifactorial including hyperammonemia, ammonia crossing the blood-brain barrier resulting in neuroinflammation, astrocyte swelling, and oxidative neuronal stress. There may be a net increase in the inhibitory neurotransmission mediated by gamma-aminobutyric acid. Systemic inflammation also occurs acting synergistically to cause HE. Placement of a TIPS may predispose patients to hepatic encephalopathy with an incidence of 5%–35% reported. HE is a clinical diagnosis and one of exclusion. Blood ammonia levels as a diagnostic criteria remain elusive according to a 2014 consensus guideline. Lactulose is the mainstay of therapy, which acts by acidification of the colon converting ammonia to ammonium. Recent studies suggest that polyethylene glycol may be superior, but further studies are needed. Antibiotics such as rifaximin in combination with other agents is the second line of therapy. There are recent reports of use of embolization of portosystemic communications as an emerging therapy.

18. **How common is HRS in the setting of cirrhosis and how is it managed?**
According to a 2007 definition, HRS is cirrhosis with ascites, a serum Cr of >1.5 mg/dL, no improvement in serum Cr despite 48 hours of diuretic withdrawal and volume resuscitation, absence of shock, no recent exposure to nephrotoxic drugs, and no signs of intrarenal disease. Acute kidney injury occurs in approximately 20% of such hospitalized patients and of these, 25% are secondary to HRS. In patients unfortunate enough to develop HRS, the 1-month mortality is 58% and the 1-year mortality is 63%. Overall, the mortality for HRS is 80% (Type 1). The only definitive treatment for HRS is liver transplantation. Bridge therapy includes initial volume expansion, pharmacologic agents (midodrine and octreotide), and the use of renal replacement therapy, which is controversial.

19. **What are the indications for use of TIPS in cirrhotic patients with recurrent variceal bleeding?**
The accepted indications for TIPS include refractory ascites, uncontrolled variceal bleeding, and recurrent variceal bleeding in patients who have failed standard initial medical and endoscopic means of control. Absolute contraindications include congestive heart failure, severe pulmonary hypertension, and severe tricuspid valve regurgitation. Early studies evaluating the role of TIPS in the prevention of recurrent variceal bleeding demonstrated that TIPS reduces the rebleeding rate, but at the expense of increasing HE without improving survival. As a result, TIPS has been recommended as rescue therapy for the up to 27% of patients who have failure to control bleeding after a variceal bleed and using conventional combined therapy of medications and EVL. More recent studies (see reference 8) have studied the effect of using coated stents in the TIPS procedure and moving to earlier (<72 hours) timing of the procedure.

20. **What are the technical aspects of TIPS placement?**
TIPS is a side-to-side portosystemic shunt created within the liver parenchyma typically between the right hepatic vein and the right portal vein. Accessing the portal vein is the most critical step of the TIPS procedure technically and is facilitated by the use of both preprocedure cross-sectional imaging as well as transabdominal ultrasound to guide needle placement into the correct portal vein branch. The procedural complication rate of TIPS may be related to intraabdominal hemorrhage and occurs in 0.6%–4.2%.

21. **Describe potential advantages of earlier use of TIPS and use of an extended polytetrafluoroethylene stent when compared with previous studies where TIPS was used only as a delayed rescue procedure with bare stents.**
Patients with Child's class C or Child's class B with recurrent bleeding who have persistent bleeding at endoscopy are at high risk for treatment failure and mortality. A recent study (see reference 8) randomized such patients to either early (<72 hours from endoscopy, preferably within 24 hours) versus continuation of medical therapy and TIPS within a conventional 3- to 5-day window. Protection from initial rebleeding, rebleeding within the first year of follow-up, and 1-year survival were all statistically significantly improved in the early TIPS group.

22. **Characterize the endothelial dysfunction (ED) in hepatic cirrhosis and how ED may contribute to liver dysfunction and PH.**
The endothelium involves >1013 cells and has multiple functions and properties. Examples include barrier function, permeability regulation, vascular tone, platelet adhesion and aggregation, prevention of thrombosis, and acting as a framework for multiple inflammatory processes. Within the hepatic circulation, ED refers primarily to the impairment of the production and release of vasodilatory factors, especially NO, considered to be a key role in the initiation and progression of liver cirrhosis. Reduced

levels of NO in the cirrhotic liver contributes to increased intrahepatic vascular resistance. In addition, increased levels of vasoconstrictor agents such as thromboxane A2 and prostanoids are important in the pathophysiology as well.

23. **Describe emerging therapies that may potentially ameliorate some of the ED, which is a component of the pathophysiology of cirrhosis.**
Experimental animal and human data (including clinical trials) have shown benefits to the use or intake of the following: Vitamins C and E (both improving NO bioavailability), folic acid and its active metabolite 5-methyltetrahydrofolate or 5-MTHF, flavonoids in the human diet that have antioxidant and vasodilatory actions including specifically resveratrol present in grapes as well as green tea polyphenol and dark chocolate.

24. **Is it possible for a cirrhotic patient to become pregnant, and if so, are there special issues or precautions?**
Pregnancy is a rare event in patients with cirrhosis; however, improvements in the treatment of chronic liver disease have resulted in both higher conception rates and successful pregnancy outcomes in such patients. Maternal complications have been described in nearly half of pregnancies affected by cirrhosis, largely as a result from variceal hemorrhage. Variceal bleeding more commonly occurs in the second and third trimesters when maternal blood volume is maximally expanded and the large intrauterine fetus compresses the inferior vena cava and collateral vasculature.

25. **Name the special treatment concerns for pregnant patients with cirrhosis.**
Upper endoscopy in general is safe during pregnancy, with the main risk being fetal hypoxia from sedative drugs or positioning. In women at high risk for bleeding, prophylaxis with nonselective ß-blockade drugs such as propranolol and nadolol, both designated as pregnancy category C drug (C+ risk cannot be ruled out; animal studies show an adverse effect, no controlled human studies available) may outweigh the potential fetal risk. Octreotide is designated as a pregnancy category B drug (B = no clear or reproducible risk shown in animal or human studies), yet theoretical concerns exist because of its vasoconstrictive properties. As of a 2008 report (see reference 9) only three cases of TIPS placement had been reported in pregnant cirrhotic patients, with one major risk being radiation exposure to the fetus. Among pregnant cirrhotic patients with known varices, up to 78% will have variceal hemorrhage during pregnancy and a mortality rate ranging between 18% and 50%.

BIBLIOGRAPHY

1. Garcia-Tsao G, Bosch J. Management of varices and variceal hemorrhage in cirrhosis. *N Engl J Med.* 2010;362(9):823–832.
2. Villanueva C, Colomo A, Bosch A, et al. Transfusion strategies for acute upper gastrointestinal bleeding. *N Engl J Med.* 2013;368(1):11–21.
3. Bleibel W, Chopra S. Portal hypertension in adults. <http://www.uptodate.com/contents/portal-hypertension-in-adults?source=search_result&search=Portal+hypertension+in+adults&selectedTitle=1~150> Accessed 20.01.16.
4. Shah NL, Banaei YP. Management options in decompensated cirrhosis. *Hepat Med.* 2015;7:43–50.
5. Garcia-Pagan JC, De Gottardi A. Review article: the modern management of portal hypertension – primary and secondary prophylaxis of variceal bleeding in cirrhotic patients. *Aliment Pharmacol Ther.* 2008;28(2):178–186.
6. Vairappan B. Endothelial dysfunction in cirrhosis: role of inflammation and oxidative stress. *World J Hepatol.* 2015;7(3):443–459.
7. Pillai AK, Andring B. Portal hypertension: a review of portosystemic collateral pathways and endovascular interventions. *Clin Radiol.* 2015;70(10):1047–1059.
8. Garcia-Pagan JC, Caca K, Bureau C, et al. Early use of TIPS in patients with cirrhosis and variceal bleeding. *N Engl J Med.* 2010;362(25):2370–2379.
9. Tan J, Surti B. Pregnancy and cirrhosis. *Liver Transpl.* 2008;14(8):1081–1091.
10. Russell MA, Craigo SD. Cirrhosis and portal hypertension in pregnancy. *Semin Perinatol.* 1998;22(2):156–165.

CHAPTER 45

GASTROESOPHAGEAL REFLUX DISEASE

Eric Bui, MD, Alden H. Harken, MD, FACS

1. **What is the most common cause of gastroesophageal reflux disease (GERD)?**
   Pregnancy. And, it's not the bowling ball in the abdomen; it's the estrogen and progesterone that relax the lower esophageal sphincter (LES).

2. **What symptoms suggest GERD?**
   Substernal burning after meals or at night, associated occasionally with regurgitation of gastric juices, is a common symptom. Discomfort is relieved by standing or antacids. Dysphagia, a late complication of GERD, is caused by mucosal edema or stricture of the distal esophagus. However, no symptom is specific for GERD. The differential diagnosis of substernal burning is wide and therapeutic decisions should not be made on symptoms alone.

3. **What is the difference between heartburn and GERD?**
   Heartburn is a lay term for mild, intermittent reflux of gastric content into the esophagus without tissue injury. It is relatively common among adults. GERD implies esophagitis with varying degrees of erythema, edema, and friability of the distal esophageal mucosa. It occurs in 10% of the population.

4. **What causes GERD?**
   The underlying abnormality of GERD is functional incompetence of the LES, which allows gastric acid, bile, and digestive enzymes to reflux into and damage the unprotected esophageal mucosa. Achalasia, scleroderma, and other esophageal motility disorders are frequently associated with GERD.

5. **Is hiatal hernia an essential defect in patients with GERD?**
   No. Not all patients with GERD have a hiatal hernia, and not all patients with a hiatal hernia have GERD. Approximately 50% of patients with GERD do have an associated hiatal hernia.

6. **What studies are useful to diagnose GERD?**
   Endoscopy with biopsy is essential in diagnosing GERD. Barium swallow with or without fluoroscopy can diagnose reflux but cannot identify esophagitis. Twenty-four-hour esophageal acid-base balance (pH) testing associates reflux with symptoms and is useful in some patients. Gastric secretory or gastric emptying tests are occasionally helpful. Manometry of the esophagus and LES is required whenever an esophageal motility disorder is suspected and before any surgical intervention.

7. **What is the initial management of a patient suspected of having GERD?**
   - Change diet to avoid foods known to induce reflux (e.g., chocolate, alcohol, and coffee).
   - Avoid large meals before bedtime.
   - Stop smoking.
   - Do not wear tight, binding clothes.
   - Elevate the head of the bed 4–5 inches.
   - Take antacids when symptomatic.
   - Weight loss can be quite effective in reducing GERD symptoms.

8. **If initial treatment fails, what should be recommended?**
   About 50% of patients show significant healing with H2 blockers, but only 10% of these patients remain healed 1 year later. Metoclopramide promotes gastric emptying but rarely relieves symptoms consistently in the absence of acid reduction.

KEY POINTS: DIAGNOSTIC WORKUP OF GASTROESOPHAGEAL REFLUX DISEASE

1. Underlying anatomic abnormality may cause functional incompetence of the LES.
2. Endoscopy and biopsy are paramount in diagnosis.
3. Swallow studies delineate possible anatomic causes.
4. Twenty-four-hour pH monitoring can link reflux to patient's symptoms.
5. Manometry of the LES is required if esophageal motility disorder is suspected.

9. **What is the role of proton pump inhibitors (PPI) in GERD?**
   PPIs (omeprazole and others) irreversibly inhibit the parietal cell hydrogen ion pump and are >80% successful in healing severe erosive esophagitis. Two-thirds of patients who continue the medication remain healed. A concern in prolonged PPI therapy is hypergastrinemia secondary to alkalinization of the antrum. Gastrin is trophic to gastrointestinal mucosa, but the initial fear of induced neoplasia has not been borne out by follow-up studies.

10. **When should operation for GERD be recommended?**
    Failure of nonoperative (medical) therapy is the primary indication for surgery. Noncompliance with prescribed treatment is a frequent cause of failure and even stricture unresponsive to dilation. With PPIs, most patients' symptoms can be controlled for long periods of time. Current recommendations for surgical intervention include (1) failed medical therapy (intractable disease, intolerance or allergy to medications, noncompliance, and recurrence of symptoms while on medical therapy), (2) complications (stricture, respiratory symptoms, cough, aspiration, premalignant mucosal changes), (3) patient preference (cost—long-term medical prescriptions can be expensive—or lifestyle issues).

11. **What is the goal of surgical treatment?**
    Operations for GERD attempt to prevent reflux by mechanically increasing LES pressure and, in most procedures, to restore a sufficient length of distal esophagus to the high-pressure zone of the abdomen. Hiatal hernia, when present, is reduced simultaneously.

12. **What procedures can accomplish this goal and how do they do it?**
    - In the Nissen fundoplication, the fundus of the stomach is mobilized, wrapped around the distal esophagus posteriorly, and secured to itself anteriorly (i.e., 360-degree wrap). The procedure alters the angle of the gastroesophageal junction and maintains the distal esophagus within the abdomen to prevent reflux. The operation is performed transabdominally by either laparotomy or laparoscopy (see Fig. 45.1).

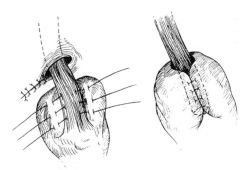

Fig. 45.1 In the Nissen fundoplication, which is used in >95% of patients, the fundus of the stomach is mobilized, wrapped around the distal esophagus posteriorly, and secured to itself anteriorly (i.e., 360-degree wrap). The procedure alters the angle of the gastroesophageal junction and maintains the distal esophagus within the abdomen to prevent reflux. The operation is performed transabdominally by either laparotomy or laparoscopy.

- The Belsey Mark IV operation accomplishes the same anatomic changes but is done via a thoracotomy (see Fig. 45.2).
- The Hill gastropexy restores the esophagus to the abdominal cavity by securing the gastric cardia to the preaortic fascia (see Fig. 45.3).
- The Toupet (partial) fundoplication is used in patients who have associated motility disorders. Because the wrap is not circumferential, the incidence of postoperative dysphagia is significantly reduced with this partial wrap compared with a full 360-degree wrap (Nissen fundoplication). However, long-term durability may not be as good as with a Nissen fundoplication. This operation can be done transabdominally by either laparotomy or laparoscopy (see Fig. 45.4).

13. **What are the success rates for such procedures?**
All of the procedures described above eliminate GERD in almost 90% of patients who are followed for 10 years, but the Nissen fundoplication wins in comparison studies. Recurrent symptoms should be thoroughly worked up because they are frequently associated with other disorders and not recurrent GERD.

14. **What are the long-term complications of such procedures?**
The repair may fail, with recurrence of reflux, after any of these operations. Incorrect placement or slippage of the stomach wrap can complicate Nissen fundoplication and the Belsey Mark IV procedure. Dysphagia and the inability to belch (i.e., gas-bloat syndrome) result from too tight a wrap.

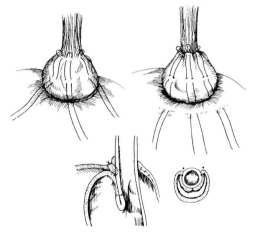

Fig. 45.2 The Belsey Mark IV operation accomplishes the same anatomic changes as the Nissen fundoplication but is done via a thoracotomy.

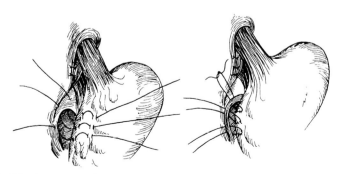

Fig. 45.3 The Hill gastropexy restores the esophagus to the abdominal cavity by securing the gastric cardia to the preaortic fascia. This is typically accomplished in conjunction with a 180-degree wrap.

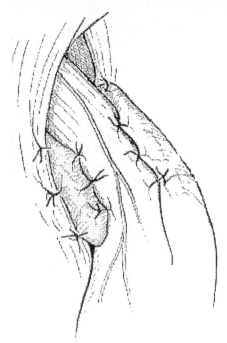

Fig. 45.4 The Toupet (partial) fundoplication is used in patients who have associated motility disorders. Because the wrap is not circumferential, the incidence of postoperative dysphagia is significantly reduced with this partial wrap compared with a full 360-degree wrap (Nissen fundoplication). However, long-term durability may not be as good as with a Nissen fundoplication. This operation can be done transabdominally by either laparotomy or laparoscopy.

15. **How can stricture from GERD be managed?**
    Pliable (unfixed) strictures can be dilated. Fixed strictures require surgical repair. A Thal patch expands the stricture by interposing a piece of stomach.

CONTROVERSIES

16. **Is GERD better treated in the long term by PPI therapy or Nissen fundoplication?**
    PPIs really work in resolving esophagitis and eliminating symptoms of GERD, but the long-term side effects are not fully known. Fundoplication potentially frees the patient from daily medicine (this has been challenged recently) and may cause morbidity in approximately 10% of patients.

17. **Should a Nissen fundoplication be performed by laparoscopy or laparotomy?**
    The same procedure can be accomplished by either approach. Postoperative morbidity and mortality is comparable. The distinct advantages of laparoscopy are less postoperative pain, shorter hospitalization, and earlier return to work.

18. **Can this disease be treated by other minimally invasive means?**
    Yes. Other endoscopic methods include:
    - Endoluminal suturing
    - Radiofrequency treatment of the LES
    - Injection of bulk-forming agents around the LES
    - Transoral incisionless fundoplication

WEBSITE

- www.emedicine.com/med/topic857.htm

Bibliography

1. Anand O, Wani S. Gastroesophageal reflux disease and Barrett's esophagus. *Endoscopy.* 2008;40(2):126–130.
2. DeMeester TR, Peters JH. Biology of gastroesophageal reflux disease: pathophysiology relating to medical and surgical treatment. *Annu Rev Med.* 1999;50:469–506.
3. Lagergren J, Bergstrom R. Symptomatic gastroesophageal reflux as a risk factor for esophageal adenocarcinoma. *N Engl J Med.* 1999;340(11):825–831.
4. Lord RV, Kaminski A, Oberg S, et al. Absence of gastroesophageal reflux disease in a majority of patients taking acid suppression medications after Nissen fundoplication. *J Gastrointest Surg.* 2002;6(1):3–9.
5. Peters JH, DeMeester TR, eds. *Minimally Invasive Surgery of the Foregut.* St. Louis: Quality Medical Publishing; 1994.
6. Roy-Shapira A, Stein HJ. Endoluminal methods of treating gastroesophageal reflux disease. *Dis Esophagus.* 2002;15(2):132–136.
7. Spechler SJ. Comparison of medical and surgical therapy for complicated gastroesophageal reflux disease in veterans. The Department of Veterans Affairs Gastroesophageal Reflux Disease Study Group. *N Engl J Med.* 1992;326(12):786–792.
8. Spechler SJ, Lee E, Ahnen D, et al. Long-term outcome of medical and surgical therapies for gastroesophageal reflux disease: follow-up of a randomized controlled trial. *JAMA.* 2001;285(18):2331–2338.
9. Strate U, Emmermann A. Laparoscopic fundoplication: nissen versus Toupet two-year outcome of a prospective randomized study of 200 patients regarding preoperative esophageal motility. *Surg Endosc.* 2008;22(1):21–30.
10. Trus TL, Laycock WS. Improvement in quality of life measures after laparoscopic antireflux surgery. *Ann Surg.* 1999;229(3):331–336.
11. Watson DI, Jamieson JG. Prospective randomized double-blind trial between laparoscopic Nissen fundoplication and anterior partial fundoplication. *Br J Surg.* 1999;86(1):123–130.
12. Huang X, Chen S, Zhao H, et al. Efficacy of transoral incisionless fundoplication (TIF) for the treatment of GERD: a systematic review with meta-analysis. *Surg Endosc.* 2017;31(3):1032–1044.

CHAPTER 46

ESOPHAGEAL CARCINOMA

Robert J. Torphy, MD, Martin D. McCarter, MD, FACS

1. **What are the presenting signs and symptoms of esophageal cancer?**
   Presenting symptoms most commonly include progressive dysphagia and weight loss. Notably, a tumor can obstruct over half of the esophageal lumen before dysphagia becomes symptomatic. Symptoms common to gastroesophageal reflux disease (GERD) such as chest or epigastric pain and regurgitation are also reported. Signs and symptoms of more advanced disease include melena and anemia from upper gastrointestinal bleeding, coughing or choking from a tracheoesophageal fistula, and hoarseness from recurrent laryngeal nerve involvement.

2. **What is the epidemiology of esophageal cancer?**
   Esophageal cancer is the eighth most common cancer in the world and sixth most common cause of cancer death in the world. Its prevalence is highest in developing nations, particularly Asia and Eastern Africa. In the United States, it is estimated that in 2016 there will be 16,910 new diagnosis and 15,690 deaths from esophageal cancer. Esophageal cancer is roughly four times more prevalent in males, and is estimated to be the seventh most common cause of cancer death in males in 2016. The incidence of esophageal cancer is highest in the seventh decade of life.

3. **What are the histological subtypes of esophageal cancer?**
   The two primary histological subtypes of esophageal cancer are adenocarcinoma and squamous cell carcinoma. Worldwide, squamous cell carcinoma is more common than adenocarcinoma, representing roughly 90% of cases. In North America and most Western European countries, adenocarcinoma is now more common than squamous cell carcinoma. The incidence of adenocarcinoma began dramatically rising in Western countries in the 1970s and may be attributed to increased rates of obesity and GERD. Conversely, the incidence of squamous cell carcinoma in Western countries has been on the decline. Squamous cell cancer is most commonly found in the upper third of the esophagus, while adenocarcinoma is most commonly found in the lower third of the esophagus. Histologic subtype is also important in treatment decisions as upper squamous cell are often treated nonsurgically with definitive chemoradiation therapy, while the treatment for adenocarcinoma involves surgical resection.

4. **What are the risk factors for developing esophageal cancer?**
   Key risk factors for developing esophageal adenocarcinoma are GERD (five- to eightfold risk increase), obesity (twofold), cigarette smoking (twofold), male sex, and white ethnicity. Key risk factors for developing squamous cell carcinoma are alcohol consumption (three- to fourfold), cigarette smoking (three- to fivefold), and male sex. Alcohol consumption and cigarette smoking also appear to have a synergistic effect on this risk.

5. **What is Barrett's esophagus and why is it important in esophageal cancer?**
   Barrett's esophagus is characterized by intestinal metaplasia in the distal esophagus with replacement of the normal squamous esophageal mucosa with metaplastic intestinal columnar cells. This diagnosis is made based on endoscopic biopsy findings of the above histology. Barrett's esophagus is a complication of GERD and is viewed as a precursor lesion to esophageal adenocarcinoma. Barrett's esophagus is thought to progress from low-grade to high-grade dysplasia, and then ultimately to cancer. The risk of progression from low-grade dysplasia to esophageal adenocarcinoma ranges from 0.1% to 0.3% per year. Under current practice guidelines, patients are typically screened for Barrett's esophagus with endoscopy when they have chronic GERD symptoms and one additional risk factor (over age 50, white, male, obese, smoking). If low-grade Barrett's esophagus is identified, patients may be screened with repeat endoscopy; however, the utility of this approach is currently in question. Findings of high-grade dysplasia carries a risk of progression to cancer of about 6% per year and warrants treatment, which is most commonly now performed with endoscopic mucosal resection or ablation.

6. **What are the steps in the diagnostic workup of esophageal cancer?**
   - History and physical examination.
   - A barium esophagram may be considered in patients presenting with dysphagia.
   - Upper gastrointestinal endoscopy and biopsies of concerning areas is necessary for diagnosis.
   - Computed tomography (CT) of the chest and abdomen with oral and IV contrast, or whole body positron emission tomography (PET/CT) to evaluate for metastatic disease.
   - Endoscopic ultrasound (EUS) to define the T stage of the primary mass and regional lymph node involvement with possible fine-needle aspiration biopsy of suspicious nodes.
   - Nutritional assessment is an important adjunct as some patients may require preoperative nutritional support.

7. **How is esophageal cancer staged?**
   Staging is based on the American Joint Committee on Cancer TNM classification. T1 tumors are confined to the lamina propria or muscular mucosae (T1a), or submucosa (T1b). T2 tumors invade the muscularis propria, and T3 tumors invade the adventitia. T4 tumors invade through the adventitia and into adjacent structures. T4a tumors invade pleura, pericardium, or diaphragm and are considered resectable, while T4b tumors invade unresectable structures (aorta, trachea, vertebrae). N stage is classified by the involvement of one to two nodes (N1), three to six nodes (N2), or seven or more regional nodes (N3). M0 is without distant metastasis and M1 is with metastatic disease to nonregional lymph nodes or distant organs. Stages I–III are defined as locoregional disease. Stage IV disease is defined by the presence of distant metastasis. Lesions that are centrally located 2–5 cm below the esophagogastric junction and infiltrate the lower esophagus from below are considered gastric cancers.

8. **What is the role for endoscopic therapies?**
   Endoscopy has evolved from a diagnostic and staging tool to a treatment modality in a highly selected group of patients with early esophageal cancer. Endoscopic treatment is an option for patients with high-grade Barrett's esophagus and T1a lesions. The risk of lymph node metastasis, recurrence, and death from esophageal cancer is low enough in this cohort of patients to avoid the added morbidity of an esophagectomy. The use of endoscopic therapy for superficial T1b lesions in the absence of nodal disease, lymphovascular invasion, or poor differentiation is currently debated. Endoscopic treatment modalities include endoscopic mucosal resection and radiofrequency ablation.

9. **When is neoadjuvant therapy used in esophageal cancer patients?**
   The Dutch chemotherapy and radiation in esophageal surgery study (CROSS) assessed the role of neoadjuvant chemotherapy versus surgery alone in patients with esophageal or esophagogastric-junction cancer. They found neoadjuvant chemoradiation therapy in esophageal cancer improved the rate of R0 resections and 5-year overall survival (47% in the neoadjuvant and surgery group versus 34% in the surgery alone group). Patients that appear to benefit most from neoadjuvant therapy are those that are clinically suspected to have any lymph node involvement (N1 or greater) or T2–T4a tumors.

10. **What are the surgical options for treatment of esophageal cancer?**
    Patients with T1a–T4a tumors with or without regional lymph node metastasis are candidates for surgical resection. T4b tumors, gastroesophageal junction tumors with supraclavicular lymph node spread, and tumors with distant metastasis are considered unresectable. Tumors within 5 cm of the cricopharyngeus muscle are typically considered unresectable and treated with definitive chemoradiation. An esophagectomy can be carried out through a variety of different approaches outlined below depending on the location of the tumor and surgeon preference. Esophagectomies can also now be performed either open or minimally invasively. Acceptable conduits to replace the esophagus include tubularized stomach, jejunum, and colon.
    - Transhiatal esophagectomy with left cervical incision and cervical anastomosis
    - Combined abdominal and right thoracic esophagectomy with intrathoracic anastomosis (Ivor Lewis esophagectomy)
    - Combined abdominal, right thoracic, and left neck incision with cervical anastomosis (McKeown esophagectomy)

11. **Which is the best operation for esophageal cancer?**
    The optimal surgical approach for esophageal cancers is still being debated. Each of the options listed above have relative pros and cons that factor into the ultimate decision. For example, a

transhiatal esophagectomy has the advantage of fewer pulmonary complications and potentially easier to manage anastomotic leaks, but it is associated with a higher anastomotic leak rate, risk of recurrent laryngeal nerve injury, and lower lymph node harvest. Conversely, a transthoracic esophagectomy may have more pulmonary complications, but it is associated with a lower anastomotic leak rate and better lymph node harvest. When the two approaches were compared in a prospective randomized trial, there was no significant difference in overall survival; however, with longer follow up there was a trend toward longer overall survival with the transthoracic approach.

12. **Key points in perioperative care following an esophagectomy**
    - Complications occur in >50% of patients. Complications include atrial fibrillation (approximately 15%), pneumonia (10%), anastomotic leak (10%), wound infection (5%), ileus (4%), chyle leak (4%), empyema requiring treatment (2%), recurrent laryngeal nerve injury, and nutritional challenges.
    - Patients should be counseled about reflux as the lower esophageal sphincter is removed with the operation.
    - High-volume centers have a mortality rate for esophagectomy of <4%.

13. **What is the long-term survival rate for patients with esophageal cancer?**
    The 5-year survival rate for esophageal adenocarcinoma ranges from close to 80% for submucosal lesions to <5% for stage IV tumors. The 5-year survival following esophagectomy alone is reported to be close to 30% and can increase to 40%–50% with neoadjuvant chemoradiation followed by esophagectomy. Outcomes are significantly better if an R0 resection is performed, meaning all gross disease is removed and all margins are microscopically negative for tumor. Adequate lymphadenectomy (with the goal of at least 15 lymph nodes evaluated) is associated with the most accurate prognostic information.

KEY POINTS: ESOPHAGEAL CARCINOMA

1. Adenocarcinoma is more common in the United States and Western countries, while squamous cell carcinoma is more common worldwide and in developing nations.
2. Important risk factors include obesity, GERD, and tobacco use for adenocarcinoma and tobacco and alcohol use for squamous cell carcinoma.
3. Diagnosis is made with upper endoscopy and biopsy.
4. Staging workup typically includes CT scan of the abdomen and pelvis or PET/CT scan, and EUS.
5. Squamous cell cancer is often treated with chemoradiation therapy alone, while adenocarcinoma is often treated with a multimodal approach including chemoradiation and surgery.
6. Neoadjuvant chemoradiation therapy is indicated for clinically suspected node positive (N1 or greater) and T2–T4a tumors.

WEBSITES

- www.nccn.org
- www.cancer.org

BIBLIOGRAPHY

1. Barnes JA, Willingham FF. Endoscopic management of early esophageal cancer. *J Clin Gastroenterol.* 2015;49(8):638–646.
2. Greenstein EJ, Litle VR. Effect of the number of lymph node sampled on postoperative survival of lymph node-negative esophageal cancer. *Cancer.* 2009;112(6):1239–1246.
3. van Hagen VP, Hulshof MC, van Lanschot JJ, et al. Preoperative chemoradiotherapy for esophageal or junctional cancer. *N Engl J Med.* 2012;366(22):2074–2085.
4. Hulscher JB, van Sandick JW, de Boer AG, et al. Extended transthoracic resection compared with limited transhiatal resection for adenocarcinoma of the esophagus. *N Engl J Med.* 2002;347(21):1662–1669.

5. Luketich JD, Pennathur A, Awais O, et al. Outcomes after minimally invasive esophagectomy: review of over 1000 patients. *Ann Surg.* 2012;256(1):95–103.
6. Merkow RP, Bilimoria KY. Use of multimodality neoadjuvant therapy for esophageal cancer in the United States: assessment of 987 hospitals. *Ann Surg Oncol.* 2012;19(2):357–364.
7. Siegel RL, Miller KD. Cancer statistics, 2016. *CA Cancer J Clin.* 2016;66(1):7–30.
8. Sihag S, Kosinski AS. Minimally invasive versus open esophagectomy for esophageal cancer: a comparison of early surgical outcomes from the Society Of Thoracic Surgeons National Database. *Ann Thorac Surg.* 2016;101(4):1281–1288.
9. Spechler SJ, Souza RF. Barrett's esophagus. *N Engl J Med.* 2014;371(9):836–845.
10. Thrift AP. The epidemic of oesophageal carcinoma: where are we now? *Cancer Epidemiol.* 2016;41:88–95.

CHAPTER 47

ACID PEPTIC ULCER DISEASE

Douglas M. Overbey, MD, Edward L. Jones, MD, MS

1. **What is peptic ulcer disease (PUD)?**
   PUD includes gastric and duodenal mucosal defects (ulcerations) extending to the muscularis mucosa.

2. **What is the incidence of PUD?**
   The lifetime risk for PUD is about 8%–14%. It usually occurs between ages 20 and 60 years, with peak incidence in the fourth decade of life. It was more common in males but is shifting toward gender equivalence. Hemorrhage is the most common cause of hospital admission, and overall hospitalization rates are decreasing with improved medical management.

3. **Explain the pathophysiology of PUD.**
   Gastric or duodenal epithelial cells secrete mucus and bicarbonate in response to irritation of the lining or cholinergic stimulation and prostaglandin stimulation respectively. The mucous acts as an impermeable barrier to acid, while the bicarbonate serves as a proximity buffer. Disruptive factors such as *Helicobacter pylori* infection and nonsteroidal antiinflammatory drugs (NSAIDs) can disrupt this equilibrium, leading to epithelial injury and ulceration. Other risk factors include cigarette smoking, blood group O, chronic pancreatitis, cirrhosis, emphysema, and α-1 antitrypsin deficiency.

4. **What is the pertinent anatomy of the foregut?**
   The foregut includes the anterior part of the alimentary canal, from the mouth to the duodenum at the ligament of Treitz. Peptic ulcers can occur throughout the length, although the majority are found in the stomach and/or duodenum and classified as follows (Fig. 47.1):
   - Type I: Ulcers along the lesser curve and incisura (most common)
   - Type II: Any gastric ulcer plus a duodenal ulcer
   - Type III: Prepyloric ulcers
   - Type IV: Ulcers at the gastroesophageal junction or proximal cardia
   - Type V: Any ulcer associated with NSAID or aspirin use

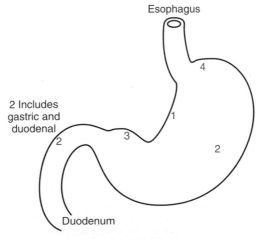

Fig. 47.1 Types of gastric ulcers.

5. **What factors cause physiologic acid secretion?**
Normal gastric acid production is 2–3 L/day. Acid production is stimulated by (1) parasympathetic action (acetylcholine from vagus nerves), (2) gastrin stimulation from G-cells in the gastric antrum, and/or (3) histamine stimulation from enterochromaffin-like cells throughout the stomach. These three factors act on parietal cells to induce insertion of K/H+ ATPase pumps on the apical surface, which then secrete hydrogen ions into the gastric lumen. Keep in mind that acid hypersecretion is only one contributory factor for PUD (40%), and type I and IV ulcers have low or normal acid levels.

6. **What is the usual presentation for PUD?**
PUD usually presents with epigastric pain that is temporally mediated by food or antacid ingestion. Nausea and vomiting may occur. Gastric ulcers typically present with pain during meals. In contrast, duodenal ulcers may initially be relieved by eating (due to closure of the pylorus during initial stimulation), but the pain returns approximately 2 hours later. Ulcers may also present with bleeding (see Chapter 53) or gastric outlet obstruction from pyloric spasm or scarring. Full thickness injury (perforation) is rare, but is classically diagnosed with peritonitis and free air on x-ray if the ulcer is located on the anterior gastric wall. Alternatively, posterior ulcers can erode in the pancreas and/or gastroduodenal artery resulting in pancreatitis or hemorrhage.

7. **What is the first diagnostic step to rule out PUD in a stable patient?**
Flexible esophagogastroduodenoscopy (EGD) is preferred although an upper GI contrast study with barium can also be done. EGD is preferred as intervention, and additional testing (biopsy for malignancy, *H. Pylori* infection, etc.) can be done at the same time. In unstable patients, after initiating resuscitation, a rapid upright chest x-ray can demonstrate free air if perforation is considered. Computed tomography scan is a more sensitive test for small perforations or in patients with unclear history to clarify a broader differential that may include pancreatitis, hepatitis, intestinal ischemia or infection, aortic aneurysm, and so on. In all patients with epigastric or chest pain, it is essential to obtain an electrocardiogram to rule out an acute coronary syndrome.

8. **What is the malignancy risk of a typical gastric or duodenal ulcer?**
In all patients, the risk of malignancy with a gastric ulcer is 2%–4%. For duodenal ulcers, the risk is <1%; thus, routine biopsy of duodenal ulcers is not recommended. For symptomatic gastric ulcers, malignancy risk can be up to 10% (as symptomatology alone increases the risk of malignancy). Giant ulcers (>2 cm in diameter) increases risk to 30%.

9. **Describe characteristics of a malignant ulcer on endoscopy.**
An uneven ulcer base, irregular shape or margin, and/or associated gastric folds with rugae interruption. Biopsy is mandatory for all gastric ulcers because up to 25% of malignant lesions have no visual abnormality. At least seven biopsies should be performed of the ulcer margin and base to ensure accuracy. Greater than 90% of benign ulcers usually heal after 12 weeks of proton pump inhibitor (PPI) therapy. Intractability should arouse further suspicion for malignancy and initiate further workup beginning with repeat endoscopy.

10. **Describe the typical management for benign initial PUD.**
Following diagnosis with biopsy for *H. pylori* and malignancy (if indicated), acid suppression with PPIs should be initiated for 8 weeks. Other risk factors such as NSAIDs, aspirin, alcohol, and nicotine should be mitigated. Histamine receptor antagonists (H2RA) can be used as a substitute in patients with allergies or intolerance to PPIs. For large, symptomatic ulcers sucralfate can be added as a barrier agent to aid in symptom relief and healing. Approximately 90% of peptic ulcers heal in 8 weeks and acid suppression therapy can be stopped. However, high-risk patients (giant ulcers, *H. pylori*- and NSAID-negative ulcers, refusal to stop NSAIDs, frequent recurrent ulcers [>2/year]) should be continued on maintenance PPI.

11. **What are side effects of short- and long-term acid suppression therapy?**
All acid suppression therapy can lead to pneumonia through nonacidic reflux. H2 receptor antagonists may induce mental status changes and gynecomastia. Cimetidine, in particular, may affect hepatic metabolism of warfarin, phenytoin, theophylline, propranolol, and digoxin, leading to abnormal serum levels. Omeprazole may cause hypergastrinemia by blocking gastric acid secretion (hence why it is important to hold if testing gastrin levels). Emerging literature suggests a possible relation to clostridium difficile infection, chronic kidney disease, dementia, and osteoporosis with prolonged PPI use.

12. **What is *H. pylori* and how is it associated with PUD?**
Helicobacter pylori is a gram-negative bacillus strongly associated with PUD. It is isolated from antral mucosa in 50% of the world's population, and in 80% of patients with PUD. *H. pylori* colonization induces chronic active gastritis, which is associated with ulcer formation and inflammation through the cag pathogenicity island-Nod1 pathway. Eradication of *H. pylori* results in near complete

resolution of ulcers (up to 98%), and the diagnosis and treatment of infection is a central part of the management of peptic ulcers. In addition, it is linked to gastric cancer and is classified as a group I carcinogen. It is also associated with mucosa-associated lymphoid tissue (MALT) lymphoma and its eradication is the mainstay of treatment for MALT lymphomas.

13. **How is *H. pylori* identified?**
Endoscopic biopsy of the gastric antrum (the most common location for colonization) can be tested for urease activity (released by *H. pylori*) most commonly via the *Campylobacter*-like organism (CLO) test. The presence of urease results in cleavage of urea to liberate ammonia, producing an alkaline pH and resultant color change in as soon as 1 hour. Histologic specimens can also be stained and/or cultured for the organisms themselves; however, this is more time consuming and costly.

Rapid urease breath tests are available with results as soon as 1 hour, and demonstrate comparable sensitivity and specificity to CLO testing. An ELISA serum test can detect anti-*H. pylori* IgA and IgG antibodies that indicate exposure (but not necessarily active infection). A stool antigen test is also available and often used for outpatient confirmation of eradication.

14. **What is treatment for confirmed *H. pylori* infection?**
First-line therapy includes "triple therapy," a 7–10 day course of antibiotics (amoxicillin and clarithromycin) along with a twice-daily PPI. In areas where resistance is common, "quadruple therapy" is recommended—bismuth, a PPI, as well as metronidazole and doxycycline.

15. **What should prompt further workup for rare causes of ulcers?**
Most commonly, failure of ulcer resolution after a 12-week trial of PPI therapy. In addition, the presence of numerous ulcers, ulcers distal to the duodenum, multiple endocrine neoplasia type I (MEN I) syndrome or a patient with recalcitrant ulcers and no additional risk factors (*H. Pylori* infection, NSAID use). The most common nonmalignant cause of recalcitrant ulcers is Zollinger-Ellison syndrome. Gastrin is secreted from a neuroendocrine tumor (gastrinoma), which is commonly found in the "gastrinoma triangle" formed by the cystic/CBD junction superiorly, the third portion of the duodenum inferiorly, and the neck/body of the pancreas medially (Fig. 47.2).

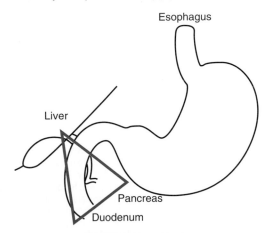

Fig. 47.2 Gastrinoma triangle.

Diagnosis is done with a fasting gastrin level and if >1000 pg/mL, it is considered positive. However, two-thirds of patients will have a nondiagnostic level and performance of the test off of a PPI is not recommended due to the high risk of ulcer bleeds when stopped abruptly. Thus, a secretin stimulation test can be performed after transition to high-dose histamine receptor antagonists (e.g., Ranitidine). Secretin (2 U/kg) are pushed over 1 minute, followed by measurements of gastrin levels at 2-, 5-, 10-, 15- and 20-minute intervals and compared to baseline. An increase of gastrin levels >120 pg/mL is diagnostic of a gastrinoma. Once diagnosed, it is important to evaluate for MEN I syndrome, as up to 50% of patients will develop a gastrinoma. Evaluation for pituitary adenomas and parathyroid hyperplasia should be completed as hypercalcemia needs to be rectified prior to treatment of gastrinoma (hypercalcemia reduces the effectiveness of PPIs in treating related peptic ulcers).

16. **What are operative indications for benign gastric or duodenal ulcer disease?**
    IHOP: Intractability, hemorrhage, obstruction, or perforation.

17. **What are the surgical options?**
    - **Graham patch:** Closure of a perforation in patients who are PPI-naïve or have untreated *H. pylori* (i.e., are likely to heal ulcers after treatment of this acute perforation) can be done by suturing the greater omentum over the perforation and widely draining the abdomen. Of note, all gastric ulcers should, at minimum, be biopsied because of the risk of malignancy. A Graham patch is the standard for small (<2 cm) perforations in the acute setting and can be performed laparoscopically or via an upper midline incision. Patient selection is important, as up to one-third of patients will require a second operation for recalcitrant disease.
    - **Antrectomy (+/– vagotomy):** If the perforation is too large for a patch or if the patient has ulcers that are refractory to medical therapy (intractable), or the patient is noncompliant with treatment, then an antrectomy (resection of the ulcerated area of the stomach) should be done. For type I and IV ulcers (low-normal acid levels), this does not require a concomitant vagotomy (ligation of the anterior vagus nerve). For type II and III ulcers in a stable patient, a highly selective vagotomy can be performed (ligation of only those vagal branches that regulate gastric parietal cells with sparing of pyloric control). As this can be difficult, if the patient is unstable, a truncal vagotomy can be quickly performed and should include a release of the pyloric muscle fibers (most commonly, Heineke-Mikulicz pyloroplasty) to avoid tonic pyloric closure and gastric outlet obstructions. A highly selective vagotomy alone can be done in the elective setting for patients with intractable ulcers without underlying gastrinoma or other treatable cause.

18. **What are reconstruction options following antrectomy?**
    Three major reconstructions are commonly performed: Billroth I, Billroth II, and a Roux-en-Y gastrojejunostomy. The Billroth procedures are named for Christian Albert Theodor Billroth (1829–1894), an Austrian surgeon who performed the first successful gastric resection in 1881. A Billroth I is the creation of an anastomosis between the duodenum and the gastric remnant (gastroduodenostomy). A Billroth II operation is constructed by sewing a loop of jejunum to the gastric remnant (gastrojejunostomy). Lastly, a Roux-en-Y gastrojejunostomy involves the creation of a "Roux" limb that is brought and connected to the stomach as well as proximal jejunum. A Billroth I has the advantage of eliminating an isolated duodenal stump and requiring one suture line instead of two or three. It allows more physiologic processing of proteins and fats but is more susceptible to gastric outlet obstruction via recurrent or marginal ulcers as well tumors and thus is not recommended after gastric resection for malignancy. It is also difficult to perform after many gastric resections because of inability to mobilize both the gastric remnant and the proximal duodenum; thus enhancing the popularity of the Billroth II. The Roux-en-Y configuration was developed to reduce reflux gastritis and esophagitis and has demonstrated consistent improvements in quality of life in comparison to both the Billroth II and Billroth I without significant increase in complications (see below).

19. **What short- and long-term complications occur with ulcer operations?**
    - **Dumping syndrome:** Resection of the pylorus can lead to uncontrolled, rapid emptying of hyperosmolar gastric contents into the proximal small bowel. This results in a rapid intravascular volume shift to the small intestine that can make patients transiently hypovolemic and produces tachycardiac and symptoms of sweating, flushing, weakness, nausea, cramping, and even syncope. This affects up to 20% of patients in the early postoperative period but is successfully managed with consumption of small, low-osmolar meals without carbohydrate-rich liquids so that just 2% of patients have chronic problems. Anticholinergic drugs can also be used for recalcitrant symptoms.
    - **Alkaline reflux:** Reflux of bile and pancreatic secretions into the stomach after a Billroth II (or more rarely, a Billroth I) can cause gastric irritation and pain. Unfortunately, few medications exist that are beneficial, and after endoscopic confirmation the preferred treatment is revision of the Billroth II to a Roux-en-Y gastrojejunostomy with at least a 40 cm efferent limb.
    - **Afferent loop syndrome:** Postprandial bilious vomiting that is typically a result of biliary and pancreatic fluid buildup in the afferent limb of Billroth II patients. Prevention is key and requires avoidance of the creation of a long or twisted afferent limb as well as maintaining a large gastrojejunal anastomosis. This is not seen in Billroth I patients but can also occur after Roux-en-Y gastrojejunostomy.

- **Duodenal stump leakage/blowout:** A highly morbid and even deadly complication after Billroth II or Roux-en-Y gastrojejunostomy. The duodenal stump is often edematous and inflamed during surgery, so the stump could begin leaking highly erosive biliary and pancreatic enzymes into the abdomen and retroperitoneal up to 1 week after surgery. Re-exploration with wide drainage and control of the leak is needed with resultant prolonged recovery.
- **Delayed gastric emptying or gastric retention:** May occur because of edema at the anastomosis or atony of the stomach after vagotomy and presents with oral intolerance or vomiting. Typically resolves as edema and inflammation subside in 4–6 weeks.
- **Bleeding/hemorrhage:** May occur from a suture line, a missed ulcer, or other gastric mucosal lesions. Maintenance of a postoperative PPI is key and, although most postgastrectomy bleeds resolve spontaneously, early endoscopic intervention may be needed.

20. **Can ulcers recur after surgical intervention?**
Yes. Ulcers typically recur at the gastric anastomosis on the intestinal side (marginal ulcers). The most common causes include incomplete vagotomy, inadequate drainage of the gastric remnant (stasis of gastric contents resulting in erosions at the anastomosis), or retained gastric antrum (gastrin-producing cells) after a Billroth II procedure.
Rate of ulcer recurrence by procedure:
    - Highly selective vagotomy: 15%
    - Truncal vagotomy and pyloroplasty: 10%
    - Antrectomy and vagotomy: 2%
    - Subtotal gastrectomy: 1%
    - Total gastrectomy: <1%

21. **What is stress gastritis and atrophic gastritis?**
Stress gastritis describes inflammation and gastric mucosal injury as a result of hypoperfusion/ischemia due to blood loss, trauma, or sepsis. Erosions typically begin in the proximal stomach and extend distally, and are eventually seen in all patients who are critically ill and can result in significant bleeding. As such, prophylaxis with acid suppression is common in high-risk (mechanical ventilation >48 hours, bleeding disorder, prior history of ulcers) intensive care unit patients.

22. **What are some unique ulcers?**
    - **Cushing's ulcer:** Named for Dr. Harvey Cushing, a neurosurgeon who described gastric ulcers in critically ill patients following a central nervous system injury. These are rare in patients receiving stress ulcer prophylaxis.
    - **Curling's ulcer:** Named for Dr. Thomas Curling, a surgeon who described gastric ulcers in critically ill patients following significant burns. These are rare in patients receiving stress ulcer prophylaxis.
    - **Cameron's ulcer:** Named for Dr. Alan Cameron after publication of his manuscript describing lesions associated with diaphragmatic hernias that can result in significant bleeding.
    - **Dieulafoy's ulcer:** Named for Dr. Paul Dieulafoy, a surgeon who described a rare arterial malformation resulting in a large submucosal branch that can erode through the mucosa resulting in abrupt hemorrhage that can be difficult to identify if not actively bleeding. Approximately 75% of these occur within 6 cm of the gastroesophageal junction and are managed endoscopically as acid suppression does not affect these lesions.

KEY POINTS: ACID PEPTIC ULCER DISEASE

1. PUD is common, and effectively treated with PPIs resulting in a significant decrease in ulcer surgery.
2. Unstable patients should be resuscitated and rapidly diagnosed with x-ray to rule out perforation and EGD to diagnose (and potentially treat) PUD.
3. All gastric ulcers should be biopsied during EGD to rule out malignancy and diagnose *H. pylori*, which can be treated with antibiotics and a PPI.
4. *H. pylori* is associated with MALT lymphomas as well as gastric carcinoma. Eradication of the infection is often the only treatment required in MALT lymphomas. Gastric cancer will require staging and possible surgical treatment.

BIBLIOGRAPHY

1. Fujishiro M, Iguchi M, Kakushima N. Guidelines for endoscopic managements of non-variceal upper gastrointestinal bleeding. *Dig Endosc.* 2016;28(4):363–378.
2. Zhang RG, Duan GC. Role of Helicobacter pylori infection in pathogenesis of gastric carcinoma. *World J Gastrointest Pathophysiol.* 2016;7(1):97–107.
3. Schwesinger WH, Page CP. Operations for peptic ulcer disease: paradigm lost. *J Gastrointest Surg.* 2001;5(4):438–443.
4. Talamini G, Tommasi M, Vantini I, et al. Risk factors of peptic ulcer in 4943 inpatients. *J Clin Gastroenterol.* 2008;42(4):373–380.
5. Gisbert JP, Calvet X, Cosme A, et al. Long-term follow-up of 1,000 patients cured of Helicobacter pylori infection following an episode of peptic ulcer bleeding. *Am J Gastroenterol.* 2012;107(8):1197–1204.
6. Chey WD, Wong BC. American College of Gastroenterology guideline on the management of Helicobacter pylori infection. *Am J Gastroenterol.* 2007;102(8):1808–1825.
7. Sung JJ, Tsoi KK. Causes of mortality in patients with peptic ulcer bleeding: a prospective cohort study of 10,428 cases. *Am J Gastroenterol.* 2010;105(1):84–89.
8. Safavi M, Sabourian R. Treatment of Helicobacter pylori infection: current and future insights. *World J Clin Cases.* 2016;4(1):5–19.
9. Ko Y, Tang J. Safety of proton pump inhibitors and risk of gastric cancers: review of literature and pathophysiological mechanisms. *Expert Opin Drug Saf.* 2016;15(1):53–63.

CHAPTER 48

SMALL BOWEL OBSTRUCTION

Emily Miraflor, MD, Amanda J. Green, MD

1. **Name three mechanisms of bowel obstruction, and give examples and incidence of each type**
   a. Extrinsic compression: Adhesions (60%), malignancy (20%), hernias (10%), volvulus and others (5%).
   b. Internal blockage of the lumen by abnormal materials (obturation): Bezoars, gallstones, worms, or foreign body (usually obstructs at the ileocecal valve).
   c. Mural disease encroaching on the lumen (inflammatory bowel disease [5%]), fibrous stricture secondary to trauma, postoperative anastomotic stricture, ischemia, radiation, intussusception).

2. **What are the most common symptoms of small bowel obstruction (SBO)?**
   a. Abdominal pain: Initially nonspecific, often colicky or crampy coinciding with waves of peristalsis trying to pass the point of obstruction.
   b. Bloating: The more distal the obstruction, the more severe the abdominal distention caused by proximal bowel dilatation.
   c. Vomiting: Bilious, frequent, and profuse with proximal obstruction; less frequent but larger volume and often feculent with distal obstruction.
   d. Obstipation: Failure to pass gas or stool; occasionally, the patient has a few loose stools early as the bowel distal to the obstruction empties.

3. **What are the pertinent questions in the patient's history?**
   • Any previous abdominal or pelvic surgery?
   • Any previous SBO?
   • Any history of cancer? What type, and how treated? Any radiation?
   • Any previous abdominal infections or inflammation (include pelvic inflammatory disease, appendicitis, diverticulitis, inflammatory bowel disease, perforation, and trauma)?
   • Any history of gallstones?
   • Any history of hernias?
   • Current medications, particularly anticoagulants, anticholinergics, chemotherapy, or diuretics?

4. **What are the findings on physical examination?**
   The patient is often dehydrated and may have a low-grade fever, postural hypotension, and abdominal distention. Inspect the abdomen for distention, scars, and hernias. Bowel sounds may be hyperactive with "tinkles and rushes" or may be totally silent if the patient has delayed seeking treatment. Percussion usually reveals diffuse tympani. Thin, elderly patients may even have visible loops of distended small bowel. Palpation may increase the abdominal pain, but localized tenderness or peritoneal signs indicate likely strangulation or another diagnosis.

5. **Is a rectal examination necessary?**
   Absolutely. The rectal examination may reveal signs of cancer, such as a rigid rectal shelf from carcinomatosis, and blood on hemoccult examination may herald ischemia or strangulation or may indicate inflammatory bowel disease. An obturator hernia can best be palpated transrectally or transvaginally. Stool in the rectal vault does not rule out an obstruction.

6. **Where should the examiner look for obstructing hernias?**
   Examine the groin near the pubic tubercle and along the inguinal floor. Check the femoral triangles for bulging or tenderness. Do a rectal examination to look for obturator hernia (see question 5). Palpate all existing incisions. Check all trocar sites from previous laparoscopic surgeries.

7. **What is the most inexpensive way to confirm the diagnosis?**
   The "four-way abdominal series" (flat and upright abdominal films, plus posterolateral and lateral chest radiographs) is diagnostic about 75% of the time. Look for:
   • Air-fluid levels in dilated small intestine (also known as stair steps or string of pearls sign).
   • Absent or minimal air in the distal colon and rectum.

- Ground glass appearance and obscuring of the psoas shadows by extraperitoneal fluid.
- Sometimes a single distended loop of small bowel with a "beak" at each end will be seen, indicating a closed-loop obstruction.
- Chest radiographs may demonstrate an infiltrate, with accompanying ileus, rather than SBO. The lateral chest radiograph is the most sensitive radiograph for identifying free air in the abdomen; a finding that necessitates an urgent laparotomy for perforated viscus.

8. **What other imaging studies can be used?**
   - **Oral contrast studies** with water-soluble contrast (Gastrografin) help to distinguish partial from complete obstruction, intraluminal tumor or foreign body, and inflammatory bowel disease; they may also define the point of obstruction. Gastrografin is both diagnostic and therapeutic in that it may actually help resolve complete and partial obstructions by its osmotic effect.
   - **Computed tomography (CT)** with intravenous (IV) contrast and with or without oral contrast can confirm the diagnosis and also predict the need for operative therapy. Free peritoneal fluid, mesenteric enhancement, decreased bowel wall enhancement, mural thickening and congestion of small mesenteric veins are concerning for ischemia and predict failure of nonoperative management, whereas fecalization of small bowel contents in the absence of a known stricture predicts successful nonoperative therapy. CT also helps identify nonadhesive causes of SBO.

9. **Which laboratory studies are indicated?**
   a. Complete blood cell count to check for leukocytosis or unexpected anemia.
   b. Urinalysis to look for urinary tract infection (UTI) (which may also cause an ileus and present with a similar picture to SBO) and to assess hydration (urine-specific gravity).
   c. Chemistry panel to check for electrolyte abnormalities such as hypokalemic or hypochloremic metabolic alkalosis (associated with vomiting of acid gastric contents), hyponatremia, and prerenal azotemia (elevated blood urea nitrogen and creatinine levels).
   d. Amylase and lipase to rule out pancreatitis; amylase can also be elevated, although not as high, with SBO or ischemic bowel.
   e. Lactate may be elevated because of dehydration, but it does not reliably predict viability of the intestine; a normal lactate does not rule out strangulation.

10. **What are the initial steps in treatment?**
    Nasogastric (NG) suction and IV fluids should be instituted to restore electrolyte and fluid balance, and a Foley catheter should be placed to monitor urine output. As soon as resuscitation is complete, prompt surgical intervention is mandatory for anyone with signs and symptoms of strangulation.

11. **How can I distinguish between a complete and partial obstruction?**
    - **Clinically:** If partial, the patient may continue to pass small amounts of gas or stool. Pain and distention decrease rapidly with NG suction.
    - **Radiographically:** Radiographs show gas moving into the colon (partial obstruction).
    - **With oral contrast studies:** Barium or water-soluble contrast agent given via the NG tube passes into the colon in partial and resolved complete obstructions. Patients with NG tube administered oral contrast that passes to the colon within 24 hours are much more likely to have successful nonoperative management of SBO.

12. **What conditions should be included in the differential diagnosis?**
    Ileus from other causes (e.g., UTI, pneumonia, hypokalemia), viral gastroenteritis, appendicitis (usually with perforation), ureteral stone, diverticulitis, mesenteric thrombosis, and obstructing colon cancer or other malignancy should be included.

KEY POINTS: SMALL BOWEL OBSTRUCTION

1. Most common cause is adhesive disease, followed by hernias.
2. Malignancy must be considered as a possible cause.
3. Treatment involves NG decompression, fluid and electrolyte repletion, and expectant management.
4. Surgical intervention is required if strangulation or closed-loop obstruction is suspected.

13. **What are the three types of SBO, based on bowel viability?**
    a. **Simple obstruction:** Nothing passes the point of obstruction, but the vascular supply is not compromised. Partial and complete SBO may resolve with nonoperative management.
    b. **Strangulated obstruction:** The mesentery is twisted or there is so much dilation of the bowel that arterial or venous flow is cut off and the bowel becomes ischemic. Urgent surgery is mandatory.
    c. **Closed-loop obstruction:** The bowel is obstructed proximally and distally, usually for a short segment, and that segment becomes massively dilated and susceptible to strangulation and perforation. Urgent surgery is mandatory.

14. **What are the five classic signs of strangulation? How accurate are they?**
    a. Continuous pain (not colicky)
    b. Fever
    c. Tachycardia
    d. Peritoneal signs (localized guarding or tenderness, rebound tenderness)
    e. Leukocytosis
    These signs usually indicate irreversible ischemia. Persistent pain, progressive fever, and leukocytosis are indications for surgery.

15. **What is the mortality rate of SBO?**
    - **Simple obstruction:** Mortality <5% if operated or resolved within 24 hours.
    - **Strangulated obstruction:** Mortality rate of 25%. The mortality depends on the patient's resiliency (comorbid disease); but strangulation escalates the mortality by fivefold.

16. **What operative interventions may be needed for treatment of SBO?**
    - Open or laparoscopic lysis of adhesions at the point of obstruction.
    - Reduction and repair of hernia.
    - Resection of obstructing lesions with primary anastomosis.
    - Resection of strangulated segment with primary anastomosis.
    - Bypass of obstructing lesions (used mostly for carcinomatosis).

17. **Describe criteria for distinguishing viable from dead bowel at the time of operation**
    Viable intestines are pink in color, have active peristalsis, and have arterial pulsations in their mesentery. In questionable cases, Doppler ultrasound can detect arterial pulsations, but the most reliable is the IV injection of fluorescein dye with use of a Wood's lamp. Viable bowel fluoresces purple.

18. **What is the risk of development of SBO after initial laparotomy? After previous laparotomy for SBO? Which operations are associated with high rates of SBO?**
    Approximately 15% of all patients undergoing laparotomy eventually develop an SBO. About 12% of patients with a prior SBO develop another. The more recurrences, the higher the recurrence rate. The highest rate of SBO is with open adnexal operations at 23%, followed by ileal-anal anastomosis at 19%. Total or subtotal colectomy has a 1-year rate of 11% and a 30% rate at 10 years. Hysterectomy also carries a high rate of SBO: about 5% for routine procedures and up to 15% after radical hysterectomy.

19. **What can surgeons do to decrease the risk of SBO?**
    - Use powderless gloves or wash off glove powder from gloves.
    - Avoid suturing through the peritoneum at closure.
    - Barrier films placed between the small bowel and the abdominal wall have been shown to decrease adhesions, though it remains to be seen if this will translate to fewer clinical SBOs.

20. **What is the role of laparoscopy in SBO?**
    Laparoscopic lysis of adhesions is usually reserved for patients who have not had multiple previous laparotomies. Approximately one-third of them can be treated successfully by laparoscopy alone, one-third require a minimal laparotomy ("lap-assisted"), and about one-third require a full open laparotomy. Recent series claim more than 80% success with laparoscopy.

21. **What should I consider if the patient has had Roux-en-Y gastric bypass (RYGB)?**
    The most common causes of SBO after RYGB are internal hernias (42%), adhesive disease (22%), jejunojejunostomy stenosis (15%), and incisional hernia (9%). Internal hernias can occur through the

transverse mesocolon, small bowel mesentery at the jejunojejunostomy, and between the jejunal mesentery and the mesocolon (Peterson's hernia). Evaluation for SBO should include upper gastrointestinal studies or CT scan, keeping a low threshold for operative exploration.

22. **What can be done for patients with multiple recurrent bowel obstructions for adhesions?**

   Long tube placement, either via NG, gastrostomy, or jejunostomy with the tube advanced through to the ileocecal valve, has been described. The long tube is left in position for approximately 7 days and reportedly allows the bowel to reform adhesions in more gentle curves. Many other techniques have been tried and abandoned, including Noble plication (i.e., suturing the bowel in orderly loops) and adding various irrigants (e.g., heparin, Dextran, saline) to the peritoneal cavity before closure.

23. **Name five complications associated with surgery for SBO**
    a. Enterotomy
    b. Prolonged ileus
    c. Wound infection
    d. Abscess
    e. Recurrent obstruction

24. **Name products purported to decrease adhesion formation**
    - Oxidized cellulose (Interceed)
    - Sodium hyaluronate and carboxymethylcellulose (Seprafilm)
    - Icodextrin (Adept; investigational)
    - 0.5% Ferric hyaluronate gel (Intergel; investigational)

BIBLIOGRAPHY

1. Beck DE, Opelka FG. Incidence of small-bowel obstruction and adhesiolysis after open colorectal and general surgery. *Dis Colon Rectum.* 1999;42(2):241–248.
2. Choi HK, Chu KW. Therapeutic value of Gastrografin in adhesive small bowel obstruction after unsuccessful conservative treatment: a prospective randomized trial. *Ann Surg.* 2002;236(1):1–6.
3. DeCherney AH, diZerega GS. Clinical problem of intraperitoneal postsurgical adhesion formation following general surgery and the use of adhesion prevention barriers. *Surg Clin North Am.* 1997;77(3):671–688.
4. Hayanga AJ, Bass-Wilins K. Current management of small-bowel obstruction. *Adv Surg.* 2005;39:1–33.
5. Helton WS, Fisichella PM. Intestinal obstruction. In: *ACS Surgery: Principles and Practice.* New York: WebMD Inc.; 2008.
6. Koppman JS, Li C. Small bowel obstruction after laparoscopic Roux-en-Y gastric bypass: a review of 9,527 patients. *J Am Coll Surg.* 2008;206(3):571–584.
7. Zerey M, Sechrist CW. The laparoscopic management of small-bowel obstruction. *Am J Surgery.* 2007;194(6):882–888.
8. Zielinski M, Eiken PW, Bannon MP, et al. Small bowel obstruction – who needs an operation? A multivariate prediction model. *World J Surg.* 2010;34(5):910–919.

CHAPTER 49

INTESTINAL ISCHEMIA

Thomas F. Rehring, MD, FACS

1. **What is the arterial supply to the gut?**

   The foregut (stomach and duodenum) receives its blood supply from the celiac artery, the midgut (jejunum to the proximal descending colon) from the superior mesenteric artery (SMA), and the hindgut (the remainder of the intraperitoneal gut) from the inferior mesenteric artery (IMA).

2. **Name the potential collateral pathways between the celiac axis and SMA, SMA and IMA, and Iliac and IMA**

   The pancreaticoduodenal arteries form the major collaterals between the celiac artery and the SMA. The gastroduodenal artery gives off the superior pancreaticoduodenal artery that encircles the head of the pancreas and anastomoses with the inferior pancreaticoduodenal artery, the first branch of the SMA.

   The SMA and IMA have two main connections. The marginal artery of Drummond lies within the mesentery of the colon and is made up of branches of the ileocolic, right, middle, and left colic arteries. The arc of Riolan (meandering mesenteric artery) is more central and connects the middle colic branch of the SMA and the left colic branch of the IMA.

   The internal iliac artery gives rise to the middle rectal artery, which can provide flow to the superior rectal and thus the IMA.

3. **For extra credit, for whom is the marginal artery of Drummond named? What about the arc of Riolan?**

   Hamilton Drummond, a British surgeon, proved the anastomotic connection that bears his name by ligating the origins of the right, middle, and left colic arteries and demonstrating flow to the sigmoidal arteries in 1913 and 1914.

   Jean Riolan (1577–1657) was a well-known French anatomist who (ironically) opposed Harvey's theory of circulation but is acknowledged to be the first person to point out the communication between the SMA and IMA.

4. **Name the common causes of acute intestinal ischemia**

   Acute SMA embolism (50% of all cases), acute SMA thrombosis, nonocclusive mesenteric ischemia (NOMI), mesenteric venous thrombosis, vasculitis, and iatrogenic causes (e.g., inotropic agents, aortic surgery).

5. **What is the mortality rate of patients with acute mesenteric ischemia?**

   Although the prognosis of embolic occlusion is somewhat better because of the dramatic presentation, the diagnosis of acute mesenteric ischemia is often made after infarction. The result is a high mortality rate (60%–80%), regardless of cause. Despite advances in diagnosis, intervention, and critical care, this figure has gone largely unchanged for more than 50 years.

6. **What is a paradoxical embolus?**

   A paradoxical embolus occurs in the setting of a venous thrombus embolizing to the arterial circulation via a cardiac defect (typically, an atrial septal defect allowing right-to-left shunting).

7. **What is the diagnostic triad of acute embolic intestinal ischemia?**

   Sudden onset of (1) severe abdominal pain, (2) bowel evacuation (vomiting or diarrhea), and (3) a history of cardiac disease (source for arterial emboli). An additional hallmark is pain out of proportion to physical findings.

8. **How does the presentation of patients with acute thrombotic occlusion differ?**

   Thrombotic occlusion typically presents in elderly patients with diffuse atherosclerotic occlusive disease or in patients with a history consistent with chronic mesenteric ischemia (see question 24). Particularly in the former group of patients, acute embolic occlusion may be indistinguishable from thrombotic occlusion.

9. **Which laboratory value is diagnostic of acute intestinal ischemia? Is acidosis?**
No laboratory values are diagnostic for acute intestinal ischemia. Metabolic acidosis is a late finding and implies advanced ischemia or infarction. Similarly, elevated lactate and elevated phosphate levels are nonspecific and frequently late findings. Although profound leukocytosis is found in the majority of patients, no laboratory studies are specific. The diagnosis is pursued on clinical suspicion alone.

KEY POINTS: DIAGNOSTIC TRIAD OF ACUTE EMBOLIC INTESTINAL ISCHEMIA

1. Sudden onset of severe abdominal pain out of proportion to physical exam.
2. Sudden bowel evacuation (vomiting or diarrhea).
3. History of cardiac disease (e.g., atrial fibrillation that accounts for embolic source).
4. No laboratory findings (e.g., lactate level) are diagnostic; metabolic acidosis is a late finding.
5. Emergent CT of the abdomen with intravenous contrast is indicated.

10. **When acute intestinal ischemia is suspected, what study is diagnostic?**
Computed tomography angiography (CTA) of the abdomen is diagnostic. It is helpful to review reconstructed sagittal views of the aorta to visualize the visceral vessels. CTA has the distinct advantages of speed, accessibility, and evaluation of the bowel in addition to other sources in the differential diagnosis of acute abdominal pain.

11. **How do the computed tomography (CT) and operative findings differ in patients with atherosclerotic occlusion versus patients with SMA embolism?**
An SMA embolus usually lodges 3–4 cm distal to the SMA origin, which is generally free of atherosclerotic plaque. As this is beyond the proximal jejunal and middle colic arteries, at laparotomy the proximal 15–25 cm of jejunum are usually spared. Thrombotic occlusion occurs directly at the ostia, where the atherosclerotic narrowing is most severe, causing ischemia of the entire midgut.

12. **What is the appropriate management of an SMA embolus? Is there a role for thrombolysis?**
Immediate heparinization, urgent exploration, embolectomy, assessment of bowel viability, and resection of any infarcted bowel. Postoperative anticoagulation is essential to avoid recurrent embolization.
Endovascular and "hybrid" open and catheter-based strategies are being increasingly utilized in the treatment of acute mesenteric ischemia. While it has clear theoretic advantages, bowel viability cannot be ascertained directly.

13. **How is visceral ischemia of thrombotic origin managed?**
The general management follows that of an embolism; however, mesenteric ischemia from thrombotic occlusion is the end stage of progressive atherosclerotic occlusion. Therefore, thrombectomy alone is not sufficient; bypass or endarterectomy of the proximal diseased vessel or vessels is necessary. Again, bowel viability is assessed after reperfusion. Endovascular techniques including pharmacomechanical thrombectomy, angioplasty, and stenting are gaining acceptance.

14. **Which intraoperative tests help surgeons determine bowel viability?**
Although systemic intravenous infusion of fluorescein, which is evaluated using a Wood's lamp, and intraoperative Doppler examination of the bowel are helpful, ultimately the decision is based on clinical judgment.

15. **When the extent of bowel viability is in question, what should be done?**
All nonviable and necrotic bowel should be resected. Continuity need not be restored initially. The surgeon should schedule a second-look operation 12–24 hours later to evaluate the bowel of marginal viability. Some segments that were initially questionable may become clearly viable or necrotic during this period.

16. **How much small intestine is required to maintain adequate nutrition?**
About 100 cm of small intestine is required to maintain adequate nutrition. The distal ileum and ileocecal valve are the most important segments to retain for vital bowel absorption and function.

17. **Should a second-look operation be canceled because a patient improves?**
Never. The decision is made in the operating room based on findings at the time of surgery. No clinical parameters within the ensuing 12–24 hours accurately indicate the status of the bowel in question.

18. **What is NOMI?**
Nonocclusive mesenteric ischemia (NOMI) historically accounts for approximately 20% of acute ischemic cases, but its incidence has been decreasing. NOMI typically occurs in critically ill patients with systemic hypoperfusion. In such low-flow states, splanchnic blood flow is reduced in an attempt to preserve perfusion to cardiac and cerebral beds. Pharmacologic agents such as ergot alkaloids, digitalis, cocaine, and vasoconstrictors may also predispose to NOMI.

19. **How is NOMI diagnosed and managed?**
Here, CTA may appear normal. Catheter angiography documents distal vasospasm in the absence of an anatomic occlusion. The right colon is most commonly affected because of its less consistent collateral blood flow. It is associated with (and may be exacerbated by) the concomitant use of digitalis in patients with systemic hypoperfusion. In severe cases associated with multisystem organ failure, the mortality rate approaches 75%. Treatment consists of hemodynamic optimization, weaning of inotropes, and selective arterial infusion of vasodilators (papaverine) through the angiogram catheter. Surgical intervention is reserved for intestinal infarction or perforation.

20. **If mesenteric vein thrombosis (MVT) is suspected, which test is best?**
The signs and symptoms of MVT are similar to those of acute intestinal ischemia, but they are often subtler. Delay in diagnosis is thought to contribute to the reported high mortality rate of 50%. Contrast-enhanced CT scan remains the gold standard for diagnosis.

21. **What are the risk factors for MVT? How is it treated?**
Approximately half of patients with MVT have an underlying hypercoagulable state. Other causes include splenectomy, portal hypertension, visceral infections, pancreatitis, malignancy, and blunt abdominal trauma.
   Treatment of MVT includes anticoagulation, broad-spectrum antibiotics, treatment of the underlying cause, and supportive measures. Surgery is reserved for resection of nonviable bowel. Venous thrombectomy has not proven to be of effective long-term benefit. The use of thrombolytic agents has been explored, but only in anecdotal reports. Furthermore, access to the splanchnic venous circulation for directed lysis is difficult.

22. **What is the primary cause of chronic mesenteric ischemia?**
Atherosclerosis. As the collateral circulation to the gut is robust, symptoms generally do not occur unless two of the three major arteries (celiac, superior mesenteric, and inferior mesenteric) are narrowed or occluded.

23. **What is the one unique risk factor for chronic mesenteric ischemia that differs from other atherosclerotic phenomena?**
It occurs more frequently in women (3:1 over men).

24. **What are the clinical features of patients with chronic mesenteric ischemia?**
Patients gradually, and sometimes unknowingly, become afraid to eat (food fear) because of postprandial pain (intestinal angina). The pain is typically described as dull, crampy, epigastric pain occurring within the first hour of consumption. Weight loss is the most consistent sign of chronic mesenteric ischemia, appearing in 80% of patients. In the absence of weight loss, the diagnosis of chronic intestinal ischemia is unlikely. Conversely, in patients with severe atherosclerosis and weight loss of unknown cause, mesenteric ischemia should be strongly considered. An epigastric bruit is present in 50% of patients with mesenteric occlusive disease.

25. **How should patients with chronic mesenteric ischemia be evaluated?**
Noninvasive ultrasound duplex scanning has a negative predictive value of 99% and may be used as a screening tool. However, it remains technician dependent, and not widely available. CTA has sensitivities and specificities exceeding 90% for the diagnosis of chronic mesenteric ischemia due to atherosclerotic lesions. In general, severe stenosis or occlusion of two of the three main mesenteric arteries must be depicted.

26. **What are the goals of arterial bypass in chronic mesenteric ischemia?**
Resolution of symptoms, improved nutrition, and prevention of visceral infarction.

27. If revascularization for chronic mesenteric ischemia is entertained, what six essential decisions must be considered?
    a. Surgical versus endovascular strategy
    b. If surgical, which approach (transabdominal, retroperitoneal, thoracoabdominal)?
    c. Which and how many vessels to revascularize?
    d. Endarterectomy, reimplantation, or bypass?
    e. If bypass, antegrade or retrograde?
    f. If bypass, what type of conduit (vein versus prosthetic)?
    (See also questions 31 and 32.)

28. What is ischemic colitis?
    Ischemic colitis is circulatory insufficiency of the colon that may result from occlusive, nonocclusive, and pharmacologic (e.g., cocaine, nonsteroidal antiinflammatory drugs) causes. Seven percent of all patients having nonemergent abdominal aortic aneurysm surgery and as many as 60% of patients who survive a ruptured abdominal aortic aneurysm suffer from ischemic colitis. Most cases are mild, typically involving only the mucosa and resulting in abdominal pain and bloody diarrhea. Severe disease (15% of cases) is characterized by transmural gangrenous infarction that presents with clear signs of peritonitis and bloody diarrhea.

29. How is ischemic colitis diagnosed and treated? What are its prognostic implications?
    The diagnosis is made by endoscopy. Mild disease is typically treated conservatively with bowel rest, vigorous hydration, and broad-spectrum antibiotics. Severe disease requires surgical resection. Overall mortality rates are about 40%, but in patients requiring colon resection, the mortality rate may exceed 85%. The high mortality in the latter group is attributed to endotoxemic shock and multisystem organ failure.

CONTROVERSIES

30. What is celiac compression syndrome (Dunbar's syndrome)?
    Celiac compression is a rare and controversial disorder most commonly described in women (female-to-male ratio = 4:1) between the ages of 20 and 50 years. Also known as median arcuate ligament syndrome, these patients appear to suffer from chronic mesenteric ischemia without angiographic evidence of atherosclerotic disease. The mechanical compression is believed to be caused by the left crus of the diaphragm (i.e., median arcuate ligament), and diagnosis occasionally is confirmed by demonstrating transient celiac compression during expiration. The associated pain is the result of a complicated and still heavily debated redirection of flow (foregut steal) away from the SMA. Effective treatment has required not only operative release of the compression but also celiac artery stent or bypass to improve the likelihood of pain resolution.

31. What is the role of percutaneous transluminal angioplasty (PTA) and stenting in chronic mesenteric ischemia?
    Endovascular treatment of chronic mesenteric ischemia has evolved over the past few years to become the initial strategy for those requiring treatment. Technical success rates approximate 80%; restenosis and recurrent symptoms are reported in 20%–50% of patients. No prospective trials have compared PTA with arterial bypass; however, retrospective reviews suggest that initial results with either technique are similar with regard to morbidity, death, and recurrent stenosis. However, symptom recurrence rates are higher with PTA.

32. Which is the preferred treatment for chronic mesenteric ischemia, antegrade or retrograde visceral artery bypass? Is it necessary to reconstruct more than one mesenteric vessel?
    As they apply to intestinal bypass, the terms antegrade and retrograde refer to the origin of the graft from the aorta as either proximal to the celiac axis or distal to the SMA, respectively. The stated advantages of antegrade bypass are less kinking of the graft and possibly better blood flow characteristics. The disadvantages are that supraceliac exposure is technically more difficult and clamping may result in renal or spinal cord ischemia. Retrograde bypass grafts are more difficult to position to avoid kinking.

    Recent series suggest that the results for single- or multiple-vessel reconstruction in either antegrade or retrograde fashion are excellent, with symptom-free survival rates >90% at 5 years.

BIBLIOGRAPHY

1. Fisher Jr DF, Fry WJ. Collateral mesenteric circulation. *Surg Gynecol Obstet.* 1987;164(5):487–492.
2. Sise MJ. Acute mesenteric ischemia. *Surg Clin North Am.* 2014;94(1):165–181.
3. Kazmers A. Operative management of acute mesenteric ischemia. Part 1. *Ann Vasc Surg.* 1998;12(2):187–197.
4. Kazmers A. Operative management of chronic mesenteric ischemia. Part 2. *Ann Vasc Surg.* 1998;12(3):299–308.
5. Menke J. Diagnostic accuracy of multidetector CT in acute mesenteric ischemia: systematic review and meta-analysis. *Radiology.* 2010;256(1):93–101.
6. Acosta S. Epidemiology of mesenteric vascular disease: clinical implications. *Semin Vasc Surg.* 2010;23(1):4–8.
7. Oderich GS. Current concepts in the management of chronic mesenteric ischemia. *Curr Treat Options Cardiovasc Med.* 2010;12(2):117–130.
8. Schermerhorn ML, Giles KA. Mesenteric revascularization: management and outcomes in the United States, 1988-2006. *J Vasc Surg.* 2009;50(2):341–348.
9. Arthurs ZM, Titus J, Bannazadeh M, et al. A comparison of endovascular revascularization with traditional therapy for the treatment of acute mesenteric ischemia. *J Vasc Surg.* 2011;53(3):698–705.

CHAPTER 50

DIVERTICULAR DISEASE OF THE COLON

Magdalene A. Brooke, MD, Gregory P. Victorino, MD, FACS

1. **What is a colonic diverticulum?**
   A protrusion of mucosa and submucosa through the muscular layers of the bowel wall. It has no muscular covering. Because these diverticula do not involve all layers of the bowel wall, they are really "false" diverticula. Diverticulum formation may be related either to weakness of the bowel wall at the sites of vessel perforation or to increased intraluminal pressure caused by low dietary fiber and constipation.

2. **What is the difference between diverticulosis and diverticulitis?**
   Diverticulosis is colonic diverticula without associated inflammation. Diverticulitis is inflammation and infection. Only 15% of patients with diverticulosis develop diverticulitis.

3. **How does a diverticulum cause pain?**
   Pain comes from inflammation or perforation of the diverticulum. If perforated, leakage may be scant and contained within pericolic fat or extensive, involving the mesentery, other organs, or the peritoneal cavity. Sigmoid diverticulitis typically causes pain in the left lower quadrant.

4. **Where in the colon are diverticula usually located?**
   In the United States, 95% of all diverticula occur in the left colon, primarily in the sigmoid colon. Diverticula, however, may occur anywhere in the colon. In Asia, right colonic diverticula are more common. The diverticula tend to occur on the mesenteric side of the antimesenteric tinea, where small perforating blood vessels create a weakness in the circular muscle of the colon.

5. **At what age is diverticulitis most common?**
   The sixth or seventh decade of life. Younger patients are more likely than older patients to have right colonic diverticulitis.

6. **What strategy may decrease diverticulitis in patients with diverticula?**
   A high-fiber diet. Large bulk in the colon decreases segmentation and intraluminal pressure.

7. **What is the best imaging test for diagnosing acute diverticulitis?**
   Computed tomography (CT) scan, which can also diagnose local complications of diverticulitis.

8. **What are the possible complications in complicated diverticulitis?**
   - Perforation
   - Inflammatory phlegmon or abscess in the bowel mesentery
   - Peritonitis
   - Intraabdominal abscess
   - Internal fistula
   - Bowel obstruction

9. **Can diverticular disease cause bleeding?**
   Yes. Diverticulosis (not -itis) is a common cause of lower gastrointestinal bleeding. Bleeding from diverticulitis is uncommon.

10. **How can the site of diverticular bleeding be localized?**
    Colonoscopy is considered first line to localize lower gastrointestinal (GI) bleeding as it also offers the opportunity to intervene using thermal coagulation, epinephrine injection, or endoscopic clipping. Patients must be adequately resuscitated prior to the procedure. If bleeding is not seen at the time of colonoscopy or a colonoscopy is not technically possible, other localization methods include CT angiography and tagged red blood cell scan.

11. **When should an operation be performed for a bleeding colonic diverticulum?**
    Replacement of 5–6 units of blood (two-thirds of a patient's blood volume) within 24 hours and rebleeding during hospitalization are standard indications for resection of the segment of colon containing a bleeding diverticulum.

12. **If bleeding is life threatening but cannot be localized within the colon, what treatment is required?**
    Subtotal colectomy with temporary ileostomy and closure of the distal sigmoid colon at the peritoneal reflection (Hartmann procedure) or total abdominal colectomy with ileorectal anastomosis is required. This operation carries a high risk of mortality.

13. **What is the clinical evidence of a vesicocolic or ureterocolic fistula after diverticular perforation?**
    Pneumaturia, fecaluria, and chronic urinary tract infections (polymicrobial).

14. **What procedure is required to repair a vesicocolic fistula?**
    A staged procedure was the standard until recently. Now most patients can be treated with a single procedure that includes sigmoid resection, colonic anastomosis, and primary repair of bladder defect with absorbable suture. A Foley catheter is usually left in place for 10 days after surgery. Some viable tissue should be placed between the colonic and bladder repairs to prevent a recurrent fistula.

15. **How is complicated diverticulitis classified clinically?**
    Diverticulitis is classified by the Hinchey classifications, originally proposed in 1978:
    - Class I – Localized, paracolonic abscess
    - Class II – Pelvic abscess
    - Class III – Purulent peritonitis
    - Class IV – Fecal peritonitis

16. **When should diverticulitis be managed operatively in the acute setting?**
    The current guidelines on management of diverticulitis recommend resection of the affected segment of colon in the setting of purulent or fecal peritonitis (Hinchey III and IV), or in the case of failure to improve with nonoperative management. There is controversy, however, regarding the best operative choice to manage the resection.

CONTROVERSIES

17. **What operation should be performed for severe diverticulitis?**
    Options for acute operative management of complicated diverticulitis include the following:
    a. Open resection with end colostomy (Hartmann procedure)
    b. Open resection with primary anastomosis, plus/minus protective ileostomy
    Classically, it has been the standard to perform option a, resection with end colostomy, because of the concern for creation of an anastomosis in an inflamed, infected setting. However, there is emerging literature supporting primary anastomosis, possibly with diverting ileostomy to protect the anastomosis. The current literature is split on the safety of this technique in the urgent or emergent setting. Guidelines recommend relying on surgeon's preference and clinical judgment to decide which is appropriate in a given clinical scenario. Option a is the safer choice in a grossly contaminated or inflamed field.

18. **Should patients with recurrent diverticulitis receive elective, prophylactic colectomy?**
    For many years the thought was that prophylactic colectomies should be performed in the setting of recurrent diverticulitis in order to prevent both future episodes and future complications requiring colostomy. Recently, this strategy has come into question. Studies overall do not find that use of elective colectomy reduces the risk of episodes of complicated diverticulitis in the future. Consensus guidelines are moving away from recommending elective resection based on age of the patient or number of episodes of uncomplicated diverticulitis, but more data is needed to assess the value of elective resection. There is still evidence to support considering elective colectomy after episodes of complicated diverticulitis requiring abscess drainage or other invasive therapy.
    The use of laparoscopic colon resection in appropriately experienced hands is supported in the literature, and recommended in current guidelines.

KEY POINTS: LOCALIZATION OF LOWER GI BLEEDING

1. In cases of hematochezia, it is important to rule out upper GI source of bleeding with placement of a nasogastric tube. Return of bile without blood is proof of lower GI source. Otherwise, EGD should be performed.
2. Common lower GI causes: Diverticulosis, cancer, angiodysplasia.
3. Tagged red blood cell nuclear scans are useful for slower GI bleeding (detects bleeding at 0.2–0.5 mL/min).

BIBLIOGRAPHY

1. Buchs NC, Mortensen NJ. Natural history of uncomplicated sigmoid diverticulitis. *World J Gastrointest Surg.* 2015;7(11):313–318.
2. Constantinides VA, Heriot A, Remzi F, et al. Operative strategies for diverticular peritonitis: a decision analysis between primary resection and anastomosis versus Hartmann's procedures. *Ann Surg.* 207;245(1):94–103.
3. Simpson J, Scholefield JH. Pathogenesis of colonic diverticula. *Br J Surg.* 2002;89(5):546–554.
4. Frattini J, Longo WE. Diagnosis and treatment of chronic and recurrent diverticulitis. *J Clin Gastroenterol.* 2006;40(suppl 3):S145–S149.
5. Feingold D, Steele S, Lee S, et al. Practice parameters for the treatment of sigmoid diverticulitis. *Dis Colon Rectum.* 2014;57(3):284–294.
6. Hinchey EJ, Schaal PG. Treatment of perforated diverticular disease of the colon. *Adv Surg.* 1978;12:85–109.
7. Moghadamyeghaneh Z, Carmichael JC, Smith BR, et al. A comparison of outcomes of emergent, urgent, and elective surgical treatment of diverticulitis. *Am J Surg.* 2015;210(5):838–845.
8. Oberkofler CE, Rickenbacher A, Raptis DA, et al. A multicenter randomized clinical trial of primary anastomosis or Hartmann's procedure for perforated left colonic diverticulitis with purulent or fecal peritonitis. *Ann Surg.* 2012;256(5):819–827.
9. Pasha SF, Shergill A, Acosta RD, et al. The role of endoscopy in the patient with lower GI bleeding. *Gastrointest Endosc.* 2014;79(6):875–885.
10. Richter S, Lindemann W. One-stage sigmoid colon resection for perforated sigmoid diverticulitis (Hinchey stages III and IV). *World J Surg.* 2006;30(6):1027–1032.
11. Schulz JK, Yaqub S, Wallon C, et al. Laparoscopic lavage vs primary resection for acute perforated diverticulitis: The SCANDIV randomized clinical trial. *JAMA.* 2015;314(13):1364–1375.
12. Simianu VV, Strate LL, Billingham RP, et al. The impact of elective colon resection on rates of emergency surgery for diverticulitis. *Ann Surg.* 2016;263(1):123–129.
13. Vennix S, Morton DG, Hahnloser D, et al. Systematic review of evidence and consensus on diverticulitis: an analysis of national and international guidelines. *Colorectal Dis.* 2014;16(11):866–878.

CHAPTER 51

ACUTE LARGE BOWEL OBSTRUCTION

Erik D. Peltz, DO, FACS, Elizabeth C. Brew, MD

1. **What are the mechanical causes of large bowel obstruction (LBO)?**
   The most common mechanical causes are carcinoma (50%), volvulus (15%), adhesions (15%), and diverticular disease (10%). Extrinsic compression from metastatic carcinoma or noncolonic neoplasms is another cause of obstruction. Less frequent causes include hernia with colonic incarceration, intussusception, benign tumor, fecal impaction, inflammatory bowel disease, ischemic colitis, adhesions, bezoars, and retroperitoneal fibrosis.

2. **How is the diagnosis made?**
   a. The patient complains of crampy abdominal pain, bloating, and obstipation. Nausea and vomiting occur later in LBO and may be feculent. An acute onset of symptoms is more consistent with volvulus compared with the gradual development of obstructive complaints from patients with colon carcinoma. Longer duration of symptoms suggest a malignant etiology for LBO.
   b. Physical examination reveals abdominal distention and high-pitched bowel sounds. Rectal examination may reveal an obstructing rectal cancer or evidence of fecal impaction. Absence of bowel sounds and localized tenderness may be signs of peritonitis. Progression of symptoms accompanied by a high fever or tachycardia requires immediate operative attention.
   c. Flat and upright abdominal radiographs reveal dilated colon proximal to the obstruction. An upright chest radiograph may show free air under the diaphragm if a perforation has occurred.

3. **How is the diagnosis confirmed?**
   Modern fast acquisition helical multidetector CT (MDCT) imaging has replaced contrast enema for confirming the diagnosis of LBO in many patients. MDCT has a reported sensitivity and specificity of 96% and 94%, respectively, in the diagnosis of LBO. Computed tomography (CT) scans may distinguish between mechanical obstruction or pseudo-obstruction and can help with the diagnosis of diverticulitis or colon carcinoma. CT scans can help distinguish between sigmoid and cecal volvulus. MDCT can show a transition point with proximal dilated colon and collapsed distal colon. An intraluminal or rectal mass can also been seen. In addition, multifocal or metastatic disease can been demonstrated. CT avoids the risk of perforation with instrumentation during enema or endoscopy, and may be of benefit in elderly or frail patients who cannot cooperate with or tolerate other diagnostic procedures.

4. **What is the role of contrast enemas in the diagnosis of LBO?**
   A contrast enema (barium or water-soluble contrast) is necessary to delineate the level and nature of an obstruction. A volvulus can be identified by a "bird's beak" narrowing at the neck of the volvulus. Sigmoidoscopy or colonoscopy is an essential part of the evaluation; it allows visualization of the colon and may be therapeutic in the case of a sigmoid volvulus.

5. **Why is tenderness in the right lower quadrant (RLQ) important?**
   The cecum is the area that is most likely to perforate. When the cecum reaches 15 cm at its widest diameter, the tension on the wall is so great that decompression is essential to prevent perforation. The larger diameter of the cecum causes more tension of the cecal wall at the same intraluminal pressure (law of Laplace). The other area at risk for perforation is the site of a primary colon cancer.

6. **Where is the obstructing cancer usually located?**
   Most obstructing colorectal carcinomas occur in the splenic flexure, descending colon, or hepatic flexure. Ten percent of patients presenting with colonic obstruction have rectal cancer, with an additional 5% with anal cancer. In contrast, lesions of the right colon usually present with occult bleeding. Cecal and rectal cancers are uncommon causes of obstruction. LBO is the initial presenting symptom of colon cancer in up to 30% of cases.

7. **What is a volvulus? Where is it located?**

A volvulus is an abnormal rotation of the colon on an axis formed by its mesentery and occurs either in the sigmoid colon (75%) or cecum (25%). **Sigmoid volvulus** occurs in an older population when chronic constipation causes the sigmoid colon to elongate and become redundant. Sigmoid volvulus is treated with initial sigmoidoscopic decompression, which can be followed with semielective surgery. **Cecal volvulus** requires a hypermobile cecum as a result of incomplete embryologic fixation of the ascending colon.

8. **When is surgery indicated?**

Surgery is performed early in colon obstruction. Urgent laparotomy is necessary in patients with suspected perforation or ischemia. Danger signs are quiet abdomen, RLQ tenderness, and increasing pain. The patient's cardiopulmonary status should be assessed and optimized preoperatively. It is essential to correct dehydration and administer perioperative antibiotics. Marking of possible stoma sites and deep venous thrombosis prophylaxis are other important preoperative considerations.

9. **Which operation should be performed for an LBO?**

The most difficult decision is whether or not to perform a primary anastomosis. Careful assessment of the patient's condition, viability of the bowel, location of the obstruction, and absence of intraabdominal contamination helps guide the decision. Specific procedures include ostomy alone for fecal diversion (initial or palliative), colectomy with primary anastomosis with or without a diverting ostomy, or colectomy with end colostomy (Hartman procedure).

An **obstructing carcinoma** may be resected satisfactorily under emergency conditions in 90% of patients. Carcinomas of the right and transverse colon (proximal to the splenic flexure) are routinely treated with resection and primary anastomosis. Recently, obstructing cancers of the descending colon have been treated either with resection and colostomy. Laparoscopic surgery for LBO has been reported to be feasible and safe, even in patients with obstructing cancers. Intraoperative lavage followed by resection and primary anastomosis has not been shown to have any advantage and has the disadvantage of increased operative time and increased contamination. Techniques for nonoperative decompression of the colon, such as balloon dilation, laser therapy, and stent placement, are under investigation. Theoretically, these techniques will allow palliation, bowel preparation, and elective colon resection.

A **volvulus** should be reduced and resected. Reduction of a sigmoid volvulus can be achieved nonoperatively by sigmoidoscopy or hydrostatic decompression with a contrast enema. The recurrence rate of volvulus after simple nonoperative reduction is 75%. Surgical therapy includes detorsion with colopexy or sigmoid colectomy. Cecal volvulus can be treated similarly with nonoperative decompression, cecopexy, or surgical resection.

The optimal treatment of **diverticular disease** is initial bowel rest; intravenous (IV) antibiotics; and percutaneous abscess drainage, if necessary. Colon resection and primary anastomosis can be performed after adequate bowel preparation.

10. **What is the role of endoluminal stenting for acute LBO?**

Colorectal stent placement may be useful for colonic decompression, bowel cleansing, and medical optimization before definitive surgical resection. In this preoperative setting colorectal stenting may allow for a single-stage surgical resection. Endoluminal stents may also be useful as an alternative to colostomy for palliative decompression in patients with unresectable malignant obstruction. Complications of stent placement include stent occlusion and migration, inadequate decompression, and bowel perforation. At this time, their limited application to a select group of patients requires careful evaluation.

11. **What are the nonmechanical causes of LBO?**

Paralytic ileus (i.e., colonic pseudo-obstruction) or toxic megacolon.

12. **What is Ogilvie's syndrome?**

Ogilvie's syndrome is an acute paralytic (adynamic) ileus or pseudo-obstruction (i.e., enormous dilation of the colon without a mechanical distal obstructing lesion). Patients present with a massively dilated abdomen and a small amount of pain. Nonoperative management, including bowel rest, IV fluids, and gentle enemas, is the therapy of choice. Gastrografin enema or colonoscopy is diagnostic and therapeutic. Neostigmine is another treatment modality in patients with colons >10 cm in diameter.

13. **What is toxic megacolon?**
Toxic megacolon is dilatation of the entire colon secondary to acute inflammatory bowel disease. This entity is commonly associated with clostridium difficile. The disease is manifested by acute onset of abdominal pain, distention, and sepsis. Initial therapy includes IV fluid resuscitation, nasogastric decompression, and broad-spectrum antibiotics. If symptoms do not resolve within a few hours, the patient requires an operation to avoid perforation. Surgical therapy most often consists of an emergency abdominal colectomy with formation of an ileostomy.

KEY POINTS: CAUSES OF LBO

1. Carcinoma (most common cause): 50%
2. Volvulus: 15%
3. Adhesions 15%
4. Diverticular disease: 10%
5. Other causes: hernia, intussusception, fecal impaction

WEBSITE

- www.emedicine.com/emerg/topic65.htm

BIBLIOGRAPHY

1. Adler DG, Baron TH. Endoscopic palliation of colorectal cancer. *Hematol Oncol Clin North Am.* 2002;16(4):1015–1029.
2. Beattie GC, Peters RT. Computed tomography in the assessment of suspected large bowel obstruction. *ANZ J Surg.* 2007;77(3):160–165.
3. Dauphine CE, Tan P. Placement of self-expanding metal stents for acute malignant large-bowel obstruction: a collective review. *Ann Surg Oncol.* 2002;9(6):574–579.
4. Frager D. Intestinal obstruction role of CT. *Gastroenterol Clin North Am.* 2002;31(3):777–799.
5. Jost RS, Jost R. Colorectal stenting: an effective therapy for preoperative and palliative treatment. *Cardiovasc Intervent Radiol.* 2007;30(3):433–440.
6. Lopez-Kostner F, Hool GR. Management and causes of acute large-bowel obstruction. *Surg Clin North Am.* 1997;77(6):1265–1290.
7. Markogiannakis H, Messaris E, Dardamanis D, et al. Acute mechanical bowel obstruction: clinical presentation, etiology, management and outcome. *World J Gastroenterol.* 2007;13(3):432–437.
8. Murray JJ, Schoetz DJ. Intraoperative colonic lavage and primary anastomosis in nonelective colon resection. *Dis Colon Rectum.* 1991;34(7):527–531.
9. Paran H, Silverberg D. Treatment of acute colonic pseudo-obstruction with neostigmine. *J Am Coll Surg.* 2000;190(3):315–318.
10. Tan SG, Nambiar R. Primary resection and anastomosis in obstructed descending colon due to cancer. *Arch Surg.* 1991;126(6):748–751.
11. Gash K, Chambers W. The role of laparoscopic surgery for the management of acute large bowel obstruction. *Colorectal Dis.* 2011;13(3):263–266.
12. Torralba JA, Robles R, Parilla P, et al. Subtotal colectomy vs. intraoperative colonic irrigation in the management of obstructed left colon carcinoma. *Dis Colon Rectum.* 1998;41(1):18–22.

CHAPTER 52

INFLAMMATORY BOWEL DISEASE

Magdalene A. Brooke, MD, Emily Miraflor, MD

1. What clinical entities encompass the diagnosis of inflammatory bowel disease (IBD)?

   Crohn's disease (CD) and ulcerative colitis (UC). A third entity called indeterminate colitis describes the situation when the clinical or pathologic features do not entirely fit the criteria for either CD or UC.

2. Although the two diseases often overlap, they usually can be distinguished by clinical criteria. What are the major clinical differences?

   Patients with CD may complain of abdominal pain and diarrhea with mucous or blood. UC patients are troubled by bloody diarrhea, but more specifically urgency that makes them hesitant to stray too far from a bathroom. An abdominal mass and a history of anorectal diseases (fissures, fistulas, abscesses) are commonly found in CD. UC patients may have perianal irritation or fissures as a result of bowel frequency but do not typically have fistulas.

3. What are the major radiologic differences between the two diseases?

   Computed tomography scans may show terminal ileal thickening, skip areas, strictures, and internal fistulas with associated phlegmons in CD. Colon wall thickening can be seen in UC.

4. What are the major histological differences?

   Granulomas in the intestinal wall and adjacent lymph nodes can occur in 60% of patients with CD. In UC, the inflammation is limited to the mucosa, whereas in CD it can be full-thickness inflammation. Crypt abscesses, crypt distortion and Paneth cell metaplasia are common histopathologic findings in UC. Granulomas associated with crypt abscesses may be seen in UC and do not necessarily indicate that the patient has CD. Additionally, severe UC can have ulcerations and erosions from the mucosa into the submucosa and can be confused with CD.

5. Crohn's colitis and UC are often difficult to distinguish clinically. What are the major differences seen at colonoscopy?

   Crohn's manifestations can be seen in any location in the GI tract from mouth to anus, and may involve noncontiguous areas. UC, however, begins in the distal large bowel and proceeds proximally in a contiguous manner.

   Crohn's colitis is focal and predominantly right sided. Aphthous ulcerations are the earliest lesions seen in CD. As the disease progresses, they may form linear or serpiginous ulcers (bear claw ulcerations) in affected areas. When these large ulcerations migrate transversely, islands of normal mucosa appear known as cobble stoning. In UC, disease begins in the rectum and progresses proximally. Skip areas are more common in CD, but be aware that UC patients treated with rectal suppositories or enemas may have a normal appearing rectum. Endoscopic findings in UC may range from simple edema of the mucosa to indurated, friable tissue that bleeds on contact.

6. Although CD may affect the gastrointestinal (GI) tract from the pharynx to the anus, what are the most common clinical patterns of GI involvement?

   Small bowel only: 28%; both ileum and colon (ileocolitis): 41%; and colon only: 27%. Crohn's involvement of the colon is also called Crohn's colitis or granulomatous colitis.

7. What are the major indications for surgery in CD?

   It depends on the site of involvement and significance of symptoms. The guiding principle is to only operate when the disease is affecting the physiology of the patient. A patient with mild diarrhea and an enteroenteric fistula does not need surgery and should be treated medically. Surgery is indicated in cases of obstruction, perforation, and when the disease process is having generalized physiologic effects such as profound diarrhea, weight loss, or sepsis. Patients may also require surgery if they do not respond to or are unable to tolerate medical therapy. Perianal disease with abscess needs urgent drainage. Approximately 80% of Crohn's patients will require surgery in their lifetime.

8. **What are the major indications for surgery in UC?**
   Acute indications for surgical intervention include severe colitis with signs of perforation or impending perforation (for example, toxic megacolon) and acute colitis that fails to improve or resolve with medical therapy alone. Chronic indications include medical intractability, severe complications such as malnutrition and failure to grow in children, and disabling extraintestinal manifestations (especially ophthalmic, skin, and joint symptoms). Approximately 20% of UC patients will require surgery in their lifetime.

9. **What is the surgical treatment of UC?**
   A total proctocolectomy provides a surgical cure for UC. Most patients do not want a permanent ileostomy, so a reconstruction to create a neorectum is performed. A pouch made out of the patient's small intestine can be fashioned and anastomosed to the anal sphincters providing fecal continence.

10. **What is the surgical procedure for an ileal stricture? What is the procedure for multiple strictures?**
    Because surgery for CD is not curative, and most patients will require multiple surgeries in their lifetimes, bowel preservation is important as repeated procedures can lead to short gut syndrome. For an isolated stricture, resection and anastomosis is the procedure of choice. One should anastomose grossly normal ileum to grossly normal colon. For those patients with multiple strictures, a procedure called a strictureplasty is performed. A longitudinal incision is made along the stricture and extended into normal bowel wall. Then the opening is closed transversely, opening the lumen so enteric contents may pass.

11. **How do you evaluate the placement of a stoma (ostomy)?**
    The location of a stoma is a major factor in patient morbidity and maintaining an acceptable quality of life. Placement of a stoma should be individualized and take into consideration the patient's abdominal contour, prior scars, belt line, and bony prominences. Creation of the stoma through the rectus abdominis muscle one-third of the way along a line drawn from the umbilicus to the superior iliac spine generally gives good results, but obese patients may need a stoma on the upper abdomen to facilitate self-care.

12. **How does one monitor a patient with UC for dysplasia?**
    After an index colonoscopy when the patient is diagnosed, surveillance colonoscopy should begin after 8–10 years of disease, and should undergo surveillance every 1–3 years depending on findings. Four quadrant biopsies every 10 cm are standard to achieve at least 35 specimens. This provides adequate sample size to detect dysplasia.

13. **Does IBD have a genetic basis?**
    About 20% of people with IBD will have an affected family member, which suggests a genetic linkage. The first Crohn's-associated mutation was the NOD2/CARD 15 gene on chromosome 16. This gene's product plays a role in immune response to certain bacterial cell wall components. A homozygous mutation of this gene increases the risk of CD by 30-fold. Well over 40 IBD-associated gene mutations have been identified, some are specific to either UC or CD, whereas other mutations can be found in either disease.

14. **What are some of the medical therapies for IBD?**
    Many first-line treatments involve the use of antiinflammatory medications that can be delivered orally or rectally. These 5-ASA compounds have minimal toxicities. Other modalities include immuno-modulating medications. Steroids are the mainstay of treatment for flares or exacerbation of disease symptoms. Immunosuppressive medications such as azathioprine, its metabolite 6-mercaptopurine, and even cyclosporine have been used in IBD. The newest class of medications used, biologics, are antibodies to specific targets (infliximab and adalimumab) such as tumor necrosis factor-a (TNF-a). Antibiotics may also be used in long-term therapy of CD patients with perianal fistulas.

15. **What is a Brooke ileostomy?**
    The Brooke ileostomy is the "rosebud" or full-thickness ileostomy folded over on itself for approximately 1 cm above the skin. This allows an adequate seal between the stoma appliance and the opening of the bowel. This prevents spillage of bowel contents onto the skin, which can cause significant skin irritation and inflammation.

16. **What is pouchitis, and which patients are likely to get it?**
    Pouchitis is defined as an inflammation of the small intestinal pouch. Of all patients who undergo a total proctocolectomy with an ileal-anal pouch, 27% will have at least one episode of pouchitis in their

lifetime. Although no cause has been found, research has focused on autoimmune possibilities, bacterial overgrowth of the small bowel, and a lack of the appropriate bacteria usually found in the colon. Most episodes are treated with antibiotics such as fluoroquinolones and metronidazole. Refractory cases are rare, and may require antiinflammatory medications or even immunosuppressive medications. Pouchitis rarely requires pouch excision. It is interesting to note that pouchitis is not seen in patients who have a pelvic pouch for other diseases, such as familial adenomatous polyposis, lending credence to theory that pouchitis may be the result of the same mechanism as IBD.

CONTROVERSIES

17. Should all patients with enteroenteral fistulas secondary to CD have surgery when the fistula is discovered?
    - **For:** Such patients ultimately do poorly, develop further intraperitoneal septic complications, and eventually require surgery.
    - **Against:** Many of these patients do well without operative treatment with medical management. Surgery is not a cure, so why subject the patient to unnecessary risk. An asymptomatic enteroenteral fistula discovered incidentally on imaging does not warrant an intervention.

18. Should all patients with UC that is documented for 10 years, whether the disease is active or not, undergo a proctocolectomy to avoid the risk of carcinoma of the colon and rectum?
    - **For:** The risk of colon cancer in UC increases by approximately 1% per year after 8–10 years of disease, so this can eliminate their risk of cancer. Of note, patients with UC and primary sclerosing cholangitis have an increased cancer risk.
    - **Against:** Using surveillance colonoscopy and biopsy, we can determine patients who are at high risk for cancer, so why subject many normal patients to the risks of surgery?

19. Is ileorectal anastomosis an acceptable operation after colectomy for UC?
    - **For:** These patients will have more normal bowel habits and avoid the higher complication rate of pelvic surgery. There is also preliminary evidence of better outcomes for female fertility compared with ileal pouch anal anastomosis.
    - **Against:** At least 50% of patients eventually require reoperation for recurrence of disease symptoms. The remaining rectum also may be a site for the development of cancer and these patients require postoperative surveillance. Additionally, using diseased rectum in the formation of an anastomosis risks anastomotic leakage. This surgical option should only be considered in patients without significant rectal inflammation.

20. Should we offer a total proctocolectomy and ileal pouch for patients with Crohn's colitis?
    - **For:** With the use of newer medications, these patients can be stoma free for many years.
    - **Against:** The rate of fistula formation and pouch failures make this surgery too risky in CD.

KEY POINTS: INFLAMMATORY BOWEL DISEASE

1. UC and CD are both inflammatory disorders featuring an abnormal immune response to both the bowel mucosa and to normal bowel flora. There is overlap between the two disorders; when the pathologic features do not clearly fit the criteria for Crohn's colitis or UC, the diagnosis of indeterminate colitis should be made.
2. CD is always a transmural process associated with noncaseating granulomas. CD can affect any part of the GI tract from the mouth to the anus. UC affects the mucosa of the colon and rectum only.
3. Because of increased rates of colon cancer in UC patients, it is recommended that screening begin 8 years after diagnosis and be repeated every 2–3 years. Random biopsies should be taken throughout the length of the colon to assess for dysplasia.
4. CD cannot be cured by surgery. Surgery is reserved for the management of complications such as obstruction, perforation, or fistulas.
5. Modern surgical management of UC consists of a total proctocolectomy with an ileal pouch reconstruction to avoid a permanent stoma. The most common long-term complication experienced by these patients is pouchitis.

BIBLIOGRAPHY

1. Khor B, Gardet A. Genetics and pathogenesis of inflammatory bowel disease. *Nature.* 2011;474(7351):307–317.
2. Michelassi F, Lee J, Rubin M, et al. Long-term functional results after ileal pouch anal restorative proctocolectomy for ulcerative colitis: a prospective observational study. *Ann Surg.* 2003;238(3):433–431.
3. Ross H, Steel SR, Varma M, et al. Practice parameters for the surgical treatment of ulcerative colitis. *Dis Colon Rectum.* 2014;57(1):5–22.
4. Strong S, Steele SR, Boutrous M, et al. Clinical practice guideline for the surgical management of Crohn's disease. *Dis Colon Rectum.* 2015;58(11):1021–1036.
5. Lichtenstein GR, Hanauer SB. Management of Crohn's disease in adults. *Am J Gastroenterol.* 2008;104(2):465–483.
6. Kornbluth A, Sachar DB. Ulcerative Colitis in adults: American college of Gastroenterology, Practice Parameters Committee. *Am J Gastroenterol.* 2010;105(3):501–523.
7. Hurst RD, Michelassi F. Strictureplasty for Crohn's disease: techniques and long-term results. *World J Surg.* 1998;22(4):359–363.
8. Konda A, Duffy MC. Surveillance of patients at increased risk of colon cancer: inflammatory bowel disease and other conditions. *Gastroenterol Clin North Am.* 2008;37(1):191–213.
9. Solomon MJ, Schmirz M. Cancer and inflammatory bowel disease: bias, epidemiology, surveillance, and treatment. *World J Surg.* 1998;22(4):352–358.
10. Zezos P, Saibil F. Inflammatory pouch disease: the spectrum of pouchitis. *World J Gastroenterol.* 2015;21(29):8739–8752.
11. Sugerman HJ, Sugerman EL. Ileal pouch anal anastomosis without ileal diversion. *Ann Surg.* 2000;232(4):530–541.

CHAPTER 53

UPPER GASTROINTESTINAL BLEEDING

Taft Bhuket, MD, Benny Liu, MD, Robert Wong, MD, MS

1. **What is upper gastrointestinal bleeding (UGIB)?**
   Bleeding from a gastrointestinal (GI) source proximal to the ligament of Treitz (i.e., from the esophagus, stomach, or duodenum).

2. **What is the ligament of Treitz?**
   It is a thin, suspensory muscle that extends from the left crus of the diaphragm to the junction of the duodenum and jejunum. It is named for the Austrian physician Wenzel Treitz.

3. **What are the most common causes of UGIB?**
   Peptic ulcer disease (PUD) is the most common cause of UGIB. Esophageal and gastric varices and esophagitis are the next most common.

4. **What are some less common causes of UGIB?**
   Upper GI cancers, vascular malformations, Mallory-Weiss tears, and Dieulafoy's lesions.

5. **What is a Dieulafoy's lesion?**
   A tortuous, submucosal artery that protrudes through the mucosa and can cause massive UGIB. It is most commonly found in the gastric fundus, but other locations throughout the GI tract have been described. It is named after the French surgeon Paul Georges Dieulafoy.

6. **What are some unusual causes of UGIB?**
   Aortoenteric fistula and hemosuccus pancreaticus.

7. **What components of the medical history can help determine the cause of UGIB?**
   - PUD: Prior history of PUD, use of aspirin or nonsteroidal antiinflammatory drugs, known *Helicobacter pylori* infection, critical illness
   - Esophageal or gastric varices: Known or suspected cirrhosis
   - Esophagitis: Gastroesophageal reflux disease or alcohol abuse
   - Malignancy: Weight loss or obstructive symptoms
   - Mallory-Weiss Tear: Recent retching or vomiting
   - Aortoenteric fistula: History of abdominal aortic aneurysm
   - Hemosuccus pancreaticus: History of pancreatitis

8. **How common is UGIB?**
   UGIB accounts for approximately 50% of all GI bleeding hospitalizations. GI bleeding is the most common cause of hospitalization due to GI disease in the United States, with more than 500,000 hospitalizations annually.

9. **What is the mortality rate for UGIB?**
   Overall mortality rates have declined over the past 2 decades and have been reported as low as approximately 2.1%–2.5% in some US studies. Mortality rates for severe UGIB, however, have not changed and remain approximately 5%–10%. This is thought to be due to an aging population with comorbid conditions and an increase in the number of patients with cirrhosis and variceal bleeding.

10. **What is severe UGIB?**
    UGIB accompanied by shock or orthostatic hypotension, a decrease in hematocrit by at least 6%, or transfusion of at least 2 units of packed red blood cells.

11. **What signs and symptoms are associated with UGIB?**
    Hematemesis or coffee ground emesis indicate UGIB. Melena (black, tarry stool) strongly suggests UGIB and is reported to be present in approximately 80% of cases. Hematochezia (bright red blood per rectum) is more commonly associated with lower GI bleeding but can be present in severe, brisk UGIB.

12. **How much GI blood does it take to cause melena?**
    Approximately 50–100 mL.

13. **What is the initial approach to a patient with a severe UGIB?**
    As in all critically ill patients, a prompt and systematic approach is warranted and should include:
    - Assessment of ABCs (airway, breathing, circulation)
    - Directed history and physical to help determine an underlying etiology
    - Placement of two large-bore intravenous (IV) catheters
    - Initial labs: Complete blood count, comprehensive metabolic profile, coagulation studies, and blood-type/cross match
    - Administer 1–2 L of IV fluids while monitoring the patient
    - Initiate appropriate pharmacotherapy (proton pump inhibitors in suspected peptic ulcer bleeding, octreotide in suspected variceal bleeding, and antibiotics in patients with cirrhosis)
    - Consult GI for diagnostic/therapeutic esophagogastroduodenoscopy (EGD)

14. **Is a nasogastric tube (NGT) helpful in patient with UGIB?**
    The role of the NGT in UGIB is controversial. Observational evidence does not suggest a clinical benefit. Further, NGT aspirates can be falsely negative in approximately 15%–20% of patients with active UGIB and standard-bore NGT probably do not allow for sufficient clearance of blood clots to improve visualization at endoscopy.

15. **What studies can be used to evaluate the source of UGIB?**
    EGD is the first and best test and can identify the source in up to 95% of cases. Angiography (computed tomography or catheter) can be considered if ongoing bleeding is suspected and EGD is either not available or cannot identify a source.

16. **What EGD techniques can be used to control bleeding?**
    EGD is highly effective at achieving hemostasis. A combination of injection, thermal, and mechanical techniques can be used to achieve hemostasis in nonvariceal bleeding. In esophageal variceal bleeding, band ligation is superior to sclerotherapy. EUS guided coil and cyanoacrylate glue injection can be used for gastric varices.

17. **What is a Sengstaken-Blakemore tube?**
    A double-ballooned tube that can be inserted into the esophagus to tamponade actively bleeding esophageal or gastric varices. It is to be used solely as a temporizing measure until definite hemostasis can be achieved. It is named for the American neurosurgeon Robert Sengstaken and the American vascular surgeon Arthur Blakemore.

18. **What are the indications for surgery in a patient with UGIB?**
    Surgery should be considered in any combination of the following circumstances:
    - Hemostasis cannot be achieved with EGD
    - Hemostasis cannot be achieved with interventional angiography
    - Persistence of hypotension or shock

KEY POINTS: UPPER GASTROINTESTINAL BLEEDING

1. UGIB is defined as bleeding coming from a site proximal to the ligament of Treitz.
2. The most common causes are PUD, esophageal/gastric varices, and esophagitis.
3. Hematemesis or coffee ground emesis indicates UGIB. Melena strongly suggests UGIB. Hematochezia might represent UGIB.
4. EGD is the initial diagnostic and therapeutic test of choice.

BIBLIOGRAPHY

1. Savides TJ, Jensen DM. Gastrointestinal bleeding. In: *Sleisenger and Fordtran's Gastrointestinal and Liver Disease.* 10th ed. Philadelphia, PA: Elsevier, 2016. [chapter 20].
2. Hwang JH, Fisher DA, Ben-Menachem T, et al. The role of endoscopy in the management of acute non-variceal upper GI bleeding. *Gastrointest Endosc.* 2012;75(6):1132–1138.
3. Laine L. Clinical Practice: Upper gastrointestinal bleed due to a peptic ulcer. *N Engl J Med.* 2016;374(24):2367–2376.
4. Lu Y, Loffroy R. Multidisciplinary management strategies for acute non-variceal upper gastrointestinal bleeding. *Br J Surg.* 2014;101(1):e34–e50.
5. Weilert F, Binmoeller KF. New endoscopic technologies and procedural advances for endoscopic hemostasis. *Clinl Gastroenterol Hepatol.* 2016;14(9):1234–1244.

LOWER GASTROINTESTINAL BLEEDING

Benny Liu, MD, Taft Bhuket, MD, Robert Wong, MD, MS,
Kathleen R. Liscum, MD

1. **Describe the initial treatment of a patient who presents with massive lower gastrointestinal (GI) bleeding.**
   Assessment of ABCs (airway, breathing, circulation). Vital signs including orthostatics should be assessed to determine the severity of blood loss. Treatment begins with resuscitation. Place two large-bore intravenous (IV) catheters (18-guage or greater) in the upper extremities. Obtain hemoglobin and hematocrit levels, blood type, and cross-match. Frequent monitoring of vital signs should be performed to assess the resuscitation efforts with the goal of normalizing blood pressure and heart rate.

2. **What is the next step in evaluating the patient?**
   In patients with massive hematochezia and hemodynamic instability, the placement of a nasogastric tube can be considered to rule out a brisk upper GI bleed. If the aspirate is bilious, the examiner can be fairly certain that the source is distal to the ligament of Treitz. However, if the aspirate reveals no bile, the test is nondiagnostic because the patient may still be bleeding in the duodenum with a competent pylorus.

3. **What are the two most common causes of significant lower GI bleeding?**
   Diverticular hemorrhage (diverticulosis) and bleeding from ischemic colitis.

4. **What are other potential causes of blood from the rectum?**
   - Colon cancer/polyps
   - Inflammatory bowel disease
   - Postpolypectomy
   - Anorectal disorders (e.g., hemorrhoids, fissure)
   - Vascular ectasia
   - Meckel's diverticulum
   - Infectious colitis

5. **After a thorough history and physical examination, what is the first step toward identifying the specific site of bleeding?**
   Digital rectal exam and anoscopy to rule out anorectal sources. Before proceeding with extensive workup of the proximal colon the clinician should feel certain that the etiology is not in the most distal portions of the GI tract.

6. **Name four options for localizing lower GI bleeding**
   - Colonoscopy
   - Tagged red blood cell scan
   - Angiography
   - Multidetector computed tomography angiography (CTA)

7. **What is the role of tagged red blood cell scan?**
   The tagged red blood cell scan can be considered in patients with overt lower GI bleeding, in which endoscopy has failed to reveal an obvious source, who continue to bleed. The tagged red blood cell scan requires a 30-minute period during which autologous red blood cells are labeled with isotope, which are then transfused back into the patient. The test detects bleeding as slow as 0.1–0.5 mL/min. Because the tagged cells stay in the patient's circulation, the patients can be rescanned up to 24 hours after the tagged red blood cells are infused, which can be helpful in localizing the source when the patient is bleeding intermittently.

8. **What is the role of angiography?**
   This study is performed in patients who have significant persistent bleeding and are hemodynamically stable enough to not require an emergent laparotomy. This test is typically performed after a positive tagged red blood cell scan or CTA, or in those patients that have failed endoscopic management.
   Angiography detects bleeding rates of 0.5–1.0 mL/min, but only if the patient is actively bleeding. When a bleeding site is identified, the angiographic appearance may provide further insight into the cause of the bleeding. Whereas diverticular bleeding is often seen as extravasation of contrast, vascular ectasia may be identified by a vascular tuft or early filling vein.

9. **What therapeutic options are available with angiography?**
   a. Embolization of the bleeding vessel
   b. Infusion of vasopressin (Pitressin) into a selected vessel (rarely performed)

10. **What role should colonoscopy play in the evaluation of patients with lower GI bleeding?**
    Almost all patients who are hemodynamically stable should undergo colonoscopy for evaluation of hematochezia. Colonoscopy, when performed within 24 hours after presentation of lower GI bleed, has been associated with shorter length of hospital stay, decreased need for blood transfusions, and lower hospitalization costs; however, there was no effect on mortality.

KEY POINTS: LOWER GASTROINTESTINAL BLEEDING

1. The most common causes of significant lower GI bleeding are diverticular hemorrhage and bleeding from ischemic colitis.
2. The most common cause of lower GI bleeding in children is Meckel's diverticulum.
3. After a thorough history and physical examination, the first steps in identifying the specific site of bleeding are digital rectal exam and anoscopy.
4. Colonoscopy, tagged red blood cell scan, CTA, and angiography are four options for localizing lower GI bleeding.
5. Indications for surgery include patients who have received 6 units of blood without resolution of bleeding and patients who continue to bleed after endoscopic management or embolization or who are too unstable to undergo any localization procedure.
6. Multidetector CT angiography can be performed in patients with overt GI bleeding where no clear source is identified on endoscopic exam. This test can detect and localize active bleeding at rates of 0.35 mL/min or greater.
7. Most lower GI bleeds spontaneously resolve. Spontaneous resolution occurs in 75% of patients with vascular ectasia, and 80%–90% of patients with diverticular bleeding.
8. Blind subtotal colectomy is limited to the small group of patients in whom a specific bleeding source cannot be identified. The procedure is associated with a 16% mortality rate. Younger patients tend to tolerate the procedure better than elderly patients. Older patients often suffer with severe diarrhea, urgency, and incontinence. However, blind segmental colectomy is associated with an even higher mortality rate (40%) and a 50% rebleeding rate.

BIBLIOGRAPHY

1. Biondo S, Kreisler E, Millan M, et al. Differences in patient postoperative and long-term outcomes between obstructive and perforated colonic cancer. *Am J Surg.* 2008;195(4):427–432.
2. Cynamon J, Atar E, Steiner A, et al. Catheter-induced vasospasm in the treatment of acute lower gastrointestinal bleeding. *J Vasc Interv Radiol.* 2003;14(2 Part 1):211–216.
3. Green BT, Rockey DC, Portwood G, et al. Urgent colonoscopy for evaluation and management of acute lower gastrointestinal hemorrhage: a randomized controlled trial. *Am J Gastroenterol.* 2005;100(11):2395–2402.
4. Lee YS, Lee IK, Kang WK, et al. Surgical and pathological outcomes of laparoscopic surgery for transverse colon cancer. *Int J Colorectal Dis.* 2008;23(7):669–673.
5. Mallant-Hent RC, van Bodegraven AA, Meuwissen SG, et al. Alternative approach to massive gastrointestinal bleeding in ulcerative colitis: highly selective transcatheter embolization. *Eur J Gastroenterol Hepatol.* 2003;15(2):189–193.
6. Schmulewitz N, Fisher DA. Early colonoscopy for acute lower GI bleeding predicts shorter hospital stay: a retrospective study of experience in a single center. *Gastrointest Endosc.* 2003;58(6):841–846.

7. Setya V, Singer JA. Subtotal colectomy as a last resort for unrelenting, unlocalized, lower gastrointestinal hemorrhage: experience with 12 cases. *Am Surg.* 1992;58(5):295–299.
8. Strate LL. Lower GI bleeding: epidemiology and diagnosis. *Gastroenterol Clin North Am.* 2005;34(4):643–664.
9. Strate LL, Syngal S. Timing of colonoscopy: impact on length of hospital stay in patients with acute lower intestinal bleeding. *Am J Gastroenterol.* 2003;98(2):317–322.
10. Zuccaro G. Management of the adult patient with acute lower gastrointestinal bleeding. *Am J Gastroenterol.* 1998;93(8):1202–1208.
11. Navaneethan U, Njei B. Timing of colonoscopy and outcomes in patients with lower GI bleeding: a nationwide population-based study. *Gastrointest Endosc.* 2014;79(2):297–306.
12. ASGE Standards of Practice Committee, Pasha SF, Shergill A, et al. The role of endoscopy in lower GI bleeding. *Gastrointest Endosc.* 2014;79(6):875–885.
13. Ghassemi KA, Jensen DA. Lower GI bleeding: epidemiology and management. *Curr Gastroenterol Rep.* 2013;15(7):333.
14. Geffroy Y, Rodallec MH. Multidetector CT angiography in acute gastrointestinal bleeding: why, when, and how. *Radiographics.* 2011;31(3):E35–E46.
15. Adams JB, Margolin DA. Management of diverticular hemorrhage. *Clin Colon Rectal Surg.* 2009;22(3):181–185.

CHAPTER 55

COLORECTAL POLYPS

Brian Hurt, MD, MS, Carlton C. Barnett, Jr., MD, FACS

1. **What are polyps?**

   A gastrointestinal (GI) polyp is an abnormal growth of tissue projecting from the mucosal layer anywhere along the GI tract. Almost half of patients with GI polyps do not complain of bowel symptoms. Bowel habit alteration is more common than abdominal pain. The majority of colorectal polyps found at screening colonoscopy are ≤5 mm. Two-thirds of polyps occur in the rectosigmoid and descending colon.

2. **What are the major types of polyps?**

   Until recently, colonic polyps were traditionally classified as either hyperplastic or adenomatous, and only the latter were believed to have the potential to progress to carcinoma.

   Polyps can be **classified by morphology** (the Paris classification)—pedunculated, sessile, flat, or depressed.

   - **Pedunculated polyps** have a head attached by a stalk to the mucosa of the colon or rectum. The stalk is usually covered with normal mucosa and <1.5 cm in length.
   - **Sessile polyps** are relatively flat where the base is attached to the colon wall.
   - **Flat polyps** have a height less than one-half of the diameter of the lesion. These account for 27%–36% of polyps.
   - **Depressed polyps** have an increased likelihood of showing high-grade dysplasia and are more often seen in Asian populations. In general, the muscularis mucosa is an important histologic landmark for differentiating invasive from noninvasive lesions because lymphatics and veins do not extend across the muscularis mucosa. Submucosal lesions such as carcinoids and lipomas may resemble colorectal polyp.

3. **At what age do polyps develop?**

   Adenomatous colorectal polyps infrequently develop under the age of 30. The incidence increases with age. Colonic screening studies in asymptomatic individuals suggest the prevalence of adenomas is 25%–30% at age 50. Autopsy studies are consistent with this clinical prevalence.

4. **Which polyps do not have malignant potential?**

   - **Hyperplastic (metaplastic) polyps** are composed of normal cellular components, do not exhibit dysplasia, and have a characteristic serrated ("saw tooth") pattern, typically <5 mm, and located in the rectosigmoid.
   - **Hamartomas** are made up of tissue elements normally found at that site, but which are growing in a disorganized mass.
   - **Inflammatory pseudopolyps** are residual, intact but inflamed colonic mucosa subject to ulcerations. They represent healing/healed islands of mucosal epithelium. Seen in ulcerative colitis, Crohn's disease, and schistosomiasis.

5. **Which polyps have malignant potential?**

   a. **Adenomatous polyps** are known to have malignant potential and are classified pathologically:

      i. **Tubular adenomas** are characterized by a network of branching adenomatous epithelium; the tubular component must be >75%. These account for more than 80% of colonic adenomas.

      ii. **Villous adenomas** have long glands extending down from the surface to the center of the polyp; the villous component must be >75% to be villous. These account for 5%–15% of adenomas.

      iii. **Tubulovillous adenomas** have 36%–75% villous component and account for 5%–15% of adenomas.

b. **Serrated polyps** are a heterogeneous group with a variable malignant potential. Histologically distinct from adenomas, the characteristic feature of all serrated polyps is the "saw-toothed" infolding of the crypt epithelium. Generally, these are broken into:

    i. **Traditional serrated adenoma** histologically display overall protuberant growth pattern with viliform projections and contain cytologically dysplastic cells with elongated nuclei and eosinophilic cytoplasm with more prevalence in the rectosigmoid colon.

    ii. **Sessile serrated adenomas** have extensions of the serrations to the crypt base and dilated L- or inverted T-shaped crypts and are more prevalent in the proximal colon.

c. There is recent evidence implicating large hyperplastic polyps, which are mostly benign, as a potential precursor to serrated polyps.

6. **What are the risk factors for high-grade dysplasia and cancer?**
Villous histology, increasing polyp size, and high-grade dysplasia are risk factors for focal cancer within an individual adenoma.

7. **What is the relationship between polyp size and risk of adenocarcinoma?**
Polyps <2 cm have a 2% risk of containing cancer, 2-cm polyps have a 10% risk, and polyps >2 cm have a cancer risk of 40%. Sixty percent of villous polyps are >2 cm, and 77% of tubular polyps are <1 cm at the time of discovery.

8. **What are juvenile polyps?**
Juvenile polyps are cystic dilations of glandular structures within the lamina propria without epithelial hyperplasia. They can be diagnosed at any age, although they are more common in childhood. Typically, these occur in the colon and rectum and are the most common cause of GI bleeding in children.

9. **How are colorectal polyps diagnosed?**
Colonoscopy is the most sensitive test for colorectal polyps and is considered the gold standard of colorectal screening methods as it should view the entire colon and it has the advantage of being both diagnostic and therapeutic. Flexible sigmoidoscopy, computed tomography (CT) colonography, barium enema, and colon capsule endoscopy can also be used to detect colorectal polyps.

10. **What are the risks of colonoscopy**
Bleeding and perforation. For screening colonoscopy, these risks continue to be extremely low, with rates of 1%–2% and 0.1%–1%, respectively. Bleeding is usually self-limited and rarely necessitates surgical intervention.

11. **How can one determine whether endoscopic polypectomy is adequate treatment?**
In general, if a margin >1 mm can be obtained, there is no invasion of the muscularis mucosa, and the histologic grade of the lesion is I or II (well to moderately well differentiated), the patient should be offered endoscopic polypectomy. Polyps with margins <1 mm, invasion into vessels or lymphatics, and histologic grade III (poorly differentiated) lesions should undergo colon resection, unless comorbid medical conditions are contraindications for surgery.

12. **What are the screening recommendations to detect polyps?**
The American Cancer Society recommends that men and women with average risk of colorectal cancer follow one of the following:
- Flexible sigmoidoscopy every 5 years
- Colonoscopy every 10 years
- Double-contrast barium enema every 5 years
- CT colonoscopy every 5 years

All positive tests should be followed up with a colonoscopy. Although in use in many health systems, the guaiac-based fecal occult blood test and the fecal immunochemical test may be controversial ways to screen for colorectal cancer, as research has shown these methods alone will miss a significant percentage of colon abnormalities.

Patients with increased risk (personal history of colorectal cancer, adenomatous polyps, inflammatory bowel disease, or a family history of colorectal cancer or polyps, or a known history of hereditary colorectal cancer syndromes) should be screened more often. Patients who have had their colorectal cancer surgically resected should have a colonoscopy 1 year after surgery, with further follow up predicated on risk factors and colonoscopic findings. If a patient has a family history of colorectal cancer, screening should start at age 40, or 10 years before the youngest case in the immediate family. High-risk individuals, those with hereditary colorectal cancer syndromes, may need to be screened even younger. Colonoscopy and sigmoidoscopy are 90% sensitive and 96% specific for polyps. Sigmoidoscopy, however, does not allow for evaluation of the proximal colon, thus lowering the overall effectiveness of this screening technique. Although highly effective, colonoscopy requires a highly trained individual to perform and comes with risks such as anesthesia, thus compromising its value as a screening tool.

13. **What are the screening recommendations for patients with known polyps?**
Patients with small hyperplastic polyps are at no increased risk and can be screened as the average population. Patients with low risk (1 or 2 tubular adenomas <1 cm with low-grade dysplasia) should have repeat colonoscopy at 5–10 years. If a patient is found to have multiple polyps or high-grade lesions, they should undergo testing at more frequent intervals (<3 years), and one should consider an underlying genetic syndrome.

14. **Which clinical syndromes are associated with colorectal polyps?**
Familial adenomatous polyposis (FAP) is an autosomal dominant disease characterized by multiple polyps throughout the GI tract accounting for <1% of colorectal cancers in the United States. The diagnosis is made clinically by observing at least 100 adenomatous polyps in the colon (>1000 in many cases). FAP is caused by a loss of function mutation in the *APC* gene located on the fifth chromosome. More than 1000 different mutations—15% from large deletions—of this gene have been implicated in FAP. Up to 25% of cases are from a sporadic, de novo mutation. Polyposis typically occurs in the second or third decade of life; 100% penetrance to colorectal cancer if untreated, diagnosed at an average age of 45. FAP is also associated with small bowel, especially periampullary polyps or cancer and mandibular osteoma.
Gardner syndrome is also associated with the loss of the *APC* gene. In addition to having polyposis like those with FAP, these patients also develop osteomas of the skull, epidermoid cysts, retinal pigmentation abnormalities, and multiple soft tissue tumors (desmoids).
Turcot syndrome is also associated with the loss of the *APC* gene, and is characterized by central nervous system tumors (gliomas) and multiple adenomatous polyps.
Peutz-Jeghers syndrome consists of multiple hamartomatous polyps throughout the alimentary tract. These polyps are associated with cutaneous melanotic spots on the lips, within the oropharynx, and the dorsum of the fingers and toes. As with hamartomatous polyps, the malignant potential is low.

15. **What is the natural history of adenomatous polyposis coli (APC)?**
A review of more than 1000 cases of APC showed that the mean age at diagnosis of polyps was 34 years, and the mean age of colorectal cancer diagnosis was 40 years. The mean age of death was 43 years. Patients should be screened annually starting at age 10–12 via flexible sigmoidoscopy or colonoscopy. Patients are also at risk of developing upper GI cancers, albeit not nearly as high a risk as colonic; based on this, the American College of Gastroenterology suggests an upper endoscopy starting at age 25.

16. **What are the surgical treatment options for FAP?**
Treatment options include total proctocolectomy with permanent ileostomy, abdominal colectomy with rectal preservation, total abdominal colectomy with ileorectal anastomosis, or proctocolectomy with ileal pouch-anal anastomosis. In patients whom the rectum is preserved (more common procedure), yearly endoscopic surveillance is necessary.

17. **What are the molecular pathways altered in the progression of colorectal polyps to adenocarcinoma?**
The altered pathways that lead to colorectal cancer are widely studied. There appear to be three molecular pathways leading to colorectal tumorigenesis. The chromosomal instability pathway is characterized by gross chromosomal abnormalities including deletions, insertions, and loss of heterozygosity. This mechanism is implicated in FAP. The second is a DNA mismatch-repair defect, which results in an accumulation of DNA defects. This is also known as microsatellite instability (MSI). MSI is what is implicated in Lynch syndrome and many sporadic cases. The third is the hypermethylation phenotype, the hyperplastic/serrated polyp pathway fits this phenotype. Colorectal cancers due to this phenotype have a particularly high frequency of methylation of mismatch-repair enzymes, silencing transcription repair, leading to accumulation of DNA defects.

18. **What role do oncogenes play in the development of adenocarcinoma from adenomatous polyps?**
Oncogenes are copies of normal genes that have been activated by mutation. Activating mutations of one allele of an oncogene can disrupt normal cell growth and differentiation, and increase the

likelihood of neoplastic transformation. Implicated genes in colorectal cancer include *Ras, src, c-myc, c-erbB-2. Ras* mutations are found in up to 50% of sporadic colorectal cancers and 50% of colonic adenomas >1 cm. *Ras* acts in a pathway transmitting extracellular progrowth signals to the nucleus. Mutations leading to colorectal cancer prevent guanosine triphosphate hydrolysis of the protein, leading to a constitutively active growth signal. The lack of mutations in smaller adenomas suggests that *ras* mutations are acquired during later adenoma progression.

19. **What role do tumor suppressors play in the development of adenocarcinoma from adenomatous polyps?**
    Tumor suppressor genes normally have an inhibitory influence on the cell cycle. If there is a mutation in a suppressor gene, the growth process proceeds relatively unchecked. Tumor suppressor genes in colorectal polyps include *APC, p53, SMAD2,* and *SMAD4.* The APC tumor suppressor gene may be the most critical gene in the early development of colorectal cancer. Somatic mutations in both alleles are present in 80% of sporadic colorectal cancers, and a single germline mutation in this gene is responsible for FAP. *p53* inactivations occur by an initial mutation of one allele followed by the loss of the remaining allele. *p53* mutations are seen in 50%–70% of colorectal cancers.

KEY POINTS: COLORECTAL POLYPS

1. A polyp is an elevation of the mucosal surface that can occur anywhere in the GI tract.
2. Hyperplastic polyps are small, constitute >90% of colorectal polyps, and are largely benign.
3. Adenomatous and sessile polyps have malignant potential. Tubular adenomas have lower malignant potential and account for 80% of colonic adenomas.
4. Major molecular pathways altered in colorectal polyps including chromosomal instability, DNA mismatch repair, and hypermethylation are implicated in the progression of colonic polyps to adenocarcinomas.
5. APC abnormalities represent major early mutations in polyps that transition to adenocarcinoma. Ras mutations occur later in this transition.

BIBLIOGRAPHY

1. Fearon ER, Vogelstein R. A genetic model for colorectal tumorigenesis. *Cell.* 1990;61(5):759–767.
2. Fukami N, Lee JH. Endoscopic treatment of large sessile and flat colorectal lesions. *Curr Opin Gastroenterol.* 2006;22(1):54–59.
3. Goel A, Nagasaka T, Arnold CN, et al. The CpG island methylator phenotype and chromosomal instability are inversely correlated in sporadic colorectal cancer. *Gastroenterology.* 2007;132(1):127–138.
4. Heitman SJ, Ronksley PE, Hilsden RJ. Prevalence of adenomas and colorectal cancer in average risk individuals: a systematic review and meta-analysis. *Clin Gastroenterol Hepatol.* 2009;7(12):1272–1278.
5. Kennedy RD, Potter DD. The natural history of familial adenomatous polyposis syndrome: a 24 year review of a single center experience in screening, diagnosis, and outcomes. *J Pediatr Surg.* 2014;49(1):82–86.
6. Leggett B, Whitehall V. Role of the serrated pathway in colorectal cancer pathogenesis. *Gastroenterology.* 2010;138(6):2088–2100.
7. Nivatvongs S, Rojanasakul A, Reiman HM, et al. The risk of lymph node metastasis in colorectal polyps with invasive adenocarcinoma. *Dis Colon Rectum.* 1991;34(4):323–328.
8. Noffsinger AE. Serrated polyps and colorectal cancer: new pathway to malignancy. *Annu Rev Pathol.* 2009;4:343–364.
9. O'Brien MJ, Winawer SJ, Zauber AG, et al. The National Polyp Study. Patient and polyp characteristics associated with high-grade dysplasia in colorectal adenomas. *Gastroenterology.* 1990;98(2):371–379.
10. Ogino S, Nosho K, Kirkner GJ, et al. CpG island methylator phenotype, microsatellite instability, BRAF mutation and clinical outcome in colon cancer. *Gut.* 2009;58(1):90–96.
11. Rex DK, Ahnen DJ, Baron JA, et al. Serrated lesions of the colorectum: review and recommendations from an expert panel. *Am J Gastroenterol.* 2012;107(9):1315–1329.
12. Sugumar A, Sinicrope FA. Serrated polyps of the colon. *F1000 Med Rep.* 2010;2:89.
13. Whitlock EP, Lin JS. Screening for colorectal cancer: a targeted, updated systematic review for the U.S. Preventive Services Task Force. *Ann Intern Med.* 2008;149(9):638–658.
14. Williams AR, Balasooriya BA. Polyps and cancer of the large bowel: a necropsy study in Liverpool. *Gut.* 1982;23(10):835–842.
15. Winawer SJ, Zauber AG, O'Brien MJ, et al. Randomized comparison of surveillance intervals after colonoscopic removal of newly diagnosed adenomatous polyps. The National Polyp Study Workgroup. *N Engl J med.* 1993;328(13):901–906.
16. Bibbins-Domingo K, Grossman DC, Curry SJ, et al. Screening for colorectal cancer: US Preventive Services Task Force recommendation statement. *JAMA.* 2016;315(23):2564–2575.

CHAPTER 56

COLORECTAL CARCINOMA

Benny Liu, MD, Taft Bhuket, MD, Robert Wong, MD, MS,
Kathleen R. Liscum, MD

1. **What are the top three causes of cancer deaths in the United States?**
   Lung, breast or prostate, and colon cancer.

2. **List a few of the presenting symptoms of patients with colorectal cancer.**
   Intermittent rectal bleeding, vague abdominal pain, fatigue secondary to anemia, change in bowel habits, constipation, tenesmus, weight loss, and perineal pain.

3. **What options are available to evaluate a patient who has hemepositive stools?**
   Colonoscopy is recommended as the preferred follow-up test for hemepositive stools.

4. **List at least five risk factors for colorectal cancer.**
   Prior adenomatous polyps, family history of colorectal cancer, age older than 50 years, inflammatory bowel disease (ulcerative colitis or Crohn's disease), personal history of colorectal cancer, exposure to pelvic radiation for cancer treatment, and inherited syndromes (i.e., familial adenomatous polyposis [FAP], Lynch syndrome, Peutz-Jeghers syndrome).

5. **What are the current US Preventative Services Task Force recommendations for colorectal cancer screening in average-risk patients?**
   Patients aged 50–75 should undergo one of these tests for colorectal cancer screening:
   - Fecal immunochemical test (FIT) or guaiac based fecal occult blood testing (FOBT) yearly
   - Flexible sigmoidoscopy every 5 years
   - Flexible sigmoidoscopy every 10 years combined with FIT yearly
   - Colonoscopy every 10 years
   - Computed tomography colonography (virtual colonoscopy) every 5 years
   - FIT-DNA testing every 1–3 years

6. **In what part of the colon or rectum are most cancers found?**
   Historically, there has been a higher incidence of cancers in the rectum and left colon. However, over the past 50 years, there has been a gradual shift toward an increased incidence of right colon cancers. This change in pattern may reflect improvement in early detection.

7. **Surgical options for colorectal cancer are dependent on the tumor location. What operation should be performed for a patient with a lesion at 25 cm from the anal verge?**
   A sigmoid colectomy.

8. **What about a lesion at 9 cm from the anal verge?**
   A low anterior resection.

9. **What about a lesion at 4 cm from the anal verge?**
   An abdominoperineal resection. This requires a permanent colostomy.

10. **What is the significance of finding adenomatous polyps in a patient's colon?**
    This patient is six times more likely to develop colorectal cancer than a patient without polyps. Evidence suggests that most colon cancers arise from adenomatous polyps. The adenoma-carcinoma sequence describes this transformational process. Patients with FAP typically harbor more than 100 polyps, which cover the colonic mucosa. If these patients go untreated, they will, without exception, develop adenocarcinoma of the colon by age 40 years.

KEY POINTS: COLORECTAL CARCINOMA

1. Presenting symptoms may include intermittent rectal bleeding, vague abdominal pain, fatigue secondary to anemia, change in bowel habits, constipation, tenesmus, and perineal pain.
2. The current recommendation of the U.S. Preventive Services Task Force for colon cancer screening in the average-risk patient aged 50–75 is to perform any one of the available approved colon cancer screening methods. The decision to perform colon cancer screening in adults 76 years of age or greater should be individualized based on the patient's overall health and prior screening history.
3. Patients with lymph node involvement should receive chemotherapy postoperatively to treat micrometastases.

11. **How does the surgeon prepare the patient's colon for an operation?**
    Bowel preparation includes both a mechanical cleansing and appropriate antimicrobial prophylaxis. This combination has resulted in significant decrease in morbidity and mortality from colon surgery. Mechanical cleansing can be accomplished by lavage with polyethylene glycol (Go-Lytely) or a combination of cathartics and enemas (Fleet's Prep).
    Antimicrobial prophylaxis should cover the expected aerobic and anaerobic flora of the gut. Significant controversy exists over whether the antibiotics should be given enterally (e.g., neomycin, 1 g, and metronidazole [Flagyl], 1 g, three times orally at 4-hour intervals the evening before surgery) or parenterally (e.g., cefotetan, 2 g intravenously within 1 hour before surgery). Many physicians give both to obtain both intraluminal and systemic protection.

12. **What is Dukes' staging system?**
    In 1932, Dr. Cuthbert Dukes described a staging system for rectal cancer. He originally described the following:
    Dukes' A: Tumor confined to bowel wall
    Dukes' B: Tumor invading through the bowel wall
    Dukes' C: Tumor cells found in the regional lymph nodes
    Since his original article was published, this classification has been modified several times. One of the most commonly used modifications is the inclusion of Dukes' D stage, which indicates distant metastases. While this system is often easier for the patients to understand, research and publications rely on the TNM staging system.

13. **Which patients with colorectal cancer require adjuvant (postoperative) therapy?**
    Patients with lymph node involvement (Dukes' C) Stage III should receive chemotherapy postoperatively to treat micrometastases. Two large studies have documented a survival advantage for these patients. However, no studies have documented a survival advantage for patients with Dukes' B Stage II disease treated with chemotherapy.
    Patients with rectal cancer with a significant chance of local recurrence (Dukes' B and C) should be treated with radiation therapy. This may be given preoperatively, postoperatively, or with a combined "sandwich" technique.

BIBLIOGRAPHY

1. Alvarez JA, Baldonedo RF. Emergency surgery for complicated colorectal carcinoma: a comparison of older and younger patients. *Int Surg.* 2007;92(6):320–326.
2. Colorectal Cancer Collaborative Group. Adjuvant radiotherapy for rectal cancer: a systematic overview of 8,507 patients from 22 randomized trials. *Lancet.* 2001;358(9290):1291–1304.
3. Jass JR. Pathogenesis of colorectal cancer. *Surg Clin North Am.* 2002;82(5):891–904.
4. Levin B, Brooks D. Emerging technologies in screening for colorectal cancer: CT colonography, immunochemical fecal occult blood tests, and stool screening using molecular markers. *CA Cancer J Clin.* 2003;53(1):44–55.
5. Lynch HT, de la Chapelle A. Hereditary colorectal cancer. *N Engl J Med.* 2003;348(10):919–932.
6. Nakamura T, Mitomi H, Ihara A, et al. Risk factors for wound infection after surgery for colorectal cancer. *World J Surg.* 2008;32(6):1138–1141.
7. Ransohoff DF. Screening colonoscopy in balance. Issues of implementation. *Gastroenterol Clin North Am.* 2002;31(4):1031–1044.
8. Saltz LB, Minsky B. Adjuvant therapy of cancers of the colon and rectum. *Surg Clin North Am.* 2002;82(5):1035–1058.
9. Scarpa M, Erroi F, Ruffolo C, et al. Minimally invasive surgery for colorectal cancer: quality of life, body image, cosmesis, and functional results. *Surg Endosc.* 2009;23(3):577–582.
10. US Preventive Services Task Force, Bibbins-Domingo K, Grossman DC. Screening for colorectal cancer US Preventive Services Task Force recommendation statement. *JAMA.* 2016;315(23):2564–2575.

CHAPTER 57

ANORECTAL DISEASE

Emily Miraflor, MD

1. **What aspect of the initial patient encounter is most important in the diagnosis of anorectal disease?**
   A careful history of anal complaints can point to the correct diagnosis even before completion of a physical exam. It is important to ask about the timeline of symptoms, characteristic of the discomfort, associated masses, bowel characteristics, sexual history, treatments attempted in the past, history of colonoscopy, and anal surgeries.

2. **What is the most common cause of painless, bright red blood per rectum?**
   Internal hemorrhoids.

3. **What are the proximal and distal anatomic landmarks of the anal canal? What is its average length?**
   Anatomists and surgeons differ on the definition of the anal canal. Anatomists consider the anal canal to be from the dentate line to the anal opening. Surgeons think bigger, and consider the anal canal to be from the anal opening to the anorectal ring, which is the most proximal portion of the external sphincter and puborectalis complex. The average length is about 3–4 cm.

4. **What is the anatomic and surgical significance of the dentate line?**
   The dentate line is the location of the anal crypts that drain the intramuscular and intersphincteric anal glands, which are the site of anorectal abscesses and fistulas-in-ano. Above the dentate line, the anal canal receives visceral innervation (involuntary control and insensate), is covered by columnar epithelium, and is the origin of internal hemorrhoids. Below the dentate line, the anal canal receives somatic innervation (voluntary control and sensate), is lined with squamous epithelium, and is the location of external hemorrhoids.

5. **What is the most common cause of anorectal abscess?**
   Ninety percent of anorectal abscesses result from infection of the anal glands that drain at the dentate line. This is often referred to as *cryptoglandular disease*.

6. **What are the four potential anorectal spaces used to classify anorectal abscesses?**
   a. Perianal (area of the anal verge)
   b. Ischiorectal (area lateral to the external sphincter muscles, extending from the levator ani muscles to the perineum)
   c. Intersphincteric (area between the internal and external sphincter muscles, continuous inferiorly with the perianal space and superiorly with the rectal wall)
   d. Supralevator (area superior to the levator ani muscles, inferior to the peritoneum, and lateral to the rectal wall)

7. **Define *fistula-in-ano***
   A fistula is an abnormal communication between any two epithelial lined surfaces. A fistula-in-ano is an abnormal communication between the anal canal and the skin of the perineum. The internal opening of the fistula-in-ano involves the anoderm, most commonly in the region of the dentate line, whereas the external orifice is located most commonly at the anal margin.

8. **What is the incidence of fistula-in-ano after appropriate surgical incision and drainage of acute anorectal abscesses?**
   It is 50%.

9. **What is the most important factor leading to the successful surgical eradication of anorectal abscesses and fistulae?**
   It is important to completely drain anorectal abscesses, thus knowledge of the perianal spaces is critical. In order to successfully treat fistula-in-ano, the course of the fistula and any of its side branches must be identified.

10. **What is Goodsall's rule?**
    Goodsall's rule is used to predict the location of the internal opening of an anorectal fistula based on the position of the external opening. An opening posterior to a line drawn transversely across the perineum originates from an internal opening in the posterior midline. An external opening, anterior to this line, originates from the nearest anal crypt in a radial direction. While this is often referred to as a rule, it is not always correct; it is more reliable for fistulas in the posterior location compared with those that have an anterior external opening.

11. **What is a seton?**
    A seton is a foreign body placed through the fistulous tract (originally a horse hair was used, but in modern practice a vessel loop or silk suture is used). Setons that are loosely placed are called draining setons. Their purpose is to allow drainage of residual purulence. In contrast a cutting seton is a seton that is serially tightened, allowing slow, controlled transection of the sphincter and extrusion of the foreign body. This slow cutting technique was thought to preserve continence while eradicating the fistula. Closer study of this technique shows that it does not necessarily preserve continence and should be used with caution.

ANAL FISSURE

12. **What is the most common location for idiopathic anal fissure?**
    Ninety percent are posterior, and 10% are anterior. Fissures in the lateral locations are rare and should prompt thoughts of alternative diagnoses such as inflammatory bowel disease (IBD), tuberculosis, or sexually transmitted diseases.

13. **What are the most common symptoms of anal fissure?**
    Patients will complain of a sensation of burning or being cut with glass during a bowel movement. This sensation will last well after the bowel movement and may be associated with small amounts of blood per rectum.

14. **What is the underlying pathophysiology of fissure?**
    Local trauma to the anal canal results in sphincter spasm. The spasm increases the pressure within the anal canal preventing blood flow to the area. Essentially, these become chronic ischemic ulcers of the anal canal.

15. **What is the differential diagnosis for anal fissure, especially if atypical in location?**
    Anorectal abscess, thrombosed hemorrhoid, IBD, or, rarely, malignancy.

16. **How do you best diagnose anal fissure?**
    The diagnosis is based on clinical history and visual inspection, not by digital rectal examination or anoscopy. A patient with the above symptoms who refuses a digital rectal exam has a fissure.

17. **What are the nonoperative treatment options?**
    The two goals of treatment are to prevent further anal trauma by improving stool consistency and to improve blood flow to the area. The first is accomplished by initiating a high-fiber diet with fiber supplementation (at least 25 g per day) and increasing hydration. Blood flow is encouraged by taking frequent warm sitz baths to relax the pelvic floor muscles and applying topical agents containing anti-inflammatory agents, local anesthetics, and vasodilators (nitroglycerin or calcium channel blockers). Injection of Botox (botulin toxin) has also been reported to be effective by relaxation of the sphincter muscles.

18. **What is the most common operation performed to treat intractable fissure?**
    Lateral internal sphincterotomy is performed to break the sphincter spasm and improve blood flow to the area. Fissurectomy is associated with loss of continence and is infrequently performed.

HEMORRHOIDS

19. **What are hemorrhoidal tissues, and what are their normal functions?**
    Hemorrhoids are cushions of vascular tissue that contribute to anal continence and protect the sphincter mechanism during defecation. Hemorrhoids are not veins, but sinusoids. Bleeding originates from presinusoidal arterioles, thus explaining the bright red bleeding.

20. **What are the most common causes of pathologic hemorrhoids?**
    Constipation, prolonged straining, pregnancy, and internal sphincter dysfunction.

21. **What is the most important difference between internal and external hemorrhoids?**
Internal hemorrhoids are above the dentate line and are insensate, whereas external hemorrhoids are below the dentate line and are sensate. Ablation of internal hemorrhoids causes a pressure sensation with an urge to defecate, but a similar approach to external hemorrhoids leads to excruciating pain.

22. **What are the most common complaints associated with pathologic internal hemorrhoids?**
Bleeding, mucus discharge, and prolapse.

23. **What are the most common complaints associated with external hemorrhoids**
Pain, inflammation, thrombosis, and anal hygiene difficulties.

24. **Are there any treatment options for symptomatic internal hemorrhoids based on identifiable physical characteristics?**
Yes. Treatment is based on the grade of the hemorrhoid, which is dependent on the degree of prolapse:
Grade 1: No prolapse. Treat with diet and stool bulking agents. Avoid prolonged straining.
Grade 2: Hemorrhoids prolapse through the anal canal but spontaneously reduce. In addition to the above measures, these patients may benefit from rubber band ligation or injection sclerotherapy.
Grade 3: Hemorrhoids prolapse, and the patient has to push them back into position. These can be treated with the above measures. Some patients may elect to undergo a stapled hemorrhoidectomy or surgical hemorrhoidectomy.
Grade 4: Hemorrhoids prolapse and cannot be reduced back into the anal canal. These typically require operative management. In severe cases, strangulation and necrosis of the hemorrhoids can occur.

PILONIDAL DISEASE

25. **What is the most common clinical presentation of a pilonidal sinus?**
Pain and swelling in the sacrococcygeal region, which typically is associated with one or more chronic draining sinus tracts. The disease occurs in hirsute individuals who often have a deep gluteal cleft. It is theorized that the disease is caused by a chronic foreign body reaction to impacted hair follicles.

26. **How is acute pilonidal abscess treated?**
When a pilonidal sinus is acutely infected, the abscess needs to be incised and drained. After resolution of the infection, definitive treatment of the sinus cavity can be undertaken. Hair removal with depilatories or by shaving may prevent future exacerbations.

27. **What is definitive therapy for pilonidal disease?**
Excision of the entire pilonidal cavity and associated sinus tracts down to the sacral fascia will remove the disease. This does create a significant wound. Closure of the wound should be done in such a way that the gluteal cleft is flattened.

28. **What is the best way to treat the wound?**
Small wounds can be closed primarily, whereas large defects may require negative pressure therapy or flap closure. Recurrence and wound care needs are lowest with flap closures.

29. **Why is pilonidal disease rare after age 40?**
Changes in body habitus are one theory.

KEY POINTS: ANORECTAL DISEASE

1. Perform a careful history and physical, with particular attention to bowel habits, before examining a patient with anorectal complaints. If a fissure is suspected, perform a limited visual inspection.
2. Be particularly familiar with the anorectal anatomy when dealing with conditions of this region.
3. Always keep in mind the location of the anal sphincter when approaching anorectal disease operatively; use a seton when in doubt.
4. Be conservative when treating hemorrhoidal disease, reserving operative therapy in most cases for the last resort.
5. Pilonidal disease should be aggressively eradicated down to the fascia at the initial operative intervention.

BIBLIOGRAPHY

1. Beck DE, Roberts PL, eds. *The ASCRS Textbook of Colon and Rectal Surgery.* New York: Springer; 2011.
2. Perry WB, Dykes SL, Buie WD, et al. Practice parameters for the management of anal fissures. *Dis Colon Rectum.* 2010;53(8):1110–1115.
3. Rivadeneira DE, Steele SR, Ternaent C, et al. Practice parameters for the management of hemorrhoids. *Dis Colon Rectum.* 2011;54(9):1059–1064.
4. Steele SR, Kumar R, Deingold DL, et al. Practice parameters for the management of perianal abscess and fistula in ano. *Dis Colon Rectum.* 2011;54(12):1465–1474.
5. Steele SR, Perry WB, Mills S, et al. Practice parameters for the management of pilonidal disease. *Dis Colon Rectum.* 2013;56(9):1021–1027.

CHAPTER 58

INGUINAL HERNIA

Magdalene A. Brooke, MD, Gregory P. Victorino, MD, FACS

1. Groin hernia refers to which three hernias?
   Direct and indirect inguinal hernias and femoral hernias.

2. Francois Poupart, a French surgeon and anatomist (1616–1708), described a ligament that bears his name. What is the anatomic name of the Poupart ligament?
   Inguinal ligament, which is a key element in most groin hernia repairs.

3. Franz K. Hesselbach, a German surgeon and anatomist (1759–1816), described a triangle that is the common site of direct hernias. What are the anatomic margins of Hesselbach's triangle?
   The triangle is defined inferiorly by the inguinal ligament, superiorly by the inferior epigastric vessels, and medially by the rectus fascia. The transversalis fascia forms the floor of the triangle. The original description used Cooper's ligament as the inferior limit, but because of the common use of the anterior approach to hernias, the more apparent inguinal ligament was substituted as the inferior limit of the triangle. With the increasing use of preperitoneal approaches to hernia repair, Cooper's ligament is again much more apparent and useful as an anatomic landmark.

4. Sir Astley Paston Cooper, an English surgeon and anatomist (1768–1841), described a ligament bearing his name. What is the anatomic name for the ligament and the proper name of Cooper's ligament repair?
   The anatomic name of Cooper's ligament is iliopectineal ligament. The Cooper's ligament repair or McVay repair was popularized by Chester McVay (1911–1987). With Barry Aston, professor of anatomy at Northwestern University, McVay provided the modern description of the groin anatomy.

5. Antonio de Gimbernat, a Spanish surgeon and anatomist (1734–1816), had his interesting name attached to the lacunar ligament, which marks the medial margin of a groin area opening. What is the opening? What hernia protrudes into this opening?
   The opening is the femoral canal, which is defined medially by the lacunar ligament, anteriorly by the inguinal ligament, posteriorly by the pectineal fascia, and laterally by the femoral vein. A femoral hernia protrudes into the femoral canal.

6. Indirect inguinal hernia (particularly in children) and hydrocele are associated with which congenital abnormality?
   Persistence of an open processus vaginalis, in the case of a hernia, allows descent of bowel into the inguinal canal. With fluid accumulation, partial obstruction presents as a hydrocele of the spermatic cord.

7. What are the diagnostic criteria for hernia in an infant or child?
   - Inguinal, scrotal, or labial lump that may or may not be reducible
   - History of a lump seen by a healthcare provider
   - History of a lump seen by the mother
   - The silk sign (the feeling of rubbing together two surfaces of silk cloth when gently rubbing together the two surfaces of a hernia sac)
   - An incarceration sometimes felt on rectal examination

8. What can be done to reduce an incarcerated hernia?
   The four-point program is easier said than done, but it is worth the effort:
   a. Sedate the patient.
   b. Place the patient in the Trendelenburg position.
   c. Apply a cold pack (over petroleum gauze to avoid skin injury) in inguinal area.
   d. In the absence of spontaneous reduction—and if the patient is quiet—use gentle manipulation.

9. **How often can incarceration be successfully reduced? What should be done next?**
   About 80% of incarcerated hernias can be reduced in children; in adults, the percentage is lower. Despite the fact that 80%–90% of inguinal hernias occur in boys, most incarcerations occur in girls. The hernia should be repaired electively within a few days after incarceration. The 20% of hernias that are still incarcerated should be operated on immediately.

10. **What is a Bassini repair?**
    The Bassini repair sutures together the conjoined tendon and the shelving edge of the inguinal ligament up to the internal ring (see Fig. 58.1). This classic procedure, introduced in 1887 at the Italian Society of Surgery in Genoa, revolutionized hernia repair. Until recently, it has been the standard of repair. After graduation from medical school and while fighting for Italian independence, Eduardo Bassini (1844–1924) was bayoneted in the groin and, as a prisoner, was hospitalized for months with a fecal fistula.

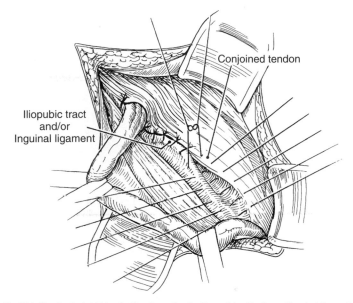

Fig. 58.1 The standard right inguinal hernia repair using the conjoined tendon and inguinal ligament.

11. **What is the recurrence rate with indirect and direct hernias that have been repaired with classic Bassini repair technique?**
    Over a follow-up period of 50 years, the recurrence rate of adult indirect hernias is 5%–10%; of direct hernias, 15%–30%.

12. **Describe a McVay hernia repair**
    The line of interrupted sutures starts at the pubic tubercle and joins the tendinous arch of the transversus abdominis muscle to Cooper's ligament up to the femoral canal. At this point, two or three transitional sutures are placed from Cooper's ligament to the anterior femoral fascia, effectively closing the medial extreme of the femoral canal. The final set of sutures joins the transversus abdominis arch and the anterior femoral fascia. The stitches usually incorporate the inguinal ligament at the upper limit of the repair, the site of the new internal inguinal ring and cord structures. About 15 years ago, McVay described laying in a mesh patch and stitching it, at its periphery, to the same anatomic structures. This application of mesh closely resembles the Lichtenstein repair (see question 17), except that it uses Cooper's ligament.

13. For what type of hernias is the McVay Cooper's ligament repair most useful?
Femoral and direct hernias.

14. What is the Shouldice repair?
The Shouldice repair, popularized at the Shouldice Clinic near Toronto, imbricates or overlays the transversalis fascia and conjoined tendon with four continuous lines, using two fine-wire sutures. The suture tract runs from the pubic tubercle to a new internal ring. Care is taken with the inferior epigastric vessels. The result is layered approximation of the conjoined tendon to the inguinal ligament tract.

15. What is the reported recurrence rate for the Shouldice repair?
The recurrence rate is 1%, the lowest reported rate for nonmesh repairs of inguinal hernias in adults.

16. For what type of groin hernia is the Shouldice repair not appropriate?
Femoral hernia.

17. Describe the Lichtenstein repair
The Lichtenstein repair consists of a sutured patch of polypropylene mesh (Marlex, C.R. Bard, Inc., Covington, GA) that covers Hesselbach's triangle and the indirect hernia area. It is considered a tension-free repair because the mesh is sutured in place without pulling ligaments or tissues together as in all other repairs. The mesh is divided at its upper end to wrap closely around the spermatic cord and its associated structures in the normal position of the internal inguinal canal (see Fig. 58.2). The Lichtenstein procedure is rapidly becoming the most widely used repair of adult inguinal hernia. The reported recurrence rate is <1%.

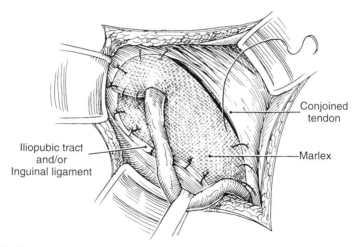

Fig. 58.2 The Marlex mesh repair of a right inguinal hernia. Note that the same structures are used but not brought together; thus, the name of the tension-free repair.

18. For what groin area is the Lichtenstein repair not appropriate?
Femoral hernia.

19. Which type of repair is acceptable for the femoral hernia?
Several different repairs can be used. Mesh in the form of a plug can be inserted into the femoral canal and fixed in place. A McVay Cooper's ligament repair can be done. A preperitoneal approach to the hernia can be used to suture or plug the defect. A suture repair or a sartorius facial flap applied from below the inguinal ligament in a femoral approach also may be used. The preperitoneal approach is increasingly used for complicated inguinal and femoral hernias.

20. What is the preperitoneal or Stoppa procedure?

The preperitoneal or Stoppa procedure is a groin hernia repair on the internal side of the abdominal wall between the peritoneum and fascial surfaces that do not open into the peritoneal cavity. The anatomic landmarks are quite different and initially quite challenging to surgeons accustomed to the external abdominal wall approach. The technique is suited for recurrent hernias in which scarring and obliterated anatomy increase the risk of cord injury and recurrence. Other problems such as large hernias and femoral hernias are corrected with this approach. Conceptually, the laparoscopic hernia repair uses the same approach (see Fig. 58.3).

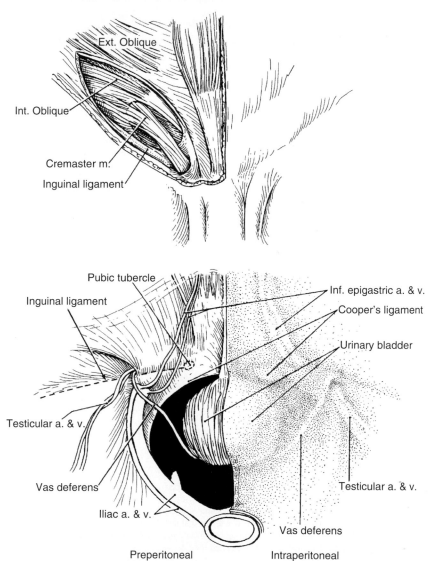

Fig. 58.3 The different appearance and landmarks are seen in the anterior view *(above)* and the posterior view *(below)* of the inguinal-femoral area. In the posterior view, the importance of the inferior epigastric vessels, bladder, and Cooper's ligament as anatomic landmarks is apparent.

21. Where are the spaces of Retzius and Bogros? Why are they increasingly important?

    Retzius' space is between the pubis and the urinary bladder. Bogros' space is between the perito-neum and the fascia and muscle planes on the posterior aspect of the abdominal wall below the umbilicus and down to Cooper's ligament. Laterally, the space goes to the iliac spines. In either the open Stoppa procedure or the laparoscopic preperitoneal repair, the spaces of Retzius and Bogros are developed for mesh placement and surgical exposure.

22. How tight around the spermatic cord should a surgically fashioned, internal inguinal ring be?

    About 5 mm, which is less than a fingertip and more than a forceps tip.

23. What is the common fascial defect of larger indirect and all direct inguinal hernias?

    Weakness or attenuation of the transversalis fascia.

24. On examination, the femoral hernia may be confused with what other inguinal hernia?

    The femoral hernia may be confused with a direct inguinal hernia because of the tendency of the femoral hernia to present at the lateral edge of the inguinal ligament.

25. What is the difference between an incarcerated and a strangulated hernia?
    - **Incarcerated:** Structures in the hernia sac still have a good blood supply but are stuck in the sac because of adhesions or a narrow neck of the hernia sac.
    - **Strangulated**: Herniated structures, such as bowel or omentum, have lost their blood supply because of anatomic constriction at the neck of the hernia. The herniated, ischemic tissue is, therefore, in various stages of gangrenous changes. Strangulated hernias are surgical emergencies.

26. Do all hernias require urgent repair?

    No. Acute incarceration or strangulation of abdominal contents in a hernia is a surgical emergency. Patients with chronic discomfort benefit from elective repair. However, recent data on men with asymp-tomatic or minimally symptomatic hernias indicates it may be safe to wait to operate until symptoms worsen. As with any surgical procedure, an individual's risk factors and baseline function need to be considered along with the risk of an operative or nonoperative approach. In the case of hernias, only a small percentage of asymptomatic patients for whom elective repair is deferred will develop acute hernia incarceration at some time in the future. Of note, in athletes, operative repair has been shown to improve quality of life and return to athletics in comparison with conservative treatment.

27. What operation is done for an uncomplicated indirect infant hernia?

    High ligation of the hernia sac.

28. What operation is done for an uncomplicated indirect hernia in young adults?

    The appropriate operation consists of high ligation and possibly one or two stitches in the transversa-lis fascia to tighten the internal ring. This is the basic Marcy technique, developed by Henry Orlando Marcy (1837–1924); it is smaller and more anatomically focused than the Bassini repair.

29. What operation is done for an uncomplicated but sizable direct hernia in elderly adults?

    Traditionally, the Bassini or McVay repair was chosen. More recently, because of the low recurrence rate, the Shouldice or Lichtenstein repair is favored.

30. What organ systems should be reviewed with particular care in the workup of patients with hernia (especially elderly patients with recent onset of hernia)?

    The gastrointestinal, urinary, and pulmonary systems should be reviewed with particular care. One is looking for causes of chronic strain or sudden forces that may have induced the hernia. Straining dur-ing defecation or urination, unusual coughing, or difficulty with breathing, if corrected, may be of great value to the patient and reduce the chance of recurrent hernia.

31. What is a sliding hernia?

    A sliding hernia is formed when a retroperitoneal organ protrudes (herniates) outside the abdominal cavity in such a manner that the organ itself and the overlying peritoneal surface constitute a side of the hernia sac.

32. **What organs can be found in sliding hernias?**
    - Colon
    - Cecum
    - Appendix
    - Bladder
    - Fallopian tubes
    - Uterus (rare)
    - Ovary

33. **What are common operative and postoperative complications of hernia repairs?**
    Intraoperative complications:
    - Injury to the spermatic cord, especially in children.
    - Injury to the spermatic vessels, resulting in atrophy or acute necrosis of testes.
    - Injury to the ilioinguinal nerve, genitofemoral nerve, and lateral femoral cutaneous nerve (the lateral femoral cutaneous nerve is uniquely vulnerable in laparoscopic and properitoneal procedures).
    - Injury to the femoral vessels.

    Postoperative complications:
    - Infection: High risk in children with diaper rash and patients with bowel injury or necrosis.
    - Hematoma: Should resolve in time.
    - Nerve injury: The nerve is not always divided and, with time, may improve. If pain persists, try lidocaine block for both diagnosis and treatment. If a nerve block is not successful, one may consider reexploration to free the nerve from scar or to excise a postsurgical neuroma.
    - Recurrence of the hernia.
    - Direct hernias often recur at the pubic tubercle. Indirect hernias recur at the internal ring. The cause is usually related to poorly placed or insufficient stitches. Other possible causes include infection, poor tissue, poor collagen formation, or too much tension at the surgical suture line. A single line of repair under moderate tension fails in a significant number of patients, regardless of adequacy of repair or healing process. Tension is almost always bad in surgery.

CONTROVERSIES

34. **What are some of the anatomic issues related to inguinal hernias?**
    At issue is the iliopubic tract, which is central to the Anson/McVay anatomic description of the inguinal area and featured in the McVay Cooper's ligament repair. Although the McVay repair is used In England, the iliopubic tract is not referred to or described in English anatomic texts.

    The term conjoined tendon, although commonly used, is considered by many to be anatomically inaccurate and misleading. The internal oblique and transversus abdominis muscles that make up the conjoined tendon are obvious and can be used surgically either alone or together. The tendinous edge of the transversus abdominis muscle and the tendinous edge of the internal oblique muscle start at their insertion on the pubic tubercle and course laterally and superiorly to the medial edge of the internal ring. At this point, the tendinous elements diminish, leaving only muscle tissues, and continue laterally and superiorly to their origins.

    Whether the lacunar ligament or the iliopubic tract defines the medial border of the femoral canal is controversial. The compromise position is that the iliopubic tract is the border, whereas in the normal unstretched state, the lacunar ligament (Gimbernat's ligament) is the border in the presence of hernia (stretched state). At surgery, it is enough to say that a palpable, visible curved ligament is present and used in some femoral repairs.

35. **How long should the patient avoid heavy lifting after a hernia repair?**
    The standard advice for decades has been 4–6 weeks. However, recent data shows no increase in recurrence rate related to early resumption of normal activities. There is no evidence to support such a long convalescent period. Recent guidelines recommend that patients should self-limit their activity as required by their postoperative pain, and that they should be reassured that physical activity does not appear to cause hernia recurrence.

36. **What are the typical indications for laparoscopic repair?**
    Hernias that are bilateral or recurrent.

37. **Is laparoscopic repair appropriate for initial, unilateral inguinal hernia?**
    Recent studies show no significant difference between laparoscopic and open repair in terms of major complications, including hernia recurrence. In addition, laparoscopic repair has the benefit of shorter recovery time, and less postoperative pain. It is important, however, to recognize that laparoscopic repair has a very gradual learning curve. The literature supports use of laparoscopic, primary, unilateral hernia repair depending on the volume of the center and surgeon's experience.

KEY POINTS: TYPES OF INGUINAL HERNIA REPAIR

1. The Bassini repair sutures together the conjoined tendon and the shelving edge of the inguinal ligament up to the internal ring.
2. The McVay repair is most useful for femoral and direct hernias.
3. The Shouldice repair imbricates the transversalis fascia and conjoined tendon with four continuous lines, using two fine-wire sutures (not appropriate for femoral hernias).
4. The Lichtenstein repair consists of a sutured patch of polyprolene mesh that covers Hesselbach's triangle and the indirect hernia sac.

BIBLIOGRAPHY

1. Avisse C, Delattre JF. The inguinal rings. *Surg Clin North Am.* 2000;80(1):49–69.
2. Avisse C, Delattre JF. The inguinofemoral area from a laparoscopic standpoint. History, anatomy, and surgical applications. *Surg Clin North Am.* 2000;80(1):35–48.
3. Bendavid R, Howarth D. Transversalis fascia rediscovered. *Surg Clin North Am.* 2000;80(1):25–33.
4. EU Hernia Trialists Collaboration. Repair of groin hernia with synthetic mesh: meta-analysis of randomized controlled trials. *Ann Surg.* 2002;235(3):322–332.
5. Bittner R, Montgomery MA, Arregui E, et al. Update of guidelines on laparoscopic (TAPP) and endoscopic (TEP) treatment of inguinal hernia (International Endohernia Society). *Surg Endosc.* 2015;29(2):289–321.
6. Fitzgibbons RJ, Ramanan B, Arya S, et al. Long-term results of a randomized controlled trial of a nonoperative strategy (watchful waiting) for men with minimally symptomatic inguinal hernias. *Ann Surg.* 2013;258(3):508–515.
7. Kockerling F, Stechemesser B. TEP versus Lichtenstein: which technique is better for the repair of primary unilateral inguinal hernias in men? *Surg Endosc.* 2016;30(8):3304–3313.
8. Miserez M, Peeters E, Aufenacker T, et al. Update with level 1 studies of the European Hernia Society guidelines on the treatment of inguinal hernia in adult patients. *Hernia.* 2014;18(2):151–163.
9. O'Reilly EA, Burke JP, O'Connell PR. A meta-analysis of surgical morbidity and recurrence after laparoscopic and open repair of primary unilateral inguinal hernia. *Ann Surg.* 2012;255(5):846–853.
10. Stroupe KT, Manheim LM, Luo P, et al. Minimally symptomatic inguinal hernias: a cost-effectiveness analysis. *J Am Coll Surg.* 2006;203(4):458–468.

BARIATRIC SURGERY

Jeffrey L. Johnson, MD, FACS, Alden H. Harken, MD, FACS

CHAPTER 59

1. **My patient weighs 250 lb (114 kg). Is he or she morbidly obese?**
   Maybe. The most widely used definition of morbid obesity uses the concept of body mass index (BMI), which is weight (kg) divided by height squared (m). This is simply a description of how heavy a patient is for his or her height. A BMI of 40 is considered morbidly obese. A patient who weighs 250 pounds and is 5'6" tall is morbidly obese (BMI = 40), but a patient who weighs 250 pounds and is 6'6" tall is simply overweight (BMI = 29).

2. **Is morbid obesity alone really all that morbid?**
   Yes. Even without overt comorbidities (such as diabetes and hypertension), individuals who are morbidly obese are at substantial risk. Many critical organ systems are affected. For example, in the cardiopulmonary system, obstructive sleep apnea, chronic hypoventilation, and pulmonary hypertension are a common finding. This translates into a higher likelihood of poor outcome after medical or surgical treatment of a wide variety of conditions. Patients who are morbidly obese have a measurably shorter life span. In many ways, it is a potentially lethal condition.

3. **What is metabolic syndrome?**
   Metabolic syndrome describes a set of changes in physiology that are associated with high cardiovascular risk. Obesity is a central feature, along with insulin resistance, elevated triglycerides, elevated low-density lipoprotein cholesterol, and hypertension.

4. **My patient has a BMI of 40. Because he or she appears so well fed, is it safe to assume his or her nutritional status and wound healing are normal?**
   No. Although the patient's total caloric intake is high, it is not uncommon for patients who are morbidly obese to have poor protein intake, poor protein stores, and vitamin deficiencies. Furthermore, concomitant diabetes may contribute to impaired wound healing.

5. **So, if patients who are morbidly obese are sick and do not heal well, why would an otherwise rational surgeon choose to do weight loss operations?**
   Because it works so well. There are few behavioral, pharmacologic, or combined approaches to the treatment of morbid obesity that are proven to promote even short-term weight loss. More pills, programs, and press have not resulted in a thinner population. Further, these nonsurgical approaches do not even approximate the amount or durability of weight loss seen in patients who undergo bariatric surgery. The weight loss after bariatric surgery is substantial and appears to be maintained for at least 15 years.

6. **Do patients who undergo bariatric surgery actually get healthier as they get thinner?**
   Yes. The majority of patients with diabetes, hypertension, urinary incontinence, and obstructive sleep apnea are essentially cured of these ills as they lose weight. Ask an internist when they last cured (not palliated) any of these conditions.

7. **If patients who are morbidly obese have decreased life expectancy, do patients who get bariatric surgery actually live longer?**
   It appears so. Two large studies have shown improved survival in patients undergoing surgery to promote weight loss.

8. **Some bariatric operations (like jejunoileal bypass) were abandoned because of metabolic complications. Are there some operations that actually work and are considered safe?**
   Yes. The Roux-en-Y gastric bypass has the best long-term safety and efficacy data. Other options include the vertical banded gastroplasty, the sleeve gastrectomy, the laparoscopic adjustable gastric band (lap band), and the duodenal switch.

9. **A Roux-en-Y gastric bypass sounds complicated. What does it entail?**
   It is not complicated. The proximal stomach is completely divided to produce a proximal pouch about 50 mL in size. The remainder of the stomach is simply left in place. The proximal small intestine (the Roux limb, or alimentary limb) is then divided and attached to the pouch. The small bowel is then reconnected downstream.

10. **Why do patients lose weight after gastric bypass?**
    There are three basic reasons. First, the patients cannot eat much at one time—50 mL is 10 tea-spoons. This is how much the patients can initially eat (or drink) at a time. It actually becomes work to get enough protein, calories, and fluids in. Second, the patients cannot (at first), tolerate concentrated sweets. The alimentary limb is made of small intestine that will react to high osmolar loads with dumping syndrome—an unpleasant combination of abdominal pain, nausea, sweating, and diarrhea. Thus, there is a significant disincentive to cheating after gastric bypass. Third, because food in the alimentary limb does not get mixed with bile and pancreatic juice until it meets the other (aptly named biliopancreatic) limb, 75 cm or more downstream, it is not efficiently absorbed.

11. **How much do patients usually lose after gastric bypass?**
    Initially, about 70% of their excess weight. This takes place over the first 12–24 months. Patients (and doctors) need to understand that it is quite unusual to get all the way down to ideal weight. These operations are not intended to produce fitness models, but rather healthier patients with improved quality of life and improved longevity.

12. **Who are the best candidates for bariatric surgery?**
    Most bariatric surgeons use Centers for Disease Control and Prevention guidelines, which include BMI (>40, or >35 with weight-related comorbidities) and the ability to understand and comply with the perioperative routine. The latter is extremely important because the patient must relearn how to eat with his or her new anatomy. This operation is not without risk and has significant health and social consequences—imagine going out to dinner when you can eat only 10 teaspoons.

13. **What are the most serious complications of gastric bypass?**
    Leak of the gastrojejunal anastomosis is the most feared complication, though it is second to pul-monary embolism as a cause of death in most series. The mortality rate is <1%, but not 0%. Wound complications (hernia, infection) are seen in about 10% of patients undergoing open surgery, and only about 1% in patients undergoing laparoscopic surgery.

14. **What is the most reliable sign of gastrojejunal leak?**
    Tachycardia. A heart rate >110 should prompt concern for a leak. Some surgeons order routine contrast studies in all patients.

KEY POINTS: BARIATRIC SURGERY

1. Morbid obesity is a serious medical condition that shortens life span.
2. Surgical weight loss promotes improved health and probably lengthens life span.
3. Although there are a number of possible surgical options, gastric bypass is the most tested.
4. Bariatric surgery requires an informed, compliant patient who understands there are significant risks.

BIBLIOGRAPHY

1. Adams TD, Gress RE, Smith SC, et al. Long-term mortality after gastric bypass surgery. *N Engl J Med.* 2007;357(8): 753–761.
2. Hutter MM, Randall S. Laparoscopic versus open gastric bypass for morbid obesity: a multicenter, prospective, risk-adjusted analysis from the National Surgical Quality Improvement Program. *Ann Surg.* 2006;243(5):657–662.
3. Madan AK, Orth W. Metabolic syndrome: yet another co-morbidity gastric bypass helps cure. *Surg Obes Relat Dis.* 2006;2(1):48–51.
4. Berbiglia L, Zografakis JG. Laparoscopic Roux-en-Y gastric bypass: surgical technique and perioperative care. *Surg Clin North Am.* 2016;96(4):773–974.

IV
ENDOCRINE SURGERY

HYPERPARATHYROIDISM

Kathryn H. Chomsky-Higgins, MD, MS, Christopher D. Raeburn,
MD, FACS, Robert C. McIntyre, Jr., MD, Barnard J. A. Palmer,
MD, MEd, FACS

CHAPTER 60

1. **How common is hyperparathyroidism (HPT)?**
   The prevalence of hyperparathyroidism is 1:1000. There are approximately 100,000 new cases of HPT annually in the United States. Seventy-four percent of all cases are in women, and the risk increases with age. Primary HPT occurs in 1 in 500 women and in 1 in 2000 men older than age 40.

2. **What are the symptoms of HPT?**
   Painful bones, renal stones, abdominal groans, psychic moans, and fatigue overtones. HPT is most commonly asymptomatic, but the classic symptoms and signs are that of hypercalcemia:
   - **Bones:** Arthralgia, osteoporosis, and pathologic fractures
   - **Stones:** Renal stones, renal insufficiency, polyuria, and polydipsia
   - **Abdominal groans:** Pancreatitis, peptic ulcer disease, and constipation
   - **Psychiatric overtones:** Fatigue, weakness, depression, memory loss, and irritability

3. **What is the most common cause of hypercalcemia in an outpatient versus an inpatient?**
   HPT is the most common cause of hypercalcemia among outpatients and the second most common cause in the hospital setting. The most common cause of hypercalcemia in hospitalized patients is malignancy. Primary HPT and malignancy account for 90% of cases of hypercalcemia.

4. **What is the differential diagnosis of hypercalcemia?**
   - Endocrine: HPT, hyperthyroidism, Addison's disease
   - Malignancy: Bone metastasis, paraneoplastic syndromes, solid tumors (squamous or small cell lung carcinoma), hematologic malignancy (multiple myeloma, leukemia, lymphoma)
   - Increased intake: Milk alkali syndrome, vitamin D intoxication
   - Granulomatous disease: Sarcoidosis, tuberculosis
   - Miscellaneous: Familial hypocalciuric hypercalcemia (FHH), thiazide diuretics, lithium

5. **How do you obtain a laboratory diagnosis of primary HPT?**
   The diagnosis of primary HPT is confirmed with an elevated serum calcium level, elevated parathyroid hormone (PTH), and the absence of low 24-hour urine calcium. An elevated serum calcium should be assessed at least twice and must be associated with elevation of intact PTH. A 24-hour urine collection for calcium >100 mg/day excludes benign FHH. Prior to the use of intact PTH levels, a chloride/phosphate ratio of >33 associated with hypercalcemia suggested primary HPT because serum phosphate levels are low in nearly 80% of patients, and serum chloride is increased in 40% of patients. Patients with elevated alkaline phosphatase associated with increased blood urea nitrogen and creatinine are at increased risk of hungry bone syndrome after parathyroidectomy.

6. **Can a patient have primary HPT and a normal PTH level?**
   Yes. A normal parathyroid response to elevated serum calcium is decreased PTH secretion. When serum calcium is high, the PTH level should be at the low end of normal. A PTH level at the high end of normal in the setting of hypercalcemia is inappropriately elevated and consistent with primary HPT. One should rule out FHH by testing 24-hour urine calcium.

7. **What is normocalcemic primary hyperparathyroidism (NPHPT)?**
   Occasionally, patients will be identified with an elevated PTH level and a normal serum calcium. This entity exists on the diagnostic spectrum of PHPT, and calcium is typically at the upper limits of the normal range. The majority of these patients will have an elevated ionized calcium. Adequate surveillance is important, as patients with NPHPT may develop hypercalcemia.

8. **What are the indications for parathyroidectomy in primary HPT?**

Symptomatic PHPT is an indication for surgery, and careful history indicates that over 90% of patients have symptoms. The indications in asymptomatic patients have broadened in the past 15 years because of the sequelae of long-term disease, low morbidity in the hands of experienced endocrine surgeons, and cure rates of over 95%. Patients with untreated primary HPT have increased death rates caused by hypercalcemia-related cardiovascular disease. Patients also have improvements in abnormal quality-of-life scores after operative success, and the costs of surgery are equivalent to that of medical follow-up at 5 years.

The 2014 Endocrine Society Fourth International Workshop for Asymptomatic Primary HPT lists the following indications for parathyroidectomy:

- Serum calcium >1.0 mg/dL above upper limit of normal
- Bones: bone mineral density (BMD) and dual-energy x-ray absorptiometry (DEXA): T-score <−2.5 at lumbar spine, total hip, femoral neck, or distal one-third radius OR vertebral fracture by x-ray, computed tomography (CT), magnetic resonance imaging (MRI), or vertebral fracture assessment (VFA)
- Renal: Creatinine clearance 60 cc/min; 24-hour urine for calcium 400 mg/day (10 mmol/day) and increased stone risk by biochemical stone risk analysis; presence of nephrolithiasis or nephrocalcinosis by x-ray, ultrasound (US), or CT
- Age <50 years
- Patients for whom medical surveillance is neither desired nor possible and in patients opting for surgery, in the absence of meeting any guidelines as long as there are no medical contraindications

9. **What are the embryologic origins and locations of the superior and inferior parathyroid glands?**

The superior parathyroid glands arise from the dorsal part of the fourth brachial pouch. In the normal position, they lie on the posterior portion of the upper half of the thyroid, cephalad to the inferior thyroid artery, and posterior to the recurrent laryngeal nerve (RLN). The superior parathyroid glands' location is more constant. The most common ectopic sites of the upper glands are posterior to the esophagus or in the tracheoesophageal groove down into the posterior superior mediastinum.

The inferior parathyroid glands arise from the dorsal part of the third brachial pouch along with the thymus. The most common location of the inferior parathyroids are on the lateral or posterior surface of the lower pole of the thyroid gland, caudal and anterior to the point where the inferior thyroid artery crosses the RLN. The inferior parathyroid glands are more commonly ectopic and may be in the thyrothymic ligament, thymus, mediastinum outside the thymus, carotid sheath, or within the thyroid (3%).

Four glands are present in 89% of patients, five in 8%, six in 3%, and less than four in 0%. The presence of as many as eight glands has been reported.

10. **What are the etiologies of primary HPT?**

Primary HPT is caused by a single adenoma in over 87% of cases; hyperplasia in 9%; double adenoma in 3%; and carcinoma in <1%. In familial HPT, multiple endocrine neoplasia (MEN) syndromes (I and II), and secondary HPT as a result of end-stage renal disease, hyperplasia is the etiology.

11. **What preoperative localization studies are available?**

The classic localization study is the sestamibi scan. Other various noninvasive localization studies include US, CT, single photon emission computerized tomography CT (SPECT/CT) and MRI. Invasive localization procedures include arteriography and venous sampling. Each of these modalities vary in sensitivity and specificity by institution and operator experience and are most accurate when a single abnormal parathyroid gland is present. Localization procedures in cases of hyperplasia may be misleading.

Preoperative localization is key to the techniques of focused parathyroid exploration or minimally invasive parathyroidectomy. Localization studies are mandatory before all reoperative parathyroidectomies for persistent or recurrent HPT and in patients with previous thyroid surgery.

12. **How is a sestamibi scan performed, and how accurate is it?**

Sestamibi is a radionuclide that is taken up by the heart, thyroid, salivary glands, and abnormal parathyroid tissue. A standard scan involves the administration of sestamibi and performance of planar imaging of the neck and upper chest at 10 and 90 minutes. The radionuclide is typically seen in multiple tissues on the early scan then typically washes out of the heart and thyroid quickly. The radionuclide is retained in the parathyroids so any remaining uptake seen on the delayed scan is specific for abnormal parathyroid tissue. The sensitivity and specificity of the sestamibi scan is approximately 85%.

Alternatively, sestamibi can be given with iodine or pertechnetate to be taken up by the thyroid. Thyroid uptake images can be subtracted from the sestamibi scan to reveal a hyperfunctioning parathyroid. SPECT and SPECT/CT provide three-dimensional information presented as cross-sectional slices through the patient and can be reformatted as needed.

13. **Outline the traditional surgical strategy of exploration for primary HPT**
The traditional parathyroid operation entails bilateral neck exploration to identify and assess all four glands. A meticulously dry, blood-free operative field must be maintained, and tissue in the region of the RLN should not be clamped or divided until the nerve is definitively identified. If a solitary adenoma and three normal glands are found, the adenoma is removed, and one of the normal glands is biopsied. Frozen-section examination confirms hypercellular parathyroid, but cannot differentiate adenoma versus hyperplasia. Four-gland enlargement (hyperplasia) is treated by subtotal parathyroidectomy (leaving approximately 50 mg of well-vascularized parathyroid tissue in the neck) or total parathyroidectomy with autoreimplantation of 50 mg of parathyroid tissue. If a remnant is left in the neck, it should be marked with a nonabsorbable suture or clip. Thymectomy in the setting of hyperplasia eliminates the possibility of thymic supernumerary glands. If more than one enlarged gland is found in association with normal-appearing glands (double adenoma), all abnormal glands should be removed.

15. **What are alternatives to the bilateral four-gland neck exploration?**
Focused parathyroidectomy, minimally invasive radio-guided parathyroidectomy (MIRP), and endoscopic neck exploration are alternative techniques that have excellent cure rates. A focused parathyroidectomy uses preoperative localization to guide a limited unilateral exploration and parathyroidectomy, avoiding bilateral exploration. This approach can be combined with intraoperative rapid PTH assay that measures PTH before the operation and 10 minutes after adequate resection. A postresection drop to <50% of the preoperative level and within the normal range predicts success. The MIRP uses sestamibi scanning the morning of surgery and an intraoperative gamma probe to guide parathyroidectomy. The ratio of ex-vivo radioactivity to background is measured to determine success at the end of the operation. Endoscopic explorations include a number of video-assisted approaches to locate abnormal glands.

15. **What should one do if an adenoma is not found in the usual locations?**
Each normal gland should be biopsied for confirmation and marked. Normal parathyroid glands should not be removed. If three normal glands are identified, the surgeon should assess whether a superior or inferior gland is missing. A missing upper gland often lies in the tracheoesophageal groove, posterior to the esophagus or in the posterior superior mediastinum (posteriorly located upper gland, or PLUG). A common mistake is inadequate mobilization of the superior thyroid gland with inadequate posterior dissection. This exploration may require ligation of the superior thyroid artery and vein. The location of missing lower glands is more variable. The thyrothymic ligament should be inspected, and the thymus then can be resected through the neck incision if necessary. The carotid sheath should be opened, and the thyroid lobe on the side of the missing parathyroid should be palpated or examined by intraoperative US for nodules. Thyroid lobectomy may be performed to remove an intrathyroidal parathyroid gland, but blind thyroid lobectomy is rarely helpful. An undescended parathyroid is rare (<1%) and is located at or superior to the carotid bifurcation. This area cannot be explored through the standard incision and requires accurate preoperative localization studies.

A sternotomy should never be done as part of an initial exploration. If the aforementioned maneuvers are unsuccessful in revealing a parathyroid adenoma, the surgeon should abort and reimage the patient. A diagram of the location of the identified glands should be made for future reference. Persistent hypercalcemia indicates the need for localization procedures.

16. **What is the outcome of surgery for primary HPT?**
The expected cure rate should be >95% for patients undergoing an initial exploration for primary HPT. Symptomatic improvement exceeds 95%. Quality-of-life scores return to normal at 6 months. After parathyroidectomy, 80% of symptomatic patients have improvement in bone density and renal function. Even in asymptomatic patients, urinary calcium and deoxypyridinoline levels decrease. Patients have fewer episodes of nephrolithiasis, gout, and peptic ulcer disease. Parathyroidectomy also appears to improve longevity in patients with primary HPT.

Recent series suggest that the cure rate is lower in patients who have negative preoperative sestamibi scans (99.3% versus 92.7%).

17. **What are the complications of parathyroidectomy?**
    Permanent RLN injury occurs in <1% of patients; however, temporary nerve paresis occurs in 3%. Temporary hypocalcemia occurs in 10% of patients, while permanent HPT occurs in only 2% of cases. An elevated preoperative alkaline phosphatase level and abnormal renal function may predict which patients are likely to have hungry bone syndrome.

18. **What are the signs and symptoms of hypocalcemia after surgery?**
    The earliest symptom of hypocalcemia is perioral numbness or paresthesias typically in the hands or feet. Untreated, severe hypocalcemia can result in carpal-pedal spasm or tetany. Chvostek's sign is spasm of the facial muscles caused by tapping the facial nerve trunk. Trousseau's sign is carpal spasm elicited by occlusion of the brachial artery for 3 minutes with a blood pressure cuff.

19. **How should patients with hypocalcemia be treated?**
    Mild hypocalcemia is treated with oral calcium supplementation. Maintaining calcium levels of 7.5–9.0 mg/dL is adequate. Oral calcium should be started as soon as possible in the form of calcium carbonate (Tums or Oscal) at 2–3 g/day in divided doses (3–4 times/day). Calcium citrate is preferred for patients with renal lithiasis because citrate can be prophylactic against renal lithiasis. In most patients, vitamin D preparations increase intestinal absorption and can be given as calcitriol (Rocaltrol), 0.25–0.75 mg/day.
    Patients with tetany caused by hypoparathyroidism require emergency treatment with intravenous (IV) calcium to prevent laryngeal stridor and convulsions. One ampule of 10% calcium gluconate (90 mg elemental calcium per 10 mL) should be given in 100-mL saline over 15 minutes, followed by an infusion of calcium (5 ampules of calcium gluconate in 500 mL of saline) at 50 mL/hr.

20. **Define persistent and recurrent HPT**
    Operative success is defined by long-term normocalcemia. Persistent HPT is defined as hypercalcemia within 6 months of surgery, while recurrent HPT is defined as hypercalcemia occurring more than 6 months after surgical intervention.

21. **What is the strategy for managing patients with persistent or recurrent HPT?**
    These patients should be reevaluated to ensure that the hypercalcemia is caused by primary HPT and not another cause. The diagnosis is confirmed and patients are evaluated for FHH, which does not warrant reoperation. The severity of disease is assessed to ensure that repeat operation is justified. Previous operative notes and pathology reports should be reviewed to assist in planning repeat therapy. Localization studies should be used extensively. When localization is successful, reoperation for persistent or recurrent HPT is curative in 85%–90%. Reexploration when localization is unsuccessful has a 50% rate of failure.
    Before reexploration, vocal cord function should be assessed in all patients. Repeat cervical exploration may be done through the previous incision, but because strap muscles are usually adherent to the thyroid, a lateral approach between the sternocleidomastoid and strap muscles may be used instead of the usual medial approach. With positive localization studies or retrospective determination of the side of the missing adenoma, the dissection may be limited if an adenoma is found.
    An alternative to repeat exploration in select patients is angiographic ablation of parathyroid tissue, which is especially useful for mediastinal adenomas because it avoids a median sternotomy. It is performed by delivering ionic contrast through an arterial catheter wedged into the feeding vessel.

22. **Define secondary and tertiary HPT**
    - Secondary HPT: Overproduction of PTH caused in response to low blood calcium that is caused by another condition. The most common causes include vitamin D deficiency, chronic renal failure, calcium deficiency, and disorders of phosphate metabolism.
    - Tertiary HPT: Autonomous secretion of PTH causing hypercalcemia. It typically occurs after long-standing secondary HPT, and is characterized by PTH secretion that does not respond to calcium or vitamin D administration.

23. **What are the indications for parathyroidectomy in end-stage renal disease (ESRD)?**
    The main indications for parathyroidectomy in ESRD are as follows:
    - Severe hypercalcemia
    - Progressive and debilitating hyperparathyroid bone disease
    - Pruritus that does not respond to dialysis
    - Progressive extra-skeletal calcification or calciphylaxis that is usually associated with hyperphosphatemia

- Otherwise unexplained symptomatic myopathy
- Renal transplant recipients with persistent HPT associated with hypercalcemia and renal insufficiency

24. **What are the options for surgical treatment of secondary and tertiary HPT?**
    Subtotal parathyroidectomy or total parathyroidectomy with autoreimplantation effectively corrects secondary and tertiary HPT. Total thyroidectomy without reimplantation is an additional option for patients who have access to regular calcium infusions.
    Subtotal parathyroidectomy is performed by excision of all identifiable parathyroid tissue except for 40–60 mg of one gland. Disadvantages of subtotal parathyroidectomy include risk of recurrent disease, which is complicated by greater morbidity if repeat neck exploration is required. Total parathyroidectomy with autotransplantation of small amounts of resected parathyroid tissue into the brachioradialis muscle in the forearm has the main advantage of the ease of removing recurrent hyperplastic glands without the added morbidity of neck reexploration.

25. **List the endocrinopathies in MEN I and II**
    MEN I (3 Ps):
    - **Hyperp**arathyroidism
    - **Pi**tuitary adenoma
    - **P**ancreatic endocrine tumor
    MEN II (3 Cs):
    - HPT (**c**alcium)
    - Medullary thyroid cancer (**c**alcitonin)
    - Pheochromocytoma (**c**atecholamines)

26. **What is the preferred operative approach for HPT in MEN patients?**
    HPT develops in over 90% of patients with MEN I. Patients typically have multiple tumors that may be asymmetric in size. The preferred operation is subtotal parathyroidectomy with transcervical thymectomy (the most likely location of supernumerary glands). Parathyroid tissue can be cryopreserved for subsequent autografting for hypoparathyroidism.
    In MEN II, 20%–30% of patients develop HPT, and multiple tumors are the norm. The HPT tends to be milder than in MEN I. All four glands should be inspected with resection of only enlarged glands or subtotal parathyroidectomy. Intraoperative PTH levels may help guide resection.

27. **Who performed the first parathyroidectomy?**
    In 1925, Felix Mendl performed the first successful parathyroidectomy at the Hochenegg Clinic in Vienna. His patient was Albert, a 34-year-old tramcar conductor who could not work because of severe osteitis fibrosa cystica.

28. **Who was Captain Martell?**
    An officer in the U.S. Merchant Marines, Captain Martell was the first patient in the United States to undergo surgery for primary HPT. Captain Martell had progressive HPT that reduced his height from 6 feet to a kyphotic 5 feet, 6 inches. After seven operations, the adenoma was finally removed from the mediastinum; however, the captain died of chronic renal failure.

29. **In what animal was the parathyroid gland first discovered?**
    The parathyroid gland was first discovered in 1852 during the autopsy of an Indian rhinoceros by the English biologist, paleontologist, and anatomist Sir Richard Owen.

KEY POINTS: HPT

1. HPT is the most common etiology of hypercalcemia in the outpatient population.
2. Elevated serum calcium with an elevated PTH without low urine calcium confirms the diagnosis of primary HPT.
3. Parathyroidectomy is indicated for primary HPT patients with symptoms or for asymptomatic patients who meet specific criteria.
4. Parathyroid location can vary considerably. Superior parathyroid glands arise from the fourth branchial (pharyngeal) pouch and lie posterior to the RLN, while Inferior parathyroid glands arise from the third branchial pouch and reside anterior to the RLN.
5. The traditional surgical procedure for primary HPT is bilateral neck exploration, but focused parathyroidectomy is a widely used alternative with excellent cure rates when localized preoperatively.

BIBLIOGRAPHY

1. Ambrogini E, Cetani F, Cianferotti L, et al. Surgery or surveillance for mild asymptomatic primary hyperparathyroidism: a prospective, randomized clinical trial. *J Clin Endocrinol Metab.* 2007;92(8):3114–3121.
2. Bilezikian JP, Brandi ML, Eastell R, et al. Guidelines for the management of asymptomatic primary hyperparathyroidism: summary statement from the fourth international workshop. *J Clin Endocrinol Metab.* 2014;99(10):3561–3569.
3. Eigelberger MS, Cheah WK. The NIH criteria for parathyroidectomy in asymptomatic primary hyperparathyroidism: are they too limited? *Ann Surg.* 2004;239(4):528–535.
4. Gil-Cardenas A, Gamino R. Is intraoperative parathyroid hormone assay mandatory for the success of targeted parathyroidectomy? *J Am Coll Surg.* 2007;204(2):286–290.
5. Kebebew E, Hwang J. Predictors of single-gland vs multigland parathyroid disease in primary hyperparathyroidism: a simple and accurate scoring model. *Arch Surg.* 2006;141(8):777–782.
6. Lambert LA, Shapiro SE, Lee JE, et al. Surgical treatment of hyperparathyroidism in patients with multiple endocrine neoplasia type 1. *Arch Surg.* 2005;140(4):374–382.
7. Lo CY, Lang BH. A prospective evaluation of preoperative localization by technetium-99m sestamibi scintigraphy and ultrasonography in primary hyperparathyroidism. *Am J Surg.* 2007;193(2):155–159.
8. Nilsson IL, Aberg J. Maintained normalization of cardiovascular dysfunction 5 years after parathyroidectomy in primary hyperparathyroidism. *Surgery.* 2005;137(6):632–638.
9. Pappu S, Donovan P. Sestamibi scans are not all created equally. *Arch Surg.* 2005;140(4):383–386.
10. Phitayakorn R, McHenry CR. Incidence and location of ectopic abnormal parathyroid glands. *Am J Surg.* 2006;191(3):418–423.
11. Richards ML, Wormuth J. Parathyroidectomy in secondary hyperparathyroidism: is there an optimal operative management? *Surgery.* 2006;139(2):174–180.

HYPERTHYROIDISM

*Kathryn H. Chomsky-Higgins, MD, MS, Robert C. McIntyre, Jr., MD,
Christopher D. Raeburn, MD, FACS, Barnard J. A. Palmer, MD, MEd, FACS*

CHAPTER 61

1. **How common is hyperthyroidism?**
   Of the 1.2% prevalence of hyperthyroidism in the United States, 0.5% is overt, while 0.7% is subclinical. The incidence of overt disease is approximately 0.4 per 1000 women, and 0.1 per 1000 men, but varies significantly by age.

2. **What are the signs and symptoms of hyperthyroidism?**
   - General: Heat intolerance, perspiration, flushing, tremor, sleep disturbance, or hair loss
   - Psychologic: Nervousness, emotional lability, anxiety, aggressiveness, or delusions
   - Cardiovascular: Palpitations, tachycardia, or supraventricular dysrhythmias
   - Respiratory: Breathlessness or hoarseness
   - Gastrointestinal: Increased appetite, weight loss, or increased frequency of bowel movements
   - Reproductive: Gynecomastia, irregular menses
   - Bone: Osteoporosis
   - Other: Ophthalmopathy, dermopathy

3. **What are the common causes of hyperthyroidism?**
   Graves' disease, toxic multinodular goiter (TMNG), and toxic uninodular goiter (Plummer's disease) are the three most common causes. Others include acute thyroiditis, subacute (de Quervain's) thyroiditis, silent thyroiditis, amiodarone-induced thyroiditis, iatrogenic thyrotoxicosis, factitious ingestion of thyroid hormone, struma ovarii, trophoblastic disease, resistance to thyroid hormone, and extensive metastases from follicular thyroid cancer.

4. **How should hyperthyroidism be investigated?**
   Serum thyroid-stimulating hormone (TSH) measurement is the most useful test in the evaluation of hyperthyroidism and should be used as an initial screening test. It has the highest sensitivity and specificity of any single blood test. A low TSH with a high serum level of free thyroxine (T_4) or triiodothyronine (T_3) is diagnostic. A high TSH with an increase in free T_4 indicates the rare patient with a thyrotropin-producing pituitary tumor. Subclinical hyperthyroidism has suppressed TSH with a high-normal T_4 or T_3.
   After the diagnosis of hyperthyroidism is made, radioactive iodine uptake (RAIU) may be used to differentiate the many causes. It is most indicated when thyroid nodules are present or when the clinical presentation of thyrotoxicosis is not diagnostic of Graves' disease. Uptake in the thyroid is usually measured at 4–6 hours then again at 24 hours.
   - High uptake: Confirms hyperthyroidism resulting from overproduction of thyroid hormone
   - Uniform uptake: Suggests Graves' disease
   - Patchy uptake: Suggests TMNG
   - Unifocal area with suppression of the remaining thyroid: Diagnostic of a toxic solitary adenoma
   - Diffuse, low uptake: Suggests thyroiditis, which can cause a self-limited course of hyperthyroidism secondary to release of preformed thyroid hormone

5. **How is the diagnosis of Graves' disease established?**
   Graves' disease can almost always be diagnosed on the basis of the clinical findings that include symmetric thyroid enlargement, recent onset ophthalmopathy, and moderate to severe hyperthyroidism. Ophthalmopathy is unique to Graves' disease and is the result of thyroid autoantibodies (particularly in smokers) that cross-react to the extraocular muscles. TSH will be low in association with an increased free T_4. If the free T_4 is normal, a free T_3 level is obtained to rule out T_3 toxicosis. RAIU shows uniform increased uptake. Because Graves' is an autoimmune disease that results in production of autoantibodies that stimulate the TSH receptor, TSH receptor antibody assays or thyroid-stimulating immunoglobulin (TSI) levels can be used to confirm the diagnosis.

6. **What are the three treatment options for Graves' disease?**
   Antithyroid drugs (ATDs), radioactive iodine (I^{131}) therapy, and surgery. Each has associated risks and benefits. In the United States, radioactive iodine (RAI) has been the preferred therapy.

7. **What are the indications for and outcomes of drug treatment?**
   The goals of medical treatment are remission of symptoms and to render the patient euthyroid as quickly and as safely as possible. They can be used alone as therapy or to attain euthyroidism before treatment with RAI or surgery.
   Beta-adrenergic blockade should be considered in all patients with symptomatic thyrotoxicosis. It should be given to all elderly symptomatic patients, those with resting heart rates greater than 90 beats per minute, or patients with coexisting cardiovascular disease.
   ATD-only treatment is preferred in patients with a high likelihood of remission (mild hyperthyroidism, a small gland, low titers), patients at high risk for surgery or RAI treatment, and those with limited longevity. Almost all patients become euthyroid within 6 weeks of initiating therapy. Long-term remission occurs in only 30% of patients, and recurrent hyperthyroidism occurs in 50% of patients when the drugs are stopped. Relapse is most common in the first 6 months after cessation of treatment.

8. **Which drugs are used for the treatment of hyperthyroidism? What are the mechanisms of action and side effects?**
   ATDs work to reduce thyroid function. They control hyperthyroidism but cannot cure Graves' disease. Therapy is usually maintained for 2 years. Beta-adrenergic receptors are used to block the symptoms of hyperthyroidism.
   Methimazole (MMI) is the mainstay of treatment, except during the first trimester of pregnancy and in thyroid storm. It inhibits the enzyme thyroperoxidase, which inhibits organification of iodine and coupling of iodothyronines. Side effects include rash, pruritus, hepatotoxicity, cholestatic jaundice, lupus-like syndrome, arthropathy, and agranulocytosis. The side effects of MMI occur at a much lower rate than propylthiouracil, except during pregnancy. MMI may cause aplasia cutis of the scalp of the newborn and a syndrome of embryonopathy that includes choanal and esophageal atresia.
   Propylthiouracil (PTU) similarly inhibits organification of iodine and coupling of iodothyronine, but also inhibits the peripheral monodeiodination of T_4 to the more physiologically active T_3. Patients should be monitored for similar side effects, which include rash, pruritus, hepatitis, cholestatic jaundice, lupus-like syndrome, arthropathy, antineutrophil cytoplasmic antibody–positive small vessel vasculitis, and the life-threatening complications of agranulocytosis or fulminant hepatic necrosis, which are rare but occur at a higher rates than with MMI. PTU is preferred during the first trimester of pregnancy and for thyroid storm.
   β-adrenergic antagonists ameliorate the signs and symptoms of disease. They should not be used alone, except for short periods before RAI or surgical therapy.
   Iodine given as Lugol's solution (5% iodine and 10% potassium iodide in water, 0.3 mL/day) or potassium iodide (60 mg three times per day) inhibits the release of thyroid hormone. It is useful for short-term therapy in preparation for surgery, after RAI therapy to hasten the fall in hormone levels, and for treatment of thyroid storm. It causes a decrease in perfusion of the thyroid, which may reduce bleeding during thyroidectomy.

9. **What are the indications and contraindications to radioactive iodine treatment?**
   RAI is preferred in patients with comorbidities that increase surgical risk, previously operated or radiated necks, or contraindications to ATDs. Pregnancy and lactation are absolute contraindications. Women of childbearing age should be evaluated with a pregnancy test before treatment and should avoid pregnancy for 6 months after treatment. Patients with coexisting or suspected thyroid cancer should avoid RAI, and RAI may exacerbate Graves' ophthalmopathy.

10. **What is the regimen of radioactive iodine treatment?**
    RAI is the most common therapy in the United States for Graves' disease. The usual dose of RAI is 10–15 mCi. TMNG is treated with slightly higher doses of 25–30 mCi. Older patients and patients with significant comorbidities should receive ATDs before RAI to prevent I^{131}-induced thyroid storm. Patients with significant eye disease and smokers should receive corticosteroids before RAI to prevent progression of ophthalmopathy.

11. **What is the outcome of radioactive iodine treatment?**
    Euthyroidism is not achieved for months after RAI treatment, but once achieved, recurrence of hyperthyroidism is rare. Hypothyroidism, the only serious side effect, is dose dependent. It occurs at a rate of 3% per year, affecting 50% of patients at 10 years and nearly 100% at 25 years.

12. **What are the indications for thyroidectomy for hyperthyroidism?**
    a. Pregnant patients who are difficult to treat medically
    b. Patients with large goiter and low RAIU
    c. Children
    d. Noncompliant patients
    e. Patients with nodules suspected to be cancer
    f. Patients with compression of the trachea or esophagus
    g. Patients with cosmetic concerns
    h. Patients with ophthalmopathy
    i. Allergy or significant side effects to ATDs
    j. Patients with significant comorbidities that require rapid achievement of a euthyroid state

13. **How should patients be prepared prior to surgery?**
    Any patient with hyperthyroidism should be rendered euthyroid before surgery. Patients may be treated with antithyroid medication plus potassium iodine. β-adrenergic antagonists also may be used alone or in combination with the above regimen.

14. **What is the extent of thyroidectomy?**
    The two surgical options for Graves' disease are near-total thyroidectomy or total thyroidectomy. The goal of near-total thyroidectomy is to preserve 4–8 g of well-vascularized thyroid tissue to avoid hypothyroidism. Because of the small risk of recurrence (8%), however, some surgeons prefer total thyroidectomy, which has a recurrence rate of close to 0%. Total thyroidectomy is preferred for patients with coexisting malignancy and patients with severe ophthalmopathy. In Plummer's disease, lobectomy or partial thyroidectomy for unilateral lesions and contralateral subtotal thyroidectomy for multiple lesions render the patient euthyroid.

15. **What is the incidence of hypothyroidism after surgery?**
    All patients who undergo total or subtotal thyroidectomy become hypothyroid and need T_4 replacement. Hypothyroidism occurs in 30% of patients following subtotal thyroidectomy, and if a significant thyroid remnant remains, immediate postoperative thyroid replacement should be provided and titrated based on subsequent thyroid function measurements.

16. **What is the appropriate treatment for toxic nodular goiter?**
    Hyperthyroidism as a result of toxic nodular goiter is permanent and without spontaneous remission; ATDs are not appropriate long-term therapy. RAI is the most common form of therapy. Larger doses (25–30 mCi) minimize the risk of persistent hyperthyroidism in such patients, who tend to be older and to have prominent cardiovascular symptoms of hyperthyroidism. Surgery is also quite effective, results in the most rapid achievement of euthyroidism, and has a low recurrence rate.

17. **What is the appropriate treatment for hyperthyroidism resulting from thyroiditis?**
    Subacute thyroiditis should be suspected if the patient has pain and tenderness in the thyroid region. A RAIU scan shows decreased uptake. The hyperthyroidism is usually mild and of short duration (weeks). Most patients do not need treatment, but a β-adrenergic antagonist and salicylates or glucocorticoids are used for symptom control. Hypothyroidism may occur but is rarely permanent.

18. **What is the appropriate treatment for thyroid storm?**
    Thyrotoxic crisis should be treated in the intensive care unit (ICU). General measures include hydration, antipyresis (acetaminophen), and nutrition. Specific measures include inhibition of T_4 synthesis and conversion to T_3 with PTU at a dose of 100 mg orally, via nasogastric (NG) tube or rectally every 6 hours. Iodides inhibit T_4 release (saturated solution of potassium iodide, SSKI, 5 drops by mouth or NG tube every 6 hours). Steroids (dexamethasone, 2 mg every 6 hours) also inhibit T_4 release and conversion to T_3. β-adrenergic antagonists (propranolol or esmolol) may control cardiovascular manifestations. Other agents that lower thyroid hormone are iopanoic acid, lithium, and potassium perchlorate. The last management option is T_4 removal by plasmapheresis, hemoperfusion, or dialysis.

19. **What surgeon won the Nobel prize for his work with thyroid disease?**
    Theodor Kocher won the Nobel Prize in Medicine in 1909 for his work on the physiology, pathology, and surgery of the thyroid gland. He was successful in reducing the high mortality rate of thyroidectomy in the late 1800s. In 1850 the mortality rate was 50%, but by 1898 the mortality rate at Kocher's clinic was 0.18%. His most significant achievement was in describing postoperative hypothyroidism as *cachexia strumipriva*.

KEY POINTS: HYPERTHYROIDISM

1. The most common etiologies of hyperthyroidism are Graves' disease, TMNG, and toxic uninodular goiter (Plummer's disease).
2. Graves' disease is diagnosed clinically, confirmed with serum thyroid testing, and treated with ATDs, radioactive iodine, or surgery.
3. TMNG should be managed with radioactive iodine or thyroidectomy; ATDs are not appropriate long-term therapy.
4. Hyperthyroidism secondary to subacute thyroiditis is usually self-limiting and rarely requires treatment beyond symptom control.
5. Thyroid storm (thyrotoxic crisis) is initially managed in the ICU with hydration, antipyresis, nutrition, PTU, iodides, and steroids.

WEBSITES

- www.endocrinesurgery.org/
- www.thyroid.org/
- www.aace.com/

BIBLIOGRAPHY

1. Bahn RS, Burch HB, Cooper DS, et al. Hyperthyroidism and other causes of thyrotoxicosis: management guidelines of the American Thyroid Association and American Association of Clinical Endocrinologists. *Thyroid.* 2011;21(6):593–646.
2. Boger MS, Perrier ND. Advantages and disadvantages of surgical therapy and optimal extent of thyroidectomy for the treatment of hyperthyroidism. *Surg Clin North Am.* 2004;84(3):849–874.
3. Cooper DS. Antithyroid drugs. *N Engl J Med.* 2005;352(9):905–917.
4. Erbil Y, Giris M, Salmaslioglu A, et al. The effect of anti-thyroid drug treatment duration on thyroid gland microvessel density and intraoperative blood loss in patients with Graves' disease. *Surgery.* 2008;143(2):216–225.
5. Kang AS, Grant CS. Current treatment of nodular goiter with hyperthyroidism (Plummer's disease): surgery versus radioiodine. *Surgery.* 2002;132(6):916–923.
6. Lal G, Ituarte P. Should total thyroidectomy become the preferred procedure for surgical management of Graves' disease? *Thyroid.* 2005;15(6):569–574.
7. Palit TK, Miller CC 3rd. The efficacy of thyroidectomy for Graves' disease: a meta-analysis. *J Surg Res.* 2000;90(2):161–165.
8. Schussler-Fiorenza CM, Bruns CM. The surgical management of Graves' disease. *J Surg Res.* 2006;133(2):207–214.
9. Vidal-Trecan GM, Stahl JE. Radioiodine or surgery for toxic thyroid adenoma: dissecting an important decision. A cost-effectiveness analysis. *Thyroid.* 2004;14(11):933–945.
10. Weetman AP. Graves' disease. *N Engl J Med.* 2000;343(17):1236–1248.
11. Witte J, Goretzki PE, Dotzenrath C, et al. Surgery for Graves' disease: total versus subtotal thyroidectomy: results of a prospective randomized trial. *World J Surg.* 2000;24(11):1303–1311.

CHAPTER 62

THYROID NODULES AND CANCER

Kathryn H. Chomsky-Higgins, MD, MS, Trevor L. Nydam, MD,
Robert C. McIntyre, Jr., MD, Barnard J. A. Palmer, MD, MEd, FACS

1. **What is the prevalence of thyroid nodules and cancer?**
   The prevalence of thyroid nodules increases throughout life and is dependent on the method of detection—by palpation 5%, by ultrasound (US) 35%, and by autopsy 50%. Thyroid nodules are four times more common in females than in males. After exposure to radiation, nodules develop at approximately 2% annually, reaching a peak at 25 years. Up to 35% of thyroid glands examined at autopsy contain occult papillary cancer (<1.0 cm). SEER database information suggests a thyroid cancer prevalence of about 637,000 in the United States and predicts 64,300 new cases in 2016.

2. **What concerns are associated with thyroid nodules?**
   Thyroid nodules are clinically relevant to patients because of the ability to grow and cause compressive symptoms, the possibility of being functional adenomas, and the small risk of malignancy.

3. **What is the importance of the distinction between solitary and multiple thyroid nodules?**
   Traditionally, multiple thyroid nodules were considered benign and solitary thyroid nodules malignant. However, multiple series suggest that a dominant nodule in a multinodular gland carries the same risk of cancer as a solitary nodule (5%). With improvements in US, each nodule should be assessed individually based on imaging characteristics.

4. **What features of the history and physical examination indicate a higher risk of cancer?**
   - Nodules occurring at the **extremes of age** are more likely to be cancerous, particularly in males.
   - **Rapid growth and local invasion** raise the possibility of malignancy, but associated symptoms (e.g., hoarseness, dysphagia) are uncommon.
   - **History of radiation exposure** increases the frequency of both benign and malignant nodules.
   - Family history of medullary or papillary thyroid cancer or Gardner syndrome (i.e., familial polyposis) increases the risk of cancer.
   - Firm, solitary nodules, fixation to adjacent structures, vocal cord paralysis, and enlarged lymph nodes also are associated with an increased risk of malignancy.

5. **What laboratory tests should be included in the evaluation of a patient with a thyroid nodule?**
   The only biochemical test that is routinely needed is a serum **thyroid-stimulating hormone (TSH)** concentration to identify patients with unsuspected hyperthyroidism.
   Thyroglobulin and serum calcitonin should not be routinely tested. Thyroglobulin can be measured in patients with differentiated thyroid carcinoma, while calcitonin should be measured only in patients with suspected medullary thyroid carcinoma (MTC). Patients with known MTC should also have **lymphocyte-derived DNA analysis for *ret* proto-oncogene mutation analysis**.
   In patients with known multiple endocrine neoplasia (MEN) 2, **serum calcium levels and 24-hour urine collection** for assessment of catecholamines and their metabolic products should be done to evaluate for hyperparathyroidism and pheochromocytoma before thyroidectomy.

6. **What imaging should be done in the evaluation of a thyroid nodule?**
   - **Thyroid US** should be performed on all patients with nodules. It determines if there is a nodule that corresponds to a palpable abnormality, evaluates for other nodules, determines if a nodule is cystic, solid, or mixed, and is the best measure of the size of a nodule. Sonographic features are superior to size for determining risk of malignancy, and suspicious characteristics include microcalcification, hypoechogenicity of a solid nodule, and intranodular hypervascularity.

US improves the accuracy of fine-needle aspiration (FNA) biopsy, which should be performed on nodules that are concerning.

- **Radioactive iodine uptake scans** are reserved for patients with suppressed TSH (<0.5 μIU/mL) to evaluate for hyperthyroidism resulting from Graves' disease, toxic multinodular goiter, or an autonomous nodule. Patients with a normal or elevated TSH do not require scanning because it cannot reliably distinguish benign from malignant nodules.

7. What is the differential diagnosis of thyroid nodules?
   - Adenoma: Macrofollicular (colloid), microfollicular, embryonal, Hürthle cell
   - Cancer: Papillary, follicular, medullary, anaplastic, lymphoma, metastatic
   - Cyst
   - Multinodular goiter with a dominant nodule
   - Other: Inflammatory diseases (e.g., Hashimoto's thyroiditis), developmental abnormalities (e.g., thyroglossal duct cyst)

8. What is the single most important test in the evaluation of thyroid nodules?
   The single best test is FNA. The overall accuracy exceeds 95% in experienced hands. If an adequate specimen is obtained, results are grouped by Bethesda Criteria (see Table 62.1) to predict the risk of malignancy and recommend a treatment plan.

Table 62.1 Bethesda FNA Thyroid Cytology

CLASSIFICATION	CATEGORIZATION	RISK OF MALIGNANCY	RECOMMENDED THERAPY
1	Nondiagnostic/unsatisfactory	1%–4%	Repeat FNA
2	Benign	0%–3%	Surveillance
3	AUS/FLUS	5%–15%	Repeat FNA
4	Suspicious for follicular neoplasm	15%–30%	Thyroid lobectomy
5	Suspicious for malignancy	60%–75%	Minimum thyroid lobectomy
6	Malignant	97%–99%	Minimum thyroid lobectomy

9. Is levothyroxine suppression treatment useful in the management thyroid nodules?
   Levothyroxine suppression treatment is generally not recommended, except in regions of the world with low iodine uptake where TSH suppression to subnormal serum levels using levothyroxine may decrease benign nodule size.

10. What are the types and distribution of thyroid cancer?
    - Papillary 80%
    - Follicular 15%
    - Medullary 5%
    - Anaplastic and lymphoma <1%

11. What are the axioms of thyroid surgery?
    - A meticulously dry operative field must be maintained.
    - Tissue in the region of the recurrent laryngeal nerve (RLN) should not be cut or clamped until the nerve is definitively identified.
    - Every parathyroid gland should be treated as if it were the last functioning gland.
    - If malignancy is suspected, the entire operation should be performed as if the lesion were cancer.

12. Define the various types of thyroid procedures
    - **Thyroid lobectomy:** Removal of a single thyroid lobe (usually with isthmus) intended to rule out the diagnosis of cancer or to treat a unilateral toxic nodule.
    - **Total thyroidectomy:** Removal of the entire thyroid gland including the isthmus and pyramidal lobe. Generally chosen as treatment for cancer or Graves' disease. This procedure has the highest risk of RLN injury and hypoparathyroidism.

- **Near-total thyroidectomy:** Removal of the entire thyroid gland except for <1 g of thyroid tissue at the ligament of Berry to avoid RLN injury. This operation has equivalent oncologic outcomes to total thyroidectomy that removes all visible thyroid tissue. However, near-total thyroidectomy may have a lower complication rate than total thyroidectomy.
- **Subtotal thyroidectomy:** Removal of the majority of the thyroid gland but leaves approximately 4–8 g of thyroid tissue to achieve an euthyroid state. Often used for Graves' disease in an attempt to avoid thyroid hormone replacement.
- **Central neck dissection:** Removal of the nodal tissue in the central or anterior neck compartment (level I), which is bordered by the hyoid bone, carotid arteries, and sternal notch.
- **Lateral neck dissection:** Removal of the nodal tissue in the lateral compartments or jugular chain, which are deep to the sternocleidomastoid muscles (levels II, III, IV).

13. What is the minimal extent of thyroidectomy for a solitary thyroid nodule?

With the exception of small lesions in the thyroid isthmus, the minimal procedure for suspected malignancy should be lobectomy including the isthmus as a diagnostic biopsy. Enucleation or nodulectomy is to be avoided. Solitary autonomous nodules should be treated with lobectomy.

14. What is the surgical therapy for thyroid carcinoma?

Thyroid carcinomas should be treated by near-total or total thyroidectomy except in young patients with small, well-differentiated tumors (<1 cm), no extrathyroidal invasion, or metastasis to lymph nodes or distant sites. In such cases, lobectomy with resection of the isthmus may be adequate therapy. Total thyroidectomy eliminates multifocal cancer in the thyroid, allows postoperative radioactive iodine for the diagnosis and therapy of metastatic disease, decreases the risk of local-regional recurrence, and improves the accuracy of serum thyroglobulin as a marker for persistent or recurrent disease. For papillary and follicular carcinomas >1 cm, total or near-total thyroidectomy improves overall survival. Enlarged cervical lymph nodes should be removed and examined by frozen section. If metastatic cancer is identified, a neck dissection is performed. "Berry picking" results in an increased rate of regional recurrence and should be avoided in favor of anatomic neck dissections.

Because medullary thyroid cancer is not responsive to radioactive iodine or levothyroxine, total thyroidectomy should be performed. A central neck dissection is mandatory to evaluate metastatic disease. If the central or lateral nodes are positive for cancer on frozen section, an ipsilateral lateral neck dissection is performed. The contralateral neck may be observed.

Surgery for anaplastic carcinoma is palliative and usually is limited to debulking and tracheostomy for relief of compressive symptoms.

15. What is the incidence of metastatic disease to the lymph nodes?

At the time of the diagnosis of well-differentiated thyroid cancer (WDTC; papillary and follicular), 20%–50% of patients will have microscopic nodal metastases if a neck dissection is done. Multiple authors advocate prophylactic central neck dissection at the time of the thyroidectomy in patients with WDTC to avoid an increased complication rate in reoperations if recurrence occurs in the central neck. However, the risk of hypoparathyroidism and nerve injury during central neck dissection is higher than that of total thyroidectomy alone, and multiple studies fail to show a significant survival benefit to prophylactic neck dissection.

In medullary thyroid cancer, 80% of patients will have positive nodes in the central and ipsilateral neck. Approximately 50% of patients will have nodal disease in the contralateral neck. Because MTC is radioactive iodine and TSH insensitive, surgery is the only therapy and neck dissection is necessary.

16. Can anything be done to identify patients with nodal disease before the initial operation?

US of the neck before thyroidectomy identifies nonpalpable node disease in 20%–30% of patients and alters the operation performed based on physical examination. US has high accuracy in the lateral neck but is not sensitive in the central neck.

17. Describe the arterial supply and venous drainage of the thyroid

The blood supply to the thyroid gland comes from the superior and inferior thyroid arteries. The superior thyroid artery is the first branch of the external carotid artery. The inferior thyroid artery arises from the thyrocervical trunk. Occasionally, a midline thyroid IMA artery arises from the aortic arch.

The three major veins are the superior, middle, and inferior thyroid veins. Superior and middle thyroid veins drain into the internal jugular vein, while the inferior vein drains into the innominate vein.

18. **Describe the anatomy of the RLNs**

The right RLN arises from the vagus and loops around the right subclavian artery. The left vagus nerve gives off the left RLN and loops around the aorta at the ligamentum arteriosus. The RLNs run obliquely through the neck, usually in the tracheoesophageal groove. Low in the neck, the nerves are more lateral and course medially as they ascend. The right nerve runs more obliquely than the left. Occasionally, the RLN branches before entering the larynx, usually on the left side. The motor fibers are contained in the anterior branch. In 1% of cases, the right RLN is not recurrent and enters the neck from a lateral and superior direction and is associated with an aberrant right subclavian artery.

19. **What defect results from injury to the RLN?**

Injury to a single RLN results in a paralyzed vocal cord causing a weak, hoarse voice. Patients may also have abnormal swallowing and problems with aspiration. Injury to both nerves causes paralysis of both cords and airflow obstruction. Bilateral RLN injury necessitates tracheostomy. RLN injury occurs in 1% of thyroidectomies.

20. **Describe the anatomy of the superior laryngeal nerve and the defect that occurs with its injury**

The superior laryngeal nerve gives off the external branch of the superior laryngeal nerve (EBSLN), which runs medial to the superior pole vessels to innervate the cricothyroid muscle. This motor nerve (i.e., Amelita Galli-Curci nerve) increases tension of the vocal cords, allowing for high notes. The internal laryngeal nerve provides the sensory innervation to the posterior pharynx. It lies superior to the thyroid cartilage. Injury to the nerve leads to a weak, low voice that fatigues easily and lacks projection. Patients may also have problems with aspiration.

21. **Do patients have voice changes independent of injury to the nerves?**

In the absence of nerve injury, 80%–85% of patients have a change in at least one voice parameter; however, only 40%–50% of patients report mild voice dysfunction. These early vocal symptoms resolve in most but may persist in approximately 15% of patients. This data is important to discuss with patients before the operation.

22. **What is the other major complication of thyroidectomy?**

Temporary hypocalcemia secondary to parathyroid injury occurs in 10%–15% of patients, whereas permanent hypoparathyroidism occurs in 3% of patients who have had thyroidectomies.

23. **What are the postoperative therapies for well-differentiated thyroid carcinoma?**

Selected patients should be treated with postoperative radioactive iodine (I[131]) ablation of remnant tissue and distal disease. All patients with WDTC should be treated with levothyroxine (Synthroid) to suppress serum levels of TSH. This three-component therapy (surgery, I[131], and levothyroxine suppression) results in the lowest recurrence rates.

24. **What are the indications for postoperative radioactive iodine (I[131]) ablation?**

RAI ablation is recommended for all tumor, node, and metastasis stage 2–4 disease and selected patients with stage 1 disease and risk factors. Risk factors include age >45 years old, male gender, tumor size, direct local invasion, nodal spread, and distant disease. Postoperative ablation and subsequent monitoring for persistent or recurrent disease requires TSH stimulation. Endogenous TSH stimulation is done with levothyroxine withdrawal. Exogenous TSH stimulation is done with recombinant human TSH (rhTSH).

25. **What is the appropriate degree of thyroid hormone suppression of TSH?**

Retrospective studies suggest that high-risk patients should have TSH suppressed to <0.1 μIU/mL. Low-risk patients should be maintained at 0.1 to 0.5 μIU/mL (normal = 0.5–5.0 μIU/mL).

26. **What is the appropriate method of following patients after their initial course of treatment?**

Patients with WDTC have a 30% risk of recurrence over 30 years of follow-up. Initially patients are followed at 6- to 12-month intervals depending on their risk stratification. A physical examination is done, and US surveillance of the neck has largely supplanted iodine scanning to detect recurrence. TSH, thyroglobulin (Tg), and thyroglobulin antibody levels should be checked with the patient on levothyroxine. An elevated Tg level with a suppressed TSH is worrisome for recurrence. If the Tg level is undetectable while on TSH suppression, endogenous or exogenous TSH stimulated Tg level is obtained. An increase in the Tg level with TSH stimulation is also worrisome for recurrence. Fifteen percent to 20% of the population has Tg antibodies that interfere with the Tg assay and can cause overmeasurement or undermeasurement.

27. **What is the appropriate management of patients with metastatic disease?**
Local or regional disease in the neck is treated by reoperation. Compartment-oriented neck dissection is advocated for regional metastasis. Distant disease should be treated with radioactive iodine if the metastases take up iodine. Pulmonary micrometastasis should be treated at 6- to 12-month intervals as long as the disease continues to respond. Radioactive iodine nonavid disease is not benefited by routine treatment. In these patients, follow-up with TSH suppressive therapy is indicated. For selected patients, metastasectomy or external beam radiation therapy (EBRT) may provide palliative benefit. Complete surgical resection of isolated bone metastasis should be considered. Alternatives, when metastases are not isolated, are radioactive iodine treatment or EBRT. Selected BRAF mutation positive lesions may be treated with kinase inhibitors to limit tumor growth. Patients with advanced progressive disease that is not radioactive iodine avid can be entered into chemotherapy clinical trials. If clinical trials are not available, cytotoxic chemotherapy consists of a doxorubicin-based regimen.

KEY POINTS: THYROID NODULES AND CANCER

1. Thyroid nodules are best evaluated by serum TSH and cervical US. FNA should be performed on any nodule that is concerning for malignancy.
2. US findings suspicious for malignancy include microcalcification, hypoechogenicity of solid nodules, and intranodular hypervascularity.
3. FNA cytology results can be classified by Bethesda Criteria to estimate risk of malignancy and direct next steps in management.
4. Thyroid nodules should be treated with thyroid lobectomy at a minimum.
5. Major complications of thyroidectomy include voice changes, hypocalcemia secondary to parathyroid injury, and expected hypothyroidism when total thyroidectomy is performed.

WEBSITES

- www.facs.org/
- www.endocrinesurgery.org/
- www.thyroid.org/
- www.aace.com/

BIBLIOGRAPHY

1. Bilimoria KY, Bentrem DJ, Ko CY, et al. Extent of surgery affects survival for papillary thyroid cancer. *Ann Surg.* 2007;246(3):375–381.
2. Brandi ML, Gagel RF, Angeli A, et al. Guidelines for diagnosis and therapy of MEN type 1 and type 2. *J Clin Endocrinol Metab.* 2001;86(12):5658–5671.
3. Cooper DS, Doherty GM, Haugen BR, et al. Management guidelines for patients with thyroid nodules and differentiated thyroid cancer. *Thyroid.* 2006;16(2):109–142.
4. Haugen BR, Ridgway EC. Clinical comparison of whole-body radioiodine scan and serum thyroglobulin after stimulation with recombinant human thyrotropin. *Thyroid.* 2002;12(1):37–43.
5. Ito Y, Miyauchi A. Lateral and mediastinal lymph node dissection in differentiated thyroid carcinoma: indications, benefits, and risks. *World J Surg.* 2007;31(5):905–915.
6. Jonklaas J, Sarlis NJ, Litofsky D, et al. Outcomes of patients with differentiated thyroid carcinoma following initial therapy. *Thyroid.* 2006;16(12):1229–1242.
7. Leboulleux S, Girard E, Rose M, et al. Ultrasound criteria of malignancy for cervical lymph nodes in patients followed up for differentiated thyroid cancer. *J Clin Endocrinol Metab.* 2007;92(9):3590–3594.
8. Lim CY, Yun JS. Percutaneous ethanol injection therapy for locally recurrent papillary thyroid carcinoma. *Thyroid.* 2007;17(4):347–350.
9. Mazzaferri EL, Robbins RJ, Spencer CA, et al. A consensus report of the role of serum thyroglobulin as a monitoring method for low-risk patients with papillary thyroid carcinoma. *J Clin Endocrinol Metab.* 2003;88(4):1433–1441.
10. Mittendorf EA, Wang X, Perrier ND, et al. Followup of patients with papillary thyroid cancer: in search of the optimal algorithm. *J Am Coll Surg.* 2007;205(2):239–247.
11. Pacini F, Molinaro E, Castagna MG, et al. Recombinant human thyrotropin-stimulated serum thyroglobulin combined with neck ultrasonography has the highest sensitivity in monitoring differentiated thyroid carcinoma. *J Clin Endocrinol Metab.* 2003;88(8):3668–3673.

12. Sawka AM, Thephamongkhol K. Clinical review 170: a systematic review and metaanalysis of the effectiveness of radioactive iodine remnant ablation for well-differentiated thyroid cancer. *J Clin Endocrinol Metab.* 2004;89(8):3668–3676.
13. Stojadinovic A, Shaha AR, Orlikoff RF, et al. Prospective functional voice assessment in patients undergoing thyroid surgery. *Ann Surg.* 2002;236(6):823–832.
14. Stulak JM, Grant CS, Farley DR, et al. Value of preoperative ultrasonography in the surgical management of initial and reoperative papillary thyroid cancer. *Arch Surg.* 2006;141(5):489–494.

CHAPTER 63

SURGICAL HYPERTENSION

Logan R. McKenna, MD, John C. Eun, MD, Robert C. McIntyre, Jr., MD

1. **What are the surgically correctable causes of hypertension?**

   Renovascular hypertension, pheochromocytoma, Cushing's syndrome, primary hyperaldosteronism (Conn's syndrome), coarctation of the aorta, and unilateral renal parenchymal disease. Surgical hypertension accounts for 5%–10% of all hypertensive patients.

2. **Which form of surgical hypertension is most common?**

   Renovascular hypertension is the most common cause of surgical hypertension (approximately 3% of patients with hypertension), followed by primary hyperaldosteronism (1.5%), Cushing's syndrome (0.5%), pheochromocytoma (0.1%–0.3%), and coarctation of the aorta (0.1%). However, in patients with resistant hypertension, defined as uncontrolled blood pressure despite the use of three or more antihypertensive agents, secondary forms of hypertension are much more prevalent. Renal artery stenosis may be present in up to 24% of patients with resistant hypertension. Also, primary aldosteronism is present 7%–20% of patients with resistant hypertension, particularly those with concurrent type 2 diabetes mellitus.

3. **What are the most common causes of renovascular hypertension?**

   The two major causes of renovascular hypertension are atherosclerosis and fibromuscular dysplasia. Atherosclerosis causes about 90% of cases and affects men twice as often as women. It usually involves the ostium and proximal third of the main renal artery, although, in advanced cases, segmental and diffuse intrarenal atherosclerosis may also be observed. The second most common cause is fibromuscular dysplasia (10%). Fibromuscular dysplasia may affect the intima, media, or adventitia, although 90% of cases involve the media. It tends to affect women between 15 and 50 years of age, frequently involves the distal two-thirds of the renal artery, and is characterized by a beaded, aneurysmal appearance on angiography.

4. **What clinical criteria support the pursuit of investigative studies for suspected renovascular hypertension?**

   Although no clinical characteristics are pathognomonic of renovascular hypertension, the following findings strongly suggest the presence of an underlying renal artery stenotic lesion:
   - Hypertension in very young individuals or in women younger than 50 years of age (suggestive of fibromuscular dysplasia)
   - Rapid onset of severe hypertension after age 50 years (suggestive of atherosclerotic renal artery stenosis)
   - Hypertension refractory to three-drug regimens
   - Accelerated or malignant hypertension
   - Deterioration of renal function after the initiation of antihypertensive agents, especially angiotensin-converting enzyme (ACE) inhibitors
   - Unilateral small kidney
   - Systolic or diastolic upper abdominal or flank bruits

5. **What is the renin-angiotensin-aldosterone system (RAAS)?**

   Renin is released from the juxtaglomerular apparatus of the kidney in response to changes in renal cortical afferent arteriolar perfusion pressure and sodium concentration. Renin acts locally and in the systemic circulation to cleave angiotensinogen, a nonvasoactive α_2 globulin that is produced in the liver, to form angiotensin I. Angiotensin I undergoes enzymatic cleavage by ACE in the pulmonary circulation to produce angiotensin II, a potent vasopressor responsible for the vasoconstrictive element of renovascular hypertension. Angiotensin II increases adrenal gland production of aldosterone with subsequent retention of sodium, which acts to increase blood volume.

6. **How do ACE inhibitors work?**

   Direct inhibition of ACE decreases concentrations of angiotensin II, which leads to decreased vasopressor activity and decreased aldosterone secretion. Removal of angiotensin II mediated negative feedback on renin secretion leads to increased plasma renin activity. A similar class of drugs, angiotensin receptor blockers (ARBs), antagonizes the action of angiotensin II at the angiotensin AT1-receptor. Because there are enzymatic pathways capable of converting angiotensin I to angiotensin II independent of ACE, there is a theoretical advantage to direct inhibition of angiotensin II using ARBs.

7. **How is renovascular hypertension diagnosed?**
The gold standard for diagnosis of renal artery stenosis remains renal arteriography, which is able to evaluate not only the degree of stenosis but also directly evaluate systolic pressure gradient. However, noninvasive methods should be used first for screening. Duplex ultrasound is the most common first study; however, it is extremely operator dependent, and lack of experienced providers may limit its use in some areas. If ultrasound is unavailable, computed tomographic angiography (CTA) is the next test of choice. Magnetic resonance angiography may be used in patients who cannot tolerate the contrast or radiation involved in CTA. Captopril renal scintigraphy, selective renal vein renin measurements, and plasma renin levels (with or without captopril administration) are **not** useful as initial diagnostic tests for renal artery stenosis. Generally, stenosis of >50%–70% is considered significant. Unfortunately, the degree of stenosis does not correlate well with severity of symptoms or predict response to therapy.

8. **Should patients with renovascular hypertension be treated medically or surgically?**
In patients with symptomatic renal artery fibromuscular dysplasia, small trials demonstrate a roughly 50% cure rate with intervention, and the current standard of care is to pursue revascularization, usually by angioplasty. Surgical or percutaneous revascularization for atherosclerotic renovascular disease is more controversial. Several large, multicenter, randomized controlled trials have shown that revascularization does not improve blood pressure reduction, cardiovascular or renal outcomes, or overall mortality compared to medical therapy. However, these studies have been criticized for excluding high-risk patients. The current American Heart Association (AHA) guidelines (2006) recommend revascularization for the following patients:
- Recurrent congestive heart failure or sudden unexplained pulmonary edema (Class I)
- Unstable angina (Class IIa)
- Accelerated hypertension, malignant hypertension, resistant hypertension (Class IIa)
- Hypertension with unexplained unilateral small kidney (Class IIa)
- Hypertension with intolerance to medication (Class IIa)

9. **Should patients with renovascular hypertension undergo surgical or percutaneous revascularization?**
Small, randomized controlled trials demonstrate similar success, morbidity, and mortality rates for percutaneous transluminal renal angioplasty (PTRA) compared to surgical revascularization, and PTRA has gradually become first-line therapy over the last 10–20 years. PTRA may be performed with or without stenting; however, PTRA alone is associated with higher restenosis rates.

10. **What findings on history and physical examination should lead to a suspicion of pheochromocytoma?**
Pheochromocytomas are neuroendocrine tumors that arise from paraganglia cells derived from the neural crest. Pheochromocytomas most often (75%–85%) arise in the chromaffin cells of the adrenal medulla. Extraadrenal pheochromocytomas most commonly occur around the inferior mesenteric artery or at the aortic bifurcation in the organ of Zuckerkandl but can occur in any chromaffin tissue in the thorax, abdomen, or pelvis. Almost all pheochromocytomas produce catecholamines autonomously. About half of patients will present with sustained hypertension, but hypertension may be paroxysmal, or the patient may even be normotensive. Classically, patients describe episodes of headache, palpitations, sweating, anxiety, and flushing.

11. **How is pheochromocytoma diagnosed?**
Initial biochemical evaluation should include measurement of either plasma-free metanephrines or 24-hour urinary fractionated metanephrines. Both tests are very sensitive, and there is no consensus on which is superior. Plasma-free metanephrines may be slightly more sensitive but less specific than urine levels, so some experts recommend measuring 24-hour urine fractionated metanephrines when suspicion for a pheochromocytoma is low (resistant hypertension, hyperadrenergic spells, or incidentaloma with imaging characteristics not consistent with pheochromocytoma) and plasma-free metanephrines when pretest probability for a pheochromocytoma is high (family history, presence of a predisposing genetic syndrome, previously resected pheochromocytoma, or adrenal mass with

imaging characteristics suspicious for pheochromocytoma). Twenty-four-hour urine samples are difficult to collect but are reliable. Plasma metanephrines are simple and convenient but must be drawn while the patient is supine, 15–20 minutes after intravenous catheter insertion to minimize false positive results. If metanephrine levels are normal, no further workup is required; if greatly elevated (>4× normal) the diagnosis of a pheochromocytoma is highly likely. Low levels of elevated metanephrines (1–3× normal) should undergo repeat testing or may be confirmed by a clonidine suppression test if required. Clonidine suppression testing is done by measuring plasma normetanephrine both before and 3 hours after clonidine administration. Elevated normetanephrine levels or a decrease of <40% from baseline confirms the diagnosis. The diagnosis of pheochromocytoma should be followed by studies to localize the tumor.

12. **What is the best test to localize a pheochromocytoma?**
Adrenal protocol computed tomography (CT) is the first-line imaging modality once the diagnosis of pheochromocytoma is established. CT scans are highly sensitive (88%–100%) and are usually the only imaging study required to localize lesions and plan for resection. Magnetic resonance imaging (MRI) should be used as the initial imaging study in patients with known metastatic disease, skull base and neck paragangliomas, the presence of surgical clips causing artifact on CT, contrast allergy, or in patients in whom radiation exposure should be limited. MRI has superior sensitivity for extraadrenal tumors with most pheochromocytomas enhancing on T2-weighted imaging. If no tumor is found in the abdomen, CT of the chest and neck should be performed. CT is preferred over MRI in this case because of better resolution in the lungs on CT. If the tumor still cannot be localized, I^{131}-metaiodobenzylguanidine (MIBG) imaging should be used. MIBG is a functional imaging modality that uses a radiolabeled norepinephrine analog that is taken up by sympathoadrenergic tissues. MIBG is recommended for patients with known metastatic disease, for patients with increased risk of metastatic disease (large tumor size, extraadrenal, multifocal, or recurrent disease), or for occult tumors that cannot be visualized on CT or MRI.

13. **Describe the perioperative management of patients with pheochromocytoma**
All patients with functional pheochromocytoma should receive appropriate preoperative medical management to block the effect of catecholamine release during surgical removal of the tumor. There is no clear consensus regarding the preferred drug and clinical practice varies widely. The main goal of preoperative management is to normalize blood pressure, heart rate, and volume status, and prevent the effects of catecholamine storm during surgery. Most commonly, alpha-blockade with phenoxybenzamine, a nonselective alpha-blocker, is employed, although selective agents such as prazosin, terazosin, or doxazosin are alternatives. Calcium channel blockers have been used as an alternative at some centers with good results. Tachyarrhythmias may be treated with beta-blocking agents but should never be given without concurrent alpha-blockade, as this will result in unopposed alpha vasoconstriction, which may precipitate worsening hypertension, end-organ malperfusion, and heart failure. Whatever the chosen agent, preoperative therapy should begin well before the operation (7–14 days) and should also include salt loading and increased fluid intake to normalize volume status prior to surgery.

14. **Should patients with pheochromocytoma be referred for genetic testing?**
Pheochromocytomas are associated with multiple genetic mutations and familial syndromes, most commonly, multiple endocrine neoplasia type 2 syndrome, von Recklinghausen disease/neurofibromatosis type 1, and von Hippel-Lindau disease. About 25% of presumably sporadic pheochromocytomas are found to have a germline mutation. While most experts do not recommend genetic testing for every patient, patients with concern for a clinical syndrome, extraadrenal tumors, multiple tumors, and age <45 years should be considered. In particular, patients with paragangliomas should be tested for mutations in succinate dehydrogenase (SDH), and patients with metastatic disease should be tested for mutations in SDH subunit B (SDH B).

15. **How is primary hyperaldosteronism (Conn's syndrome) diagnosed and treated?**
Conn's syndrome, which results from autonomous mineralocorticoid hypersecretion, is characterized by hypertension, hypokalemia, hypernatremia, metabolic alkalosis, and periodic muscle weakness and paralysis. It is most often caused by an aldosterone-secreting adenoma but may also be caused by bilateral adrenal hyperplasia. Initial evaluation should include measurement of morning plasma aldosterone concentration (PAC) and plasma renin activity (PRA). The diagnosis of primary aldosteronism is suspected if the PAC/PRA ratio is >20 and PAC is >15 ng/dL. In patients with spontaneous hypokalemia, undetectable PRA, and PAC >20 ng/dL, the diagnosis is confirmed. However, in most

patients, the diagnosis must be confirmed by further testing, such as an oral sodium loading test or saline infusion test. Persistently high aldosterone levels despite a large sodium challenge confirm the diagnosis. Once the diagnosis of primary aldosteronism is confirmed, patients should undergo adrenal CT to differentiate unilateral versus bilateral primary aldosteronism. Adrenal vein sampling (AVS) is done to confirm unilateral disease amendable to surgery. Some experts advocate for selectively performing AVS. In young patients (<35 years) with marked aldosterone excess and unilateral adrenal lesions, no further workup is necessary. However, most advocate for routinely performing AVS, and certainly patients over 35 years old with bilateral adrenal abnormality should undergo AVS. Patients with unilateral disease should undergo adrenalectomy when possible. Patients with bilateral disease, or those unable or unwilling to undergo surgery should be treated with a mineralocorticoid antagonist, most commonly spironolactone.

16. **Why does Cushing's syndrome cause hypertension?**
In the cardiovascular system, glucocorticoids produce increased cardiac chronotropic and inotropic effects, along with an increased peripheral vascular resistance. Receptors in the distal renal tubules respond to glucocorticoids by increasing tubular resorption of sodium. These receptors belong to a different class from receptors that mediate the more potent actions of aldosterone.

17. **What findings suggest aortic coarctation?**
Lower blood pressure in the legs than in the arms and diminished or absent femoral pulses may suggest coarctation of the aorta. Rib notching may be evident on chest radiograph in patients with longstanding, hemodynamically significant coarctation. Bruits may be heard over the chest or abdominal wall. Adults may even develop congestive heart failure and renal failure.

18. **How does aortic coarctation cause hypertension?**
No single cause has been identified. Mechanical obstruction to ventricular ejection is one component that leads to upper extremity hypertension. Hypoperfusion of the kidneys with resulting activation of the RAAS probably contributes. Abnormal aortic compliance, variable capacity of collateral vessels, and abnormal setting of baroreceptors have also been implicated.

KEY POINTS: SURGICAL HYPERTENSION

1. The causes of surgically correctable hypertension include renovascular hypertension, pheochromocytoma, Cushing's syndrome, Conn's syndrome, coarctation of the aorta, and unilateral renal parenchymal disease.
2. The most common cause of renovascular hypertension is atherosclerosis.
3. The diagnosis of pheochromocytoma is confirmed by measurement of plasma-free or 24-hour urine fractionated metanephrines.
4. Conn's syndrome is characterized by hypertension, hypokalemia, hypernatremia, metabolic alkalosis, and periodic muscle weakness and paralysis.

BIBLIOGRAPHY

1. Bloch MJ, Basile J. Diagnosis and management of renovascular disease and renovascular hypertension. *J Clin Hypertens (Greenwich)*. 2007;9(5):381–389.
2. Vongpatanasin W. Resistant hypertension: a review of diagnosis and management. *JAMA*. 2014;311(21):2216–2224.
3. Anderson GH, Blakeman N. The effect of age on prevalence of secondary forms of hypertension in 4429 consecutively referred patients. *J Hyperten*. 1994;12(5):609–615.
4. Safian RD, Textor SC. Renal-artery stenosis. *N Engl J Med*. 2001;344(6):431–342.
5. Hirsch AT, Haskal ZJ, Hertzer NR, et al. ACC/AHA 2005 Guidelines for the management of patients with peripheral arterial disease (lower extremity, renal, mesenteric, and abdominal aortic): a collaborative report from the American Association for Vascular Surgery/Society for Vascular Surgery, Society for Cardiovascular Angiography and Interventions, Society for Vascular Medicine and Biology, Society of Interventional Radiology, and the ACC/AHA Task Force on Practice Guidelines (Writing Committee to Develop Guidelines for the Management of Patients With Peripheral Arterial Disease) endorsed by the American Association of Cardiovascular and Pulmonary Rehabilitation; National Heart, Lung, and Blood Institute; Society for Vascular Nursing; TransAtlantic Inter-Society Consensus; and Vascular Disease Foundation. *J Am Coll Cardiol*. 2006;47(6):e1–e192.
6. Herrmann SM, Saad A. Management of atherosclerotic renovascular disease after cardiovascular outcomes in renal atherosclerotic lesions (CORAL). *Nephrol Dial Transplant*. 2015;30(3):366–375.
7. Mousa AY, Gill G. Renal fibromuscular dysplasia. *Semin Vasc Surg*. 2013;26(4):213–218.

8. Kiernan CM, Solórzano CC. Pheochromocytoma and paraganglioma: diagnosis, genetics, and treatment. *Surg Oncol Clin N Am*. 2016;25(1):119–138.
9. Mittendorf EA, Evans DB. Pheochromocytoma: advances in genetics, diagnosis, localization, and treatment. *Hematol Oncol Clin North Am*. 2007;21(3):509–525.
10. Lenders JW, Duh QY, Eisenhofer G. Pheochromocytoma and paraganglioma: an endocrine society clinical practice guideline. *J Clin Endocrinol Metab*. 2014;99(6):1915–1942.
11. Rossi GP, Pessina AC. Primary aldosteronism: an update on screening, diagnosis and treatment. *J Hypertens*. 2008;26(4):613–621.
12. Funder FW, Carey RM, Mantero F. The management of primary aldosteronism: case detection, diagnosis, and treatment: an Endocrine Society clinical practice guideline. *J Clin Endocrinol Metab*. 2016;101(5):1889–1916.
13. Torok RD, Campbell MJ, Fleming GA, Hill KD. Coarctation of the aorta: management from infancy to adulthood. *World J Cardiol*. 2015;7(11):765–775.

CHAPTER 64

ADRENAL INCIDENTALOMA

Maria B. Albuja-Cruz, MD, FACS, Christopher D. Raeburn, MD, FACS,
Robert C. McIntyre, Jr., MD

1. **What is the arterial and venous anatomy of the adrenal gland?**
   There are two adrenal glands, each located in the retroperitoneum superior to the kidneys. The blood supply consists of three arteries: The superior adrenal artery that is a branch of the inferior phrenic artery, the middle adrenal artery that is a branch of the abdominal aorta, and the inferior adrenal artery that is a branch of the renal artery. The main central vein on the right usually exits the upper one-third of the gland and drains directly to the vena cava. The left central vein is longer and drains to the left renal vein. In addition to the central veins, a series of small veins parallels the arteries.

2. **What are the layers of the adrenal and what hormones are produced in each layer?**
   The cortex has three distinct zones: The zona glomerulosa adjacent to the outer capsule where aldosterone is produced; the zona fasciculata that produces glucocorticoids (cortisol) and some sex steroids; and the zona reticularis that is adjacent to the medulla and produces cortisol, androgens, and estrogens.
   - **G**lomerulosa salt (aldosterone)
   - **F**asciculata sugar (cortisol)
   - **R**eticularis sex (androgens and estrogens)
   The medulla is derived from neural crest cells, acts as a sympathetic ganglion, and secretes catecholamines, specifically, norepinephrine, epinephrine, and dopamine.

3. **What is an adrenal incidentaloma?**
   An incidental adrenal tumor (incidentaloma) is an unsuspected adrenal mass of 1 cm or more in diameter discovered by imaging performed for another indication. Adrenal incidentalomas are found in approximately 5% of patients undergoing abdominal imaging, with peak prevalence in the sixth and seventh decades of life. The definition of incidentaloma excludes patients undergoing imaging procedures as part of staging and workup for cancer. Detection of an adrenal incidentaloma warrants clinical, biochemical, and radiologic evaluation to establish its secretory status and risk of malignancy.

4. **What three questions should be answered when an adrenal tumor is identified?**
   a. Is the tumor hormonally hyperactive?
   b. Does it have imaging characteristic concerning for primary adrenal malignancy (adrenocortical carcinoma [ACC])?
   c. Does the patient have a history of a prior malignancy?

5. **What is the differential diagnosis of an incidental adrenal tumor?**
   The differential diagnosis of an adrenal incidentaloma are as follows:
   - Nonfunctioning adenomas (80%)
   - Cortisol-producing adenoma (5%)
   - Pheochromocytoma (PHEO) (5%)
   - Aldosterone-producing adenoma (1%)
   - ACC (<5%)
   - Metastatic lesion (2.5%)
   - If past history of cancer 32%–73%
   - Other: Ganglioneuromas, myelolipomas and benign cysts

6. **What is the initial biochemical workup to determine if an incidentaloma is hormonally hyperfunctioning?**
   1. Plasma metanephrines and normetanephrines or 24-hour urine metanephrines and fractionated catecholamines
      Diagnostic of PHEO if greater than fourfold above upper reference range

2.   Serum potassium and ratio of plasma aldosterone concentration (PAC) to plasma renin activity (PRA) **only** if patient has hypertension with or without hypokalemia
     Suggestive of an aldosterone-producing tumor if PAC >15 ng/dL and PAC/PRA >20
3.   One-milligram overnight dexamethasone suppression test
     Suspicious for a cortisol-producing tumor if a.m. serum cortisol >5 μg/dL

7. **What is the next step in management of a nonhyperfunctioning adrenal incidentaloma?**
   Adrenal incidentalomas >4 cm should undergo adrenalectomy. Adrenal incidentalomas <4 cm should be reimaged in 3–6 months and then annually for 1–2 years; functional studies should be repeated annually for 5 years. If mass grows more than 1 cm or becomes hormonally hyperactive then adrenalectomy is recommended. The risk of an adrenal mass becoming hormonally hyperactive during 1, 2, and 5 years is 17%, 29%, and 47%, respectively. The most common hormonally active lesions in patients with previously nonhyperfunctioning incidentalomas is subclinical Cushing's syndrome.

8. **What are the common clinical features of PHEO?**
   PHEOs are rare neuroendocrine tumors that arise from the chromaffin cells of the adrenal gland and produce excessive amounts of one or more catecholamines: norepinephrine, epinephrine, and dopamine. Paragangliomas (PGLs), the extraadrenal counterparts of PHEO arise from ganglia along the sympathetic and parasympathetic chain. The five Ps of the paroxysm are:
   * Pressure (high blood pressure)
   * Pain (headaches)
   * Perspiration (profuse)
   * Palpitations
   * Pallor

   PHEO/PGL are a rare cause of secondary hypertension, with an incidence in hypertensive patients of about 0.2%–0.6%. About 15% of patients with a PHEO have no history of hypertension.

9. **Does the rule of 10 in relation to PHEO still hold true?**
   No. Based on new research findings, it is now known that up to 35% of PHEO/PGL are hereditary, and therefore genetic testing is recommended for all patients with PHEO/PGL.
   Also, it has been found that up to 17% of PHEO/PGL are malignant. Mutations in the gene encoding succinate dehydrogenase subunit B (SDHB) can lead to metastatic disease in >40% of patients. For these reasons, lifelong annual biochemical testing to assess for recurrent or metastatic PHEO is recommended. Furthermore, up to 20% of PHEO/PGL arise in childhood.

10. **What are the most common genetic disorders associated with PHEO/PGL?**
    * **Multiple endocrine neoplasia type 2 (MEN2)** is caused by mutations in the rearranged during transfection protooncogene.
    * Medullary thyroid cancer (MTC) is usually the presenting diagnosis for MEN2 patients. MEN2 is subdivided into MEN2A, MEN2B, and familial MTC.
    * MEN2A have a 95% chance of developing MTC, a 50% chance of PHEO and a 15%–30% chance of primary hyperparathyroidism. (Three Cs: catecholamines, calcium, calcitonin.)
    * MEN2B have a 100% chance of developing MTC and a 50% chance of PHEO, but also present with marfanoid body habitus and mucosal ganglioneuromas.
    * Familial MTC have no risk of developing PHEO.
    * **von Hippel-Lindau (VHL) syndrome** is caused by mutations in the VHL tumor suppressor gene.
    * Patients with this syndrome are predisposed to multiple types of tumors. VHL is subclassified based on the risk of PHEO/PGL.
    * VHL type 1 is the most common form, and patients have no risk of developing PHEO/PGL. Patients with VHL type 1 develop retinal angiomas, central nervous system (CNS) hemangioblastomas, renal cell carcinomas (RCC), islet cell tumor of the pancreas, endolymphatic cell tumors, cyst or cystadenomas of the kidney, pancreas, epididymis, or broad ligament.
    * VHL type 2 patients have a 10%–20% chance of PHEO/PGL and are further subdivided into type 2A (without RCC and infrequent type 1 tumors), type 2B (with RCC or any type 1 tumors) and type C (only PHEO/PGL).
    * **Neurofibromatosis type 1 (NF1) syndrome** is caused by germline mutation in the NF1 gene.
    * Patients with NF1 have <6% chance of developing PHEO/PGL. NF1 syndrome is characterized by neurofibromas and multiple café au lait spots, iris hamartomas (Lisch nodules), and CNS gliomas.

- **Familial PGL syndrome** is caused by mutation in one of the succinate dehydrogenase (SDH) subunit (A, B, C, D) genes.
- Patients with this syndrome are predisposed to develop PGL throughout the body. Succinate dehydrogenase subunit B mutations are the most common and are associated with more aggressive tumors (SDH**B** = bad), younger age at presentation, and higher rate of metastasis.

11. **What is the biochemical workup for a PHEO/PGL?**

The biochemical diagnosis of PHEO/PGL is made by measuring plasma-free metanephrines or 24-hour urinary fractionated metanephrines. The blood sample for plasma metanephrines should be obtained in a supine position after patient has been fully recumbent for at least 30 minutes. Elevated more than threefold above upper limit of normal is highly diagnostic of PHEO/PGL.

Medications such as acetaminophen, antidepressant medications, some antihypertensive medications, cocaine, and other common medications can result in mildly or markedly raised values in biochemical testing (false positive results). It is recommended to stop these medications, if possible, for 2 weeks and then repeat the biochemical testing. Also, foods such as caffeine can cause elevations in catecholamines and metanephrines and should be avoided before repeating testing.

Clonidine suppression test is a useful method for patients with equivocal results in plasma and/or urine metanephrines as it distinguishes true-positive from false-positive borderline elevations. Clonidine normally suppresses the release of norepinephrine from sympathetic nerve endings but does not affect the catecholamine secretion from a PHEO. Clonidine suppression test is indicative of PHE/PGL, if plasma normetanephrines remain elevated 3 hours after the administration of clonidine and there is <40% decrease in normetanephrines level compare to baseline.

Chromogranin A (CgA) is a nonspecific marker of neuroendocrine tumors and is commonly measured in patients with PHEO/PGL. CgA is a valuable marker for monitoring disease, and it is elevated in 91% of patients with PHEO/PGL.

12. **What biochemical testing should be done first: Plasma metanephrines or 24-hour urine fractioned metanephrines?**

The choice of biochemical testing for PHEO/PGL should be directed by the pretest level of suspicion for disease.

- **Twenty-four–hour urine fractionated metanephrines** is the test of choice for low-risk patients (low pretest probability) for PHEO/PGL. Low-risk patients are those who are being tested for sporadic PHEO based on having poorly control hypertension, flushing spells, palpitations, and/or an incidental adrenal mass with imaging characteristics consistent with a adrenocortical mass. In these settings, the 24-hour urine metanephrines have a good sensitivity and a significantly better specificity than plasma-free metanephrines.
- **Plasma-free metanephrines** is the test of choice for high-risk patients (high pretest probability) for PHEO/PGL. High-risk patients are those who are being tested for PHEO/PGL because the presence of a vascular adrenal mass, genetic syndrome (MEN2, VHL, NF1, familial PGL syndrome), past history of PHEO/PGL, family history of PHEO/PGL, imaging study suspicious for PHEO. In these settings, the plasma metanephrines have a good specificity and a significantly higher sensitivity than 24-hour urine metanephrines. For pediatric patients, plasma-free metanephrines is the test of choice because of the difficulties in collecting a 24-hour urine sample.

13. **What imaging studies should be obtained to localize a PHEO/PGL?**

Once there is clear biochemical evidence of PHEO/PGL, contrast computed tomography (CT) scan of the abdomen and pelvis should be the first-choice imaging modality. MRI is recommended in patients with metastatic PHEO/PGL, for detection of skull-base and neck PGLs. MRI is also useful in patients with surgical clips, patients allergic to CT contrast, and patients in whom radiation exposure should be limited (pregnant women, children, patient with known germline mutations).

In patients with biochemical proof of PHEO/PGL and a negative abdominal imaging, consider CT of the neck and chest.

14. **How should a patient with a PHEO/PGL be prepared for surgery?**

All patients with hormonally hyperfunctioning PHEO/PGL should undergo preoperative alpha adrenergic blockade for 7–14 days in order to avoid profoundly unstable intraoperative blood pressure. Classic nonselective long-acting alpha-adrenergic blockade is phenoxybenzamine. Therapy is started at 10 mg twice daily and the dosage is titrated up to achieve goals of treatment. Short-acting alpha-adrenergic blockade (prazosin, doxazosin, terazosin) and calcium channel blockers (nicardipine) are alternative options.

Preoperative beta-adrenergic receptor blockers are indicated for those patients who have tachycardia, only after the administration of alpha-adrenergic blockade. Propranolol (10–40 mg every 6–8 hours) is the most commonly used beta-blocker in this scenario.

Goals of treatment are a blood pressure <130/80 seated and more than 90 systolic blood pressure when standing; heart rate of 60–70 seated and 70–80 standing.

Liberal fluid and salt intake is another important component in the preoperative management of patients with PHEO/PGL because they have intravascular volume depletion.

15. What are the surgical options for the management of PHEO/PGL?
Surgical resection is the only chance for cure for patients with PHEO/PGL. For unilateral PHEO <6 cm, minimally invasive adrenalectomy is recommended. Minimally invasive adrenalectomy can be performed transperitoneally or retroperitoneally depending on surgeon's preference and expertise.

For unilateral PHEO >6 cm or invasive PHEO, open adrenalectomy is recommended to assure complete resection of tumor, prevent tumor rupture, and avoid local recurrence.

For bilateral PHEOs or recurrent PHEO in contralateral adrenal gland after prior adrenalectomy, cortical-sparing adrenalectomy is a good option with a low risk of recurrence (approximately 7%).

For PGLs, laparoscopic resection is a good option for small tumors that are in favorable locations and noninvasive.

16. What are the major complications during the perioperative and postoperative period for patients undergoing surgical resection of PHEO/PGL?
The major potential complications in the perioperative and postoperative period are hypertension, hypotension, and hypoglycemia. During the perioperative period, it is paramount to have great communication with anesthesia when manipulating the tumor and when ready to ligate adrenal vein so they are prepared to manage possible severe blood pressure changes. Hypertension can be managed with antihypertensive medications such as nitroprusside, nicardipine, nitroglycerin, or phentolamine. Severe hypotension is managed primarily with large-volume intravenous fluid; some patients may require alpha-adrenergic agonist such as epinephrine. Postoperatively, blood pressure, heart rate, and plasma glucose levels should be closely monitored for 24–48 hours.

17. What is the function of aldosterone?
Aldosterone is the principle mineralocorticoid. It increases sodium (Na) and water resorption by the kidney in exchange for potassium or hydrogen. Aldosterone release is stimulated by angiotensin II, which is derived from the renin-mediated conversion of angiotensinogen to angiotensin I that is converted to angiotensin II by angiotensin-converting enzyme (ACE). Renin release from the kidney is stimulated by hypovolemia, beta-adrenergic stimulation, and prostaglandins. Hyponatremia and hyperkalemia directly stimulate aldosterone secretion. Aldosterone secretion is also stimulated by adrenocorticotropic hormone (ACTH). Because ACTH has diurnal variation, aldosterone and cortisol levels vary depending on the time of the day.

18. What is primary hyperaldosteronism?
Primary hyperaldosteronism (PA), also known as Conn's disease, is a clinical syndrome characterized by drug resistance and refractory hypertension (need >3 antihypertensive agents) along with spontaneous hypokalemia (serum potassium <3.5 mEq/L) or severe (<3 mEq/L) diuretic-induced hypokalemia. However, the majority of patients with PA have normal serum potassium levels and only a minority (9%–37%) are hypokalemic. Most patients with PA have either an aldosterone-producing adenoma (APA; 30%–40%) or bilateral adrenal hyperplasia (60%–65%). Less common causes include unilateral hyperplasia (2%), ACC (<1%), and rare familial form of PA (<1%).

19. Who should be screened for PA?
- Any patient with hypertension and hypokalemia (spontaneous or diuretic-induced hypokalemia).
- All patients with drug-resistant hypertension.
- Patients with hypertension and an adrenal incidentaloma. It is not necessary to screen normotensive patients with an adrenal incidentaloma for PA.
- Any patient in whom the physician is considering secondary hypertension.

20. **How do you screen for PA?**

Determining the ratio of plasma aldosterone concentration (PAC; ng/dL) to plasma renin activity (PRA; ng/mL). A PAC/PRA ratio >20 and a PAC >15 ng/dL is suggestive of PA. Patients must be off diuretics, beta-blockers, and ACE inhibitors for 4 weeks. Prior to blood sample, patients should have liberalization of sodium intake and be given potassium supplements to correct hypokalemia if present. Sample should be collected in the morning after patient has been up for 2 hours and seated for 5–15 minutes.

21. **What is the confirmatory testing for PA?**

If a positive screening test is obtained, PA can be confirmed by demonstrating lack of suppression of aldosterone levels after salt loading. This can be done in one of the following ways:

a. **Saline suppression test:** PAC is measured after 2 L/4 h of IV 0.9% NS. A PAC >10 ng/dL is confirmatory of PA.

b. **Oral salt loading test:** Patients are instructed to add one flat teaspoon of salt to their daily food intake and consume salty foods for 72 hours. During the third day, 24-hour urine is performed for aldosterone, sodium, and creatinine measurement. Twenty-four–hour urine aldosterone >12 μg/day is diagnostic of PA.

22. **How do you image the patient with primary hyperaldosteronism?**

Once the biochemical diagnosis of PA has been made, the priority is to distinguish between unilateral versus bilateral sources of aldosterone excess. Adrenal protocol CT scan provides anatomic information important for surgical planning and may demonstrate a unilateral adenoma. However, anatomic imaging is incapable of determining the functionality of each gland and therefore is unable to discriminate between unilateral versus bilateral sources of aldosterone excess. The gold standard test, and an essential step to make this discrimination, is adrenal vein sampling (AVS). AVS changes the management of PA based on CT in up to 25% of patients. AVS is done under cosyntropic stimulation. Then the corrected aldosterone/cortisol ratios (aldosterone/cortisol ratio of one side to aldosterone/cortisol ratio of the other side) of >4:1 are indicative of a unilateral source of aldosterone excess.

23. **What is the treatment of PA?**

Patients who are appropriate surgical candidates with unequivocal unilateral source of aldosterone excess (as determined by AVS) should undergo unilateral laparoscopic adrenalectomy.

Large aldosterone-producing tumors (>4 cm) should raise concern for ACC and therefore undergo open adrenalectomy.

Patients with bilateral involvement should be managed with medical therapy, as they respond poorly to surgery (even with bilateral adrenalectomy, cure rates are <20%). Spironolactone (12.5–50 mg/day) is the first-line therapy and the most effective treatment.

24. **What are the outcomes of unilateral adrenalectomy for PA?**

Patients with unilateral source of aldosterone excess can expect a 100% cure of hypokalemia, >90% will show significant improvement in hypertension, and 30%–60% will be able to discontinue all antihypertensive medications. Factors that suggest a favorable outcome include young age, shorter duration of hypertension, fewer antihypertensive medications, a good response to spironolactone, female, and less severe hypertension.

25. **How can one predict the resolution of hypertension after adrenalectomy for PA?**

The Aldosterone Resolution Score (ARS) accurately identifies individuals at low (ARS ≤1) or high (ARS ≥4) likelihood of complete resolution of hypertension without further need of lifelong antihypertensive medications after adrenalectomy for aldosteronoma.

	Points	
Predictor	**Present**	**Absent**
No. antihypertensive medications <2	2	0
Body mass index <25	1	0
Years of hypertension <6	1	0
Female	1	0
Total[a]	5	0

[a]Possible score range 0– 5.

26. **What is Cushing's syndrome?**
Cushing's syndrome results from chronic exposure to excess glucocorticoids from either exogenous pharmacologic doses of corticosteroids or from an endogenous source of cortisol. Clinical features include:
    - Obesity, especially truncal, moon facies, and buffalo hump (dorsocervical fat pad)
    - Thin skin, striae, and hirsutism
    - Muscle weakness and wasting
    - Hypertension
    - Menstrual irregularity
    - Osteoporosis
    - Pancreatitis
    - Increased infection risk
    - Depression

27. **How is Cushing's syndrome different from Cushing's disease?**
Cushing's disease is a pituitary tumor releasing ACTH that stimulates the release of cortisol from the adrenal gland. Cushing's syndrome is the clinical manifestation of the excess cortisol despite the etiology.

28. **What are the causes of Cushing's syndrome?**
    - Exogenous steroid administration. Overall this is the most common cause of Cushing's syndrome.
    - Endogenous Cushing's syndrome is divided between ACTH-dependent (about 80%) and ACTH-independent (about 20%).
        - ACTH-dependent form includes:
            - ACTH-secreting pituitary adenoma (Cushing's disease), by far most common
            - Ectopic (nonpituitary) ACTH producing tumors (small cell lung carcinoma, lung carcinoid, MTC, PHEO)
        - ACTH-independent form includes:
            - Unilateral cortisol-producing adrenal adenomas
            - ACCs
            - Bilateral macronodular adrenal hyperplasia
            - Primary pigmented nodular adrenocortical disease
            - Isolated micronodular adrenocortical disease.

29. **What is the diagnosis modality for Cushing's syndrome?**
Testing is based on demonstrating three pathophysiologic derangements typical of Cushing's syndrome.
    a. Loss of a normal diurnal pattern (late-night salivary cortisol): Elevated nighttime cortisol levels appear to be the earliest and most sensitive marker for Cushing's syndrome. Sensitivity and specificity >90%–95%.
    b. Loss of sensitivity to glucocorticoid negative feedback (low-dose dexamethasone suppression test): 1 mg of dexamethasone is given orally at 11:00 p.m. and serum cortisol is measured at 8:00 a.m. the next morning. Suppression of plasma cortisol to <1.8 μg/dL has the best negative predictor value for Cushing's syndrome. Positive test should be followed by 24-hour urine cortisol, late-night salivary cortisol, or 2-day low-dose dexamethasone suppression test.
    c. Excess production of cortisol (24-hour urine free cortisol): 24-hour urinary-free cortisol that is more than four times the normal value is considered diagnostic of Cushing's syndrome. Up to threefold elevations can be associated with pseudo-Cushing's syndrome (chronic anxiety, depression, alcoholism, obesity), therefore confirmatory testing is needed.

    Next, ACTH is measured in the plasma. A suppressed plasma ACTH is sufficient to identify patients with an autonomous cortisol-secreting adrenal tumor. After ACTH-independent Cushing's syndrome is confirmed, a CT scan should be performed to determine the source of adrenal cortisol hypersecretion.

30. **What considerations should be taken when performing adrenalectomy for cortisol-producing adrenal adenomas?**
Preoperatively, one should assure that patients' diabetes and hypertension are adequately treated. Patients with Cushing's syndrome have an increased relative risk for thromboembolic complications, thus measures should be implemented to prevent this complication.

There is no need for glucocorticoid replacement intraoperatively in patients with Cushing's syndrome. However, patients with Cushing's syndrome have a suppressed hypothalamic-pituitary-adrenal (HPA) access leading to atrophy of the contralateral gland. Therefore, after adrenalectomy for cortisol-producing adrenal adenomas, patients may require glucocorticoid replacement to prevent sudden and potentially lethal adrenal insufficiency. Cosyntropin stimulation test can be done on postoperative day 1 to determine the need for glucocorticoid replacement after adrenalectomy. On postoperative day 1, a basal cortisol level and ACTH should be checked, and a serum cortisol level should be drawn 60 minutes after administration of cosyntropin 250 μg IV. Patients do not need glucocorticoid replacement if basal cortisol is >5 μg/dL, stimulated cortisol is >18 μg/dL, and the patient has no clinical symptoms of adrenal insufficiency. On the other hand, the patient will need glucocorticoid replacement if basal cortisol is ≤5 μg/dL, or stimulated cortisol is ≤18 μg/dL, or patient has clinical symptoms of adrenal insufficiency.

The time for the HPA axis to recover varies from 6–18 months. Cosyntropin stimulation studies are done every 3–6 months to determine when steroids can be discontinued.

31. **What is the outcome of resection of adrenal cortisol-producing adenomas?**
Adrenalectomy results in excellent improvement in the symptoms of Cushing's syndrome and improves patient quality of life. Hypertension and diabetes will resolve in 65%–80% of patients. The physical changes of Cushing's syndrome will resolve in 85%. These improvements take 6–12 months to occur.

32. **What are the determinants of long-term survival for patients with ACC?**
ACC is a rare and highly aggressive malignancy. Tumor stage at presentation and curative resection by an experienced surgeon are the two determinants of long-term survival.

33. **What is the clinical presentation of patients with ACC?**
Most patients with ACC (50%–60%) seek medical advice because of evidence of adrenal steroid hormone excess. In functional ACC, signs and symptoms of Cushing's syndrome are the most frequent presentation. Cushing's syndrome develops rapidly and dramatically over a few months. A high percentage of women with ACC develop signs and symptoms of androgen excess (which leads to virilization with acne, hirsutism, and oligomenorrhea) with or without concomitant Cushing's syndrome. Estrogen (which leads to feminization with gynecomastia, loss of libido, and testicular atrophy) or aldosterone (hypertension, hypokalemia) excess occurs in <10% of cases. Patients with nonsecreting tumors may present with abdominal pain or only an incidental adrenal mass (>15% of ACC).

34. **What imaging features are concerning for ACC?**
Size of an adrenal mass remains the single best indicator of malignancy. Tumors <4 cm have a 2% risk of malignancy; from 4.1–6 cm a 6% risk of malignancy, and >6 cm a 25% risk of malignancy.

ACC have irregular boards and are inhomogeneous with evidence of necrosis or hemorrhage. ACC have an attenuation of >10 Hounsfield units (HU) on unenhanced CT scan, and delayed postcontrast CT scan typically shows an enhancement washout of <50% and a delayed (after 10–15 min) attenuation of >35 HU. By MRI, they are hyperintense compared to the liver on T2 images.

Evidence of metastatic disease to liver plus a large adrenal mass should raise concern for ACC.

35. **What is the role of percutaneous biopsy in the evaluation of an adrenal tumor?**
There is almost no role for percutaneous biopsy in the diagnostic workup of an adrenal tumor because it cannot differentiate an adrenal adenoma from a carcinoma, and the violation of the tumor capsule may promote needle track metastases. Therefore, percutaneous biopsy is reserved for patients who have a prior history of cancer to evaluate for metastasis and is performed only if the result will influence therapy. It is always necessary to exclude PHEO first.

36. **What is the treatment of ACC?**
Complete surgical resection is the treatment of choice for nonmetastatic ACC, and it is virtually the only chance for cure. Open adrenalectomy is the procedure of choice. En-bloc resection of involved adrenal gland and surrounding tissues (kidney, liver, inferior vena cava, pancreas, stomach, or spleen) should be performed as well as lymphadenectomy. It is paramount to leave the tumor capsule intact during resection to reduce local recurrence. Recurrence rate is high in patients undergoing primary resection, 30%–50% with complete resection (R0), and up to 80% in patients with incomplete resection (microscopic disease at surgical margins, R1).

Adjuvant mitotane treatment after complete resection is recommended for patients with potential residual disease (R1 or RX resection), and in patients with R0 resection but high-risk disease (ki-67 index >10%).

Adjuvant external beam radiation therapy of the tumor bed is recommended for patients with incomplete surgical resection (R1/RX).

Surgery is also recommended in patients with metastatic ACC if radical resection seems feasible.

In patients not amenable to surgery, mitotane (alone or in combination with cytotoxic drugs) remains the treatment of choice. Commonly used cytotoxic agents include etoposide, doxorubicin, cisplatin, and streptozotocin.

Overall, 5-year survival for patients with ACC is 37%–47%, approximately 65% for patients with stage I and II, and 24% and 0% for patients with stages III and IV, respectively.

37. **What type of tumors metastasize to the adrenal gland?**
Metastatic disease to the adrenal gland is rarely found in patients without a history of a known malignancy. Lung, breast, stomach, kidney, melanoma, and lymphoma commonly metastasize to the adrenal glands.

38. **What are the causes of adrenal hemorrhage (AH)?**
AH is a rare yet potentially life-threatening event. It is classically associated with the Waterhouse-Friderichsen syndrome of meningococcal septicemia, but it has occurred in Pseudomonas infection, *Staphylococcus aureus*, Klebsiella species, *Escherichia coli,* and *Proteus bacteremia*. The most common cause of AH is trauma (accounts for 80% of cases of AH), yet the incidence of traumatic AH is 0.03%–4.95%. AH may also result from acute stress (surgery, sepsis, burns, hypotension, and pregnancy), anticoagulation, coagulopathy, neonatal stress, idiopathic disease, or underlying adrenal tumor. PHEO is the most common cause of massive bleeding from a primary adrenal tumor and can be lethal in up to 50% of the cases. Most cases of HA are unilateral and carry a benign clinical course. However, it is important to recognize cases of massive bilateral AH that have the potential to cause adrenal insufficiency.

BIBLIOGRAPHY

1. Libe R, Dall'Asta C. Long-term follow-up study of patients with adrenal incidentalomas. *Eur J Endocrinol.* 2002;147(4):489–494.
2. Ioachimescu AG, Remer EM. Adrenal incidentalomas: a disease of modern technology offering opportunities for improved patient care. *Endocrinol Metab Clin North Am.* 2015;44(2):335–354.
3. Yip L, Tublin ME, Falcone JA, et al. The adrenal mass: correlation of histopathology with imaging. *Ann Surg Oncol.* 2009;17(3):846–852.
4. Zeiger M, Thompson G, Duh Q-Y, et al. American Association of Clinical Endocrinologists and American Association of Endocrine Surgeons medical guidelines for the management of adrenal incidentalomas. *Endocr Pract.* 2009; 15(suppl 1):1–20.
5. Lenders JW, Duh QY, Eisenhofer G, et al. Pheochromocytoma and paraganglioma: an Endocrine Society clinical practice guideline. *J Clin Endocrinol Metab.* 2014;99(6):1915–1942.
6. Martucci VL, Pacak K. Pheochromocytoma and paraganglioma: diagnosis, genetics, management, and treatment. *Curr Probl Cancer.* 2014;38(1):7–41.
7. Hodin R, Lubitz C. Diagnosis and management of pheochromocytoma. *Curr Probl Surg.* 2014;51(4):151–87.
8. Kudva YC, Sawka AM. The laboratory diagnosis of adrenal pheochromocytoma: the Mayo Clinic experience. *J Clin Endocrinol Metab.* 2003;88(10):4533–4539.
9. Sawka AM, Jaeschke R. A comparison of biochemical tests for pheochromocytoma: measurement of fractionated plasma metanephrines compared with the combination of 24-hour urinary metanephrines and catecholamines. *J Clin Endocrinol Metab.* 2003;88(2):553–558.
10. Carey RM. Primary aldosteronism. *J Surg Oncol.* 2012;106(5):575–579.
11. Harvey AM. Hyperaldosteronism: diagnosis, lateralization, and treatment. *Surg Clini North Am.* 2014;94(3):643–656.
12. McKenzie TJ, Lillegard JB. Aldosteronomas–State of the art. *Surg Clin North Am.* 2009;89(5):1241–1253.
13. Rossi GP, Auchus RJ, Brown M, et al. An expert consensus statement on use of adrenal vein sampling for the subtyping of primary aldosteronism. *Hypertension.* 2014;63(1):151–160.
14. Utsumi T, Kawamura K, Imamoto T, et al. High predictive accuracy of aldosteronoma resolution score in Japanese patients with aldosterone-producing adenoma. *Surgery.* 2012;151(3):437–443.
15. Zarnegar R, Young WFJ, Lee J, et al. The aldosteronoma resolution score: predicting complete resolution of hypertension after adrenalectomy for aldosteronoma. *Ann Surg.* 2008;247(3):511–518.
16. Lacroix A, Feelders RA. Cushing's syndrome. *Lancet.* 2015;386(9996):913–927.
17. Raff H, Carroll T. Cushing's syndrome: from physiological principles to diagnosis and clinical care. *J Physiol.* 2015;593(3):493–506.

18. Ortiz DI, Findling JW, Carroll TB. Cosyntropin stimulation testing on postoperative day 1 allows for selective glucocorticoid replacement therapy after adrenalectomy for hypercortisolism: results of a novel, multidisciplinary institutional protocol. *Surgery.* 2016;159(1):259–266.
19. Fassnacht M, Kroiss M. Update in adrenocortical carcinoma. *J Clin Endocrinol Metab.* 2013;98(12):4551–4564.
20. Lacroix A. Approach to the patient with adrenocortical carcinoma. *J Clin Endocrinol Metab.* 2010;95(11):4812–4822.
21. Fassnacht M, Libé R. Adrenocortical carcinoma: a clinician's update. *Nat Rev Endocrinol.* 2011;7(6):323–335.
22. Stigliano A, Chiodini I, Giordano R, et al. Management of adrenocortical carcinoma: a consensus statement of the Italian Society of Endocrinology (SIE). *J Endocrinol Invest.* 2015;39(1):103–121.
23. Hoff AO, Berruti A. 5th International ACC Symposium: future and current therapeutic trials in adrenocortical carcinoma. *Horm Cancer.* 2016;7(1):29–35.
24. Simon DR, Palese MA. Clinical update on the management of adrenal hemorrhage. *Curr Urol Rep.* 2009;10(1):78–83.
25. Vella A, Nippoldt TB. Adrenal hemorrhage: a 25-year experience at the Mayo Clinic. *Mayo Clin Proc.* 2001;76(2):161–168.
26. Kawashima A, Sandler CM, Ernst RD, et al. Imaging of nontraumatic hemorrhage of the adrenal gland 1. *Radiographics.* 1999;19(4):949–963.

V
BREAST SURGERY

CHAPTER 65

BREAST MASSES

Christina A. Finlayson, MD

1. **What are evidenced-based components of breast screening?**
   Screening mammography has the most evidence to support it as a breast cancer screening tool.
   A screening study has value when:
   a. The incidence of the disease is high.
   b. The risks from the screening study are low.
   c. There are disease-specific treatments that can be administered when the disease is caught early that will improve the patient outcome more than waiting to treat the disease if it is identified later.
   Screening mammography detects breast cancer before it causes clinical symptoms. The incidence of breast cancer is high; one in eight women will develop breast cancer in their lifetime. Screening mammography is relatively low risk and low cost. The most common risk is false-positive findings that might require further imaging or biopsy. There are many excellent treatments for breast cancer, including surgery, chemotherapy, hormonal therapy, biologic therapy, and radiation therapy. Breast cancers treated at an early stage do better than breast cancers that are diagnosed at a late stage.

2. **When should routine screening mammography begin?**
   There is quite a bit of controversy surrounding the optimum mammography screening schedule for women at average risk of developing breast cancer. There is controversy about when screening should start, how often it should be done, and when it should stop. The options include:
   a. Starting screening between age 40 and 50 years
   b. Screening interval of 1–2 years
   c. Stopping screening between age 75 and 90 years
   The greatest benefit in screening programs occurs when a patient goes from no screening to some screening. Further modifications to the screening schedule will provide smaller incremental benefits in disease diagnosis. These incremental benefits are accompanied with a proportional increase in risk. Each woman can identify the risk:benefit ratio at a level comfortable to her. At minimum, a woman at average risk should begin screening no later than 50 and no less often than every 2 years, continuing until she is at least 75 years old.
   For women at high risk because of family history or other circumstances, screening may begin earlier, but not before age 30, and be done more often, but not more frequently than annually.

3. **What about breast self-examination or clinical breast exam?**
   Many large studies done in multiple countries have failed to show a survival benefit to regularly scheduled breast self-examination. Women should be familiar with their breasts and report any changes to their healthcare provider.
   Clinical breast examination done by a healthcare provider has also been shown to create more false positives than true positives and not improve outcomes.

4. **Does a normal or negative mammogram guarantee that no cancer is present?**
   No. Mammography has a false-negative rate of at least 15%. For a breast cancer to be detected on mammography, it must have tissue characteristics that are different from the surrounding tissue. Some tumors, particularly lobular carcinoma, invade the surrounding breast tissue in a way that does not alter the characteristics of the breast tissue. Such tumors are often not visible on mammogram.

5. **What is the role of screening magnetic resonance imaging (MRI) as an adjunct to mammography?**
   American Cancer Society guidelines published in 2007 recommend screening MRI for women with a >20% lifetime risk of developing breast cancer. This includes women who have a known gene mutation that predicts for the development of breast cancer, a strong family history of breast or ovarian cancer that suggests a genetic mutation, and women who have received chest radiation for Hodgkin's disease as teenagers or young adults. Gene abnormalities that predict for early breast cancer include *BRCA1*, *BRCA2*, Li-Fraumeni, Cowden, or Bannayan-Riley-Ruvalcaba syndromes. With expanded

genetic testing now being easily available, additional gene mutations are being identified regularly and should be included in high-risk screening recommendations.

MRI is quite sensitive for identifying breast cancer but is criticized for having a lower specificity that leads to additional imaging and biopsies. MRI should be used in conjunction with mammography and is not an independent screening modality for breast cancer.

6. **What is the role of ultrasound (US) in the diagnosis of breast cancer?**
US is used during the diagnostic evaluation of a breast mass or mammographic finding but is not used as a screening tool. If a patient with a complaint of a palpable mass has benign characteristics on physical examination and has a negative targeted US, the negative predictive value for cancer is 99.8%.

7. **A woman calls her healthcare provider to report a new breast mass. What type of mammography should be ordered?**
If there is a clinical finding, a diagnostic mammogram should be ordered.

8. **What is the difference between a screening and a diagnostic mammogram?**
Screening mammography is done in asymptomatic women to look for an occult breast cancer. Two views of each breast are obtained.

When a woman has a breast complaint, such as a mass or an abnormal screening mammogram, diagnostic mammography is performed.

A diagnostic mammogram pays particular attention to the area of clinical concern. Additional views taken at multiple angles or compression views taken with increased magnification of the abnormality help to distinguish between benign and malignant changes. US is usually included in a diagnostic evaluation. A radiologist is immediately available during diagnostic imaging.

9. **How are breast imaging abnormalities characterized?**
The American College of Radiography has developed a standard interpretation score to decrease ambiguity with breast imaging reporting. This applies to mammography, breast US, and MRI.
Bi-Rads
0   Requires further evaluation
1   Negative (normal examination without any findings)
2   Benign (normal examination with a definitely benign finding)
3   Probably benign (<3% chance of malignancy)
4   Suspicious (30% chance of malignancy)
5   Highly suspicious or malignant
6   Known malignancy
   - Category 0 is a temporary designation that requires further evaluation. This can be comparison to old films or diagnostic imaging. After further evaluation, such mammograms are reclassified into one of the other categories.
   - Categories 1 and 2 require no further evaluation; the usual mammographic schedule is not altered.
   - For category 3, a short-interval (6-month) diagnostic mammogram of the affected breast is recommended. Alternatively, a biopsy may be performed.
   - Categories 4 and 5 require a biopsy.

10. **What are the characteristics of a dominant breast mass?**
Identification of a dominant mass, especially in premenopausal women, can be challenging. Typically, a dominant mass can be palpated in three dimensions, and its density is distinct from surrounding breast tissue. Symptoms of equal importance are nodule, lump, thickening, and asymmetry. Breast cancer cannot be excluded by physical examination alone. "Failure to be impressed by physical examination findings" is the most common reason cited for a delay in the diagnosis of breast cancer.

11. **What are the four most frequently encountered palpable breast masses?**
Most dominant masses are benign. Examples include cysts, fibroadenomas, and fibrocystic masses. Carcinoma, although not the most common form of breast mass, is the reason that all persistent, dominant masses require a diagnosis. Other less common causes of palpable breast masses are lipomas, granulomas, fat necrosis, epidermal inclusion cysts, lactational adenomas, or phyllodes tumors.

12. **What are the differential characteristics of the most common palpable masses?**
A cyst is a regular, mobile mass that may be tender. It may be quite firm or fluctuant. A fibroadenoma is usually smooth, firm, elongated (longer than it is wide), and mobile with discrete borders.

Fibrocystic changes often are described as "lumpy-bumpy" breast tissue. There may be a discrete focal area of fibrosis that is more dominant than the background irregular tissue.

Carcinoma is usually an irregular, hard, painless mass. In advanced stages it may become fixed to the chest wall or be associated with overlying skin changes. Although this is the classic presentation, carcinoma may present in a form similar to benign lesions. Lobular carcinoma often appears as a soft mass or area of thickening. Because physical examination alone is unreliable in definitively excluding breast cancer, a biopsy must be obtained for all persistent, dominant solid masses.

13. **A 32-year-old woman presents with the complaint of a breast lump. Which questions about the patient's history are important in the evaluation of the mass?**
The size of the mass, whether it has changed in size, how long it has been present, whether it is painful, skin changes, nipple discharge, or changes in relation to the menstrual cycle may be helpful. Evaluation of any breast condition includes an assessment of risk factors for breast cancer, including personal or family history of breast, ovarian, or other cancers; age at menarche; age at first full-term pregnancy; age at menopause, if applicable; birth control or hormone replacement use; and history of previous breast biopsy.

14. **The mass identified in question 10 is discrete, not tender, easily palpable, and has gradually increased in size. What is the most appropriate next step?**
Breast imaging will further define the characteristics of a breast mass. US of a discrete mass can determine if it is cystic or solid. There are specific US criteria for defining a simple cyst. A simple cyst can be aspirated or observed. A complex cyst must be further evaluated by aspiration (to see if it completely resolves) or by biopsy. A solid mass that is not clearly a benign lesion requires a tissue diagnosis.

Mammography is also done for appropriate age women. A negative mammogram, however, does not exclude a breast cancer.

15. **How is a cyst aspiration performed?**
A 22-gauge needle is inserted into the cyst, and fluid is withdrawn. Generally, a 10-mL syringe is adequate, although occasionally cysts contain larger amounts of fluid. If the cyst is quite deep and difficult to fix between the physician's fingers, the aspiration can be performed under US guidance. Aspiration of a cyst is both diagnostic and therapeutic. After aspiration, the mass should resolve completely. If a mass persists or recurs after two aspirations, it should be excised. Cyst fluid may be clear or cloudy yellow, green, gray, or brown. A purely blood aspirate or an aspirate of what appears to be old blood should be sent for cytology, and excision of the lesion should be performed.

16. **What techniques are available for diagnosis of a palpable, solid breast mass?**
Fine-needle aspiration (FNA), core biopsy, incisional biopsy, and excisional biopsy have a role in diagnosing palpable breast masses. Which technique is used depends on the nature of the lesions and available technical support.

FNA recovers cells from the mass and requires a dedicated cytopathologist for accurate interpretation. Several benign and malignant lesions can be characterized accurately by FNA, but FNA cannot discriminate between invasive and in situ carcinoma. To be used effectively, it must be correlated with physical examination and breast imaging.

Core biopsy is also a sampling technique that removes 14- to 18-gauge pieces of tissue for histologic evaluation by the pathologist. Because it is a sampling, there is a risk of missing the lesion and obtaining a false-negative result. Again, correlation with physical examination and imaging is important to avoid failure to diagnose a breast cancer.

Incisional biopsy is rarely used today. It has a role when a highly suspicious lesion that is a candidate for neoadjuvant treatment fails to be definitively diagnosed on core biopsy.

Excisional biopsy completely removes the target lesion. It provides the most tissue for pathologic evaluation and, in benign disease, is both diagnostic and therapeutic.

BIBLIOGRAPHY

1. *American Cancer Society Breast Cancer Screening Guidelines.* http://www.cancer.org/cancer/news/specialcoverage/american-cancer-society-breast-cancer-screening-guidelines; 2015 Accessed 04.03.16.
2. *United States Preventive Services Task Force.* http://www.uspreventiveservicestaskforce.org/Page/Document/UpdateSummaryFinal/breast-cancer-screening1?ds=1&s=breast cancer screening; 2016 Accessed 04.03.16.
3. Scalia-Wilbur J, Colins BL. Breast cancer risk assessment: moving beyond BRCA 1 and 2. *Semin Radiat Oncol.* 2016;26(1):3–8.
4. Sable, MS. Clinical manifestations and diagnosis of a palpable breast mass. In: UpToDate, Post, TW, ed, *UpToDate*: Waltham, MA; 2016.

CHAPTER 66

PRIMARY THERAPY FOR BREAST CANCER

Kristine E. Calhoun, MD, Benjamin O. Anderson, MD

1. **How is breast cancer diagnosed?**

   A breast cancer diagnosis requires tissue confirmation by needle sampling or less commonly by surgical biopsy. Historically, excisional biopsy was the gold standard, but needle sampling has become the preferred initial diagnostic method most often using core needle biopsy. Needle sampling is desirable because it does not create skin incisions that adversely affect surgical planning in the event a therapeutic surgical procedure is needed. Needle sampling is also desirable for long-term follow-up in the case of benign biopsies because it does not distort the breast shape or architecture for future clinical breast examination (CBE) and breast imaging. While surgical excision can be used for diagnosis, it is often undesirable as an initial step for cancers because the operation generally will not be adequate as a therapeutic procedure and also requires the creation of skin incisions that may be undesirable for subsequent lumpectomy or mastectomy planning.

2. **What are the limitations of needle sampling?**

   The two options for needle sampling are fine-needle aspiration (FNA) and core needle biopsy. FNA may be used when core sampling is not feasible, but FNA provides more limited information about the sampled lesion. Both FNA and core needle biopsy can have false-negative results caused by sampling error. As a result, comprehensive diagnostic evaluation requires triple test evaluation where needle sampling results are compared with clinical evaluation (history and physical exam) and breast imaging (mammogram and ultrasound [US]) to determine if further tissue sampling is warranted or if the patient may be followed clinically. If the needle sampling diagnosis is negative for cancer and these findings correlate with the clinical presentation and breast imaging findings (mammogram and US), all of which suggest a benign breast process (concordance), the patient may have clinical follow-up examination without further intervention. However, if the needle sampling results do not match the findings from clinical examination or breast imaging (discordance), additional tissue sampling with a surgical excisional biopsy should be considered.

3. **How do fine needle aspiration and core needle biopsy differ?**

   FNA cytology is technically simple to perform, can be read immediately, and is cheap. By comparison, core needle biopsy, like surgical biopsy, requires that the specimen sit in fixative overnight. However, core needle sampling can allow complete operative planning, including decisions about lumpectomy versus mastectomy and/or the use of sentinel node mapping or complete axillary node dissection for staging. Because FNA is cytologic rather than histologic sampling, it cannot distinguish between invasive and in situ cancers. FNA cytology requires an expert cytologist for correct interpretation. Centers with specialized cytology expertise can set up effective systems where women are promptly and effectively evaluated, often with same-day diagnosis at significantly lower cost. However, the perceived complexity of FNA-based diagnostic systems have led most United States-based centers to base their diagnostic workup on core needle biopsy.

   By contrast to FNA, core needle biopsy (using standard 14-gauge or large-bore 8-gauge vacuum-assisted sampling) obtains true histology specimens that functionally resemble miniature surgical biopsies. Core needle samples do not distort the breast tissue nor do they leave large scars after healing, making them clearly preferable to surgical biopsy. Core biopsy can distinguish invasive from noninvasive cancer, ductal from lobular histology, and high-grade from low-grade disease. Special sections of core needle biopsy specimens can be prepared for immunohistochemistry staining to determine estrogen receptor (ER), progesterone receptor (PR), and Her-2/neu oncogene overexpression status. A pathologist skilled in reading standard surgical breast slides should also be comfortable reading breast core needle slides but may not be comfortable interpreting a breast FNA. Because of its versatility and the relative paucity of breast cytology expertise, core needle biopsy has become the most commonly accepted diagnostic standard for tissue sampling of the breast in the United States.

4. **Why should the breast be imaged before performing a breast biopsy?**
   Breast cancer generally begins as clinically occult disease that evolves to become palpable as the cancer grows and induces fibrosis in the breast. Even experienced surgeons can be surprised to find that seemingly small palpable cancers can be much more extensive in the breast than anticipated based on CBE alone. Preoperative imaging helps surgeons optimize surgical outcomes by avoiding these surprises and correctly assessing the extent of disease in the breast and/or axilla prior to embarking on surgical treatment. In some settings, breast imaging can allow the clinician to forego tissue sampling (e.g., simple cysts seen on breast US).
   Specific breast imaging tools include mammography, US, and magnetic resonance imaging (MRI):
   - The mammogram is the surgeon's road map, illustrating the distribution of fatty and dense tissues within the breast and simultaneously identifying additional lesions in the same or opposite breast that might warrant surgical attention. Screening mammograms are used in asymptomatic patients as part of a population-based screening program intended to increase the fraction of cancers diagnosed at earlier stage. Diagnostic mammogram is used when there is a clinical complaint or when the screening images have demonstrated a finding that needs additional investigation.
   - Diagnostic breast US is a powerful tool for visualizing mammographically detected localized breast masses or palpable findings and can be used to guide needle sampling. Screening whole-breast US has been evaluated and can increase the number of screen-detected cancers but is generally not used routinely because of the large number of false-positive US findings warranting US-guided biopsy and/or interval follow-up.
   - Breast MRI is used for breast cancer screening among women at significantly increased breast cancer risk on the basis of strong family history, especially when they have dense breasts on mammographic imaging. Many cancer centers use MRI with newly diagnosed breast cancers to assess extent of disease beyond what is seen on standard imaging. Surgeons can have a "love-hate" relationship with MRI because on the one hand it can give excellent delineation of the extent of existing cancers, but on the other hand it has a high false-positive rate of 20%–30%, requiring additional evaluation or even MRI-guided biopsy. MRI sometimes finds very small foci of breast cancer at some distance from the known primary, a disease that most likely would respond to radiation therapy and/or systemic therapy, but once found needs to be removed.

5. **Does a delay between biopsy and definitive treatment adversely affect cure?**
   Generally no, as long as the delay is only for days or weeks. Breast cancers typically evolve slowly, so treatment should be initiated within 3–4 weeks of initial diagnosis, if possible. Delays of longer than 3–6 months should be avoided. There is more urgency with pregnancy-associated breast cancer, in which tumor growth can be much more rapid. It is not appropriate to postpone the treatment of a breast cancer until the end of pregnancy, unless the pregnancy is almost to term. The standard of care for breast cancer diagnosed during the second or third trimesters is to start neoadjuvant chemotherapy. Some chemotherapeutic agents such as doxorubicin (Adriamycin) can be safely given during the second and third trimesters of pregnancy because it does not cross the placental barrier.

6. **How is breast cancer staged?**
   See Table 66.1.

7. **Why is staging of breast cancer important?**
   Breast cancer stage correlates with likelihood of relapse and mortality. Tumor, node, and metastasis staging summarizes data about tumor size, axillary node metastases, and distant metastases. Stage 0 cancers are noninvasive cancers (e.g., ductal carcinoma in situ [DCIS]); stage I breast cancers are small node-negative invasive cancers; stage II cancers are intermediate-sized cancers with or without axillary nodal metastases; stage III cancers are locally advanced cancers, usually with axillary nodal metastases; and stage IV cancers are those that have already metastasized to distant sites.
   Staging is important because it is a framework for planning adjuvant drug therapy and radiation treatment, both of which are critical to reducing breast cancer recurrence rates. Randomized trials that have proven treatment efficacy use stage as a basis for selected patient groups that are reasonably uniform. The staging framework also gives clinicians a standardized shorthand vocabulary for presenting clinical scenarios that are intuitively clear and understandable. For example, a T3N0 cancer is large but node negative, while a T1aN2 cancer is very small but has significant nodal burden.

Table 66.1 Staging of Breast Cancer

TNM	HISTOLOGY	TUMOR SIZE	NODAL METASTASES	DISTANT METASTASES
0	Noninvasive	Any	—	—
IA	Invasive	<2 cm (T1)	No (N0)	No
IB	Invasive	<2 cm (T1)	Yes, micro (N1mi)	No
IIA	Invasive	<2 cm (T1)	Yes, 1–3 (N1)	No
		2–5 cm (T2)	No (N0)	No
IIB	Invasive	2–5 cm (T2)	Yes, 1–3 (N1)	No
		>5 cm (T3)	No (N0)	No
IIIA	Invasive	<2 cm (T1)	Yes, 4–9 (N2)	No
		2–5 cm (T2)	Yes, 4–9 (N2)	No
		>5 cm (T3)	Yes, 1–3 (N1)	No
		>5 cm (T3)	Yes, 4–9 (N2)	No
IIIB	Invasive	Involved muscle or skin (T4)	No/Yes (N0, N1, N2)	No
IIIC	Invasive	Any size (Any T)	Yes, 10þ (N3)	No
IV	Invasive	Any size	Yes or no	Yes

8. **What is the overall survival rate after definitive multimodality treatment with curative intent?**
   Stage 0 (DCIS): Nearly 100% 10-year overall disease-specific survival rate
   Stage I: 90% 10-year overall disease-specific survival rate
   Stage II: 75% 10-year overall disease-specific survival rate
   Stage III: 40% 10-year overall disease-specific survival rate
   Stage IV: Cancer with distant metastases
   A gradual incremental improvement in breast cancer survival over recent years has been attributed to earlier detection and improved systemic therapy. Cytotoxic chemotherapy (e.g., CMF, Adriamycin, paclitaxel [Taxol]) for hormone-receptor negative cancers, hormonal therapy (e.g., tamoxifen, aromatase inhibitors) for hormone-receptor positive cancers, and biologic therapy (e.g., Herceptin for Her-2/neuoncogene overexpressing cancers) have improved disease-free and overall survival in breast cancer patients, even those with advanced disease.
   The management of metastatic (stage IV) breast cancer represents a fundamental therapeutic shift from that of stage 0–III disease. Instead of treating with curative intent, metastatic breast cancer receives tailored minimally morbid therapeutic regimens with the goal of stabilizing disease rather than permitting progression. The goal is to optimize quality of life, and some prolongation of life can be achieved in some circumstances. While cures can, on rare occasions, occur because of unusually favorable biologic response to treatment, stage IV breast cancer is generally assumed to be incurable and will eventually take the patient's life.

9. **What is the difference between noninvasive (in situ) and invasive breast cancers?**
   Noninvasive (in situ) cancers are lesions in which the malignant cells remain confined to the ductal tree or segment in which they originated. In situ cancers have minimal chance of spreading to nodes or distant sites. Invasive cancers have infiltrated through the basement membrane of their originating duct or lobule and concomitantly may have developed metastatic potential. In situ cancers have cells that are largely biologically incompetent and are unable to establish growth in distant tissues, so even if cells from these early cancers "escape" from the duct or are pushed into surrounding tissues during needle sampling, they remain unable to create metastatic disease. Thus, the primary reason for treating in situ cancer is to stop it from transforming into invasive cancer that does have the potential to spread to distant sites.

While DCIS and lobular carcinoma in situ (LCIS) are both in situ lesions, DCIS is generally treated surgically, while LCIS generally is not. DCIS has a higher risk of progression to invasive disease at the site where it is occurring in the breast, making local control of disease an appropriate intervention in most cases. LCIS, by contrast, is associated with an increased risk of subsequent invasive cancer, but that subsequent invasive disease following LCIS diagnosis is likely to be somewhere else in the breast or even in the opposite breast. For this reason, DCIS is generally considered preinvasive cancer, while LCIS is considered a breast cancer risk factor.

Complete axillary lymph node dissection (ALND) is not warranted for staging DCIS because the risk of nodal metastasis is remote. However, selective "sentinel lymphadenectomy," in which node mapping techniques are used to find and remove the "first upstream" node or nodes, may be used in conjunction with surgical treatment of DCIS, especially when a total mastectomy is planned. Sentinel node biopsy can only be performed with the breast in place and is no longer possible following mastectomy. If a mastectomy is performed for presumed DCIS and then occult invasive cancer is found, minimally invasive axillary staging is no longer possible. Surgeons need to think ahead to avoid this situation.

10. **Where does invasive breast cancer spread (other than to lymph nodes)? Which diagnostic tests are useful for identifying such metastases?**
Breast cancer can spread to the bones, lung, liver, peritoneal surfaces, and brain. Bone scans are quite sensitive but less specific for bone metastases. Standard radiographs help distinguish metastases from benign inflammatory conditions. Lung metastases are identified by chest radiographs or computed tomography (CT) scan with or without PET scan. Liver metastases can be identified using liver function tests (LFTs), but these tests are neither specific nor sensitive, with 25% of breast cancer patients with documented liver metastases having normal LFT results. Liver imaging tests (abdominal CT with or without PET scan, US, or MRI) are more expensive but more reliable. Brain metastases are imaged by head CT or MRI scanning, but only in the symptomatic patient.

11. **Which tests should be obtained before surgery to screen for metastases?**
All patients with symptoms suggesting metastatic disease (bone pain, pulmonary symptoms, jaundice, seizures, or focal neurologic symptoms) should be fully evaluated after invasive breast cancer has been diagnosed. In high-risk patients (nodal disease at diagnosis or large tumors), staging studies can be done on an individual basis in the asymptomatic patient, especially those with a very advanced clinical stage. In asymptomatic patients with lower clinical stage, staging studies should be postponed until surgical staging is complete.

A standard minimal preoperative workup for invasive disease consists of a chest radiograph and LFTs. In reality, the utility of these tests among early-stage cancers is low. Routine chest radiography identifies unsuspected lung metastases in <1% of patients. Chest radiography often is justified for preoperative planning and is useful as a baseline test for future comparison. The measurement of circulating tumor markers (CEA, CA-125, etc.) is of little or no value in most circumstances and should be discouraged.

12. **What are the alternatives for primary surgical treatment of invasive breast cancer?**
   - Mastectomy
      a. Modified radical mastectomy (MRM): Modified radical mastectomy (removal of the breast and the level 1, level 2 axillary lymph nodes), has replaced radical mastectomy (removal of breast, lymph nodes, and pectoralis muscle) as the standard of care for patients with node-positive disease who undergo mastectomy. The pectoralis minor muscle can be removed with minimal morbidity in a modified radical mastectomy to facilitate dissection of the highest (level III) lymph nodes (if involved), although most surgeons are not trained in this technique today.
      b. Total, or simple, mastectomy: This variation of mastectomy involves removal of the whole breast but eliminates routine axillary node dissection. It is often coupled with sentinel node biopsy in those with clinically node-negative breast cancers, because once the breast is removed, sentinel node biopsy is no longer possible.
   - Partial mastectomy (lumpectomy or quadrantectomy): Breast conservation therapy requires the removal of the tumor with a margin of normal breast tissue (negative margins) and is followed by postoperative breast irradiation. Trials with 20-year follow-up have shown that survival is equivalent for patients treated with lumpectomy and radiation, total mastectomy, and radical mastectomy. Mastectomy is preferred when negative margins cannot be achieved. Lumpectomy can be coupled with sentinel node biopsy if the patient is clinically node-negative or with axillary node dissection if the patient has documented nodal disease and such dissection is indicated.

13. **What is the National Surgical Adjuvant Breast and Bowel Program?**

The National Surgical Adjuvant Breast and Bowel Program (NSABP) is a United States-based trials group that performed many of the classic randomized trials that shaped our modern approach to breast cancer multimodality therapy. The NSABP helped demonstrate that breast cancer can be a systemic problem at the time of diagnosis and that smaller operations are equivalent to larger ones for curative potential. The NSABP has reported that tamoxifen can decrease the chances that a woman with a high risk of developing breast cancer will do so and has demonstrated that sentinel node biopsy is a safe procedure for axillary staging. Currently, NSABP is evaluating the efficacy of accelerated partial breast irradiation in which the radiation course is significantly shortened by just radiating the lumpectomy site for small node-negative invasive cancers.

14. **What is the significance of the NSABP B-06 trial?**

NSABP B-06 was a multicenter study initiated in the 1970s, and now with more than 20 years of follow-up, that randomized nearly 2000 women with stage I and II tumors (<4 cm) to one of three treatment arms: segmental mastectomy (SM; a.k.a., lumpectomy) alone, SM with radiation, and total mastectomy (TM). All patients underwent axillary dissection, and patients with positive nodes received adjuvant chemotherapy. There were no differences in overall survival rates among any of the three treatment groups, indicating that breast conservation therapy is effective for achieving both local and distant disease control. However, radiation therapy decreased local recurrence in patients treated with lumpectomy from almost 40% at 12 years without radiotherapy to <10% with whole-breast radiation, meaning that lumpectomy alone is generally an inadequate strategy for managing invasive cancers because of inadequate local control of disease.

15. **What is the difference among quadrantectomy, lumpectomy, and partial mastectomy?**

The differences are minimal because they all refer to removing part of the breast, just in varying amounts, for the purposes of treating breast cancer. The original quadrantectomy promoted by the Italians included excision of the entire involved breast quadrant, along with the overlying skin. Standard lumpectomies remove less tissue and may or may not involve skin removal, but they still demand negative surgical margins for both invasive cancer and DCIS. In these cancer operations, the surgeon is intending to achieve negative or free margins. What constitutes an adequate lumpectomy margin is controversial. A consensus statement from the Society of Surgical Oncology and the American Society of Radiation Oncology in 2013 endorsed the position that no tumor at ink was an adequate margin following lumpectomy for stage I and II cancers.

This stands in contrast to surgical biopsy, in which the surgeon is trying to remove as little tissue as possible to make a histologic diagnosis of a questionable lesion, and there is no intention to remove excess tissue or achieve negative margin status.

16. **Are some patients poor candidates for breast conservation therapy?**

Contraindications (relative or absolute) to breast conservation include (1) cancers that cannot be excised with negative margins without mastectomy, (2) cancers that are too large relative to the breast to obtain acceptable cosmetic results, (3) multicentric cancers, and (4) patients who do not desire or who have a specific contraindication to adjuvant radiation therapy (e.g., scleroderma, history of prior breast or chest wall radiation). The use of multiple lumpectomies for multicentric tumors in the same breast is considered investigational at this time and being studied in clinical trials.

17. **What is oncoplastic surgery?**

This is a collection of procedures that use combined oncologic and reconstructive principles in performing a partial mastectomy. Large, full-thickness segments of breast are excised, usually in conjunction with the overlying skin. Using mastopexy techniques, the gland is remodeled on the chest wall to preserve the breast's natural shape and appearance without creating an unsightly tissue divot under the skin.

18. **After mastectomy, which patients may undergo immediate breast reconstruction (i.e., during the same operation)?**

Patient selection for immediate reconstruction can be controversial. Most agree that those with noninvasive (in situ) or early invasive (stage I and selected stage II) breast cancers may be offered immediate reconstruction using a myocutaneous flap, a temporary tissue expander that is replaced by an implant, or a combination of both. Immediate reconstruction in patients with locally advanced (stage III) breast cancers should be taken on a case-by-case basis because these patients may ultimately require postmastectomy chest wall irradiation. Radiation adversely affects the cosmetic outcome in reconstructed tissue flaps, may lead to tissue flap loss, and can promote capsular contracture around implants.

19. **When is chest wall radiation therapy indicated after mastectomy?**
   The majority of mastectomy patients do not require radiation therapy. Exceptions are those at heightened risk of locoregional recurrence in the mastectomy bed. Postmastectomy radiation therapy (PMRT) is indicated with significant nodal burden (four or more positive nodes, or 1–3 nodes with other features of biologic aggression such as extranodal extension). PMRT may be indicated for large T3 (>5 cm) primary invasive cancers, although the need for PMRT for large but node-negative cancers is less clear. A less consistent indication is a positive or close mastectomy margin; PMRT is considered on a case-by-case basis in these situations.

20. **How has sentinel lymph node mapping changed breast cancer management?**
   The historic gold standard for staging the axilla in patients with invasive breast cancer was a level 1 and 2 ALND, which provides important staging information, but can be associated with morbidity, the most notable of which is lymphedema of the arm (20%–30% risk). Sentinel lymph node mapping, where a radioactive tracer (technetium labeled sulfur colloid), blue dye (Lymphazurin or methylene blue), or combination of both are injected into the breast to identify the first upstream axillary node(s) to which a primary breast cancer drains, was introduced in the mid-1990s and has become the standard of care for axillary staging in the node-negative patient and selectively in node-positive patients. If the sentinel lymph nodes are negative for cancer, it is not necessary to perform a completion node dissection. When axillary surgery is confined to sentinel node mapping and biopsy, lymphedema risk is reduced to 3%–5%.

21. **What was the ACOSOG Z-11 trial, and how did it change the management of the axilla in early stage breast cancers?**
   Traditionally, axillary sentinel node was performed to determine whether the axillary nodes were positive for metastases. If the SLNs were negative, no additional nodes were removed. If the SLNs were positive, a completion ALND was indicated. The Z-11 trial established that for patients having a lumpectomy followed by whole-breast radiation and the indicated systemic therapy, patients can have one or two positive SLNs and still not undergo a completion ALND because the outcomes were the same, whether or not the ALND was performed, including axillary bed recurrence rates of <1%. The trial did not include patients undergoing mastectomies, neoadjuvant chemotherapy, or partial breast radiation, so ALND is still standard of care for these individuals, even if one SLN is positive. Clinical trials are ongoing to see if ALND is still necessary in these other clinical situations.

22. **Are there risks of axillary staging by sentinel lymph node mapping?**
   Sentinel node mapping appears most appropriate for breast cancers with clinically node-negative axillae. The technique may be less reliable with large (T3) cancers, nodes extensively replaced with cancer, or possibly after neoadjuvant chemotherapy. Thus, the primary risk of sentinel node mapping is that it may understage a patient by suggesting that the cancer is node negative when, in fact, nodal metastases are present in other nonsentinel lymph nodes (i.e., a false-negative result). As a result, the patient may be treated with less aggressive therapy than is appropriate to minimize cancer mortality. The risk of a false-negative sentinel node biopsy is <5% for surgeons trained in the procedure.
   Traditionally, patients with node positive disease (core biopsy proven) who undergo neoadjuvant chemotherapy were treated with ALND. SLN following neoadjuvant therapy to see if the chemotherapy downstaged the axillary disease, with elimination of ALND if the SLN is negative, is being investigated. In these patients, if the SLN remains positive after neoadjuvant therapy, ALND is still being performed.

23. **Which tests should be obtained after surgery to screen for metastases or as baseline studies for future comparison?**
   The usefulness of metastatic screening tests correlates with the locoregional tumor and nodal (TN) staging determined at surgery. Patients with more advanced cancers are at higher risk for developing cancer recurrence with metastases, making additional diagnostic studies valuable. Bone scan, CT scan (chest, abdomen, pelvis), and/or PET scan are used among higher risk patients and occasionally reveal previously unappreciated metastatic disease. Some physicians also use circulating tumor markers such as CEA CA-27, 29 to follow treatment results and monitor for evidence of cancer recurrence, although the value of these studies is debatable.

Conversely, baseline studies are best avoided in asymptomatic patients with early cancers because the chance of a false-positive test is higher than the chances of finding clinically occult distant metastases. For example, with stage I breast cancer, the likelihood of a false-positive result on bone scans vastly exceeds the likelihood of a true-positive result. Similarly, brain imaging (CT or MRI) should be reserved for those patients with neurologic symptoms because of low yield in asymptomatic patients.

24. **What is neoadjuvant therapy for breast cancer?**

Locally advanced but operable (stage IIIA, B, C, and some stage II) cancers have a higher likelihood of recurrence after surgery. Neoadjuvant therapy (before surgery), also referred to as primary chemotherapy, is used to decrease the local tumor burden and begin treatment of presumed micrometastatic systemic disease at the earliest possible time. It does not appear that the timing of chemotherapy relative to surgery influences survival time from diagnosis, although this continues to be studied. Neoadjuvant chemotherapy may downstage some cancers that are otherwise marginal for breast conserving therapy into successful lumpectomy candidates but is generally not used to convert a patient who requires mastectomy at presentation into a lumpectomy candidate. Finally, neoadjuvant therapy may be offered to higher risk tumors regardless of stage, including those that are ER/PR negative and/or Her2 positive.

25. **What is inoperable breast cancer?**

Inoperable breast cancer has advanced beyond the boundaries of surgical resection. The spread may be regional (involving large amounts of the chest wall skin) or distant (distant metastases, stage IV). Ipsilateral supraclavicular lymph node metastases are a poor prognostic indicator but are currently staged as stage III, not stage IV, disease. Primary therapy for such advanced cancers is systemic treatment (chemotherapy or hormonal therapy) rather than surgery. Surgery combined with radiation therapy becomes an adjuvant therapy for local control of disease after a good response to systemic treatment.

There is still controversy regarding surgical resection of the primary lesion or axillary nodes in stage IV disease, so these individuals should be treated in a multidisciplinary clinic and on a case-by-case basis. Many will only offer surgical therapy to those patients whose disease improves with systemic treatment, or at least disease that remains stable. Patients with evidence of disease progression should not proceed to surgery, unless it is for palliative wound care reasons.

26. **How is DCIS treated?**

As the earliest form of breast cancer requiring treatment, DCIS has the widest range of treatment choices. Also called intraductal carcinoma, DCIS can be safely treated by breast conservation therapy (lumpectomy plus adjuvant radiation), provided that the disease is excised with negative margins. If negative margins cannot be achieved, then mastectomy is recommended for disease control. Although axillary dissection for staging is not indicated, sentinel lymph node biopsy may be offered if mastectomy is the operation of choice. Because it lacks metastatic potential, DCIS does not require systemic drug treatments beyond endocrine therapy. Tamoxifen may play a role in breast cancer prevention, and it lowered local recurrence after lumpectomy and radiation in the NSABP B-24 trial. There are some who believe DCIS should be managed more like a risk factor lesion, with primary medical therapy and watchful waiting, not surgery or radiation, but this is controversial and should be considered investigational at this time. One concern of watchful waiting is that by leaving DCIS in the breast, the lesion will transform into invasive cancer, which can then metastasize.

27. **Can some cases of DCIS be treated by lumpectomy without radiotherapy?**

Using carefully collected retrospective data, Silverstein and colleagues developed a prognostic index (scoring system) for DCIS based on histologic grade, tumor size, and margin width. Their data suggest that small (<1 cm) non–high-grade DCIS lesions excised with wide surgical margins do not require radiation therapy in addition to lumpectomy. However, eliminating radiation treatment after lumpectomy for DCIS remains controversial. Several phase III randomized studies have shown the benefits of local control with radiation therapy. In addition, one recent group demonstrated a 12% local recurrence rate at 5 years, following only local excision, leading the authors to conclude that the elimination of radiation resulted in unacceptably high recurrence rates. A gene profiling assay providing a DCIS score has been developed that helps identify DCIS cases at lower risk of local recurrence when treated with surgical excision alone, but the actual utility of this system is still be assessed in clinical practice.

28. **How does DCIS management differ from that for LCIS?**
DCIS is considered a preinvasive, or noninvasive, malignancy. It is traditionally treated surgically with lumpectomy or mastectomy, with or without radiation therapy, similar to how invasive breast cancer is managed. The overall goal is negative margin resection to prevent recurrence, which can be either a DCIS or an invasive cancer recurrence. By contrast, LCIS is viewed as a risk-factor lesion for the development of subsequent breast cancer and is generally not thought to be cancer per se. If diagnosed on a core needle biopsy, a subsequent excisional biopsy is recommended to rule out the concurrent existence of either DCIS or an invasive cancer. If LCIS is identified on a surgical specimen, negative margin resection is not required.

29. **Why are patients with LCIS not treated surgically?**
LCIS does not invariably degenerate into invasive cancer, although women with biopsy-proven LCIS have an 8- to 10-fold increased risk of developing breast cancer during their lifetimes. The cancer may be ductal or lobular and may develop in either breast. LCIS is, therefore, considered to be a marker for high breast cancer risk, warranting careful surveillance with serial mammography, physical examination, and possibly MRI. Because future breast cancer risk is the same for both breasts, bilateral mastectomy would be the only logical surgical procedure for this condition. Such aggressive therapy is not warranted in the majority of patients, although it may be considered in high-risk individuals on a case-by-case basis.
Pleomorphic LCIS (pLCIS) is an unusual LCIS variant exhibiting cellular and molecular features resembling DCIS. Experts debate whether this should be managed as LCIS or DCIS. If percutaneous needle biopsy demonstrates pLCIS, excisional biopsy is warranted because a significant fraction will upgrade to DCIS or invasive carcinoma. Excising pLCIS to clear margins is problematic as it would be associated with a high mastectomy rate of unclear benefit.

30. **Can drugs be used to prevent breast cancer among women at high risk?**
In the NSABP P-01 Tamoxifen Prevention Trial, women at heightened risk for the development of breast cancer (>1.66% 5-year risk) developed fewer breast cancers when given tamoxifen versus placebo. For women with LCIS, the 5-year breast cancer incidence was 6.8% in the placebo group and 2.5% in the tamoxifen group, representing a 56% absolute reduction in breast cancers. However, the number of breast cancers that were prevented rivaled the number of tamoxifen-associated complications, including endometrial cancers and thrombotic events.
No survival benefit to tamoxifen prophylaxis has yet been observed. At this time, women with LCIS and no major medical contraindications may be offered tamoxifen as an option for cancer prevention, although they may reasonably decline when presented with the complete data. The use of tamoxifen alternatives and aromatase inhibitors remains less defined for risk reduction.

KEY POINTS: PRIMARY THERAPY FOR BREAST CANCER

1. Historically, excisional biopsy was the gold standard for the diagnosis of breast cancer.
2. Now, the preferred initial diagnostic method is core needle biopsy (FNA if core sampling is not available).
3. The surgical alternatives for treatment of primary invasive breast cancer are modified radical mastectomy, total mastectomy, or partial mastectomy. Total mastectomy and partial mastectomy can be coupled with SLN for axillary staging.
4. The NSABP B-06 trial found no difference in overall survival in women with stage I and II breast cancer who underwent either SM, SM with radiation, and TM, but radiation decreased local recurrence in the lumpectomized breast.

BIBLIOGRAPHY

1. Anderson BO, Calhoun KE. Evolving concepts in the management of lobular neoplasia. *J Natl Compr Canc Netw.* 2006;4(5):511–522.
2. Mougalian SS, Soulos PR, Killelea BK, et al. Use of neoadjuvant chemotherapy for patients with stage I to III breast cancer in the United States. *Cancer.* 2015;121(15):2544–2552.
3. Burke EE, Portschy PR. Prophylactic mastectomy: Who needs it, when and why. *J Surg Oncol.* 2015;111(1):91–95.
4. Chen CY, Calhoun KE, Masetti R, et al. Oncoplastic breast conserving surgery: a renaissance of anatomically-based surgical treatment. *Minerva Chir.* 2006;61(5):421–434.

5. Fisher B, Anderson S, Bryant J, et al. Twenty-year follow-up of a randomized trial comparing total mastectomy, lumpectomy, and lumpectomy plus irradiation for the treatment of invasive breast cancer. *N Engl J Med.* 2002;347(16):1233–1241.
6. Fisher B, Costantino JP, Wickerham DL, et al. Tamoxifen for prevention of breast cancer: current status of the National Surgical Adjuvant Breast and Bowel Project P-1 Study. *J Natl Cancer Inst.* 2005;97(22):1652–1662.
7. Lehman CD, Gatsonis C, Kuhl CK, et al. MRI evaluation of the contralateral breast in women with recently diagnosed breast cancer. *N Engl J Med.* 2007;356(13):1295–1303.
8. Lyman GH, Temin S, Edge SB, et al. Sentinel lymph node biopsy for patients with early-stage breast cancer: American Society of Clinical Oncology clinical practice guideline update. *J Clin Oncol.* 2014;32(13):1365–1383.
9. Lyman GH. Appropriate role for sentinel node biopsy after neoadjuvant chemotherapy in patients with early-stage breast cancer. *J Clin Oncol.* 2015;33(3):232–234.
10. Morrow M, Strom EA, Bassett LW, et al. Standard for breast conservation therapy in the management of invasive breast carcinoma. *Ca Cancer J Clin.* 2002;52(2):277–300.
11. Saslow D, Boetes C, Burke W, et al. American Cancer Society guidelines for breast screening with MRI as an adjunct to mammography. *CA Cancer J Clin.* 2007;57(2):75–89.
12. Silverstein MJ. The University of Southern California/Van Nuys prognostic index for ductal carcinoma in situ of the breast. *Am J Surg.* 2003;186(4):337–343.
13. Truong PT, Olivotto IA. Selecting breast cancer patients with T1-T2 tumors and one to three positive axillary nodes at high postmastectomy locoregional recurrence risk for adjuvant radiotherapy. *Int J Radiat Oncol Biol Phys.* 2005;61(5):1337–1347.
14. Rakovitch E, Nofech-Mozes S, Hanna W, et al. A population-based validation study of the DCIS Score predicting recurrence risk in individuals treated by breast-conserving surgery alone. *Breast Cancer Res Treat.* 2015;152(2):389–398.
15. Veronesi U, Cascinelli N, Mariani L, et al. Twenty-year follow-up of a randomized study comparing breast-conserving surgery with radical mastectomy for early breast cancer. *N Engl J Med.* 2002;347(16):1227–1232.
16. Yen TW, Kuerer HM, Ottesen RA, et al. Impact of randomized clinical trial results in the national comprehensive cancer network on the use of tamoxifen after breast surgery for ductal carcinoma in situ. *J Clin Oncol.* 2007;25(22):3251–3258.
17. Giuliano AE, Hunt KK, Ballman KV, et al. Axillary dissection vs no axillary dissection in women with invasive breast cancer and sentinel node metastasis: a randomized clinical trial. *JAMA.* 2011;305(6):569–575.
18. Moran MS, Schnitt SJ, Giuliano AE, et al. Society of Surgical Oncology-American Society for Radiation Oncology consensus guideline on margins for breast-conserving surgery with whole-breast irradiation in stages I and II invasive breast cancer. *J Clin Oncol.* 2014;32(14):1507–1515.
19. Boughey JC, Suman VJ, Mittendorf EA, et al. Factors affecting sentinel lymph node identification rate after neoadjuvant chemotherapy for breast cancer patients enrolled in ACOSOG Z1071 (Alliance). *Ann Surg.* 2015;261(3):547–552.
20. Flanagan MR, Rendi MH, Calhoun KE. Pleomorphic lobular carcinoma in situ: radiologic-pathologic features and clinical management. *Ann Surg Oncol.* 2015;22(13):4263–4269.

VI
OTHER CANCERS

CHAPTER 67

WHAT IS CANCER?

Jeffrey C. Liu, MD, FACS, John A. Ridge, MD, PhD

1. **What is a neoplasm?**
   A neoplasm, or tumor, is any new mass of cells, where they grow under conditions that normally should not give rise to new cell growth. Benign neoplasms grow, but they do not spread; they disrupt adjacent tissues through mass effect. A malignant neoplasm, or cancer, is composed of cells that invade adjacent tissues and spread. Cancer can spread through lymphatics or through the blood stream (hematologic).

2. **What kinds of cancer are there?**
   Cancers are defined by their tissue of origin. Cancers of epithelial origin, such as skin cancer, tongue cancer, breast cancer, or colon cancer, are called carcinomas. Malignant tumors of mesenchymal origin largely arise from connective tissue and are called sarcomas. Cancers are usually solid groups of cells, but some, like leukemia, are "liquid" tumors. Hematologic malignancies, such as leukemia and lymphoma, are also of mesenchymal origin. Some cancers, like melanoma, arise from cells of the neural crest.
   Different types of cancer can arise within a single organ and each may be treated differently. For example, adenocarcinoma, small cell carcinoma, and squamous cell carcinoma all arise within the lung and each is treated differently.

3. **Are all cancers life threatening?**
   Yes. With enough time, every cancer is a fatal disease. However, different cancers progress at different rates. Some cancers, such as adenocarcinoma of the pancreas, are aggressive, difficult to treat, and kill quickly. Other cancers, such as most thyroid and prostate cancers, can be slow growing and often years will pass before patients succumb.

4. **How are cancers diagnosed?**
   Diagnosing cancer requires taking a sample of the tumor for microscopic examination; this is called a biopsy. Several histologic tests are performed. These can include specimen staining, most commonly using a hematoxylin and eosin (H&E) stain. Immunohistochemistry, using an antibody to a protein of interest, can be used to identify proteins found in cancers of a given type. In situ–hybridization DNA can detect DNA sequences of viral origin (e.g., human papilloma virus or Epstein-Barr virus), and gene arrangement studies demonstrate mutations for causing a disease (e.g., the *BCR-ABL* gene rearrangement is associated with chronic myelogenous leukemia).

5. **After diagnosis, what comes next?**
   After proving the presence of cancer, testing is performed to ascertain the extent of disease—this is called staging. The physical examination may help assess both the primary tumor and nearby lymph node basins. Loss of function can indicate deep tumor spread or tumor invasion of nerve pathways. An enlarged liver may be a sign of hepatic metastases, changes in percussion and auscultation may reflect pleural effusions and obstructing tracheal lesions, and abdominal distention is a sign of ascites or of bowel obstruction. Examination of the primary site (such as the larynx or colon) may require endoscopy.
   Nowadays, imaging is almost invariably performed, which may include a computed tomography (CT) scan or magnetic resonance imaging. Functional imaging, such as fluorodeoxyglucose-positron emission tomography, may show lesions that use more sugar than surrounding normal tissues.

6. **Why and how are cancers staged?**
   Cancer staging employs a common language for describing a cancer's extent, suggests the right treatment for a cancer based on the size and spread of the disease, and may help to predict a patient's prognosis. Staging is an essential aspect of cancer evaluation and treatment of solid tumors. For almost all cancers, staging employs the tumor, node, and metastasis (TNM) system, where T describes the primary tumor extent, N describes the presence and extent of regional nodal

metastases, and M reflects distant metastatic cancer. The TNM categories are combined to assign stages between I and IV, where IV is the most advanced. Most cancers are staged according to the methods described by the American Joint Committee on Cancer in a staging manual (see reference 1).

7. How do cells become cancerous?

In a word, mutations. Cancer is a derangement of cells resulting from changes in DNA that alter cellular programming and behavior. When such mutations result in cells that destroy nearby tissues and spread, that is cancer. Mutations in DNA can have effects in many different ways. Mutations in genes can result in loss of function or even gain of function. For example, mutations in the *p53* gene resulting in loss of function are seen in a majority of cancers (see reference 2). Mutations within promoter regions, splice sites, microRNA, or regulatory elements can all affect cell function. Chromosomal breaks, deletions, and duplications also alter cellular regulation. Mutations may arise spontaneously, be facilitated by inherited genetic variation, result from viral infection, or be caused by carcinogenic agents (including drugs, toxins, and ionizing radiation).

8. What cell behaviors are affected to cause cancer?

While some mutations may have little to no effect on cell function, other mutations have significant sequelae. While mutations in DNA are at the core of cancer development, studies show that other changes to key functional parts of cell function are required for the development of cancer (see reference 3). Individual mutations are usually less important than the sum total of mutations and the pathways they affect.

There are at least six major hallmarks that are important for cancer development. They are (1) sustaining proliferative signaling, (2) resisting cell death, (3) evading growth suppressors, (4) inducing angiogenesis, (5) enabling replicative immortality, and (6) activating invasion and metastasis. Other major features of cancer progression include reprogramming energy metabolism and evading immune destruction. Though some cancers seem to have a simple cause, it is the accumulation of mutations that turns normal cells into cancerous ones.

9. What is a metastasis?

A metastasis is a mass of cancer cells resulting from spread from the original tumor location to another place in the body. A metastasis is not contiguous with the location of the primary cancer. This spread can be through the bloodstream or lymphatic channels. Metastatic cells are similar to those of the original tumor but have the capacity to travel and to grow where they arrive.

10. Do all cancers spread?

About 25% of patients with solid tumors have detectable metastases at the time of diagnosis. However, fewer than 50% of the remainder develop metastases during the course of treatment. Metastases are usually more common from advanced primary cancers than from early ones. Some cancers rarely spread, such as basal cell carcinoma of the skin and some types of sarcomas.

11. How is cancer treated?

Surgery, radiation treatment, and chemotherapy can be used to treat cancer. Most modern cancer treatments involve one or more of these techniques. If a cancer has not spread, then removing it during an operation is very effective treatment. Radiation treatment entails killing the cancer in place through transfer of energy to the cancer cells, resulting in fatal cell damage. Chemotherapy largely employs the administration of medicines that interfere with tumor metabolism to kill cancers or slow their progression. Recent advances in medical treatment of cancers include treatment with agents that increase the body's response to the presence of cancer cells (which are no longer truly "self").

12. When is surgery, radiation, or chemotherapy chosen for treatment?

Treating most cancers is complex. Treatment of each cancer should be unique, but there are common threads. Decades of experience, the patient's needs, and extent of the cancer all direct choice of treatment. Some cancers are treated with only a single modality, while others are treated with a combination of them. The choice of treatment is influenced by the type and stage of cancer. Small or early cancers may often be treated with only surgery, or occasionally by radiation alone. Some cancers, like lymphoma, are primarily treated with only chemotherapy. Control of more advanced cancers may require treatment with two or more approaches. Widespread cancers are likely to be treated only with chemotherapy. The National Comprehensive Cancer Network guidelines suggest the best ways to treat cancers of most sites and stages (see reference 1).

13. How is surgery used to treat cancer?

Surgery sounds easy: Cut out the cancer! However, cancer operations should be chosen carefully and designed for a specific tumor. In general, surgery works to treat the primary cancer (the T in the TNM staging), as well as regional lymph nodes (the N in the TNM staging). Surgery may be employed to treat distant metastasis, but only in the proper setting. Complete resection of the primary cancer site is a key part of curative surgery. Depending on the cancer type, removal of lymph nodes may also be performed, either as part of treatment for metastatic lymph nodes or as a diagnostic procedure to learn more about the tumor's extent. Thus, pathologic results of node removal may direct subsequent treatment.

Some cancers are not treated with surgery at all. For example, lymphoma is a cancer of lymph nodes, and surgery is used primarily in the diagnosis, not treatment, of this disease. Surgery has little or no role in the treatment of leukemia.

14. What are surgical margins?

For most cancers treated with surgery, it is very important to remove the entire cancer in order to reduce the risk that it returns where it began. Removing a "cuff" of normal tissue around the primary tumor helps to ensure the surgeon has removed all of the original tumor. This cuff of normal tissue is called a margin.

15. What is sentinel lymph node biopsy?

For some cancers, finding out whether a cancer has spread to regional lymph nodes helps to guide treatment. However, removing all of the lymph nodes to which a cancer may spread sometimes has serious side effects. For example, with a melanoma of the arm, the lymph nodes of the axilla may be at highest risk for regional spread. Removing these lymph nodes for examination can determine whether the cancer has spread, but axillary lymph node dissection has significant long-term side effects, such as chronic swelling (lymphedema) of the arm. The nodes guarding the rest of the body from spread are called sentinel nodes, and they are the first to which cancer spreads. Usually only one or two lymph nodes actually trap the first cells spreading through the lymph channels. Studying those few lymph nodes permits pathologists to find even small amounts of metastatic cancer (by careful study that is impossible for many lymph nodes). Identifying the sentinel nodes permits better pathologic examination and also means that the patient does not sustain the side effects of complete lymph node removal.

16. How does radiation treat cancer?

Radiation treats cancers by delivering energy to them, leading to damage to their DNA. The DNA strands may be broken, the DNA may be damaged in a way that prevents the cell from dividing, and DNA damage may alert cell control mechanism to injury, leading the cell to commit suicide (apoptosis). When a cell is sufficiently damaged, it cannot replicate and dies.

17. Are there multiple types of radiation?

There are several types of radiation treatment for cancer. Most radiation treatment involves delivering energy to the cancer with high-energy photons, but other forms may be used. The radiation energy can come from a variety of accelerators, from radioactive elements, or even from heat and light. Most radiation treatment is delivered as photons, with energy similar to gamma rays from the nucleus, but generated by a linear accelerator.

18. How does chemotherapy treat cancer?

Chemotherapy agents are usually given through the bloodstream to reach all parts of the patient with the cancer. There are many types of chemotherapy. Some are cytotoxic, meaning that the drugs damage the cells and prevent them from replicating or increasing in number. Examples are platinum compounds (e.g., cisplatin), taxanes, and topoisomerase inhibitors.

Another category of chemotherapy treatment is hormonal. Some cancers grow better with hormonal stimulation. Reducing those hormone levels can arrest growth in a cancer and even lead to programmed cell death. Examples of this are tamoxifen for breast cancer, which blocks the effects of estrogen, and leuprolide for prostate cancer, which affects testosterone production.

19. What is targeted therapy (biologics)?

All forms of cancer treatment are directed to a target of some kind (such as surgery to remove the primary tumor, radiation to a bone metastasis, or chemotherapy to damage tumor DNA). However, the term *targeted therapy* has come to refer to a class of systemic treatments whose greatest effect is on mechanisms of tumor growth that are less important to the growth of normal cells. There are many types of targets. For example, cetuximab is a monoclonal antibody binding to the epidermal growth factor receptor, which is overexpressed on the surface of some cancer types (see reference 4). Imatinib is a small molecule that specifically inhibits the *BCR-ABL* translocation tyrosine kinase in chronic myelogenous leukemia, and in tumors that express c-kit (see reference 5). Other "-ibs" (e.g., sorafenib) interfere with tyrosine kinases important to tumor growth (and less important for normal cells), and other "-mabs" bind to targets important to angiogenesis (e.g., Bevacizumab).

20. **What is immunotherapy?**

Immunotherapy is an increasingly promising area of cancer treatment that utilizes the patient's immune system to attack cancers. So far, two major strategies have been employed. The first is extraction of immune cells from the patient, priming them in the laboratory to attack the patient's cancer, and then reintroducing them to destroy it. This has had some dramatic results (see reference 6). Another strategy has been the development of immune checkpoint inhibitors. These drugs release the brake that shuts down the immune system after stimulation. In part, cancer cells are able to grow into tumors by avoiding attack by the immune system. When the brake is released, the immune system is sometimes able to identify the cancer again and to target it for destruction. Ipilimumab and pembrolizumab are monoclonal antibody immune checkpoint inhibitors that have recently shown impressive activity in melanoma (see references 7 and 8). Their use in other cancers is currently under investigation, and new drugs and immune mechanisms are under active investigation.

21. **How are surgery, radiation, and chemotherapy combined for treatment?**

As mentioned previously, treatment of cancer can involve one or more strategies for treatment. Combining therapy can be synergistic, with greater effects on the cancer than each modality alone. Giving chemotherapy during the course of radiation (concomitant chemoradiation) can increase the potency of radiation treatment.

In addition, there are different ways to sequence treatments. Adjuvant therapy is added on to improve cancer control after definitive treatment has been delivered. For example, after surgical excision of a cancer, radiation or chemotherapy may be given afterward as additional treatment. Neoadjuvant, or induction, refers to giving a treatment prior to definitive therapy. For example, chemotherapy may be given to a patient to shrink the tumor prior to a definitive therapy such as surgery. This technique may be used to shrink a breast cancer before surgical treatment of the primary tumor, and it may also be employed to deliver earlier systemic treatment to microscopic distant metastases.

KEY POINTS: CANCER

1. Cancer is a growth of abnormal cells in the body, which develop from accumulating mutations.
2. Staging is a critical part of cancer evaluation to determine options for treatment.
3. Surgery, radiation, and chemotherapy are the three main ways to treat cancers. The right treatment may involve giving one or more treatments in combination.

BIBLIOGRAPHY

1. *National Comprehensive Cancer Network.* Clinical guidelines in oncology. <https://www.nccn.org/professionals/physician_gls/f_guidelines.asp#site>; 2017 Accessed 01.03.17.
2. Muller PA, Vousden KH. p53 mutations in cancer. *Nat Cell Biol.* 2013;15(1):2–8.
3. Hanahan D, Weinberg RA. Hallmarks of cancer: the next generation. *Cell.* 2011;144(5):646–674.
4. Mendelsohn J, Baselga J. The EGF receptor family as targets for cancer therapy. *Oncogene.* 2000;19(56):6550–6565.
5. Capdeville R, Buchdunger E. Glivec (STI571, imatinib), a rationally developed, targeted anticancer drug. *Nat Rev Drug Discov.* 2002;1(7):493–502.
6. Maude SL, Frey N, Shaw PA, et al. Chimeric antigen receptor T cells for sustained remissions in leukemia. *New Engl J Med.* 2014;371(16):1507–1517.
7. Hodi FS, O'Day SJ, McDermott DF, et al. Improved survival with ipilimumab in patients with metastatic melanoma. *New Engl J Med.* 2010;363(8):711–723.
8. Robert C, Schachter J, Long GV, et al. Pembrolizumab versus ipilimumab in advanced melanoma. *New Engl J Med.* 2015;372(26):2521–2532.

CHAPTER 68

MELANOMA

Martin D. McCarter, MD, FACS

1. **What is melanoma?**
   The term *melanoma* implies a malignant tumor that arises from melanocytes. The most malignant of all skin cancers, melanoma usually forms from a preexisting nevus or mole but may develop de novo. It accounts for <1% of all skin cancers, but the vast majority of skin cancer deaths.

2. **What is the incidence of melanoma?**
   It is the sixth most common cancer in the United States and currently is the cancer with the most rapid rise in incidence in the United States. The overall incidence is approximately 20/100,000 population, with a lifetime risk of approximately 1 in 75. Over 76,000 new cases of melanoma are reported each year, with more than 10,000 deaths from the disease.

3. **What are the types of moles (nevi)?**
   Intradermal: The most benign form
   Junctional: The junctional component may be the site of melanoma formation
   Compound: Intradermal and junctional together; intermediate activity
   Spitz: Once called juvenile melanoma, it is actually a spindle cell epithelioid nevus that is quite benign
   Dysplastic: The most likely to turn malignant (especially in dysplastic nevus syndrome)

4. **What are the risk factors in melanoma formation?**
   - Large number of moles (>50 moles >2 mm in diameter)
   - Changing nevi
   - History of melanoma
   - Family history of melanoma
   - Light, poorly tanning skin; blonde or reddish-brown hair
   - History of episodic, acute, severe sunburns
   - Dysplastic nevus syndrome, or familial atypical multiple mole melanoma syndrome (FAMMM)

5. **What is the familial melanoma syndrome?**
   The inherited FAMMM syndrome has been defined as the occurrence of melanoma in one or more first- or second-degree relatives and the presence of >50 moles of variable size, some of which are atypical, histologically. The risk of melanoma in this syndrome runs as high as 100% in the person's lifetime. People with FAMMM frequently have a mutation in p16 mapped to chromosome 9.

6. **What are common sites of melanoma development?**
   The most common sites are the posterior trunk in men and lower extremities in women. All sun-exposed areas are possible sites. Less common sites for melanoma formation are the soles of the feet, palms, and genitalia. Unusual noncutaneous sites for melanoma formation are the eye, anus, and gastrointestinal tract.

7. **What are the warning signs of melanoma?**
   Skin lesions that display:
   A = **A**symmetry
   B = Irregular **b**order
   C = **C**olor: Variable, spotted, often very black with irregular tan areas, red or pink spots, ulcerated when advanced (bleeds easily)
   D = **D**iameter (>5–6 mm)
   E = **E**nlargement or **E**levation

8. **What are the main types of melanoma and their incidence?**
   Superficial spreading: 75% of all cases; most common
   Nodular: 15% of cases; most malignant, well circumscribed, deeply invasive

Lentigo maligna melanoma: 5% of cases; relatively good prognosis.
Acral lentiginous: 5% of cases; most common type in people of color; appears on the soles, palms, subungual sites.
Other rare types include desmoplastic, ocular, and mucosal melanomas

9. **Which moles should be considered for removal?**
Growing and darkening nevi should be excised, especially in sun-sensitive patients. Itching is a sign of early malignant change. Ulceration is a late sign. Because melanoma may be familial in origin, children of patients with melanoma should be carefully screened for very dark nevi.

10. **How should suspicious nevi be biopsied?**
Total excision of the lesion with a narrow (1-mm) margin of normal skin plus primary repair should be done. Partial incisional biopsy is acceptable if the lesion is large or if total excision would require reconstructive surgery. Punch biopsy, incisional biopsy, or saucerization are all appropriate as long as a **full-thickness** specimen is obtained. Expert pathologic study is essential.

11. **Do melanomas spontaneously regress or even disappear?**
Remarkably, some melanomas can regress or even disappear. Approximately 10% of melanoma patients with metastasis present with metastasis from an unknown primary site.

12. **What are the Breslow and Clark classifications of melanoma invasion?**
The **Breslow depth** has become the preferred classification because it is a more standardized method to measure melanoma depth. It requires an optical micrometer fitted to the ocular position of a standard microscope. Lesions are classified as follows:
- ≤1.0 mm
- 1.01–2.0 mm
- 2.01–4.0 mm
- ≥4.0 mm

Lesions <1 mm include melanoma in situ and thin invasive tumors. The cure rate in the latter is over 95% with excision. Tumors of 1.01–4.0 mm are called intermediate but involve risk of metastasis. Lesions >4.0 mm are high-risk lesions with a poor cure rate.

The **Clark** level refers to penetration of the melanoma through the layers of the skin. This is largely used for historical reference now:
- Level I: Intradermal melanoma that does not metastasize; may be better termed *atypical melanotic hyperplasia*: A benign lesion.
- Level II: Melanoma that penetrates the basement membrane into the papillary dermis.
- Level III: Melanoma that fills the papillary dermis and encroaches on the reticular dermis in a pushing fashion.
- Level IV: Melanoma that invades the reticular dermis.
- Level V: Melanoma that works its way into the subcutaneous fat. Measurement of thickness is important, and the tumor should be measured from the total height of the lesion vertically at the point of maximal thickness. In addition, if ulceration is present, the measurement should be from the bottom of the ulcer crater down to the deepest margin of the lesion (see Fig. 68.1).

13. **What is the tumor, node, metastasis (TNM) staging system for melanoma?**
The TNM staging system is the most comprehensive classification of melanoma. Using established risk factors for advanced disease, it stratifies patients based on the thickness of the melanoma, ulceration, micrometastases or nodal metastases, and distant metastatic disease. Last revised in 2007, it more accurately predicts overall prognosis. See Table 68.1.

14. **Can the Breslow depth of invasion be used to predict the relative risk of nodal metastasis?**
See Table 68.2.

15. **What are the characteristics of a subungual melanoma?**
Subungual lesions are often mistaken for a chronic inflammatory process; therefore, most patients present quite late. They are usually older than patients with other forms of cutaneous melanoma. The great toe is the most common site of origin. Amputation at or proximal to the metatarsal phalangeal joint and sentinel lymph node (SLN) biopsy is advised for those without evidence of regional or systemic spread of disease.

16. **Describe the technique of SLN biopsy**

The SLN biopsy is based on the theory that lymph from a solid neoplasm initially drains to a central sentinel node. These sentinel nodes are the first nodes at risk for metastatic disease. The nodes can be biopsied and examined with serial sectioning and immunohistochemical staining. The SLN identification technique requires the cooperation of a surgeon, radiologist, and pathologist. Lymphoscintigraphy with the injection of radioactive technetium sulfur colloid (99mTeSC) is performed around the site of the primary melanoma. This identifies the regional nodal basins at risk. In the operating room, an intradermal injection of blue contrast dye (lymphazurin 1% or methylene blue) is performed around the primary site. A handheld gamma detector identifies the hot spot, and a small incision is made over this area for removal of the SLN. A combination of blue contrast dye and radiocolloid provides the highest yield of sentinel node identification.

17. **Why is SLN biopsy an important tool in the treatment of melanoma?**

The presence of metastasis in the SLN is a powerful independent predictor of overall survival. SLN biopsy has relatively minimal morbidity, yet identifies patients who are at high risk for recurrence. The

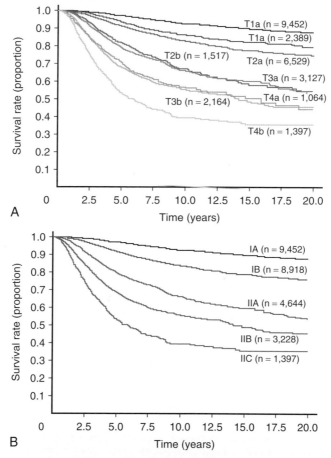

Fig. 68.1 Survival curves from the American Joint Committee on Cancer Melanoma Staging Database comparing (A) the different T categories and (B) the stage groupings for stages I and II melanoma. For patients with stage III disease, survival curves are shown comparing (C) the different N categories and (D) the stage groupings. *(From Balch CM, Gershenwald JE, Soong SJ, et al. Final version of 2009 AJCC melanoma staging and classification. J Clin Oncol. 2009;27(36):6199–6206. Reprinted with permission from the American Society of Clinical Oncology.)*

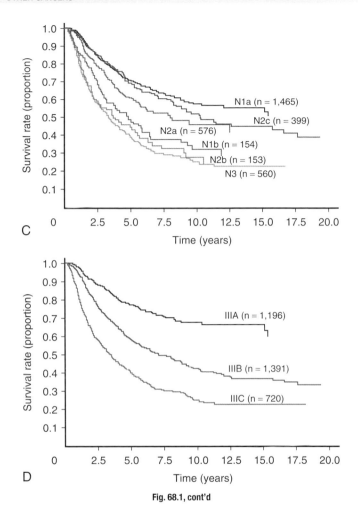

Fig. 68.1, cont'd

status of the SLN helps select patients who may benefit from regional node dissection or adjuvant therapy.

18. **Does a regional lymph node dissection improve survival in patients with melanoma?**
   No. In general, a regional lymph node dissection does not improve survival in all comers with melanoma. However, retrospective studies and subgroup analysis from the MSLT-1 study suggests some patients may benefit from a regional node dissection, so it is still offered to patients with limited nodal disease.

19. **What is the accuracy of sentinel lymph node biopsy for melanoma?**
   In general, the procedure is 95% accurate in predicting the presence of additional nodal metastasis in the region sampled. There is a 5% false-negative rate. Of those with a completion lymph node dissection, approximately 20% will have additional positive nodes. One advantage of the SLN technique is enhanced pathologic analysis with multiple fine cuts of only a few select nodes.

Table 68.1 Tumor, Node, and Metastasis Classification Cutaneous Melanoma

CLASSIFICATION	THICKNESS (MM)	ULCERATION STATUS/MITOSES
T		
Tis	NA	NA
T1	≤1.00	a. Without ulceration and mitosis $< 1/mm^2$ b. With ulceration or mitoses $\geq 1/mm^2$
T2	1.01-2.00	a. Without ulceration b. With ulceration
T3	2.01-4.00	a. Without ulceration b. With ulceration
T4	>4.00	a. Without ulceration b. With ulceration
N	No. of Metastatic Nodes	Nodal Metastatic Burden
N0	0	NA
N1	1	a. Micrometastasis* b. Macrometastasis†
N2	2-3	a. Micrometastasis* b. Macrometastasis†
N3	4+ metastatic nodes, or matted nodes, or in transit, or satellites with metastatic nodes	
M	Site	Serum LDH
M0	No distant metastases	NA
M1a	Distant skin, subcutaneous, or nodal metastases	Normal
M1b	Lung metastases	Normal
M1c	All other visceral metastases	Normal
	Any distant metastasis	Elevated

Abbreviations: NA, not applicable; LDH, lactate dehydrogenase.
*Micrometastases are diagnosed after sentinel lymph node biopsy.
†Macrometastases are defined as clinically detectable nodal metastases confirmed pathologically.

20. **What are the unfavorable features of melanoma in predicting prognosis and metastatic risk?**
   Tumor thickness (Breslow), anatomic invasion of dermis (Clark), nodal status, angiolymphatic invasion, regression, microsatellitosis, neurotropism, head and neck or trunk versus extremities, ulceration, and male gender are unfavorable.

21. **What are acceptable surgical margins for treating primary melanoma?**
   Surgical science is alive and well! Through a series of prospective randomized trials, the following guidelines have been established (Table 68.3).

22. **What is the significance of a *BRAF* mutation in melanoma?**
   A mutation in the signaling kinase *BRAF* occurs in approximately 50% of metastatic melanomas. It is a so-called driver mutation that promotes metastasis. For those patients with BRAF V600E mutations, targeted oral therapies have shown a significant improvement in survival, though most tumors eventually develop secondary mutations that are refractory to treatment.

Table 68.2 Anatomic Stage Groupings for Cutaneous Melanoma

	Clinical Staging*				Pathologic Staging†		
	T	N	M		T	N	M
0	Tis	N0	M0	0	Tis	N0	M0
IA	T1a	N0	M0	IA	T1a	N0	M0
IB	T1b	N0	M0	IB	T1b	N0	M0
	T2a	N0	M0		T2a	N0	M0
IIA	T2b	N0	M0	IIA	T2b	N0	M0
	T3a	N0	M0		T3a	N0	M0
IIB	T3b	N0	M0	IIB	T3b	N0	M0
	T4a	N0	M0		T4a	N0	M0
IIC	T4b	N0	M0	IIC	T4b	N0	M0
III	Any T	N > N0	M0	IIA	T1-4a	N1a	M0
					T1-4a	N2a	M0
				IIB	T1-4b	N1a	M0
					T1-4b	N2a	M0
					T1-4a	N1b	M0
					T1-4a	N2b	M0
					T1-4a	N2c	M0
				IIIC	T1-4b	N1b	M0
					T1-4b	N2b	M0
					T1-4b	N2c	M0
					Any T	N3	M0
IV	Any T	Any N	M1	IV	Any T	Any N	M1

*Clinical staging includes microstaging of the primary melanoma and clinical/radiologic evaluation for metastases. By convention, it should be used after complete excision of the primary melanoma with clinical assessment for regional and distant metastases.

†Pathologic staging includes microstaging of the primary melanoma and pathologic information about the regional lymph nodes after partial (i.e., sentinel node biopsy) or complete lymphadenectomy. Pathologic stage 0 or stage IA patients are the exception; they do not require pathologic evaluation of their lymph nodes.

(From Balch CM, Gershenwald JE, Soong SJ, et al. Final version of 2009 AJCC melanoma staging and classification. *J Clin Oncol.* 2009;27(36):6199–6206. Reprinted with permission from the American Society of Clinical Oncology.)

Table 68.3 Estimated Risk of Sentinel Lymph Node Metastasis Based on Tumor Thickness

TUMOR THICKNESS	RELATIVE RISK OF SENTINEL LYMPH NODE METASTASIS
≤1.0 mm	<5%
1.01–2.0 mm	10%–20%
2.01–4.0 mm	25%–35%
≥4 mm	35%–55%

23. **What other treatments have been shown to improve survival in melanoma patients?**

    Immunotherapy with so-called checkpoint inhibitors (such as anti-CTLA-4 and anti-PD-1 antibodies) are used in the metastatic setting to improve response rates (20%–40%) and increase overall survival. Local injection of oncolytic virus (Tvec) may also improve survival in select patients with localized unresectable disease. IL-2 can result in significant durable responses, but in only about 5% of patients.

24. **When should amputation be used in the management of locally advanced melanoma?**
    Rarely. With the development of isolation limb perfusion, the indications for major limb amputation are rare. Amputation does not affect survival and as such should be used only for local control of disease that cannot be managed in a limb-preserving manner. Partial digital amputation is the recommended therapy for subungual melanoma to achieve local control.

25. **What is the treatment of a patient with metastatic nodes confined to a single area when the primary site is unknown?**
    Approximately 10% of patients with isolated regional nodal metastasis present with an unknown primary. If careful workup reveals no other foci of melanoma, regional lymph node dissection should be carried out.

26. **What is the incidence of lymphedema following a regional lymph node dissection, and how do you manage it?**
    The incidence varies from approximately 10% to 30%. Early recognition is the key. Physical therapy and custom compressive garments may help reduce the severity of the edema.

27. **What are the indications for a SLN biopsy?**
    In general, patients with a primary melanoma >1 mm in Breslow depth are considered for a SLN biopsy. The incidence of a positive sentinel node is approximately 5% for melanomas of 1 mm Breslow depth and increases to nearly 50% for the highest risk melanomas. Other indications include melanomas with a positive deep margin on shave biopsy, ulceration, or lymphovascular invasion.

28. **Is there a role for surgery in patients with stage IV (metastatic) melanoma?**
    Absolutely. In selected patients (generally a long disease-free interval, single site of disease), up to 30% who undergo a resection will be alive at 5 years (compared to <5% who do not undergo resection).

KEY POINTS: MELANOMA

1. The term *melanoma* implies a malignant tumor.
2. Melanoma is the sixth most common cancer in the United States and the fastest rising cancer in men.
3. The warning signs of melanoma are skin lesions that display asymmetry, irregular borders, color changes, diameter >5–6 mm, and enlargement or elevation (A, B, C, D, E).
4. The surgeon's role is to provide local control with adequate margins (1–2 cm) and assess prognosis (SLN biopsy).

WEBSITES

- www.nccn.org
- www.cancer.org

BIBLIOGRAPHY

1. Balch CM, Gershenwald JE, Soong SJ, et al. Final version of 2009 AJCC melanoma staging and classification. *J Clin Oncol.* 2009;27(36):6199–6206.
2. Larkin J, Chiarion-Sileni V, Gonzalez R, et al. Combined nivolumab and ipilimumab or monotherapy in untreated melanoma. *N Engl J Med.* 2015;373(1):23–34.
3. Blazer 3rd DG, Sondak VK. Surgical therapy of cutaneous melanoma. *Semin Oncol.* 2007;34(3):270–280.
4. Jakub JW, Reintgen DS. Regional node dissection for melanoma: techniques and indication. *Surg Oncol Clin N Am.* 2007;16(1):247–261.
5. Morton DL, Thompson JF, Cochran AJ, et al. Sentinel-node biopsy or nodal observation in melanoma. *N Engl J Med.* 2006;355(13):1307–1317.
6. Noorda EM, Vrouenraets BC. Isolated limb perfusion in regional melanoma. *Surg Oncol Clin N Am.* 2006;15(2):373–384.

7. Flaherty KT, Robert C, Hersey P, et al. Improved survival with MEK inhibition in BRAF-mutated melanoma. *N Engl J Med*. 2012;367(2):107–114.
8. Tsao H. Atkins MB.Management of cutaneous melanoma. *N Engl J Med*. 2004;351(10):998–1012.
9. Thompson JF, Scolyer RA. Surgical management of primary cutaneous melanoma: excision margins and the role of sentinel lymph node examination. *Surg Oncol Clin N Am*. 2006;15(2):301–318.
10. Young SE, Martinez SR. The role of surgery in treatment of stage IV melanoma. *J Surg Oncol*. 2006;94(4):344–351.

CHAPTER 69

NONMELANOMA SKIN CANCER

Tiffany L. Tello, MD, Sarah Tuttleton Arron, MD, PhD

1. **What are the most common types of nonmelanoma skin cancer (NMSC)? Which type is the most prevalent?**
   The most common types of NMSC are the keratinocyte carcinomas, basal cell carcinoma (BCC), and squamous cell carcinoma (SCC). BCC represents nearly 80% of NMSCs, while squamous cell carcinoma represents approximately 20% of NMSCs. There are several rare types of NMSC, such as Merkel cell carcinoma, sebaceous gland carcinoma, dermatofibrosarcoma protuberans, and cutaneous lymphoma, that comprise a small percentage of NMSCs.

2. **How common is NMSC?**
   NMSC is the most prevalent malignancy in the United States. There are more cases of NMSC each year than all other cancers combined. In 2012, there were an estimated 5.4 million cases of NMSC, and the incidence continues to rise. It is estimated that one in two men and one in three women in the United States will develop NMSC.

3. **What are the risk factors for developing NMSC?**
   - Cumulative ultraviolet (UV) radiation exposure
   - History of severe sunburn
   - Tanning bed use
   - Red hair, fair skin, freckles
   - Poor tanning ability
   - North European ancestry
   - Family history of skin cancer
   - Immunosuppression (including HIV, alcoholism, chronic lymphocytic leukemia, organ transplantation, and chronic immunosuppressive medications)
   - Smoking
   - Arsenic exposure
   - History of long-term voriconazole therapy
   - History of radiation therapy
   - Human papillomavirus infection
   - Chronic ulcers, sinus tracts, and scars
   - Genetic polymorphisms, such as those in the melanocortin 1 receptor, common in patients with red hair
   - Certain genetic syndromes, including Gorlin syndrome, albinism, epidermolysis bullosa, epidermodysplasia verruciformis, xeroderma pigmentosum, and other rare genetic conditions of DNA repair

4. **What are the major subtypes of BCC? Which are the more aggressive subtypes?**
   - Superficial
   - Nodular
   - Micronodular
   - Infiltrative
   - Morpheaform
   - The most aggressive subtypes are micronodular, infiltrative, and morpheaform

5. **What features of SCC are associated with a higher risk of recurrence and metastasis?**
   - Location on the lip, ear, and genitalia
   - Size >2 cm in diameter
   - Depth >4 mm or extending into the subcutaneous fat
   - Poorly differentiated histology
   - Recurrent lesions
   - SCC arising in an immunosuppressed patient
   - SCCs arising within scars, chronic ulcers, sinus tracts, or areas of chronic inflammation

6. **Does BCC metastasize?**
BCC very rarely metastasizes, though when advanced, these tumors can invade locally into soft tissue, cartilage, and bone. BCC can also spread along nerves (perineural spread) into the skull base.

7. **What is the incidence of lymph node metastases in cutaneous SCC?**
Unlike BCCs, cutaneous SCCs carry risk of metastatic disease, primarily to the lymph nodes. The 5-year rate of metastasis encompassing all cutaneous SCC is 5%, though high-risk lesions can have significantly higher rates. The 5-year survival drops to approximately 50%–70% after surgery and adjuvant radiation therapy when lymph node metastases are present.
Lesions at higher risk for lymph node metastases:

High risk feature	Rate of lymph node metastases
Lesions >2 cm in diameter	30%–42%
Depth >2–4 mm	4%–45%
Location on the lip or ear	10%–14%
SCCs arising in scars, sinus tracts, or chronically inflamed skin	20%–38%
Recurrent tumors	16%–45%
SCCs in solid organ transplant recipients	8%–12%
Poorly differentiated histology	32%–58%

8. **How is cutaneous SCC staged?**
The American Joint Committee on Cancer staging for cutaneous squamous cell carcinoma (8th ed., 2017):

Stage	T: Primary Tumor Characteristics	N: Nodal Involvement	M: Metastases
0	In situ	N0	M0
I	T1	N0	M0
II	T2	N0	M0
III	T3	N0 or N1	M0
	T1 or T2	N1	M0
IV	T1, T2, or T3	N2	M0
	Any T	N3	M0
	T4	Any N	M0
	Any T	Any N	M1

T0	No evidence of primary tumor
Tis	Carcinoma in situ
T1	Tumor <2 cm in greatest dimension
T2	Tumor ≥2 cm, but <4 cm in greatest dimension
T3	Tumor ≥4 cm in greatest dimension or the presence of minor bone erosion, perineural invasion, or deep invasion.[a]
T4a	Tumor with gross cortical bone/marrow invasion
T4b	Tumor with skull base invasion and/or skull base foramen involvement
N0	No regional lymph node metastasis
N1	Metastasis in a single ipsilateral lymph node ≤3 cm in greatest dimension without extranodal extension (ENE)[b]
N2	Metastasis in a single ipsilateral lymph node >3 cm but <6 cm in greatest dimension; or involvement of multiple ipsilateral, contralateral, or bilateral lymph nodes, none >6 cm in greatest dimension and without evidence of ENE[b]
N3	Metastasis in lymph node that is >6 cm in greatest dimension or metastasis in any node(s) that is ENE[b] positive
M0	No distant metastasis
M1	Distant metastasis present

[a]Deep tumors are defined as those with invasion beyond the subcutaneous fat or depth >6 mm (as measured from the granular layer of adjacent normal epidermis to the base of the tumor)
[b]ENE = Extranodal extension (through the lymph node capsule into the surrounding tissue, with or without associated stromal reaction)

9. **How do you treat cutaneous SCC and BCC?**

Modality of treatment depends on the tumor subtype, location, and presence of high-risk features. Most tumors are treated with wide local excision or Mohs micrographic surgery. Topical immuno-modulators, topical chemotherapeutic agents, and electrodessication and curettage are suitable for some low-risk NMSCs. Each treatment option will be discussed in more detail in the following questions. Occasionally, radiation therapy is considered for patients who are poor surgical candidates or as adjuvant therapy for invasive or metastatic disease.

10. **What margin is appropriate for wide local excision of cutaneous SCC and BCC?**

A 4–5 mm margin is appropriate for wide local excision of BCCs and SCCs. Some large SCCs require a 1 cm margin.

11. **What is Mohs micrographic surgery?**

Mohs surgery is a tissue sparing technique for the complete removal of skin cancer with histologic evaluation of 100% of the surgical margin. After the tissue is removed, a map is created with corresponding ink marking of the tissue edges for orientation. The tissue is frozen and placed on slides for hematoxylin and eosin staining and subsequent evaluation by the Mohs surgeon. If the tumor remains at any margin, another layer of tissue is removed in that specific location and again evaluated microscopically for evidence of residual tumor. This process is repeated until the entire tumor is removed. Mohs surgery can be considered for any tumor with a contiguous growth pattern.

12. **When should a patient be referred to a Mohs micrographic surgeon?**

The Appropriate Use Criteria (AUC) for Mohs surgery is a set of guidelines created by a joint committee in 2012 to help prevent the overuse of Mohs surgery, while appropriately triaging those patients who would benefit from this technique. The following is a summary of AUC indications for Mohs surgery:
- Tumors larger than 1 cm on the face or 2 cm on the trunk or extremities
- Tumors occurring on the "mask" or "H-zone" of the face (eyelids, nose, ears, lips, chin, temple, and central face) or tumors on the hands, feet, or genitals
- Tumors with aggressive histology, perineural invasion, or perivascular involvement
- Recurrent or incompletely excised tumors
- Tumors in immunocompromised patients
- Tumors that arise in previously irradiated skin, scars, or sites of chronic inflammation/ulceration
- Genetic conditions with increased risk of skin cancer (basal cell nevus syndrome or xeroderma pigmentosum)

13. **What are the advantages of Mohs micrographic surgery compared to wide local excision?**
- Histologic margin control with evaluation of 100% of the tumor margin by horizontal sectioning (standard vertical bread-loaf technique offers <1% of the true surgical margin for evaluation by the pathologist). This allows for histologic confirmation of tumor removal while the patient is still in clinic and before closing the wound.
- Preservation of tissue, as the surgeon can cut very close to the clinically evident margin of the tumor rather than taking a margin of normal tissue.
- Mohs micrographic surgery offers a cure rate of 98% at 5 years for primary BCCs and SCCs. This is the highest cure rate among all treatment options for cutaneous neoplasms that grow in continuity.

14. **What topical therapies can be considered for cutaneous SCC and BCC? How do they work?**

Topical imiquimod and topical 5-fluorouracil are FDA approved for the treatment of superficial BCCs. They are commonly used off-label for the treatment of SCC in situ (SCCIS) as well.

Imiquimod is a topical immunomodulator that works as a Toll-like receptor 7 agonist, thereby activating the immune system locally. This medication should be applied to the tumor (plus a 1-cm margin) 5 days per week for 6 weeks. The cure rate is 81%–88% for superficial BCCs, and 73%–88% for SCCIS. This is not FDA-approved for use in immunocompromised hosts.

Topical 5-fluorouracil is a pyrimidine analog that interferes with DNA synthesis. The 5% cream should be applied to the tumor plus a 1-cm margin twice daily for 3–6 weeks. The cure rate is 90%–93% for superficial BCCs and 48%–85% for SCCIS.

15. **When is electrodessication and curettage used to treat NMSCs? How is this procedure performed?**
    Electrodessication and curettage is an effective treatment option for small primary superficial and nodular BCCs as well as SCCIS. This treatment will leave a round scar and should only be used in noncosmetically sensitive areas. After injection with local anesthetic, the tumor is debulked with the cutting edge of a curette until the coarse resistance of normal tissue is appreciated. Electrocautery or electrodessication should then be performed over the entire curetted area plus a 2 mm margin. The process of curetting and electrodessication should be repeated three times. The cure rate for small primary BCCs with nonaggressive histology is around 92% at 5 years.

16. **When should you avoid repairing a defect with a flap?**
    If there is concern for development of recurrent disease (i.e., high-risk tumor in an immunosuppressed patient) you should not repair the defect with a flap as it will be more difficult to monitor for tumor recurrence.

17. **What is the relative risk of a patient with a solid organ transplant developing cutaneous SCC and BCC? Which transplant patients are at highest risk?**
    There is a 65-fold increased risk of cutaneous SCC and a 10-fold increased risk of BCC in solid organ transplant patients. The 4:1 ratio of BCC to SCC incidence seen in the general population is reversed in transplant recipients. Transplant recipients should be referred to dermatology for regular full-body skin examination.
    Heart and lung transplant recipients are at highest risk as they tend to require higher levels of immunosuppressant medication. Other risk factors include white race, male sex, and older age at the time of transplantation.

18. **When should sentinel lymph node biopsy be considered in cutaneous SCC?**
    The role of sentinel lymph node biopsy in cutaneous SCC has not yet been well defined. However, there is a subset of patients who may benefit from sentinel lymph node biopsy. Some authors suggest considering patients who are categorized as T2 or higher, as they have >10% risk of lymph node metastases. This includes patients with SCCs >2 cm in greatest dimension or tumors <2 cm with two or more high-risk features (depth >2 mm, perineural invasion, anatomic site on the ear or lip, and poorly differentiated histology). Immunosuppressed patients with high-risk tumors could also be considered for sentinel lymph node biopsy.

19. **What syndrome is characterized by numerous BCCs, frontal bossing, and medulloblastoma? Which gene is mutated in this condition?**
    Gorlin syndrome (basal cell nevus syndrome) is an autosomal dominant condition characterized by a mutation in the *PTCH1* gene. *PTCH1* is a tumor suppressor in the Hedgehog signaling pathway, and loss of this gene leads to tumor proliferation. These patients develop BCCs starting in adolescence. They also have palmar pits, frontal bossing, medulloblastomas, odontogenic keratocysts of the jaw, and abnormalities of the vertebrae and ribs.

20. **What systemic medication can be considered for patients with locally advanced BCC, those who are poor surgical candidates, or those with numerous BCCs?**
    Vismodegib and Sonidegib are targeted molecular inhibitors of the Hedgehog signaling pathway. Activating mutations in this pathway are present in over 90% of BCCs, and therefore inhibition can lead to regression of tumor. This medication carries significant side effects of muscle cramps, alopecia, and dysgeusia. It is teratogenic and so should not be used in women of childbearing potential.

21. **What is the precursor lesion to cutaneous SCCs?**
    The precursor lesion to cutaneous SCC is the actinic keratosis. Actinic keratoses are rough pink papules in sun-exposed areas that represent in-situ dysplasias. Approximately 60% of cutaneous SCC arise in sites of preexisting actinic keratoses, though only a small percentage of actinic keratoses actually progress to SCC.

22. **What topical treatments can be considered for patients with numerous actinic keratoses to prevent development of cutaneous SCCs?**
    Field treatment to the most severely affected areas should be considered in patients with numerous actinic keratoses. Options include cryotherapy, topical 5-fluorouracil, imiquimod, ingenol mebutate, or photodynamic therapy. These treatments are similar in efficacy for the treatment of actinic keratoses.

23. **What systemic treatment option is available for patients with numerous SCCs? What are the side effects?**
    Acitretin is a systemic retinoid that can be considered for patients with numerous SCCs. It decreases the development of new primary lesions and is commonly used in solid organ transplant patients with numerous SCCs. The major side effects include teratogenicity, transaminitis, hyperlipidemia, and dryness of the eyes, lips, mouth, and skin.

24. **After treatment of an NMSC, how should the patient be followed? How should they be counseled?**
    Patients should have a full-body skin examination by a dermatologist every 6 months for the first 2 years after an NMSC. If no additional skin cancers are found during that period, exams can then be spaced annually. Note that once a patient develops one NMSC, the risk of developing a second NMSC is increased 10-fold.
    Strict photoprotection will decrease the development of new primary NMSC, and the patient should be counseled accordingly. The patient should wear broad-spectrum sunscreen (with SPF >30) daily, wide-brimmed hats, long sleeves, and avoid midday sun when UV irradiation is at its peak.

KEY POINTS: NONMELANOMA SKIN CANCER

1. NMSC is the most prevalent malignancy in the United States, with more cases each year than all other cancers combined.
2. The appropriate margin for excision of an NMSC is typically 4–5 mm.
3. High-risk NMSCs, particularly large lesions, those on the face, or those in immunosuppressed patients, should be referred for Mohs micrographic surgery. The AUC for Mohs surgery is an excellent guide of when to place a referral.
4. Solid organ transplant patients are at particularly high risk for developing skin cancers (and have a higher rate of lymph node metastases). These patients should be referred to a dermatologist for regular skin examinations.

BIBLIOGRAPHY

1. Rogers HW, Weinstock MA, Feldman SR, Coldiron BM. Incidence estimate of nonmelanoma skin cancer (keratinocyte carcinomas) in the US Population, 2012. *JAMA Dermatol.* 2015;151(10):1081–1086.
2. American Cancer Society, Inc. *Cancer Facts & Figures 2017.* American Cancer Society, Surveillance Research, 2017. https://www.cancer.org/research/cancer-facts-statistics/all-cancer-facts-figures/cancer-facts-figures-2017.html. Accessed March 2017.
3. Agnew KL, Bunker CB. *Fast Facts: Skin Cancer.* 2nd ed. Health Press Limited; 2013.
4. Alessi SS, Sanches JA. Treatment of cutaneous tumors with topical 5% imiquimod cream. *Clinics (Sao Paulo).* 2009;64(10):961–966.
5. Romagosa R, Saap L, Givens M, et al. A pilot study to evaluate the treatment of basal cell carcinoma with 5-fluorouracil using phosphatidyl choline as a transepidermal carrier. *Dermatol Surg.* 2000;26(4):338–340.
6. McGillis ST, Fein H. Topical treatment strategies for non-melanoma skin cancer and precursor lesions. *Semin Cutan Med Surg.* 2004;23(3):174–183.
7. Love WE, Bernhard JD. Topical imiquimod or fluorouracil therapy for basal and squamous cell carcinoma: a systematic review. *Arch Dermatol.* 2009;145(12):1431–1438.
8. Miller DL, Weinstock MA. Nonmelanoma skin cancer in the United States: incidence. *J Am Acad Dermatol.* 1994;30(5 Pt 1):774–778.
9. Alam M, Ratner D. Cutaneous squamous-cell carcinoma. *N Engl J Med.* 2001;344(13):975–983.
10. Rowe DE, Carroll RJ. Prognostic factors for local recurrence, metastasis, and survival rates in squamous cell carcinoma of the skin, ear, and lip: implications for treatment modality selection. *J Am Acad Dermatol.* 1992;26(6):976–990.
11. American Academy of Dermatology, American College of Mohs Surgery, American Society for Dermatologic Surgery Association, et al. AAD/ACMS/ASDSA/ASMS 2012 appropriate use criteria for Mohs micrographic surgery: a report of the American Academy of Dermatology, American College of Mohs Surgery, American Society for Dermatologic Surgery Association, and the American Society for Mohs Surgery. *Dermatol Surg.* 2012;38(10):1582–1603.
12. Navarrete-Dechent C. High-risk cutaneous squamous cell carcinoma and the emerging role of sentinel lymph node biopsy: a literature review. *J Am Acad Dermatol.* 2015;73(1):127–137.
13. Califano JA, Lydiatt WM. Cutaneous squamous cell carcinoma of the head and neck. In: Amin MB, Edge SB, eds. *AJCC Cancer Staging Manual.* 8th ed. New York: Springer; 2017:171–179.
14. James WD, Berger TG. *Epidermal nevi, neoplasms, and cysts. Andrews' Diseases of the Skin: Clinical Dermatology.* 12th ed. Philadelphia: Elsevier; 2016:634–635.
15. Farasat S, Yu SS, Neel VA, et al. A new American Joint Committee on Cancer staging system for cutaneous squamous cell carcinoma: creation and rationale for inclusion of tumor (T) characteristics. *J Am Acad Dermatol.* 2011;64(6):1051–1059.

CHAPTER 70

PAROTID TUMORS

Michael L. Lepore, MD, FACS

1. **Describe the location and characteristics of the parotid gland.**

   The paired parotid glands are the largest of the three major salivary glands. The parotid gland is triangular in shape bounded superiorly by the zygomatic arch; posteriorly by the external auditory canal; inferiorly by the styloid process, the styloid muscle, and the jugular and internal carotid vessels; and anteriorly by the masseter muscle. The tail of the parotid gland may extend inferior-posterior to the level of the sternocleidomastoid muscle and mastoid process. Its main histologic feature consists of clusters of acinar cells that are mainly serous secreting.

2. **What is the salivary gland unit?**

   The parotid salivary gland units consist of the acinar cells of the parotid gland and a transport system. The transport system consists of the following: the intercalated ducts, the striated ducts, and the excretory ducts. These ducts are all interconnecting, emptying into the oral cavity via Stenson's duct. Contractile myoepithelial cells surrounding both the acinous cell units and the intercalated ducts force the watery secretions through the duct system into the oral cavity.

3. **What is the relationship of the facial nerve to the parotid gland?**

   The facial nerve divides the parotid gland into a superficial and deep lobe. The facial nerve enters the temporal bone at the anterior superior portion of the internal auditory canal. The nerve then travels through the mastoid bone in the fallopian canal exiting the skull base at the stylomastoid foramen. The nerve lies lateral to the styloid process and posterior belly of the digastric muscle and medial to the mastoid tip. As the nerve exits the stylomastoid foramen, it immediately gives off three motor branches: one to the stylohyoid muscle, one to the posterior belly of the digastric muscle, and the third to the three postauricular muscles of the pinna. The nerve then proceeds anteriorly for a short distance and at the pes anserinus divides into two major divisions—the temporofacial and cervicofacial divisions. After dividing, the nerve will then turn laterally to enter the posterior aspect of the parotid gland. The temporofacial division subsequently divides into the temporal, zygomatic, and buccal branches. The cervicofacial division divides into the marginal mandibular and cervical branches. The deep parotid lobe lies between the temporofacial and cervicofacial divisions. There are numerous variations in the division of the nerve, and careful identification of each division and branch must occur to avoid injury to the nerve.

4. **What branches of the facial nerve are at major risk of injury during parotid gland surgery?**

   The temporal and marginal mandibular branches of the facial nerve are at major risk of injury because of their small size and lack of anastomotic connections. Careful identification and dissection is extremely important.

5. **What is the significance of the salivary gland unit in tumor development?**

   There are currently two theories of tumor development based on the salivary gland unit.
   a. Bicellular theory: Tumors arise from stem cells. The intercalated duct reserve cells give rise to the pleomorphic adenoma, oncocytomas, adenoid cystic carcinomas, adenocarcinomas, and acinic cell carcinomas. The excretory duct reserve cells will give rise to squamous cell and mucoepidermoid carcinomas.
   b. Multicellular theory: Each tumor type is associated with a specific differentiated cell of origin within the salivary gland unit. Therefore, excretory duct cells give rise to squamous cell carcinomas, intercalated duct cells give rise to pleomorphic adenomas, striated ducts give rise to oncocytomas, and acinar cells give rise to acinic cell carcinomas.

6. **What are the four most common benign tumors of the salivary gland origin and their characteristics?**

   a. The pleomorphic adenoma (mixed tumor) accounts for approximately 80% of all benign parotid tumors. They are slow growing and are not well encapsulated. The recurrence rate is 1%–5% with appropriate excision. Malignant degeneration may occur in approximately 2%–10% of cases.

b. Warthin's tumor (papillary cystadenoma lymphomatosum or adenolymphoma). This tumor occurs later in life. It is the second most common tumor representing approximately 5% of all benign tumors. There is a male predominance. Approximately 12% of Warthin's tumors occur bilaterally.

c. Oncytoma occur in the sixth decade of life and are composed of large oxyphilic cells. Oncocytes found in these tumors and Warthin's tumors are responsible for concentration of technetium 99m pertechnetate.

d. Monomorphic adenoma includes the following: Basal cell adenoma, clear cell adenoma, glycogen-rich adenoma. The most common of the three is the basal cell adenoma. These tumors are well circumscribed and encapsulated.

7. **What is the treatment for benign tumors of the parotid gland?**
The treatment is a superficial parotidectomy with preservation of the facial nerve. After the gland is removed and sent to the frozen section lab, it should be properly oriented and tagged for the pathologist. If there is a close margin, then patients should be observed for recurrence, particularly in the case of a pleomorphic adenoma.

8. **Describe the five most common malignant parotid tumors and their characteristics.**
   a. Mucoepidermoid carcinoma is the most common malignant tumor of the parotid gland, accounting for 30% of all parotid malignancies. They are classified as either low-grade or high-grade malignancies. The low-grade form has a higher ratio of mucous cells to epidermoid cells and behaves like benign tumors. In the case of high-grade tumors, there is a higher portion of epidermoid cells resembling a squamous cell carcinoma. The latter have a high propensity for metastasis.

   b. Adenocarcinomas represent approximately 15% of parotid gland tumors. The neoplasms present as firm or hard masses attached to the surrounding tissue. Adenocarcinomas lack keratin and therefore are easily differentiated from mucoepidermoid carcinomas.

   c. Adenoid cystic carcinoma (cylindromas) account for 6% of all salivary gland neoplasms. It is the most common malignancy of the submandibular and minor salivary glands. Adenoid cystic carcinomas are unpredictable and may remain quiescent for years. These tumors grow along perineural planes and have a high incidence of distant metastasis, particularly to the lungs. There are three histologic types—cribriform, solid, and tubular. The solid form has the worst prognosis, and the cribriform is considered the most benign of the group.

   d. Malignant mixed tumors (carcinoma expleomorphic adenoma) are believed to develop from a preexisting pleomorphic adenoma. It appears to represent 2%–5% of parotid malignancies.

   e. Lymphomas of the parotid gland most commonly occur in elderly males. They account for 0.6%–5% of parotid tumors. The entire parotid gland is enlarged as well as regional lymph nodes. Fine-needle aspiration (FNA) with flow cytometry may assist in diagnosing this condition because the treatment consists of chemotherapy followed by radiation therapy.

9. **What are the most common salivary gland neoplasms in children?**
Salivary gland neoplasms in the very young are rare. Approximately 65% of tumors are benign, the most common being hemangiomas. The remaining 35% of salivary gland tumors in children are malignant. The most common is the mucoepidermoid carcinoma.

10. **What is the role of intraoperative facial nerve monitoring in parotid gland surgery?**
Facial nerve monitoring is a useful means of identifying the facial nerve, particularly during difficult parotid gland surgery. Multiple peripheral probes are normally placed at four locations—at the region of the temporal branch that innervates the frontalis muscle, the region of the zygomatic branch that innervates the orbicularis oculi muscle, the region of the buccal branch that innervates the orbicularis oris muscle, and the region of marginal mandibular nerve that innervates the muscle of the depressor muscle of the lower lip. When the major divisions of the facial nerve are stimulated distally, facial movement will be evident. If the pes anserinus is stimulated, all distal branches of the nerve will fire simultaneously. Because this monitoring equipment is readily available at most institutions, one should consider its use, particularly from a medicolegal standpoint.

11. **What is the significance of a dumbbell tumor?**
Occasionally, deep lobe parotid tumor may present, on examination, as a mass in the lateral pharyngeal wall. This is primarily the result of a weakness in the stylomandibular membrane.

12. **Of all the three paired major salivary glands, which gland has the highest incidence of salivary gland tumors?**
   The parotid gland has the highest incidence of salivary gland tumors. Approximately 80% of all tumors located in this gland are benign. A good rule of thumb to remember with respect to malignant tumors is the 25/50/75 rule. As the salivary gland gets smaller, the incidence of malignancies increases. Thus in the parotid gland, the incidence of malignancies is 25%, in the submandibular gland it is 50%, and in the sublingual gland it is 75%.

13. **What is the significance of facial nerve weakness or paralysis in association with parotid gland enlargement?**
   Involvement of the facial nerve in the presence of a parotid mass is usually an indication that a malignant process is present. The degree of paralysis should be noted clinically, and preoperative photos should be taken for documentation.

14. **What is the workup for a mass in the parotid space?**
   The workup is based on the clinical history and physical findings on examination of the patient. Classically, patients with a tumor involving the parotid gland will complain of a painless mass that is slow growing in the preauricular region in 80% of cases, or at the angle of the mandible (tail of the parotid gland). In 30% of cases, the mass may be painful, and in 7%–20% of cases, there may be facial nerve involvement. In these patients, one should suspect a high index of suspicion for a parotid malignancy. Approximately 80% of patients with facial nerve paralysis have nodal metastasis at the time of diagnosis. A careful examination of the oral cavity, scalp, larynx, base of tongue, and pharynx by means of a flexible endoscopic exam should be performed to rule out other primary sites. A thorough examination of the neck is important in order to determine if metastatic disease has spread beyond the parotid gland. FNA may be easily performed in the clinical setting. Contrast computed tomography (CT) and magnetic resonance imaging are helpful in determining the location and extent of the mass; however, benign pathology can give similar findings—poorly defined borders as well as enhancement.

15. **What is the role of fine-needle aspiration biopsy (FNAB) in the diagnosis of parotid gland enlargement?**
   FNAB is a useful diagnostic adjunct in the evaluation of masses in the head and neck. FNAB is highly dependent on the experience of the pathologist. Therefore, its role in the evaluation of salivary gland tumors is somewhat controversial. It has a sensitivity of >90% and a specificity of >95%. It has a positive predictive value of approximately 84% and a negative predictive value of approximately 77%. It is an excellent method of differentiating between a benign (lymphadenopathy) and a malignant process.

16. **Are there any lymph nodes present in the parotid gland?**
   There is anywhere between 1 and more than 20 lymph nodes randomly distributed within the parotid gland. Occasionally, you may see either salivary gland ducts or acini (Neisse Nicholson rest) within the nodal tissue.

17. **Describe the current tumor, node, and metastasis classification of malignant parotid gland tumors.**
   Primary Tumor
   TX Tumor extent unknown or cannot be assessed
   T0 No evidence of a primary tumor
   Tis Carcinoma in situ
   T1 Tumor <2 cm in greatest diameter
   T2 Tumor >2 cm but <4 cm in greatest diameter
   T3 Tumor >4 cm and/or tumor having extraparenchymal extension
   T4a Tumor invades skin, mandible, ear canal, and/or facial nerve
   T4b Tumor invades skull base and/or pterygoid plates or encases the carotid artery
   All categories are subdivided into (a) no local extension and (b) local extension.
   Lymph nodes
   NX Regional lymph nodes cannot be assessed
   N0 No regional lymph node metastasis
   N1 Metastasis to a single ipsilateral node equal to 3 cm
   N2 Metastasis to a single ipsilateral lymph node between 3 and 6 cm or in multiple

ipsilateral nodes, none >6 cm, or bilateral or contralateral lymph
nodes none >6 cm
N2a Metastasis to a single ipsilateral node >3 cm, but not >6 cm
N2b Metastasis in multiple ipsilateral lymph nodes, none >6 cm in its greatest dimension
N2c Metastasis in bilateral or contralateral lymph nodes, none >6 cm in its greatest dimension
N3 Metastasis in a lymph node >6 cm in its greatest dimension
Metastasis
MO No distant metastasis
M1 Distant metastasis

18. **How are parotid tumors staged?**
There are six stage groupings for parotid tumors.

	Primary tumor	*Nodal involvement*	*Distant Metastasis*
Stage I	T1	N0	M0
Stage II	T2	N0	M0
Stage III	T3	N0	M0
	T1, T2, T3	N1	M0
Stage IV A	T1, T2, T3	N2	M0
	T4a	N0, N1, N2	M0
Stage IV B	T4b	Any N	M0
	Any T	N3	M0
Stage IV C	Any T	Any N	

19. **How are parotid tumors managed?**
If the histopathologic diagnosis is unknown prior to surgery, the minimum surgical procedure
that should be performed is a superficial parotidectomy with dissection and preservation of the
facial nerve with intraoperative frozen sections. Enucleation of a parotid tumor mass should
not be performed because of the high incidence of recurrence. If the frozen section diagnosis
returns positive for a malignant tumor, there are multiple treatment options available depending
on the type of tumor identified, the presence of lymph nodes, distant metastasis, and facial nerve
involvement.
Group 1: T1 or T2N0 low-grade malignancies (acinic cell carcinoma and low-grade mucoepidermoid
carcinomas). A superficial parotidectomy is performed with preservation of the facial nerve.
Group 2: T1 or T2N0 high-grade features (high-grade mucoepidermoid carcinoma, adenocarcinoma,
adenoid cystic carcinoma, squamous cell carcinoma, carcinoma expleomorphic, and malignant
mixed tumors).
  a. Total parotidectomy should be performed (removal of the superficial and deep lobes).
  b. If the facial nerve is not involved it should be preserved. If the nerve is involved, it should be
  resected and cable grafted with a sural nerve graft.
  c. A modified or selective neck dissection should be performed.
  d. Patient should receive postoperative radiation therapy to the parotid bed and the neck.
Group 3: T3N0 or and N1 high-grade cancers and recurrent cancers.
  a. The treatment of choice is aggressive radical surgical resection, including the deep lobe of the
  parotid.
  b. If branches of the facial nerve are involved, they should be removed and grafted at the time of
  surgery. If the tumor involves the facial nerve at the stylomastoid foramen, then a mastoidec-
  tomy with exposure of the facial nerve within the fallopian canal and resection of the nerve until
  negative margins are obtained.
  c. Cable grafting of the facial nerve should be considered.
  d. A modified neck dissection is performed in all T3N0 categories, and a radical neck dissection in
  T3N+ categories.
  e. The patient should receive postoperative radiation therapy to the primary parotid area and the
  neck.
Group 4: T4 category.
  a. In this group, a radical parotidectomy is performed to include the surrounding tissue involved
  (buccal fat, skin, ear canal, mastoid bone, and mandible).

b. The facial nerve is usually involved and sacrificed, and primary reconstruction of all involved areas must be performed at the time of surgery.

c. The patient will need postoperative radiation therapy to the primary parotid site, surrounding area, and the neck.

20. **What are the potential complications of parotid gland surgery?**
Skin flap necrosis
Bleeding (hematoma)
Infection
Salivary gland fistula
Facial nerve paresis; temporary in 10% of patients, usually the result of a stretched nerve, or permanent paralysis in <2% of patients.
Frey's syndrome or gustatory sweating (flushing and sweating of the skin overlying the surgical site). This is the result of inappropriate autonomic reinnervation of sweat glands in the skin from parotid parasympathetic nerve branches to the parotid into the more superficial sweat glands of the skin.

21. **Is there a role for chemotherapy in the treatment of parotid gland malignancies?**
Parotid gland tumors normally respond very poorly to chemotherapy. Adjuvant chemotherapy is currently indicated only for palliation. Platinum-based agents are most commonly used because they induce apoptosis and cell death. On the other hand, doxorubicin-based agents promote cell arrest.

22. **Why should you be careful when dealing with cystic lesions of the parotid gland?**
Cystic lesions of the parotid gland were once thought to be rare lesions. However, in the last 20 years, the incidence of cystic lesions has increased, particularly in the HIV population. When a mass is noted in the parotid gland in an HIV-positive patient, one must think of the presence of a lymphoepithelial cyst. Huang et al. recommend a CT scan and an FNA to rule out other types of cystic lesions and not to operate on these patients. On multiple occasions, needle aspiration of the fluid built up is necessary to relieve pain; however, the fluid only returns, and in some instances the cyst enlarges. In this group of patients, performing a superficial parotidectomy with facial nerve sparing may be indicated.

23. **Are intraoperative frozen sections reliable in order to differentiate between benign and malignant parotid tumors, and would you resect the facial nerve on the basis of a frozen section?**
At times, it is difficult for pathologists to make a conclusive diagnosis based on frozen sections; consequently, they will have a tendency to defer the diagnosis until an adequate histologic workup is performed. Therefore, most surgeons will hesitate performing a major destructive procedure until the final pathologic diagnosis is received in writing. In this instance, the surgeon should only perform a superficial lobe parotidectomy. In the event that the patient must return to the operating room, the procedure becomes more difficult and facial nerve injury rates are higher. One extremely important point, at the time of the original surgery, is to tag the parotid tissue along its superficial, deep, anterior, superior, inferior, and posterior margins, before it is sent to the pathologist. This will enable the pathologist to accurately determine where positive margins are located. This will also aid the surgeon in accurately assessing these areas at the time of reoperation.

24. **What role does vascular endothelial growth factor (VEGF) play in salivary gland neoplasms?**
Neovascularization in salivary gland neoplasms has been recently studied. There appears to be a direct correlation with an increase angiogenesis and the progression of salivary gland tumors. The VEGF is expressed in half of the salivary glands tested. It also appears to correlate well with clinical staging, metastatic rate, recurrence rate, and patient survival.

25. **Which oncogenes have been implicated in the molecular mechanism by which tumorigenesis occur in salivary gland tumors?**
The following oncogenes are known to be associated with a wide variety of human cancers and also may play a role in parotid cancer development: *p53, Bcl-2, P13K/Akt, MDM2,* and Ras.
For example, *p53* oncogene has been found in both benign and malignant salivary gland tumors. The presents of p53 mutations appears to correlate with a higher rate of tumor recurrence.
Ras is a G protein involved in growth signal transduction. Derangements in ras signaling have been implicated in a wide variety of solid tumors. For example, H-Ras mutations have been noted in several types of parotid tumors including pleomorphic adenomas, adenocarcinomas, and mucoepidermoid carcinomas.

KEY POINTS: PAROTID TUMORS

1. The most common benign tumor of the parotid gland is a pleomorphic adenoma.
2. The most common malignant tumor of the parotid gland is a mucoepidermoid carcinoma.
3. Adenoid cystic carcinoma has the highest incidence of perineural invasion.
4. FNAB is a useful diagnostic tool that may assist the surgeon in the preoperative evaluation avoiding a surgical procedure that is unnecessary (e.g., lymphoma).
5. The most common parotid malignant tumor in children is a mucoepidermoid carcinoma.
6. The most common benign tumor in children is a hemangioma.
7. The presence of facial nerve paresis or paralysis is a strong indication of an underlying malignant process. Pleomorphic adenomas should not be enucleated from the parotid gland tissue because of the high incidence of recurrence.

BIBLIOGRAPHY

1. Arabi Mianroodi AA, Sigston EA. Frozen section for parotid surgery: should it become routine? *ANZ J Surg.* 2006;76(8):736–739.
2. Balakrishnan K, Castling B, McMahon J, et al. Fine needle aspiration cytology in the management of a parotid mass: a two centre retrospective study. *Surgeon.* 2005;3(2):67–72.
3. Brennan JA, Moore EJ. Prospective analysis of the efficacy of continuous intraoperative nerve monitoring during thyroidectomy, parathyroidectomy, and parotidectomy. *Otolaryngol Head Neck Surg.* 2001;124(5):537–554.
4. Carlson GW. The salivary glands. Embryology, anatomy, and surgical applications. *Surg Clin North Am.* 2000;80(1):261–273.
5. Hollander L, Cunningham MP. Management of cancer of the parotid gland. *Surg Clin North Am.* 1973;53(1):113–119.
6. Huang RD, Pearlman S. Benign cystic vs. solid lesions of the parotid gland in HIV patients. *Head Neck.* 1991;13(6):522–526.
7. Koyuncu M, Sesen T, Akan H, et al. Comparison of computed tomography and magnetic resonance imaging in the diagnosis of parotid tumors. *Otolaryngol Head Neck Surg.* 2003;129(6):726–732.
8. Lee JH, Lee JH. Unique expression of MUC3, MUC5AC and cytokeratins in salivary gland carcinomas. *Pathol Int.* 2005;55(7):386–389.
9. Lin CC, Tsai MH. Parotid tumors: a 10-year experience. *Am J Otolaryngol.* 2008;29(2):94–100.
10. Medina JF. Neck dissection in the treatment of cancer of major salivary glands. *Otolaryngol Clin North Am.* 1998;31(5):815–822.
11. Rabinov JD. Imaging of salivary gland pathology. *Radiol Clin North Am.* 2000;38(5):1047–1057.
12. Spiro RH. Diagnosis and pitfalls in the treatment of parotid tumors. *Semin Surg Oncol.* 1991;7(1):20–24.
13. Zbaren P, Schar C. Value of fine-needle aspiration cytology of parotid gland masses. *Laryngoscope.* 2001;111(11 Pt 1):1989–1992.

CHAPTER 71

NECK MASSES

Nathan W. Pearlman, MD, Michael L. Lepore, MD, FACS

1. **What is a reasonable differential diagnosis for masses/lumps in the ipsilateral neck?**
   Nonspecific lymphadenopathy
   Salivary gland tumor
   Viral or bacterial infectious process
   Lymphoma
   Carotid body tumor/chemodectoma
   Metastatic carcinoma
   Tuberculosis or a fungal disease
   Prominent normal anatomy

2. **Could normal anatomy be a lump?**
   Yes. The right and left neck are usually mirror images, and normal anatomy on one side is occasionally more prominent than its counterpart on the other. The most common example of this is a prominent posterior belly of the omohyoid in the posterior triangle or unilateral enlargement of a submaxillary or parotid gland. The key finding is a similar but less prominent structure in the same location in the contralateral neck.

3. **Other than normal anatomy, is there any way to narrow this list of possibilities?**
   a. Eighty percent of enlarged lymph nodes in the anterior triangle are benign, whereas the situation is reversed in the posterior triangle.
   b. Other than location, nonspecific lymphadenopathy is generally asymptomatic or mildly tender, usually of recent onset, mobile, soft, usually <3 cm, and overlying skin is normal.
   c. Nodes reflecting a more serious viral or bacterial process are often multiple, bilateral, tender, generally soft, and overlying skin may be erythematous.
   d. A carotid body/glomus tumor may or may not be tender (usually not), of rubbery consistency, and depending on its size may be fixed to the carotid bifurcation and cannot be separated from the carotid pulse.
   e. Submaxillary and parotid gland tumors are rubbery, relatively immobile, nontender, and cannot be separated from the gland. Of note, tumors in the tail of the parotid gland often enlarge and obliterate the angle of the mandible.
   f. Nodes involved by metastatic carcinoma may be single or multiple, hard, nontender, often >3 cm, present for some time, and may involve overlying skin.
   g. Lymphoma nodes are relatively nontender, usually >3 cm, soft, unilateral or bilateral, and often accompanied by recurring fevers, night sweats, and enlarged nodes in the axilla or groin.
   h. Tuberculosis and/or fungal diseases (actinomycosis, etc.) can mimic all of the above.

4. **What are the next steps to evaluate this situation?**
   First is a complete history and physical examination, with particular emphasis on the mouth, pharynx, thyroid, and other lymph node basins. In about 50% of cases, this will narrow the differential diagnosis to two or three likely possibilities. The next step is either a computed tomography (CT) scan or magnetic resonance imaging (MRI) if the mass cannot be separated from important structures (carotid pulse, etc.), or ultrasound (US)-guided fine-needle aspirate (FNA). US-guided FNA is 80%–90% accurate in providing a rapid diagnosis, and is probably the most cost-effective next step.

5. **What if the history and physical examination are noncontributory, but the FNA shows metastatic cancer. Where did it come from?**
   If the enlarged node is in the anterior triangle, the most likely spots are somewhere in the mouth, naso-/hypopharynx, or larynx. If the node is in the posterior triangle, the primary is more likely nasopharynx, esophagus, or thyroid. However, nodes that lie just above the clavicle usually represent cancer of the lung or other sites (stomach, prostate, etc.) in the chest or abdomen. To further evaluate

these possibilities, the next step becomes examination of the mouth, pharynx, larynx, esophagus, and tracheobronchial tree under anesthesia. If examination of the above areas is difficult while the patient is awake, the above areas may be reexamined under general anesthesia. If something is noted, then biopsies should be performed. If nothing is noted, then blind biopsies should be performed of the base of the tongue and the nasopharynx. In about 10%–15% of cases, this will either detect the primary or find a second, synchronous, cancer of the aerodigestive tract.

6. **This seems like a time consuming and expensive approach. Why not just excise the node, find out what the problem is, and go from there?**
Excisional biopsy should never be the initial diagnostic maneuver, unless absolutely necessary. If lymphoma or an unusual infection is present, but not suspected, the node may be mishandled when sent to pathology or microbiology. If metastatic cancer is the problem, the biopsy creates scarring in the field, complicates subsequent management, and may be detrimental to survival. Open biopsy is a particularly bad choice if the lump is a carotid body tumor and not metastatic cancer.

7. **All right, the patient is found to have metastatic squamous cancer, but the primary cannot be found. What is the treatment algorithm?**
First, the patient should undergo a CT, CT-positron emission tomography, or MRI scan to determine other sites of disease, both above and below the clavicles. Then, if nothing else is found other than the involved cervical node, there are basically two choices. One is a functional or modified neck dissection, followed by postoperative irradiation to the neck and likely primary site(s). The other choice is primary irradiation alone to the same areas, with close follow-up, reserving surgery for emergence of disease at a later time. Prognosis in such patients is primarily determined by the presence of metastatic disease and much less so by the primary tumor.

8. **If the FNA shows only lymphocytes, how do we proceed?**
The lymphocytes probably represent benign inflammation but could represent lymphoma or Warthin's tumor of the parotid (cystadenoma lymphomatosum). So, to be sure, one should reexamine the patient in 6–8 weeks to make sure the initial diagnosis was sound. Alternatively, if only lymphocytes are found, it may **now** be reasonable to excise the node for final diagnosis.

KEY POINTS: NECK MASSES

1. Eighty percent of enlarged lymph nodes in the anterior triangle of the neck are benign, whereas the situation is reversed in the posterior triangle.
2. Following a history and physical and a CT or MRI, the most efficient next step is a fine needle aspiration of a node.
3. When the FNA reveals metastatic cancer, the next step is panendoscopy (evaluation of the mouth, pharynx, larynx, esophagus, and tracheobronchial tree under anesthesia).
4. When the FNA reveals metastatic squamous cell cancer, but the primary neoplasm cannot be found, either modified surgical neck dissection with postoperative radiation or radiation alone, saving surgery for regional recurrence, would be an acceptable option.
5. Never biopsy a pulsatile mass in Zone III of the neck or in the tonsillar region or nasopharyngeal area because this may represent a carotid body tumor or an abnormal course of the internal carotid artery, respectively.
6. If purulent material is discovered when aspirating a lymph node, the material should be submitted for acid-fast bacilli workup, particularly in children, AIDS patients, and the immigrant population.

BIBLIOGRAPHY

1. Attie JN, Setzon M. Thyroid cancer presenting as an enlarged cervical lymph node. *Am J Surg.* 1993;166(4):428–430.
2. Chau I, Kelleher MT, Cunningham D, et al. Rapid access multidisciplinary lymph node diagnostic clinic analysis of 550 patients. *Br J Cancer.* 2003;88(3):354–361.
3. Gleeson M, Herbert A. Management of lateral neck masses in adults. *BMJ.* 2000;320(7248):1521–1524.
4. King AD, Ahuja AT, Young DKW, et al. Malignant cervical lymphadenopathy: diagnostic accuracy of diffusion-weighted MR imaging. *Radiology.* 2007;245(3):806–813.
5. Mallon DH, Kostalas M, MacPherson FJ, et al. The diagnostic value of fine needle aspiration in parotid lumps. *Ann R Coll Surg Engl.* 2013;95(4):258–262.

6. Rice DH, Spiro RH. Metastatic carcinoma of the neck, primary unknown. In: *Current Concepts in Head and Neck Cancer*. Atlanta: American Cancer Society; 1989.
7. Smith OD, Ellis PDM. Management of neck lumps–a triage model. *Ann R Coll Surg Engl*. 2000;82(4):223–226.
8. Troost EG, Vogel VW, Merkx MA, et al. 18-FLT PET does not discriminate between reactive and metastatic lymph nodes in primary head and neck cancer patients. *J Nucl Med*. 2007;48(5):726–735.

VII
VASCULAR SURGERY

CHAPTER 72

WHAT IS ATHEROSCLEROSIS?

Craig Selzman, MD, FACS

1. **Do you have to be old to have atherosclerosis?**
   No. The initial (or type I) lesion, consisting of lipid deposits in the intima, has been well characterized in infants and children.

2. **What is a fatty streak?**
   Fatty streaks or type II lesions are visible as yellow-colored streaks, patches, or spots on the intimal surface of arteries. Microscopically, they are characterized by the intracellular accumulation of lipid.

3. **What is a foam cell?**
   A foam cell is any cell that has ingested lipids, thus giving the histologic appearance of a sudsy vacuole. In general, a foam cell refers to a lipid-laden macrophage; however, other cells that uptake lipids, particularly vascular smooth muscle cells, also may be considered foam cells.

4. **Describe the progression of atherosclerosis.**
   Although the sequence of events is not always consistent, fatty streaks progress to type III or intermediate lesions. This growth is characterized by extracellular pools of lipid, which are generally clinically occult. However, when the pools coalesce to create a core of extracellular lipid (type IV lesion or atheroma), the blood vessel architecture has been altered sufficiently to become clinically overt. With smooth muscle cell (SMC) proliferation and collagen deposition, the atheroma becomes a fibroatheroma (type V). The fibroatheroma is characterized by thrombogenic surface defects that provoke intramural hemorrhage or intraluminal thrombus (type V lesion), resulting in vessel occlusion, which, in the case of a coronary artery, results in myocardial infarction (MI).

5. **Of 100 medical student volunteers, how many have significant atherosclerosis?**
   In 1953, Enos reported autopsy findings from 300 United States male battle casualties in Korea (average age, 22 years). He noted that 77% of the hearts had some gross evidence of coronary atherosclerosis. About 39% of the men had luminal narrowing, estimated at 10%–90%, and 3% had plaques causing complete occlusion of one or more coronary vessels. However, a subsequent study evaluating 105 combat casualties in Vietnam demonstrated that only 45% exhibited atherosclerosis, and fewer than 5% were considered severe. Finally, a recent study looking at 105 trauma victims corroborated the Korean War study by demonstrating a 78% incidence of atherosclerosis, with left main or significant two- and three-vessel involvement in 20%.

6. **What are the classic risk factors for atherosclerotic cardiovascular disease?**
   The classic risk factors include tobacco use, hyperlipidemia, hypertension, diabetes mellitus, and family history of cardiovascular disease. More recent evidence suggests the importance of obesity, emotional stress (weaker), and physical inactivity (that's you).

7. **How do such diverse risk factors produce similar disease?**
   That is the million-dollar question. Do parallel pathways lead to a final atherosclerotic lesion, or do the apparently dissimilar risk factors activate signals that converge to a few dominant events, promoting the development of atherosclerosis? Certainly, this question has broad therapeutic implications. It would be a lot easier to inhibit a single proximal point in this process rather than to treat multiple divergent, more distal cellular pathologic events.

8. **What is the response to injury?**
   The premise that atherogenesis represents an exaggerated inflammatory, fibroproliferative response to injury has evolved into an attractive unifying hypothesis of vascular disease and repair. Mechanical, metabolic, and toxic insults may injure the vessel wall. The common denominator is endothelial injury. Disruption of the endothelium not only results in endothelial cell dysfunction but also allows adhesion and transmigration of circulating monocytes, platelets, and T lymphocytes. Within the developing lesion, the activated cells release potent growth-regulatory molecules that may act in both a paracrine

335

and autocrine manner. Under the influence of cytokines and growth factors, vascular smooth muscle cells (VSMCs) adapt to a synthetic phenotype and begin proliferation and migration across the internal elastic lamina into the intimal layer. Stimulated VSMCs allow the deposition of extracellular matrix, thus converting the initial lesion to a fibrous plaque.

9. **What is C-reactive protein (CRP)? Is it just another random, nonclinically relevant marker of inflammation?**
   CRP is one of many acute phase proteins elaborated from hepatocytes on inflammatory stimulation. Originally isolated from the serum of patients with pneumonia, it has a high binding affinity for pneumococcal C-polysaccharide. Although CRP is best known as an active peptide by neutralizing foreign antigens, controlling tissue damage, and promoting tissue repair, it is increasingly considered a sensitive marker of inflammation. Unlike other markers of inflammation, CRP levels are stable over long periods of time, have no diurnal variation, can be measured inexpensively with available high-sensitivity assays, and have shown specificity in predicting risk of cardiovascular events. Indeed, elevation of CRP levels might be more predictive of cardiac events than elevation of low-density lipoprotein (LDL) levels. These observations may influence therapy because nonhyperlipidemic patients with elevated CRP levels might benefit from aggressive statin (3-hydroxyl-3-methylglutaryl [HMG]-reductase inhibitors) therapy.

10. **Does vascular injury mean only direct physical injury, as with an angioplasty catheter?**
    No. Injury is a catch-all word that includes physical injury, such as angioplasty, hypertension, shear forces (atherosclerotic lesions typically occur at bifurcations), and other diverse insults, including viruses, bacteria, nicotine, homocysteine, and oxidized LDLs.

11. **Are lipids important?**
    The lipid hypothesis of atherosclerosis suggests that the cellular changes in atherosclerosis are reactive events in response to lipid infiltration. Indeed, antilipid therapy is one of the few strategies that has induced regression of atherosclerosis in randomized, prospective clinical trials. Strong evidence also derives from patients with genetic hyperlipidemias; homozygotes rarely live beyond age 26 years.

12. **What is metabolic syndrome?**
    Often referred to as syndrome X, metabolic syndrome is a phenomenon in older, sedentary people who have hyperinsulinemia associated with elevated blood sugar, high blood pressure, and increased triglycerides with decreased high-density lipoprotein (HDL) cholesterol levels. The prevalence in the United States is estimated to be nearly 25% of the population. Clinically, such patients develop premature cardiovascular disease. Insulin resistance with elevated insulin levels, with or without overt diabetes, fuels important aspects of atherogenesis, including dyslipidemias, endothelial dysfunction, hypertension, and SMC proliferation. For the trivia fans, and not to be confused with your in-laws, a similar condition has been observed in overweight horses known as equine metabolic syndrome.

13. **What is leptin? What is its association with atherosclerosis?**
    Leptin is a hormone secreted by adipocytes that maintains homeostasis between energy stores and energy expenditure through regulation of appetite and food intake. Alterations in the signaling pathway of leptin, whether through leptin resistance or leptin depletion, can result in excessive food intake and obesity. Leptin is also proatherogenic. It signals proliferation of monocytes, promotes oxidative stress in the endothelial cell, and prompts hypertrophy and proliferation of vascular smooth muscle cells.

14. **Why would vitamin E be (even theoretically) protective against cardiovascular disease?**
    Antioxidant therapy with vitamins C and E and beta-carotene is intuitively sound. In vitro, these agents afford resistance of LDL to oxidation and reduce elaboration of vessel-injuring reactive oxygen species. Reactive oxygen metabolites (as much as 5% of oxygen), such as superoxide and hydrogen peroxide, directly injure vascular cells, impair endothelial vasomotor function, promote platelet aggregation and leukocyte adhesion, and stimulate VSMC proliferation. Although descriptive, case-control, and prospective cohort studies have found inverse associations between the frequency of coronary artery disease (CAD) and dietary intake of antioxidant vitamins, randomized therapeutic trials thus far have exhibited no benefit of doing so.

15. **What is homocysteine?**
This amino acid intermediate in the metabolism of methionine is an essential amino acid in the synthesis of both animal and plant proteins. Excessive homocysteine in the vessel wall reacts with low-density proteins to create damaging reactive oxygen species. Epidemiologic evidence correlates elevated levels of homocysteine and decreased levels of folate with cardiovascular disease.

16. **How does homocysteine rank as a risk factor for atherosclerosis?**
It is estimated that 10% of the risk of CAD in the general population is attributable to homocysteine. An increase in 5 μmol/L in plasma homocysteine concentration (normal, 5–15 μmol/L) raises the risk of coronary disease by as much as an increase of 20 mg/dL in the cholesterol concentration.

17. **Should everyone take folate supplements?**
Folic acid, vitamins B_{12} and B_6, and pyridoxine are important cofactors for the enzymatic processing of homocysteine. Indeed, the reduction in mortality from cardiovascular causes since 1960 has been correlated with the increase in vitamin B_6 supplementation in the food supply. Although these supplements may decrease homocysteine levels, the expected decrease in cardiovascular events has not yet been documented in prospective, randomized clinical trials. In fact, the results of the HOPE-2 study concluded that in patients with vascular disease or diabetes over 55 years old, dietary supplementation with folic acid, B_6, and B_{12} for 5 years did not reduce the risk of major cardiovascular events.

18. **What microorganisms have been implicated in atherosclerosis?**
Bacteria include *Chlamydia pneumoniae, Helicobacter pylori,* streptococci, and *Bacillus typhosus.* Viruses include influenza, herpes virus, adenovirus, and cytomegalovirus.

19. **Are individuals with sexually transmitted diseases (STDs) at greater risk for cardiovascular disease?**
The initial epidemiologic description linking *Chlamydia* species to atherosclerosis was reported by venereologists in South America in the 1940s. *C. pneumoniae,* a ubiquitous respiratory organism, is the predominant species subsequently identified in cardiovascular lesions. More than 50% of the population has antichlamydial antibodies (ACAs) by age 50 years; yet this 50% of the population does not have this STD.

20. **Is there an *H. pylori* peptic ulcer equivalent in atherosclerosis? Should we all take a macrolide a day?**
The jury is still out. It is unlikely that eradication of *Chlamydia* species will have the same profound effect on disease as eradication of *H. pylori.* However, *C. pneumoniae* may be another factor, exacerbating the response to injury. Evidence suggests that antibiotic therapy decreases the number of cardiovascular events in patients with elevated ACA titers.

21. **If you have multiple cavities, should you electively schedule your coronary artery bypass surgery?**
In several cohort studies, chronic periodontitis was associated with a 15% greater risk of developing coronary heart disease. Closer evaluation suggests that this link is actually much weaker. The major problem of existing studies is the high incidence of tobacco abuse in patients with dental disease. Interestingly, when you maximize oral hygiene by full dental extraction, edentulous people had a similar risk of heart disease with those with chronic periodontitis.

22. **What is the role of the endothelium?**
A healthy blood vessel wall is lined by a monolayer of phenomenally metabolically active endothelial cells. The surface area of the endothelium is approximately 5000 m^2 but comprises only 1% of the total body weight. While acting as a physical barrier to protect the underlying vessel and allowing formed blood elements to flow freely, thus preventing thrombosis, this seemingly bucolic layer is a central control center of vascular physiology. The endothelium is a key docking point for monocytes, neutrophils, and lymphocytes by virtue of its ability to express sticky, cell-specific adhesion molecules. The endothelium is a source for cytokines and peptide growth factors that act in both autocrine and paracrine fashion to promote atherogenesis.

23. **What are some of the products of endothelial cells that govern vasomotor tone?**
Factors that favor vascular relaxation include nitric oxide and prostacyclin. Conversely, factors favoring vascular constriction include thromboxane, leukotrienes, free radicals, endothelins, and cytokines (e.g., tumor necrosis factor and interleukin-1).

24. **What is the importance of vascular thrombosis?**
Thrombosis is central to the pathogenesis of acute arterial insufficiency and acute coronary or cerebrovascular syndromes, including unstable angina, non–Q-wave MI, acute (ST-elevation) MI, and vessel occlusion after vascular intervention (angioplasty).

25. **Describe the three main phases of platelet involvement with thrombus formation.**
The three main phases of platelet involvement in thrombus formation are platelet adhesion, activation, and aggregation. With exposure of the subendothelial space after vascular injury, platelets adhere to exposed basement membrane proteins such as proteoglycans, collagen, fibulin and laminin, and molecules secreted locally, such as von Willebrand factor (VWF), through their membrane glycoprotein receptors. Platelet activation occurs following adhesion, enhancing the ability of nearby platelets to attach to the developing thrombus. This process is energy dependent, requiring adenosine triphosphate. The predominant stimulators of activation include collagen, VWF, epinephrine, and thromboxane A2. Lastly, platelet aggregation occurs, in which platelets collect in an amplified manner leading to final thrombus formation. This step is mediated by the glycoprotein IIb/IIIa receptor and its interaction with VWF, fibronectin, and fibrinogen. This process takes only minutes. Pharmacologic blockade of the glycoprotein IIb/IIIa receptor is actively used by our cardiology colleagues for treatment of acute coronary syndromes.

26. **What is the mechanism of plaque rupture?**
The structural support for an atherosclerotic plaque is the fibrous cap, an organized layer of SMCs and connective tissue. This cap serves as a subendothelial barrier between the vessel lumen and the atherosclerotic necrotic core, filled with lipid droplets, inflammatory cells, and calcium salts. When the fibrous cap is thin, it can be damaged by inflammatory cytokines and proteases released by macrophages, T cells, and mast cells. Once destroyed, the contents of the necrotic core are exposed, prompting thrombosis and near or total artery occlusion. This process occurs in up to 70% of coronary artery thrombosis.

27. **What are some of the clinical complications of atherosclerotic plaque formation?**
Aneurysmal dilatation, arterial stenosis and occlusion, arterial wall rupture, and thromboembolic events leading to MI and stroke.

28. **If atherosclerosis is an inflammatory disease, should we all be taking an aspirin a day?**
Maybe. Strategies aimed at limiting the inflammatory cascade offer promise as antiatherosclerosis therapy. Examples in daily use include aspirin, fibrinolytics, HMG-reductase inhibitors, and estrogens. Others in the preclinical arena include gene therapy, anticytokine therapy, and antigrowth factor therapy. Certainly, primary prevention is important in limiting the initial injury stimulus. However, the smoldering inflammation involved with atherosclerosis may best be attacked by modifying the vascular cells' response to these insults.

BIBLIOGRAPHY

1. Ayada K, Yokota K. Chronic infections and atherosclerosis. *Ann NY Acad Sci.* 2007;1108:594–602.
2. Davi G, Patrono C. Platelet activation and atherothrombosis. *N Engl J Med.* 2007;357(24):2482–2494.
3. Enos WF, Holmes RH. Coronary disease among United States soldiers killed in action in Korea. *J Am Med Assoc.* 1953;152(12):1090–1093.
4. Fruchart JC, Nierman MC. New risk factors for atherosclerosis and patient risk assessment. *Circulation.* 2004;109(23 suppl 1):III15–III19.
5. Hansson GK. Inflammation, atherosclerosis, and coronary artery disease. *N Engl J Med.* 2005;352(16):1685–1695.
6. Selzman CH, Miller SA. Therapeutic implications of inflammation in atherosclerotic cardiovascular disease. *Ann Thorac Surg.* 2001;71(16):2066–2074.
7. Lonn E, Yusuf S, Arnold MJ, et al. Homocysteine lowering with folic acid and B vitamins in vascular disease. *N Engl J Med.* 2006;354(15):1567–1577.
8. Zimmerman MA, Selzman CH. Diagnostic implications of C-reactive protein in atherosclerosis. *Arch Surg.* 2003;138(2):220–224.
9. Libby P, Bornfeldt KE. Atherosclerosis: successes, surprises, and future challenges. *Circ Res.* 2016;118(4):531–534.

CHAPTER 73

ARTERIAL INSUFFICIENCY

Lisa S. Foley, MD, Charles J. Fox, MD, FACS

1. **Describe claudication and its physiology.**

   Intermittent claudication consists of reproducible lower extremity muscular pain induced by exercise and relieved by short periods of rest. It is caused by arterial obstruction, which restricts the normal exercise-induced increase in blood flow, producing transient muscle ischemia. Studies have shown that more than half of patients with intermittent claudication have never complained of this symptom to their physicians, assuming that difficulty with walking is a normal consequence of aging. Finally, only one-third or less of patients with peripheral arterial disease (PAD) have typical claudication; others have atypical leg pain or are asymptomatic because medical comorbidities limit ambulation. Claudication is a marker of systemic atherosclerotic disease, with associated cardiovascular mortality rates at 5 and 10 years of roughly 42% and 65%, respectively.

2. **List the different nonoperative therapies for intermittent claudication.**

   Risk factor modification, exercise, and pharmacologic therapies. Smoking cessation reliably doubles walking distances and reduces the need for eventual amputation in patients with PAD. Exercise (defined as walking until onset of leg pain, resting, and then resuming walking) for 30–60 minutes, 3 days per week for 6 months has also been demonstrated in multiple randomized trials to increase walking distance by more than 100%. Currently, the only Food and Drug Administration–approved drugs for the treatment of claudication are Pentoxifylline (minimally effective) and Cilostazol (more effective). Pharmacologic therapy should also target dyslipidemia, hypertension, and glycemic control. In addition, lifelong antiplatelet therapy is essential. Of note, the benefits of lifestyle modification, especially smoking cessation, are also imperative following operative intervention on PAD. Graft failure rates in patients who continue to smoke after peripheral arterial bypass are threefold higher than their nonsmoking equivalents. Nicotine inhalation promotes PAD and graft failure by increasing platelet aggregation, decreasing prostacyclin, and increasing thromboxane, promoting vasoconstriction and thrombosis.

3. **Define critical limb ischemia (CLI).**

   CLI potentially threatens the viability of the limb. Symptoms include rest pain, typically occurring at night when the patient is supine and gravity contribution to foot arterial pressure is no longer present. This pain is relieved with foot dependency. Peripheral circulation in CLI is not sufficient to heal minor skin breakdown caused by incidental trauma. These patients develop ischemic ulcers that are frequently painful and can progress to gangrene. CLI implies chronicity and should be distinguished from acute limb ischemia, which is due to sudden (defined as 2 weeks or less) reduction in limb perfusion.

4. **What is the ankle brachial index (ABI)?**

   ABI is the highest ankle pressure (anterior tibial or posterior tibial artery) divided by the higher of the two brachial pressures. The normal ABI is slightly >1 (1.10). An ABI of 0.5–0.8 is typical of patients with claudication. Even in the absence of symptoms, an ABI of <0.9 is 95% sensitive for PAD confirmed by angiography. Patients with rest pain have an ABI <0.5, and patients with tissue necrosis often have an ABI much lower.

5. **Describe the natural history of claudication.**

   Multiple natural history studies have documented the benign nature of claudication. The cumulative 10-year amputation rate is 10%. One-third of patients experience symptom deterioration, and half of these patients require some sort of revascularization. Continued smoking and diabetes are major risk factors for progression. Of note, however, is that PAD is a marker of overall cardiovascular disease status. Patients with PAD have a 20% risk of myocardial infarction (MI) or stroke and a 10% risk of death in 5 years. Given the relatively low 10-year amputation rate, higher cardiovascular mortality rate, and poor compliance with smoking cessation in these patients, many vascular surgeons are increasingly reluctant to perform a major open revascularization for claudication alone.

6. **Describe the natural history of CLI.**

   CLI often requires revascularization or primary amputation. Percutaneous interventions are increasingly used as the primary therapy with surgical procedures or amputation used if they fail. A subgroup of patients with CLI cannot be effectively treated with surgical or endovascular revascularization. Meticulous wound management and intermittent pneumatic compression therapy can help patients with uncomplicated chronic nonhealing ulcers. Again, the presence of CLI is a harbinger of grave overall health status. About 40% of patients with CLI will have an amputation, and 20% will die within 6 months of diagnosis.

7. **What are segmental limb pressures? How are they used?**

   Just as the ABI is recorded at the ankle, cuffs at the high thigh, above knee, below knee, and toe level can record pressures. Noting the location of decreases in arterial pressure can determine the level of the vascular obstruction. Typically, a reduction in pressure of 20 mm Hg or greater between segments is considered significant and will help determine the level of obstruction.

8. **Describe the natural history of vein graft occlusions.**

   Although bypass grafts can dramatically improve lower extremity circulation, they have a limited life expectancy and may require maintenance for longevity. In the first 1–2 years, lesions intrinsic to the graft are often the primary threat to graft patency. After 2 years, inflow and outflow disease are common sources of reduced flow through the graft, which can lead to occlusion. When these grafts fail, the limb involved frequently has poorer perfusion than before the bypass. This is because of division of major arterial collateral pathways during the operation and thrombus propagation or embolization to occlude distal arteries at the time of graft occlusion.

9. **What is the prognosis of young patients with vascular disease?**

   Significant atherosclerosis in young patients (age <40 years) is infrequent. These patients are often heavy smokers with a high incidence of diabetes, renal failure, and/or hypercoagulable states (defective fibrinolysis, anticardiolipin antibodies, homocysteinemia, or deficiencies in natural anticoagulants). Those with limb-threatening conditions frequently progress to limb loss despite attempts at revascularization. Reconstructive procedures have limited success and require frequent revision in this population.

10. **Describe the anatomic distribution of vascular disease in diabetes.**

    Patients with diabetes are unique. They have a predilection for calcification of the arterial wall, rendering noninvasive diagnostic studies (ankle pressure, ABI) unreliable because of false elevation. The digital arteries are usually spared, and the great toe pressure can be used to approximate the ankle pressure. The inflow arteries (i.e., aorta, iliac, common femoral) are also often spared. Intermittent disease is common in the superficial femoral and popliteal arteries. Significant occlusive disease frequently affects the profunda femoris, posterior and anterior tibial, and pedal arteries, with relative sparing of the peroneal artery.

11. **What are the implications of renal failure on outcomes?**

    Patients with end-stage renal failure who have CLI are at the end of life, with 3-year survival rates of <30%, similar to patients with metastatic cancer. In addition, the healing potential for partial foot amputations after successful revascularization is limited.

    Reconstructions in these patients are technically difficult because of calcified distal targets. The combination of these problems reduces efficacy of vascular reconstructions, which is an important consideration when discussing goals for management in these patients.

12. **Discuss the concept of inflow versus outflow.**

    The limb is thought of as a circulation network when planning revascularization procedures; it requires blood to enter the leg from the heart (inflow) and reach the foot from the thigh (outflow). In the normal limb, the inflow to the leg arises from the aortoiliac tree and continues into common and deep femoral arteries. The normal outflow to the foot is the popliteal and three tibial arteries (anterior, posterior, and peroneal). For bypasses to remain patent, they need adequate blood coming into them and a vascular bed to supply). Treatment of inflow and outflow may be accomplished through hybrid procedures that use both endovascular and open surgical procedures to treat the critical lesions. For example, an iliac stenosis may be treated with endoluminal therapy and a popliteal occlusion with surgical bypass.

13. **What are the choices for autogenous conduits?**

The success of infrainguinal bypass is highly dependent on the conduit. The best choices for conduit in order of preference would be a single segment greater saphenous vein, spliced pieces (composite) of saphenous vein, lesser saphenous veins, arm veins, spliced lesser saphenous or arm veins, and prosthetic material with a distal vein patch with or without fistula. Autologous veins should have a 3mm diameter and a soft, blue appearance and distend easily under hydrostatic pressure. Sclerotic or narrow segments of vein should be avoided. Cryopreserved cadaver veins are expensive and are generally of limited durability. Vein grafts outlive prosthetic grafts, even in the above-knee position. However, in patients with no autologous vein conduit, heparin-bonded polytetrafluoroethylene (PTFE) grafts have been used for above-knee bypass with slightly reduced 5-year patency rates (52%) compared to that of autologous vein grafts (76%).

14. **What are the indications for arteriography?**

Arteriography is performed to plan future operations or at the time of planned interventions. Diagnostic arteriography without intervention is rarely used in PAD, as computed axial tomography angiography with lower extremity runoff can provide sufficient information to plan intervention.

15. **What are the patency rates of inflow procedures?**

The durability of vascular reconstructions is measured by patency. Patency has three types, measured with a life table method, which accounts for all-cause mortality occurring in vascular patients over time. Patency can be primary (the graft is functioning without any intervention), assisted primary (the graft has required intervention to keep it functioning), or secondary patency (restored patency period after thrombosis). The four most common procedures to improve inflow are iliac angioplasty, aortofemoral bypass, femorofemoral bypass, and axillofemoral bypass. The most durable is the aorto-femoral bypass, which has a 10-year primary patency of 80%. Five-year primary patency rates for iliac stent-grafting, axillofemoral, and femorofemoral bypass are all roughly 70%. Five-year patency of iliac stent-grafting can be improved to roughly 90% with concomitant common femoral endarterectomy, and thus this technique has been widely applied to treat sole iliac lesions or iliac lesions that limit inflow to a planned distal bypass.

16. **What are the patency rates of infrainguinal bypass procedures?**

Infrainguinal bypasses include grafts to the above-knee popliteal, below-knee popliteal, the tibial, and the pedal arteries. Five-year primary patency rates for above-knee popliteal grafts with saphenous vein and prosthetic are 80% and 65%, respectively. Five-year primary patency rates for below-knee saphenous vein popliteal grafts are 75%. Five-year primary patency rates for tibial bypasses are 65%. The five-year primary patency rate for pedal bypass is 50%. Autologous greater saphenous vein is the conduit of choice for these bypasses. Heparin bonded PTFE grafts is a potential alternative for patients who do not have suitable vein for conduit.

17. **Name the primary cause of perioperative mortality.**

The majority (>90%) of all peripheral vascular disease patients have underlying coronary artery disease (CAD). Because of the ambulatory limitations of their peripheral vascular disease, many patients' CAD is asymptomatic. The most common cause of perioperative mortality in vascular surgery is MI. The decision to work up and revascularize (surgically or with angioplasty and stenting) CAD in these patients before the vascular operation is recommended in patients undergoing a major elective vascular operation.

18. **Name the primary cause of perioperative morbidity.**

Wound complications occur in about 25% of patients undergoing lower extremity bypass for CLI. Postoperative lymphedema, ischemic neuropathy, and prolonged (often measured in months rather than weeks) wound healing are all important issues for these patients.

19. **What are the causes of graft failure?**

About 30% of patients undergoing infrainguinal bypass surgery will experience graft failure by 2–3 years. Early failure (within 30 days) is caused by technical problems with the operation (graft kinking or twisting, narrowing of the anastomosis, bleeding, infection, intimal flaps, or embolization). Graft failure at months 2–18 is most often caused by fibrointimal hyperplasia at distal anastomoses or venous valve sites within the graft. Late graft failure (>18 months) is most frequently caused by recurrent atherosclerosis of the inflow and outflow vasculature. Hypercoagulable states are an unusual cause of graft failure.

20. **What therapeutic options are available for graft failure?**

If a vein graft fails postoperatively, the patient is immediately returned to the operating room to perform angiography, explore the distal and/or proximal anastomosis, and identify the technical problem. If no identifiable problem is found and thrombectomy alone is performed, there is a high likelihood of repeated failure. In those instances, evaluation should broaden to assess inflow, outflow, and the quality of conduit and consider harvesting new conduit or treating concomitant disease to improve flow through the bypass. If a graft fails several weeks or months later, the optimal management strategy is more controversial. Graft exploration and open surgical thrombectomy stenosis may be less effective than thrombolytic therapy and/or mechanical thrombectomy. Determination of the cause of failure is a necessity to maintain patency. Replacing the vein graft with a new bypass provides the most durable alternative when it is technically possible and the patient is an operative candidate. The main challenges in replacing the vein graft are finding appropriate inflow and outflow vessels and appropriate bypass graft conduit.

21. **What method of graft surveillance should be used?**

Because of the limited options for occluded vein bypass grafts, ultrasound studies are used to detect stenosis within the graft before occlusion. Various criteria have been championed to accurately detect >50% narrowing within the graft or native inflow and outflow arteries.

Examinations of the graft are conducted at 1, 3, 6, 9, and 12 months postoperative and yearly thereafter. Natural history data indicate that grafts with >50% stenosis left untreated are associated with high intermediate-term failure rates. Recurrent symptoms and changes in the ABI are too insensitive to detect these lesions.

22. **What therapeutic options are available for graft stenosis?**

The majority of vein graft stenosis are caused by fibrointimal hyperplasia of sclerotic portions of the graft or valve sites. These lesions are a firm rubber consistency and less amenable to long-term success with percutaneous angioplasty, although focal lesions are usually initially treated in this manner with cutting percutaneous balloon angioplasty (cPTA). Open techniques (resection and interposition vein grafting or vein patch angioplasty) are more durable but are reserved for long segment lesions that are not amendable to cPTA. As a general rule, the results of intervention on failing grafts are superior to the results of intervention on those that have thrombosed.

23. **What is the role of iliac angioplasty and stenting?**

Iliac artery atherosclerotic lesions that respond best to balloon angioplasty are of short length (<3 cm) and are confined to the common iliac artery. Patients without diabetes fare better than patients with diabetes. Current reports of initial success are >90%, which has improved with the use of stents to treat iatrogenic arterial dissections. Newer endovascular techniques combining angioplasty and stents have long-term patency rates (6–8 years) of more than 80% in well-selected patients. Most patients with aortoiliac disease without complete long segment occlusions are initially managed with endovascular techniques. Increasingly, longer segment and less favorable anatomic lesions are being managed with endoluminal therapies as endovascular technologies for aortoiliac disease expand.

24. **How is viability determined in cases of acute ischemia?**

The five Ps of acute ischemia are pain, pallor, pulselessness, paresthesia, and paralysis. Early findings with acute ischemia include absent pulse, pain, and pallor. Paresthesia and paralysis are later findings. Recent basic science reports argue against the classical teaching that irreversible muscle ischemia occurs after 6 hours and suggest early and permanent histologic changes begin within a 1–2 hours of arterial occlusion. Perhaps the most sensitive finding that indicates limb nonviability is muscle rigor in the calf. The vast majority of ischemic limbs can be managed with initial heparin therapy followed by thrombolytic therapy or open surgical thrombectomy depending on the arterial tree and clinical scenario.

25. **How is thrombus distinguished from embolus in acute ischemia?**

The diagnosis of acute thrombotic versus embolic lower extremity arterial occlusion is distinguished primarily through history, exam, and imaging. Findings suggestive of embolus include a history of recent MI, cardiac arrhythmias, or known cardiac thrombus. Patients with embolus frequently have rather profound leg ischemia because of the sudden and proximal nature of the occlusion (aortic or femoral bifurcation) and the absence of any developed collaterals. These patients lack a history of PAD that would otherwise suggest a thrombotic rather than embolic event. Thrombotic events are more commonly seen in patients with known cardiovascular disease risk factors such as smoking, dyslipidemia, and diabetes. Occasionally, arteriography may be required to differentiate between thrombotic and embolic events. Patients with acute limb ischemia from a thrombotic source will likely have a reduced ABI on the unaffected side, and imaging will reveal underlying atherosclerosis.

26. **When is thrombolysis indicated?**
Thrombolytic therapy is indicated in patients without contraindications (age >80, recent surgery, relative bleeding risks) and a recent venous or arterial thrombotic occlusion (<2 weeks). The thrombus is crossed with a guidewire, and the lytic medication (urokinase, streptokinase, or tissue plasminogen activator) is administered directly within the thrombus under catheter direction. The patients are admitted to an intensive care unit and returned frequently to the angio suite over 1–3 days to assess the response. Patients who are severely limb threatened may be best served with immediate restoration of circulation by open surgical thrombectomy.

27. **What is compartment syndrome?**
Reperfusion after acute ischemia can lead to profound tissue swelling in the involved extremity. Edema of the involved muscle increases the pressure within the fascia bound calf muscle compartments (i.e., anterior, lateral, deep posterior, and superficial posterior) to a level that exceeds the capillary perfusion pressure (>30 mm Hg). Nerve and muscle necrosis is inevitable unless the pressure is relieved by a four-compartment fasciotomy. Patients may complain of intense pain with foot dorsiflexion, calf swelling, and paresthesia in the webspace between the first and second metatarsals. Pedal pulses can remain palpable and are not a reliable examination finding. Severe pain with passive range of motion at the ankle is highly concerning for compartment syndrome and should prompt measuring compartment pressures or proceeding to fasciotomy depending on the clinical picture.

28. **What is the role of endovascular therapy in infrainguinal occlusive disease?**
Endovascular therapy is increasingly being used to treat infrainguinal occlusive disease in patients with claudication and CLI. This includes angioplasty and stenting for stenosis and recanalization for long segment occlusions. In addition, atherectomy devices have been used for treating stenosis in the femoral, popliteal, and tibial arteries. Results are favorable and these techniques are employed widely.

KEY POINTS: ARTERIAL INSUFFICIENCY

1. ABI is the highest ankle pressure divided by the higher of the two brachial pressures.
2. CLI threatens the viability of the limb and requires urgent surgical revascularization when possible.
3. Patients with end-stage renal failure who have CLI have limited lifespan with estimated 3-year survival rates <30%.
4. If a vein graft fails immediately postoperatively, immediate reexploration is recommended.

WEBSITES

- http://apds.org/physician-resources/acs-surgery-principles-and-practice/
- www.vascularweb.org

BIBLIOGRAPHY

1. Amonkar SJ, Cleanthis M, Nice C, et al. Outcomes of intra-arterial thrombolysis for acute limb ischemia. *Angiology.* 2007;58(6):734–742.
2. Gerhard-Herman M, Gardin JM, Jaff M, et al. Guidelines for noninvasive vascular laboratory testing: a report from the American Society of Echocardiography and the Society for Vascular Medicine and Biology. *Vasc Med.* 2006;11(3):183–200.
3. Hiatt WR, Krantz MJ. Masterclass series in peripheral arterial disease. Antiplatelet therapy for peripheral arterial disease and claudication. *Vasc Med.* 2006;11(1):55–60.
4. Klein WM, van der Graaf Y, Seegers J, et al. Dutch iliac stent trial: long-term results in patients randomized for primary or selective stent placement. *Radiology.* 2006;238(2):734–744.

5. Landis GS, Faries PL. New techniques and developments to treat long infrainguinal arterial occlusions: use of reentry devices, subintimal angioplasty, and endografts. *Perspect Vasc Surg Endovasc Ther.* 2007;19(3):285–290.
6. Lau H, Cheng SW. Eighteen-year experience with femoro-femoral bypass. *Aust N Z J Surg.* 2000;70(4):275–278.
7. Nehler MR, Hiatt WR. Exercise therapy for claudication. *Ann Vasc Surg.* 1999;13(1):109–114.
8. Novo S, Coppola G. Critical limb ischemia: definition and natural history. *Curr Drug Targets Cardiovasc Haematol Disord.* 2004;4(3):219–225.
9. Taylor SM, Kalbaugh CA, Blackhurst DW, et al. Postoperative outcomes according to preoperative medical and functional status after infrainguinal revascularization for critical limb ischemia in patients 80 years and older. *Am Surg.* 2005;71(8):640–645.
10. Wind J, Koelemay MJ. Exercise therapy and the additional effect of supervision on exercise therapy in patients with intermittent claudication. Systematic review of randomised controlled trials. *Eur J Vasc Endovasc Surg.* 2007;34(1):1–9.
11. Cull DL, Langan EM. Open versus endovascular intervention for critical limb ischemia: a population-based study. *J Am Coll Surg.* 2010;210(5):555–563.
12. Mills JL. Mechanisms of vein graft failure: the location, distribution, and characteristics of lesions that predispose to graft failure. *Semin Vasc Surg.* 1993;6(3):78–91.
13. Kalbaugh CA. Contemporary outcomes of iliofemoral bypass grafting for unilateral aortoiliac occlusive disease: a 10-year experience. *Am Surg.* 2008;74(6):555–559.
14. Patel SD. Hybrid revascularization of complex multilevel disease: a paradigm shift in critical limb ischemia treatment. *J Cardiovasc Surg (Torino).* 2014;55(5):613–623.
15. Bradbury AW, Adam DJ, Bell J, et al. Bypass versus angioplasty in severe ischemia of the leg (BASIL) trial: a survival prediction model to facilitate clinical decision making. *J Vasc Surg.* 2010;51(suppl 5):52S–68S.
16. Fox CJ. Pathogenesis of Vascular Injury. In: Rasmussen T, Tai N, eds. *Vascular Trauma.* 3rd ed. Philadelphia, PA: Elsevier; 2015.

CHAPTER 74

CAROTID DISEASE

Melissa K. Suh, MD, Bernard Timothy Baxter, MD

1. **What primary diseases affect the carotid arteries?**
   Atherosclerosis is by far the most common disease affecting the carotid arteries, accounting for 90% of lesions in the Western world. The carotid artery also can be affected by kinking secondary to arterial elongation, fibromuscular dysplasia, extrinsic compression (e.g., neoplasm), radiation-induced changes, trauma (causing bleeding, occlusion, or dissection), and inflammatory arteriopathies (e.g., temporal arteritis, Takayasu's arteritis).

2. **What are the histologic features of atherosclerotic plaques?**
   Plaques are likely formed according to the response to injury hypothesis. Plaques begin in the intima and media through a complex series of events. Initially, smooth muscle cells are recruited and connective tissue proteins are produced in excess. Incorporation of low-density lipoprotein cholesterol, monocytes, and platelets leads to formation of the mature plaque consisting of a lipid core and a fibrotic cap covering the core. Hemorrhage into the plaque (intraplaque hemorrhage) may cause sudden growth, acutely increasing the degree of stenosis or causing occlusion.

3. **What are the clinical sequelae of atherosclerotic disease?**
   Thrombosis and embolization are the most common complications of atherosclerotic plaques. Thrombosis and embolization typically occur when the outer fibrous layer of the plaque is degraded by enzymes from inflammatory cells exposing the lipid core. This core is highly thrombogenic and friable, predisposing to thrombosis and embolization of lipids and platelet aggregates. Atherosclerosis may also be a factor in development of carotid artery aneurysms, although this is controversial because they may occur without atherosclerosis.

4. **What are the most common symptoms of carotid artery disease?**
   - Transient ischemic attack (TIA)
   - Cerebrovascular accident (CVA)
   - Amaurosis fugax

5. **Define TIA, CVA, and amaurosis fugax.**
   These clinical terms describe a spectrum of cerebral or retinal ischemic syndromes. A TIA is a neurologic deficit that lasts <24 hours, but it typically last only minutes. Clinically, a CVA, or acute stroke, is defined by a persistent neurologic deficit lasting >24 hours. Amaurosis fugax is an episode of transient (minutes to hours) monocular blindness, often likened to a window shade being pulled across the eye. It is caused by an acute decrease in blood flow secondary to embolization through the ophthalmic artery to the retina. When this occurs, blood flow to the periphery of the retina is lost first, with the ischemia (loss of vision) working its way toward the center of the retina, hence the sensation of a shade being pulled down.

6. **What are Hollenhorst plaques?**
   Hollenhorst was an ophthalmologist who first described refractile plaques of cholesterol in the retinal vessels. They are usually seen at branch points in the vessel and are the result of arterial to arterial emboli. The most common source is a carotid bifurcation plaque, but they may originate from disease in the common carotid or the ascending aorta.

7. **What mechanisms produce neurologic deficits?**
   - Embolization from proximal atherosclerotic arteries (ascending aorta, aortic arch, carotid arteries), the heart, the venous system in the case of a right to left cardiac shunt (paradoxical emboli)
   - Reduced cerebral blood flow from shock causing global ischemia
   - Atherosclerotic occlusive disease of intra- or extracranial arteries to the brain that reduce flow below a critical level
   - Intracranial hemorrhage

8. **What is the natural history of a TIA?**
   The natural history of a TIA is defined by the pathology of the ipsilateral carotid artery. Based on past data from prospectively randomized patients with severe stenosis (>70%), the risk of ipsilateral stroke within 24 months is 26%. For those with moderate disease (50%–69%), the risk is 22% at 5 years. With minimal stenosis (<30%), the risk is 1% at 3 years. The medical therapy at the time of this study did not routinely include statins and dual antiplatelet therapy. The risks may be less with current best medical therapy, and this is being addressed in new randomized trials.

9. **What is the effect of medication on TIA and stroke?**
   Antithrombotics: Acetylsalicylic acid (aspirin) has long been the mainstay for stroke prevention. It is a cyclooxygenase inhibitor that decreases platelet stickiness and inflammation. It lowers the incidence of stroke in women. Although it has not been shown to lower stroke incidence as a single endpoint in men, it has been shown to lower the incidence of myocardial infarction (MI) and stroke when these endpoints are combined. Clopidogrel (Plavix) inhibits adenosine diphosphate-dependent platelet aggregation. It has been shown to decrease the risk of stroke, MI, or death compared to aspirin. When stroke alone is considered as the endpoint, combination therapy with aspirin and clopidogrel does not provide significant benefit and can increase bleeding risk. Dual therapy is typically used after TIA or minor stroke thought to be caused by atheroemboli and after carotid stenting, but the optimal duration of therapy is still unknown.
   Aspirin plus dipyridamole, a phosphodiesterase and adenosine deaminase inhibitor, has been shown to be significantly more effective than aspirin alone for stroke prevention. This combination has similar beneficial effects to clopidogrel.
   Statins: Statins are 3-hydroxy-3-methylglutaryl-coenzyme A reductase inhibitors that decrease cholesterol production and lower serum lipid levels. Statin treatment can lower the cardiovascular event risk by 20%–30% and reduce the risk of recurrent stroke in hyperlipidemic patients. Statin therapy is approved and recommended for stroke prevention in patients with TIAs, stroke, or significant carotid stenosis. The indications for statin therapy are rapidly evolving and currently extend to normolipidemic patients at high risk for atherosclerosis.
   Antihypertensives: Treating hypertension with a goal blood pressure <140 systolic and <90 diastolic reduces CVD risk and has been shown to decrease morbidity and mortality from stroke. Recent data suggest that a target systolic blood pressure is associated with decreased cardiovascular events but did not lower the risk of stroke.

10. **What does a carotid bruit signify?**
    A carotid bruit is a general marker for atherosclerosis that lacks specificity; it indicates an increased risk of both cardiac and cerebral vascular events. Absence of a bruit does not indicate absence of disease.

11. **Does the sound of a bruit correlate with the degree of stenosis?**
    Typically, a higher degree of stenosis will produce a higher pitch up to a certain point. Beyond that, flow may be reduced to a point that the bruit may actually diminish or disappear.

12. **What preliminary test should be ordered to evaluate a cervical bruit or carotid stenosis based on clinical findings such as TIA or CVA?**
    Duplex ultrasound is accurate and inexpensive. To confirm carotid disease or look for other sites of disease when carotid duplex does not correlate with symptoms, magnetic resonance angiography or computed tomography angiography are now used; importantly they add valuable information about arch vessels and intracranial circulation. Because cerebral angiography is invasive and associated with additional risk, including embolic stroke, it is reserved for cases where specific, additional anatomic information is required.

13. **When is intervention indicated for symptomatic carotid artery disease?**
    Intervention is strongly indicated for symptomatic carotid artery disease associated with >70% stenosis. The absolute risk reduction of stroke is 17% at 2 years. There is a smaller benefit in patients with symptomatic stenosis of 50%–69% (6.5% risk reduction at 5 years). Symptomatic patients with stenosis of <50% do not benefit from intervention.

14. **Should a patient with asymptomatic stenosis undergo surgery?**
    In a large randomized trial, absolute reduction in risk of stroke is 6% over a 5-year period in asymptomatic patients with >60% stenosis who undergo carotid endarterectomy (CEA) plus aspirin versus patients treated with aspirin alone (5.1% versus 11%). Thus, CEA should be considered in asymptomatic carotid disease when the patient is expected to live at least 3 years, is at low risk of a cardiac event, and when the CEA can be performed with a combined stroke and mortality rate of <3%. Because of the small benefit and the known risk of MI associated with CEA, risk stratification is important in this group.

15. **What is the role of carotid artery stenting (CAS)?**
    CEA has typically been seen as the standard of care for carotid artery disease with percutaneous angioplasty with stenting as an alternative for high-risk symptomatic patients. Multiple randomized control trials looking at CEA versus stenting have been published along with long-term follow-up data. Overall, the stroke risk is higher in the perioperative period for CAS, while CEA has a higher risk of MI. When the combined endpoints of stroke, MI, and death are taken together, outcomes appear similar. Outcomes for CAS are worse in the most elderly.

16. **Should a protective device be used for carotid stenting?**
    Distal embolization, when carefully measured, is common with CAS. Studies have established that some type of cerebral protection device can decrease the risk of embolization with CAS. The most commonly used devices are filters placed distal to the stenosis to capture debris released during angioplasty and stenting.

17. **What are the important anatomic considerations for CAS?**
    Aortic arch anatomy can vary within the general population. It is important to understand the arch configuration and the branching pattern of the main arch vessels prior to intervention. The takeoff of the left common carotid as a common trunk with the brachiocephalic or high on the brachiocephalic are the most common variations. With increasing age, the aorta elongates and the arch becomes more tortuous, making access more challenging. This may be the reason that CAS is associated with worse outcomes in the very elderly.

18. **Which cranial nerves may be injured during CEA? What are the clinical signs of injury?**
    - Marginal mandibular branch of the facial nerve (cranial nerve [CN] VII): Droop of ipsilateral corner of mouth
    - Glossopharyngeal nerve (CN IX): Difficulty in swallowing both solids and liquids
    - Recurrent laryngeal nerve (branch of vagus, CN X): Hoarseness, loss of effective cough
    - Superior laryngeal nerve (branch of vagus, CN X): Voice fatigue, loss of high-pitch phonation
    - Hypoglossal nerve (CN XII): Deviation of tongue to ipsilateral side, difficulty with speech and chewing

19. **What is the danger of wound hematoma after surgery?**
    The main danger is airway compromise, which may necessitate emergent decompression by opening of the wound. Whether drains placed in the wound bed prevent hematoma formation is not clear.

20. **When do neurologic events occur during CEA?**
    - Dissection: Dislodgement of material from the arterial wall with embolization
    - Clamping: Ischemic infarct
    - Postoperatively: Reperfusion, intimal flap

21. **What is a shunt? When is it used?**
    A shunt is a small plastic tube that loops around the surgical field and provides blood flow during the CEA. A shunt is used to avoid intraoperative cerebral ischemia. Many surgeons routinely use shunts, but others use them selectively, if at all. The decision to use a shunt is based on known absence of collateral circulation or intraoperative assessment. Intraoperative assessment can be done a number of ways including assessment of (1) neurologic status in an awake patient when the CEA is done under local anesthesia or with a block, (2) electroencephalogram or cerebral blood flow changes after clamping, or (3) stump pressure. None of these methods is 100% sensitive.

22. **What is stump pressure?**
    Stump pressure is the residual pressure in the internal carotid artery after clamping the external and common carotid arteries. It is used to assess the adequacy of cerebral perfusion. The safe pressure varies, but mean pressure should be at least 40 mm Hg.

23. **Does stenosis recur after stenting or CEA or CAS?**
    Yes. The long-term risk of restenosis is similar between CEA and CAS, with the overall incidence at 10 years between 8% and 12%. The rate of restenosis is highest in the first 2 years after intervention and decreases to <1% per year thereafter. During the first 24 months after operation or stenting, restenosis is thought to be secondary to myointimal hyperplasia. Beyond this time, it is caused by disease progression (atherosclerosis).

24. **What is the best treatment for restenosis after endarterectomy?**
Cranial nerve injury is more common with redo CEA (reported incidence 2%–20%). Most injuries are transient, however, and surgery remains an option. If the arch anatomy is acceptable, stenting has become the preferred treatment modality. Given that the lesion may be primarily hyperplasia, the risk of embolization, in comparison to a primary, atherosclerotic lesion, would appear to be less, lending further support to this approach.

25. **In which layer of the artery is the CEA performed?**
The outer layers of the tunica media.

26. **When the internal carotid artery is occluded, which branches of the external carotid artery form collaterals and reestablish circulation in the circle of Willis?**
The periorbital branches of the external carotid artery form communications with the ophthalmic artery, a branch of the internal carotid.

27. **What are the functions of the carotid sinus and the carotid body?**
Both are located at the carotid bifurcation and are innervated by the glossopharyngeal and vagus nerves, respectively. The function of the carotid sinus is regulation of blood pressure. Hypertension stimulates efferent impulses to the vasomotor center in the medulla, inhibiting sympathetic tone and increasing vagal tone. The carotid body regulates respiratory drive and acid-base status via chemoreceptors. It also induces bradycardia when manipulated (this is your target during carotid massage for cardiac dysrhythmias).

28. **When was the first successful surgical procedure of the extracranial carotid artery performed? Who is credited with it?**
In 1954 by Felix Eastcott.

KEY POINTS: CAROTID DISEASE

1. The symptoms of carotid disease include TIA, CVA, and amaurosis fugax.
2. A carotid bruit is a general marker for atherosclerosis, including both coronary artery and cerebrovascular disease.
3. Intervention is strongly indicated for symptomatic carotid artery disease associated with >70% stenosis.

BIBLIOGRAPHY

1. Bhatt DL, Fox KA, Hacke W, et al. Clopidogrel and aspirin versus aspirin alone for the prevention of atherothrombotic events. *N Engl J Med.* 2006;354(16):1706–1717.
2. Brott TG, Hobson 2nd RW, Howard G, et al. Stenting versus endarterectomy for treatment of carotid-artery stenosis. *N Engl J Med.* 2010;363(1):11–23.
3. Brott TG, Howard G, Roubin GS, et al. Long-term results of stenting versus endarterectomy for carotid-artery stenosis. *N Engl J Med.* 2016;374(11):1021–1031.
4. Diener HC, Bogousslavsky J, Brass LM, et al. Aspirin and clopidogrel compared with clopidogrel alone after recent ischaemic stroke or transient ischaemic attack in high-risk patients (MATCH): randomised, double-blind, placebo-controlled trial. *Lancet.* 2004;364(9431):331–337.
5. ESPRIT Study Group, Halkes PH. Aspirin plus dipyridamole versus aspirin alone after cerebral ischaemia of arterial origin (ESPRIT): randomised controlled trial. *Lancet.* 2006;367(9523):1665–1673.
6. Halliday A, Mansfield A, Marro J, et al. Prevention of disabling and fatal strokes by successful carotid endarterectomy in patients without recent neurological symptoms: randomised controlled trial. *Lancet.* 2004;363(9420):1491–1502.
7. Mas JL, Chantellier G, Beyssen B, et al. Endarterectomy versus stenting in patients with symptomatic severe carotid stenosis. *N Engl J Med.* 2006;355(16):1660–1671.
8. Paraskevas KI, Hamilton G. Statins: an essential component in the management of carotid artery disease. *J Vasc Surg.* 2007;46(2):373–386.
9. Ridker PM, Danielson E, Fonseca FA, et al. Rosuvastatin to prevent vascular events in men and women with elevated C-reactive protein. *N Engl J Med.* 2008;359(21):2195–2207.
10. SPRINT Research Group, Wright Jr JT, Williamson JD, et al. A randomized trial of intensive versus standard blood-pressure control. *N Engl J Med.* 2015;373(22). 2103–2016.
11. Yuan K, Kim AS. When a single antiplatelet agent for stroke prevention is not enough: current evidence and future applications of dual antiplatelet therapy. *Curr Treat Options Cardiovasc Med.* 2016;18(4):26.

CHAPTER 75

ABDOMINAL AORTIC ANEURYSM

Lisa S. Foley, MD, Charles J. Fox, MD, FACS

1. **What is an abdominal aortic aneurysm (AAA)?**
   The aorta tapers in size from roughly 2.8 cm in the thorax to roughly 2.0 cm in the abdomen of adult men. Aneurysms are defined by a 50% increase in normal vessel diameter. The normal infrarenal aortic diameter is 2.0 cm, and, therefore, it is considered aneurysmal at 3.0 cm.

2. **What is the incidence of AAA?**
   - Three percent in unselected adult patients screened with ultrasound (US)
   - Five percent in patients with known coronary artery disease (CAD)
   - Ten percent in patients with known peripheral vascular disease

3. **What is the etiology of AAA?**
   Degenerative, rather than atherosclerotic, pathologic changes account for more than 90% of aneurysms in the infrarenal aorta. Elastin is the primary load-bearing element of the aorta. In the normal human aorta, there is a gradual reduction in the amount of elastin present in the distal compared with the proximal aorta. Elastin fragmentation and degeneration are observed histologically in AAA walls. These observations help explain the predilection of AAAs in the infrarenal aorta. Absence of vasa vasorum in the infrarenal aorta has led to the suggestion of a nutritive deficiency. The degradation of aortic media in aneurysmal disease implies a disrupted balance between proteolytic enzymes and their inhibitors.

4. **Do AAAs have a genetic component?**
   Multiple reports describe a familial subgroup of AAAs. Prospective studies using ultrasound screening of AAA patients' siblings >50 years old demonstrate that ~25% of male siblings and 7% of female siblings will have an infrarenal aortic diameter >3.0 cm. This screening yield is even higher when the index family member is female. Therefore, screening of AAA patients' first-degree relatives who are 50 years old and older makes sense. The proposed genetic defect has been linked to abnormal type III collagen. Additionally, more recent population-wide genomic studies have revealed an association between a genetic variant of low-density-lipoprotein receptor-related protein 1 and patients with AAA.

5. **Are patients with AAA prone to aneurysms in other vascular beds?**
   Yes. Forty percent of patients with a popliteal artery aneurysm will have an AAA. Seventy-five percent of patients with a femoral artery aneurysm also have an AAA. Patients with thoracic aneurysms have a 20% chance of having a simultaneous AAA. Five percent of patients develop aortic aneurysms proximal to their graft at 5 years following infrarenal AAA repair.

6. **Can AAAs reliably be detected on physical examination?**
   No. The aortic bifurcation is at the level of the umbilicus, and, therefore, the pulsatile mass of an AAA is located in the epigastrium. Gastric and bowel contents may obscure the abdominal exam, thus only relatively large AAAs can be detected in thin patients. There is also a tendency to overestimate the size of the aorta in a thin patient with a large pulse pressure, thus physical exam is not sufficient for a diagnosis but can identify the need for imaging.

7. **Can AAAs be detected by radiography?**
   Plain abdominal or lumbar spine radiographs can detect occult AAA in about 20% of cases. A thin rim of calcification identifies the aneurysmal aortic wall. The majority of AAAs contain insufficient calcium to be visualized by radiography.

8. **Which imaging method is the best for screening patients for AAA?**
   Abdominal ultrasound permits measurement accuracy within 0.3 cm and data in both cross-sectional and longitudinal dimensions. This modality is commonly used for asymptomatic screening because of cost efficiency and lack of radiation exposure.

9. **What is the best single imaging modality to plan AAA repair?**
   The arterial phase contrast-enhanced computed tomography (CTA) scan is the single best imaging modality. Diameter measurements are accurate within 0.2 cm. Venous anomalies (i.e., retroaortic or circumaortic left renal vein, inferior vena cava [IVC] duplication, and left-sided IVC) may alter the operative approach when visualized on CT. Additionally, size and patency of access vessels available on CTA can provide essential information when endovascular aneurysm repair (EVAR) is being considered. CTA is also excellent at detecting aneurysmal rupture or leak (92% accuracy and 100% specificity).

10. **What is the manifestation of a symptomatic AAA?**
    Acute low back pain is the most common presenting symptom (82%), but only one-third of symptomatic AAAs are diagnosed before rupture. A hypotensive elderly man with acute onset of low back pain has a leaking AAA until proven otherwise. Less common presenting symptoms include early satiety (duodenal compression), hydronephrosis (ureteral compression), and iliocaval thrombosis (venous obstruction).

11. **What is the appropriate management of a patient suspected of a ruptured AAA?**
    If the patient is hemodynamically stable with intact distal pulses, large-bore intravenous access should be obtained and blood immediately cross-matched. Additionally, a femoral arterial line and sheath may be placed for urgent balloon occlusion of the aorta, should the patient become unstable. If the patient is stable for imaging, a stat CTA chest/abdomen/pelvis with bilateral lower extremity runoff should be obtained with surgical team at bedside. If any hemodynamic instability occurs, emergent surgical exploration is warranted. In patients who are hemodynamically unstable with a pulsatile abdominal mass, only an electrocardiogram is required prior to proceeding to the operating room (OR) to rule out myocardial infarction (MI). Uncross-matched blood and femoral arterial access are priorities but should not delay transport to the OR. Additionally, a patient with suspected rupture should not be intubated in the ED. The patient should be prepped and draped awake as even brief hypotension that accompanies anesthesia induction can precipitate cardiac arrest. In cases where EVAR is appropriate, the entire procedure can be done under local anesthesia in cooperative patients, without the need for general anesthesia.

12. **Should all patients presenting with AAA rupture undergo repair?**
    Patients in profound shock, with a concomitant MI, or cardiac arrest at the time of presentation have little chance of survival. Extreme age, dementia, metastatic cancer, and other severe end-stage medical problems should prompt an emergent discussion with the patient and/or family regarding prognosis and goals of care.

13. **Do all patients with ruptured AAAs make it to surgery?**
    Approximately half of patients with a ruptured AAA die before reaching the hospital (and many of those do not attempt reaching the hospital—diagnosis is made at autopsy for patients with sudden death). One-fourth of all patients with ruptures who reach a medical facility alive will die before they can be brought to the OR. Therefore, only 25% of patients survive long enough to have definitive aortic repair following a rupture.

14. **How is a ruptured AAA treated operatively?**
    The patient should not be anesthetized until completely prepped, draped, and ready for immediate incision because any brief hypotension caused by induction medications can cause cardiac arrest. Rapid proximal aortic control is the key to successful outcome of operations for ruptured AAA. Retrograde aortic balloon occlusion has become a popular mechanism by which proximal control can be gained rapidly by those familiar with this technique. For unstable patients, proximal aortic control can be obtained at the diaphragm. As soon as control is obtained, the patient is resuscitated and clamps or balloons are moved to an infrarenal location to improve visceral circulation. The transected aorta should be prepared using the technique described as a Creech endoaneurysmorrhaphy, in which the posterior wall is left intact. For heavily calcified arteries, the use of pledgeted sutures and large bites of healthy aorta wall is advised to prevent anastomotic leakage.

15. **How should patients with symptomatic nonruptured AAAs be managed?**
    Symptomatic AAAs are rapidly expanding and at high risk for rupture. Therefore, most vascular surgeons agree that symptomatic but intact AAAs should be repaired expeditiously (as early as is conveniently possible).

16. **Are there any alternatives to open surgical repair for ruptured AAA?**
    Endovascular prosthetic grafts are frequently and successfully placed in high-risk patients with either free intraperitoneal or contained ruptures.

17. **What are the rupture rates of AAAs?**
    A 5-cm diameter AAA has an annual rupture risk of <1%. The risk of AAA rupture increases logarithmically with size. Annual rupture risk is 10% for a 6-cm AAA and 30% for AAAs >7 cm.

18. **How fast do AAAs enlarge?**
    The average expansion rate of all AAAs is 0.4 cm per year. A general rule of thumb is that AAAs will expand by up to 10% of their diameter every year. The larger the aneurysm, the larger size change is expected. However, 20% of all AAAs demonstrate no change in size over time. Conversely, 20% expand at a rate >0.5 cm per year. Rapid expansion (0.5 cm/6 months) is considered to be predictive of rupture and an indication for repair.

19. **When are angiograms helpful in the diagnostic workup for AAA?**
    Traditionally, angiography has been indicated in patients when there is concern regarding the extent of the proximal neck, concomitant visceral occlusive disease, renal artery anomalies, a prior colectomy with need to visualize the visceral circulation, or lower extremity occlusive or aneurysmal disease. More recently, thin slice (<3 mm) CTA are used to plan for the endovascular repair of an AAA (EVAR). Standard angiography is rarely used unless the patient is too unstable for CTA.

20. **What is the difference between extraperitoneal and transabdominal approach?**
    Elective aortic graft placement can be carried out equally well via a transperitoneal or extraperitoneal approach. The former provides easier iliac vessel exposure according to some reports. The extra peritoneal approach provides expeditious exposure of the suprarenal aorta and facilitates postoperative pulmonary and gastrointestinal recovery.

21. **What are endografts? Are they durable?**
    Endovascular grafts are graft-covered stents with metallic support that are placed via the femoral artery by fluoroscopic methods to exclude the aneurysm without the need for an abdominal incision or cross-clamping the aorta. Multiple different series of successful endovascular AAA repair have established EVAR as the preferred method when anatomic factors allow for this option. Successful endograft placement has been reported in a wide variety of high-risk operative candidates. The major drawbacks are late leaks migration and repressurization of the aneurysm sac with the potential for late rupture or reintervention. This may ultimately increase the cost of the procedure and require compliant long-term patient follow-up.

22. **What are the advantages and disadvantages of an EVAR?**
    Numerous studies report that EVAR has demonstrated a trend toward reduced operative mortality over open AAA repair in anatomically suitable circumstances. Moreover, when endovascular teams and protocols are established, institutions show superior results with EVAR over open repair for the management of ruptured AAAs. However, EVAR requires ongoing surveillance and lifelong follow-up compared with open AAA repair, and reintervention rates are higher.

23. **What are the complications of EVAR? How are they treated?**
    There may be aneurysm expansion from continued arterial perfusion of the aneurysm sac after EVAR. This is termed *endoleak*, and it occurs in 15%–20% of EVARs. Type I endoleak results from antegrade flow at the stent graft attachment site. These are treated with re-ballooning and possibly proximal or distal extension grafts at the time of discovery. Type II endoleaks result from retrograde flow in a collateral vessel feeding the aneurysm such as the lumbar arteries or inferior mesenteric artery. Because most of these endoleaks are self-limiting, observation is appropriate when the AAA is not increasing in size. However, type II endoleaks can be treated with percutaneous coil embolization or open ligation of the culprit if the AAA increases in size by more than 20%. Type III endoleaks result from antegrade flow at the junction point between graft components. These are repaired with a secondary endograft. Type IV endoleaks result from graft wall porosity and can be treated with secondary stenting or with observation. Aortic CT scans are conducted at regular intervals post-EVAR to identify late type II endoleaks that can lead to delayed AAA rupture.

24. Describe the evaluation needed for a patient receiving EVAR.

A history and physical examination with a careful focus on the cardiopulmonary system is essential along with appropriate laboratory data to assess comorbidities and renal function. A CTA with fine cuts and three-dimensional reconstructions can help measure the diameter and evaluate the neck length, angulation, and thrombus. It will also provide valuable data on vessel diameter (iliac and femoral arteries), calcification, and tortuosity to determine the suitability of the patient and the type of device that will best seal the aneurysm. In general, the proximal aortic neck diameter below the lowest renal artery should be between 18 and 32 mm with at least 10–15 mm in neck length depending on the device selected.

25. What are the technical aspects of EVAR?

Percutaneous femoral access is obtained bilaterally, and percutaneous closure devices are placed at the start of the case. Significantly calcified femoral arteries or if there is a need for iliac vessel access because of size constraints, longitudinal or oblique incisions in the groin/iliac fossa expose the arteries for proximal and distal control and subsequent introduction of conduits, may be needed for the introduction of sheaths, wires, and the endovascular device to repair the AAA. The patient receives systemic heparinization before arterial puncture. An aortogram confirms the anatomical landmarks needed for graft deployment and the distance from the renal arteries to the common iliac artery bifurcation to accurately select the graft length for the main body and iliac limbs. The location of the renal arteries must be precisely noted. In most cases, after deployment of the aortic graft, sealing is accomplished using a compliant balloon. A contra-lateral limb within the iliac artery is deployed and overlaps the main graft to achieve a good seal and avoid a type III endoleak. A repeat angiogram confirms placement and identifies type I, II, and III endoleaks. After deployment of the grafts, suture mediated closure devices are deployed, or femoral arteriotomies are closed with nonabsorbable suture following open femoral exposure.

26. At what size should asymptomatic AAAs be repaired electively?

They should be repaired electively when the AAA reaches 5.5 cm in diameter. The only benefit for repair of an asymptomatic AAA is to prevent subsequent rupture and death. Therefore, candidates for elective repair should be expected to live at least 2 years.

27. What are the technical aspects of open AAA surgery?

The two important decisions are the location of arterial clamps and the type of graft to place. The majority of cases can be managed by placing the arterial clamp below the renal arteries. This avoids prolonged ischemia to the kidneys. The aneurysm is opened after clamping proximally and distally. Lumbar artery orifices are oversewn to prevent bleeding from collateral arteries. The inferior mesenteric artery is often occluded, but when it is patent with vigorously back-bleeding, reimplantation should be considered.

28. What are the major noncardiac complications of AAA repair?

Renal failure (elevation in creatinine) and intestinal ischemia (bloody diarrhea).

KEY POINTS: ARTERIAL INSUFFICIENCY

1. An AAA is defined as a >50% increase in normal aortic diameter.
2. Forty percent of patients with a popliteal artery aneurysm harbor an AAA.
3. CTA is the single best imaging modality to plan an AAA repair.
4. AAA should be repaired electively when the size reaches 5.5 cm in diameter.
5. Neck length, angulation, and presence of circumferential mural thrombus of the AAA determine if EVAR is feasible.

WEBSITES

- http://apds.org/physician-resources/acs-surgery-principles-and-practice/
- www.vascularweb.org

BIBLIOGRAPHY

1. Harkin DW, Dillon M. Endovascular ruptured abdominal aortic aneurysm repair (EVRAR): a systematic review. *Eur J Vasc Endovasc Surg.* 2007;34(6):673–681.
2. Tambyraja A, Murie J. Predictors of outcome after abdominal aortic aneurysm rupture: Edinburgh Ruptured Aneurysm Score. *World J Surg.* 2007;31(11):2243–2247.
3. EVAR Trial Participants. Endovascular aneurysm repair versus open repair in patients with abdominal aortic aneurysm (EVAR trial 1): randomised controlled trial. *Lancet.* 2005;365(9478):2179–2186.
4. Greenhalgh RM, Brown LC. Comparison of endovascular aneurysm repair with open repair in patients with abdominal aortic aneurysm (EVAR trial 1), 30-day operative mortality results: randomised controlled trial. *Lancet.* 2004;364(9437):843–848.
5. EVAR Trial Participants. Endovascular aneurysm repair and outcome in patients unfit for open repair of abdominal aortic aneurysm (EVAR trial 2): randomised controlled trial. *Lancet.* 2005;365(9478):2187–2192.
6. Faries PL, Cadot H. Management of endoleak after endovascular aneurysm repair: cuffs, coils, and conversion. *J Vasc Surg.* 2003;37(6):1155–1161.
7. Lecroy C, Passman MA. Should endovascular repair be used for small abdominal aortic aneurysms? *Vasc Endovascular Surg.* 2008;42(2):113–119. discussion, 120–121.
8. Powell JT, Brown LC, Forbes JF, et al. Final 12-year follow-up of surgery versus surveillance in the UK Small Aneurysm Trial. *Br J Surg.* 2007;94(6):702–708.
9. Alonso-Perez M, Segura RJ, Sanchez J, et al. Factors increasing the mortality rate for patients with ruptured abdominal aortic aneurysms. *Ann Vasc Surg.* 2001;15(6):601–607.
10. Lederle FA, Johnson GR, Wilson SE, et al. Rupture rate of large abdominal aortic aneurysms in patients refusing or unfit for elective repair. *JAMA.* 2002;287(22):2968–2972.
11. Lederle FA, Wilson SE, Johnson GR, et al. Immediate repair compared with surveillance of small abdominal aortic aneurysms. *N Engl J Med.* 2002;346(19):1437–1444.
12. Wieker CM, Spazier M. Indications for and outcome of open AAA repair in the endovascular era. *J Cardiovasc Surg (Torino).* 2016;57(2):185–190.
13. Tsilimparis N, Saleptsis V. New developments in the treatment of ruptured AAA. *J Cardiovasc Surg (Torino).* 2016;57(2):233–241.
14. Kauvar DS, Martin ED. Thirty-day outcomes after elective percutaneous or open endovascular repair of abdominal aortic aneurysms. *Ann Vasc Surg.* 2016;31:46–51.
15. Chang DC, Parina RP. Survival after endovascular vs open aortic aneurysm repairs. *JAMA Surg.* 2015;150(12):1160–1166.
16. Karkos CD, Papadimitriou CT, Chatzivasileiadis TN, et al. The impact of aortic occlusion balloon on mortality after endovascular repair of ruptured abdominal aortic aneurysms: a meta-analysis and meta-regression analysis. *Cardiovasc Intervent Radiol.* 2015;38(6):1425–1437.

CHAPTER 76

VENOUS DISEASE

Steven R. Shackford, MD, FACS

1. **What is deep venous thrombosis (DVT)? What initiates it, and what causes it to propagate?**

   DVT means thrombosis in the deep veins of the extremities and neck, as opposed to the superficial veins. In the lower extremity, DVT includes thrombus found in any of the following veins—iliac, femoral, popliteal, tibial, and peroneal. The soleal and gastrocnemius venous plexuses are also considered to be part of the deep system. In the upper extremity, DVT includes thrombus in the axillary, subclavian, and brachial veins. Thrombus in the jugular vein, when it occurs, is often reported when the upper extremity is interrogated with duplex ultrasound and is considered by many to be DVT.

   Factors that initiate and propagate DVT (originally proposed by Ludwig Aschoff and Rudolf Virchow, circa 1856) are reduced or negligible venous flow or stasis, mechanical injury to the vein wall, and hypercoagulability. Recently, it has become recognized that a fourth element is also important, inflammation. Normally, the venous endothelium expresses a nonthrombogenic or anticoagulant phenotype, but this can change in the presence of inflammatory stimuli, which can evoke a procoagulant phenotype. Any single factor or all four may be present in a patient with DVT. In most patients, at least two are operative in the pathogenesis and propagation of thrombus.

2. **What causes stasis of venous blood flow?**

   Stasis is common in hospitalized patients. It occurs during bedrest; during anesthesia when patients are often pharmacologically paralyzed; after certain types of trauma, such as spinal cord injury with paralysis; following a stroke that results in a paralyzed extremity; and during positive pressure ventilation, which periodically produces stasis by impeding venous flow into the chest. Stasis also occurs when a healthy person is immobile for prolonged periods of time, such as occurs during prolonged air or ground travel (>8–10 hours).

   Stasis can initiate endothelial activation. When blood is static in the vein, erythrocyte hemoglobin rapidly becomes desaturated. Vein endothelium, which is dependent on venous luminal oxygen, becomes hypoxic. The endothelial response to hypoxia is activation and a change from the normally anticoagulant phenotype to the procoagulant phenotype. Activation results in the expression of P-selectin and the attraction of leukocytes and platelets, which predispose to thrombus formation.

3. **What can cause venous wall injury?**

   Mechanical trauma to the vein wall can result from indwelling catheters, from a gunshot wound or stabbing, from a splinter of bone accompanying a fracture, or from a retractor injury during surgery. Also, venous distention, as a result of muscular relaxation during anesthesia and surgery, may produce microscopic intimal tears and stasis. The injured venous intima exposes the subendothelial matrix, which is rich in tissue factor, thus activating the coagulation cascade.

4. **What are the causes of hypercoagulability?**

   Hypercoagulability can occur as a result of the normal physiologic responses to surgical stress and trauma, or it can be due to genetic factors. It has been repeatedly shown that surgery and injury produce a hypercoagulable state, which is best demonstrated by tests examining the viscoelastic properties of whole blood, such as thromboelastography.

   Genetic factors producing hypercoagulability include Factor V Leiden mutation, antithrombin deficiency, protein C deficiency, protein S deficiency, lupus anticoagulant, antiphospholipid syndrome, and prothrombin 20210A mutation. The most common of these is the Factor V Leiden mutation (resulting in resistance to activated protein C), which occurs in about 5% of American Caucasians.

5. **What are the clinical risk factors for DVT?**

   There is general agreement that the following factors place patients at particularly high risk: A known hypercoagulable state or a suggestive family history of same, coexisting solid organ malignancy (which characteristically produces migratory or recurrent episodes of deep or superficial venous thrombophlebitis, originally described by Armand Trousseau, circa 1860), history of prior DVT or pulmonary embolism (PE), spinal cord injury with paralysis, obesity (BMI >30 kg/m^2), major surgery lasting longer than 2 hours, lower extremity or pelvic fracture, pregnancy, age greater than 40 years, prolonged (>72 hours) bedrest, mechanical ventilation for a period exceeding 3 days, and inflammatory bowel disease. The list is by no means exhaustive. The clinician should maintain a high index of suspicion whenever the Aschoff/Virchow triad may be present. For example, the risk should be high in any patient with a repair of a vein injury due to a stab wound or gunshot wound.

6. **What signs and symptoms suggest DVT? How can DVT be accurately diagnosed?**
The signs and symptoms suggestive of DVT are calf or thigh pain, swelling, pedal or ankle edema, tenderness to palpation (in some cases a palpable "cord" is present), and increased skin temperature. None of these signs is specific for DVT, and in many cases none are present (particularly with DVT involving the veins distal to the popliteal). In fact, most cases of DVT in surgical and trauma patients are asymptomatic. Even the well-known Homan's sign (i.e., calf pain with dorsiflexion of the foot) is unreliable; its accuracy is only 50%.

    Diagnosis requires imaging. Duplex ultrasound examination, using both B-mode and color flow analysis, is the diagnostic test of choice, replacing phlebography. Duplex has sensitivity and specificity rates of >95%.

7. **What is the incidence of DVT in surgical patients?**
The reported incidence of DVT in surgical patients, including those undergoing elective or urgent procedures and those who suffer significant injury, is extremely variable dependent upon whether only symptomatic DVT is reported or both symptomatic and asymptomatic DVT are reported. Asymptomatic cases are found by using surveillance (usually duplex ultrasound) of moderate or high-risk patients. Thus, the reported incidence of DVT is prone to surveillance bias, which means that the routine use of a sensitive diagnostic test, such as duplex ultrasound or venography, in all patients (i.e., those with and without symptoms) will detect more cases of DVT. The incidence is also dependent on the type of procedure and whether or not the patient has received prophylaxis. In postoperative general surgery patients without prophylaxis the incidence of DVT detected by routine screening is reported to be as high as 30%. In patients undergoing general and vascular surgery, the incidence of **symptomatic** DVT ranges from 0.14% for carotid endarterectomy to 0.94% for colectomy. In severely injured trauma patients without prophylaxis, the incidence of DVT detected by routine screening venography is as high as 58%. In patients undergoing either total hip replacement or total knee replacement and receiving prophylaxis, the incidence of **symptomatic** DVT is 2.7 % and 1.8%, respectively. The incidence of **asymptomatic** DVT in similar patients with prophylaxis is 13.2% and 38.1%, respectively. The difference in the magnitude of the reported incidence in these two groups is due to surveillance bias. In summary, patients who are injured, undergoing cavitary elective or emergency surgery, and having either total knee or hip arthroplasty should be considered at high risk for DVT, and appropriate prophylaxis should be initiated.

8. **What is the natural history of DVT?**
DVT usually begins in the calf, either in the valve cusps of the tibial veins or in the venous plexus of either the gastrocnemius or the soleus muscle. Approximately 20%–40% of these will resolve in 48 hours, but the remainder will persist. Of the persistent calf DVT, 25%–30% propagate into the popliteal vein and become above-knee DVT. If untreated, approximately 25% of these (or about 6% of the originally persistent calf vein DVT) are associated with a PE. Of those patients who are symptomatic for above-knee DVT, approximately 20% will have recurrent DVT, and 20%–25% will develop postthrombotic syndrome within 2 years. Of those medical patients with a PE, 15% are dead within 1 year. Given the significant morbidity and mortality associated with DVT, effective prophylaxis and effective treatment are essential to high-quality patient care.

9. **What is the usual source of a pulmonary embolus?**
Calf vein thrombus propagates proximally into the popliteal, femoral, or iliac veins (or a combination of veins). These proximal DVTs are responsible for >90% of true PE. Thrombus in the subclavian vein is thought to embolize in 10%–12% of cases of upper extremity DVT.

10. **What is de novo pulmonary thrombosis (DNPT)?**
DNPT has recently been described in trauma patients, and is thought to be secondary to chest trauma or local inflammation and not associated with either lower or upper extremity DVT. In fact, the majority of cases of PE now being reported in trauma patients are not associated with any evidence of DVT. The identification of DNPT is likely related to the frequency with which chest CT is ordered in trauma

patients, either to rule out a pulmonary embolus or discovered incidentally during a CT obtained for another suspected diagnosis. There is ongoing debate as to whether or not DNPT should be aggressively treated as a true PE.

11. **Is there any value to D-dimer testing?**
Measurement of D-dimer cross-linked fibrin degradation products (FDPs), formed by the action of plasmin on cross-linked fibrin, has been proposed as an alternative to initial noninvasive testing for either DVT or PE. A sensitivity of 96.8% and a specificity of 35.2% have been reported for the enzyme-linked immunosorbent assay (ELISA) test, making it theoretically possible to limit noninvasive testing to those with positive D-dimer testing. Unfortunately, the ELISA test is time consuming and impractical as a screening test. In addition, false-positive results are a problem in patients with malignancy, infection, pregnancy, trauma, hemorrhage, or recent surgery. Thus, D-dimer testing has little utility is surgical patients or those with injury, who are known to be at high risk for DVT.

12. **What methods of perioperative DVT prophylaxis should be used and in which surgical patients?**
Perioperative DVT prophylaxis is strongly recommended in all high-risk patients who are older than 40 years and undergoing major, general, or orthopedic procedures. In general surgical patients, well-applied prophylactic measures decrease the relative risk of DVT by 67%. The best prophylaxis for DVT includes preoperative and postoperative ambulation. Intermittent pneumatic compression stockings and pharmacologic prophylaxis (low-dose unfractionated heparin [LDUH] or low molecular weight heparin [LMWH]) are recommended in high-risk patients.

13. **How does LDUH work?**
LDUH binds to antithrombin (AT), rendering it more active. Low-dose heparin (5000 U administered subcutaneously every 8 hours until the patient is fully ambulatory) activates AT, inhibits platelet aggregation, and decreases the availability of thrombin.

14. **What is LMWH?**
LMWH is a fragment of heparin produced by enzymatic cleaving of the heparin molecule. It exerts its anticoagulation effect by binding with AT and inhibiting several coagulation enzymes, principally factor Xa. It has a longer half-life than unfractionated heparin and can be administered once daily. LMWH gives a more predictable anticoagulant response at high doses, and thus can be administered without monitoring (it is not necessary to follow the partial thromboplastin time).

15. **Should the placement of an inferior vena cava (IVC) filter ever be considered?**
An IVC filter should be considered in a patient with a PE who is adequately anticoagulated at the time of the embolus. It should also be considered in a patient with a known proximal DVT who has an absolute contraindication to anticoagulation.

16. **What is the treatment for proximal DVT?**
Anticoagulation is the treatment. Until recently, the only option was a vitamin K antagonist (VKA) preceded by therapeutic anticoagulation with either UFH or LMWH (the heparin bridge is given to immediately block the activated coagulation system and possibly neutralize a disproportionate effect of the VKA on proteins C). LMWH is recommended as initial parenteral therapy. A recent metaanalysis indicated that LMWH was associated with fewer deaths, a lower incidence of significant hemorrhage, and lower rates of recurrent VTE.

Direct factor Xa inhibitors are now available (i.e., rivaroxaban), which can be given as monotherapy (without the need for a heparin bridge) and have been shown to be noninferior to the combination of LMWH and VKA. In addition, they do not require monitoring and have no dietary restrictions. Currently, there is no reversal agent for Xa inhibitors.

17. **How long should anticoagulation be continued following an episode of DVT?**
Patients with a transient risk factor (e.g., trauma, surgery) should be anticoagulated for 3 months. Treatment should be extended for greater than 3 months for an initial DVT of unknown origin. If the bleeding risk is high, anticoagulation should be extended to 6 months; if bleeding risk is low to moderate, anticoagulation can be extended indefinitely. Risk factors for recurrent DVT include personal or strong family history of DVT or a thrombophilic state (e.g., cancer, hypercoagulable syndrome). In the presence of one of these risk factors, the physician must weigh the risks and benefits of lifelong anticoagulation in consultation with the patient. Patients with malignancy require extended therapy. Long-term treatment with LMWH is more effective than VKA in preventing recurrent VTE in cancer patients.

18. **What is the treatment for distal DVT?**
The clinical significance of isolated calf vein thrombosis is controversial. Asymptomatic ambulatory outpatients require no initial treatment, but serial imaging is recommended (usually within 72 hours) to detect propagation. Patients who have significant symptoms or who have evidence of propagation on repeat imaging should be therapeutically anticoagulated and be treated similarly to those with proximal DVT. Distal DVT has been associated with a 3%–6% incidence of PE following trauma.

19. **What are the causes and characteristics of chronic venous insufficiency and postphlebitic or postthrombotic syndrome?**
The primary cause is venous valvular incompetence or persistent venous obstruction producing an impediment to venous return resulting in ambulatory venous hypertension. After DVT, involved venous segments eventually recanalize to some degree. The process of recanalization damages the venous valves. The loss of valvular function disables the gastrocnemius/soleus muscle pump resulting in venous pooling and stasis resulting in venous hypertension. Protein-rich fluids, fibrin, and red blood cells are extravasated as a result of the increased venous pressure. This process leads to inflammation, scarring, fibrosis of the subcutaneous tissues, and discoloration by hemosiderin deposition (brawny edema in the gaiter area). The resultant inflammatory reaction, scarring, and interstitial edema create a further barrier to capillary flow and diffusion of oxygen resulting in inadequate nutrition to the skin. These changes may lead to tissue atrophy and ulceration (i.e., a venous stasis ulcer). Even without stasis ulceration, postphlebitic syndrome can be very disabling.

20. **Do all patients with DVT develop postphlebitic or postthrombotic syndrome?**
Approximately 20%–25% of patients with a proximal symptomatic DVT will develop a clinically relevant postphlebitic syndrome within 2 years. Recent epidemiologic studies suggest that the incidence of venous ulceration is about 5%. Of interest, 50% of patients with venous ulcers have no history of DVT (probably because of previous asymptomatic calf vein DVT).

21. **What is the treatment of postphlebitic syndrome?**
With proper patient education and compliance with a treatment and prevention regimen, postphlebitic stasis sequelae can be controlled by nonoperative means in 90% of patients. Nonoperative treatment consists of graded elastic compression stockings to retard swelling and periodic leg elevation during the day. Patients must be taught to elevate their legs above the heart (toes above your nose) at regular intervals (e.g., 10–15 minutes every 2 hours). Severe stasis dermatitis and ulceration can be effectively managed with an Unna's boot (compression with gauze impregnated with zinc oxide and calamine lotion) and elastic support.

22. **What is the difference between phlegmasia alba dolens and phlegmasia cerulea dolens?**
These two entities occur following iliofemoral venous thrombosis, 75% of which occur on the left side presumably because of compression of the left common iliac vein by the overlying right common iliac artery (May-Thurner syndrome). Iliofemoral venous thrombosis is characterized by unilateral pain and edema of an entire lower extremity, discoloration, and groin tenderness. In **phlegmasia alba dolens** (literally, painful white swelling), the leg becomes pale. Arterial pulses remain normal. Progressive thrombosis may occur with propagation proximally or distally and into neighboring tributaries. The entire leg becomes both edematous and mottled or cyanotic. This stage is called **phlegmasia cerulea dolens** (literally, painful purple swelling). When venous outflow is seriously impeded, arterial inflow may be reduced secondarily by as much as 30%. Limb loss is a serious concern and aggressive management (i.e., venous thrombectomy, catheter-directed lytic therapy, or both) is necessary.

23. **What is venous claudication?**
When venous recanalization fails to occur after iliofemoral venous thrombosis, venous collaterals develop to bypass the obstruction to venous outflow. These collaterals usually suffice while the patient is at rest. However, walking induces increased arterial inflow that exceeds the capacity of the venous collaterals resulting in progressive venous hypertension and venous distention. This results in calf pain commonly described as tight, heavy, or bursting (venous claudication). Relief is obtained with rest and elevation.

24. **How can one distinguish between primary and secondary varicose veins?**
Primary varicose veins result from uncomplicated saphenofemoral venous valvular incompetence and have a greater saphenous distribution, a positive tourniquet test, no stasis sequelae (dermatitis or ulceration), and no morning ankle edema. **Secondary varicose veins** are a consequence of deep and perforator venous incompetence secondary to postphlebitic syndrome.

25. **What are the indications for treatment of varicose veins? What is the treatment?**
Varicose veins should be treated when they produce symptoms of aching and discomfort (i.e., itching, heaviness). Initial treatment is conservative with the use of support stockings. Compliance with the use of support hose is generally poor, particularly in warmer environments as the tight knit of the stocking does not allow for heat exchange. Failure of conservative therapy, as evidenced by persistent symptoms or intolerance of support stockings, is an indication for more invasive treatment. Ligation of incompetent perforators, high saphenous vein ligation, injection sclerotherapy, greater saphenous stripping or radiofrequency ablation, and selective stab phlebectomy are the treatment options available. The choice of which therapy or combination of therapies is best is dependent on the severity of the symptoms and the severity of the disease. The best results are obtained with early treatment before continuous retrograde pressure and flow down the superficial system and into communicating perforating veins (whenever the patient is standing) cause secondary, irreversible perforator incompetence.

KEY POINTS: VENOUS DISEASE

1. More than 95% of DVTs develop in the deep veins of the lower extremities; the majority originates in the valve sinuses of the calf veins.
2. The Aschoff/Virchow triad consists of hypercoagulability, disruption of an intact venous intimal lining, and stasis of venous blood flow.
3. The best prophylaxis for DVT includes preoperative and postoperative walking. Prophylactic anticoagulation should be considered for surgical patients who have significant risk factors for DVT.
4. The complications of DVT are PE, recurrent DVT, and postthrombotic syndrome.
5. The treatment of DVT and PE is therapeutic anticoagulation.
6. Studies comparing the effectiveness of prophylactic or therapeutic regimens for DVT **must** include some method of surveillance because most DVT is asymptomatic and can only be detected using surveillance imaging.

BIBLIOGRAPHY

1. Wakefield TW, Dalsing MC. Venous disease. In: Mulholland MW, Lillemoe KD, eds. *Greenfield's Surgery: Scientific Principles and Practice.* 4th ed. Philadelphia, PA: Lippincott Williams & Wilkins; 2006:1791–1800.
2. Knudson MM, Gomez D. Three thousand seven hundred and thirty-eight pulmonary emboli: a new look at an old disease. *Ann Surg.* 2011;254(4):625–632.
3. Van Gent JM, Zander AL, Olson EJ, et al. Pulmonary embolism without deep venous thrombosis: de novo or missed deep venous thrombosis. *J Trauma Acute Care Surg.* 2014;76(5):1270–1274.
4. Brandjes DPM. Hei Acenocoumarol and heparin compared with acenocoumarol alone in the treatment of proximal-vein thrombosis. *New Engl J Med.* 1992;327(21):1485–1489.
5. Wells P, Forgie MA. Treatment of venous thromboembolism. *JAMA.* 2014;311(7):717–728.
6. Kearon C, Akl EA, Camerota AJ, et al. Antithrombotic therapy for VTE disease; Antithrombotic therapy and prevention of thrombosis, 9th edition: American College of Chest Physicians Evidence-based Clinical Practice Guidelines. *Chest.* 2012;141(suppl 2):419S–494S.
7. Olson E, Zander AL, Van Gent J-M, et al. Below-knee deep vein thrombosis: an opportunity to prevent pulmonary embolism? *J Trauma Acute Care Surg.* 2014;77(3):459–463.
8. Kahn SR. The post-thrombotic syndrome: progress and pitfalls. *Br J Haematol.* 2006;134(4):357–365.
9. Masuda EM, Kistner RL. The controversy of managing calf vein thrombosis. *J Vasc Surg.* 2012;55(2):550–561.
10. Bandle J, Shackford SR, Kahl JE, et al. The value of lower-extremity duplex surveillance to detect deep vein thrombosis in trauma patients. *J Trauma Acute Care Surg.* 2013;74(2):575–580.

CHAPTER 77

NONINVASIVE VASCULAR DIAGNOSTIC LABORATORY

Jessica L. Williams, MD, Jason Q. Alexander, MD, FACS,
Tony Nguyen, DO

1. **What is the role of the vascular diagnostic laboratory (VDL) in the assessment and treatment of patients with suspected vascular disease?**
   Although traditional evaluation by an experienced physician remains the foundation of vascular diagnosis, clinical assessment has its limitations. For example, only one-third of cervical bruits are associated with significant carotid artery disease; conversely, as many as two-thirds of patients with severe carotid disease present without a cervical bruit. Half of patients with extensive deep venous thrombosis (DVT) of the lower extremity lack signs and symptoms referable to the lower extremities, and more than half of patients presenting with clinical signs of DVT are venographically normal. As many as 40% of patients with diabetes have no large-vessel peripheral arterial occlusive disease. The VDL provides objective, quantitative, and functional status data to delineate the severity of extracranial cerebrovascular disease, peripheral arterial occlusive disease, and acute and chronic venous disease.

2. **What differentiates the VDL from diagnostic radiology and ultrasound (US)?**
   The VDL provides functional information rather than or in addition to the morphologic data provided by radiology tests and general US images. This information is particularly important for peripheral arterial occlusive disease, chronic venous insufficiency, and postoperative surveillance of vascular interventions. Anatomic information about the site of stenosis or occlusion is of limited value without knowledge of the functional significance when assessing peripheral arterial disease. Treatment options for patients with chronic venous insufficiency are dependent on the function of the deep and superficial venous systems rather than ultrasonographic evidence of blockages. Early identification of narrowing in the postoperative period may allow early intervention to extend durability of repair.

CEREBROVASCULAR DISEASE

3. **Which noninvasive tests should be used to diagnose extracranial carotid artery disease?**
   Duplex US has a sensitivity of 99% in detecting carotid artery disease and an accuracy of 95% in correctly classifying carotid stenoses as ≥70% reduction in diameter. Although catheter-based angiography is the gold standard for evaluation of carotid artery occlusive disease, this procedure is associated with a 1% stroke rate. Computed tomography angiography (CTA) and magnetic resonance angiography (MRA) also demonstrate high sensitivity and specificity for carotid occlusive disease, but to obtain these results requires the administration of contrast agents (usually either Renografin or gadolinium) that carry a risk of nephropathy or systemic fibrosis. These risks are not associated with duplex US.

4. **What is duplex US?**
   Duplex US uses both image and velocity data (hence the name duplex) in a nearly simultaneous presentation of US echo images (often referred to as grayscale or B-mode US) and blood velocity waveforms obtained by Doppler US. The Doppler signals are obtained from a single small region of the blood vessel. Average velocities can be estimated for multiple such regions over a large area of the vessel. By assigning colors to the velocities, blood flow can be visually represented. Such a presentation, called color-flow duplex US, aids the duplex examination but cannot replace the information obtained from the Doppler velocity waveform.

5. **Why is blood velocity important in assessing the degree of carotid artery stenosis?**
   It is often difficult to measure the arterial lumen accurately on a B-mode US image because the acoustic properties (and hence the image) of noncalcified plaque, thrombus, and even blood may

Table 77.1 University Of Washington Criteria

Stenosis Criteria

STENOSIS (%)	PSV (CM/S)	EDV (CM/S)	FLOW CHARACTERISTICS
1–15	<125	<140	No spectral broadening
16–49	<125	<140	Minimal spectral broadening
50–79	≥125	<140	Marked spectral broadening
80–99	≥125	>140	Marked spectral broadening
Occlusion	N/A	N/A	No internal carotid flow signal

Table 77.2 Carotid Consensus Panel Criteria

Stenosis Criteria

STENOSIS (%)	PSV (CM/S)	EDV (CM/S)	ICA/CCA RATIO
Normal	<125	<40	<2
<50	<125	<40	<2
50–69	125–230	40–100	2–4
>70	≥230	>100	>4
Near Occlusion	High, low, or undetectable	Variable	Variable
Occlusion	Undetectable	N/A	N/A

be similar. Arterial narrowing forces blood through a narrower channel, which increases the blood velocity. This velocity can characterize the degree of arterial narrowing. Current practice classifies the degree of internal carotid stenosis based exclusively on the Doppler velocity data.

6. **What are the velocity criteria and categorical ranges of carotid artery stenosis?**
The criteria developed at the University of Washington (Table 77.1) were the original thresholds. However, in 2003 the Carotid Consensus Panel developed criteria that are widely used today (Table 77.2). Note that progressive carotid stenosis increases the flow velocity signal as the volume of blood is squeezed through the gradually smaller orifice. However, ultrasonography is dependent on each individual ultrasonographer and each type of machine. Furthermore, variation in patient comorbidities can affect velocity. For example, patients with improved ejection fraction (EF) will have elevated velocities compared with patients having lesser EF but similar narrowing. Thus, any noninvasive VDL must continually evaluate the criteria that they employ and compare to gold standard measurements (catheter-based angiography) to verify their criteria.

7. **Is duplex US capable of determining whether the internal carotid is occluded?**
As the stenosis in a vessel becomes tighter, the velocity of blood flow increases. At a critical point, however, the diameter of the stenosis becomes so narrow that blood can no longer traverse at a high speed and will actually slow down. When the stenosis approaches occlusion, the velocity of the blood flow will slow down to the point that it is no longer in the range of the US machine. The duplex study may then interpret an internal carotid artery as occluded when in fact there is trickle flow or a string sign. This is an important differentiation. Internal carotid artery occlusion rarely requires intervention, but a critical stenosis associated with trickle flow or a string sign carries a significant risk of stroke.

8. **How accurate is duplex US of the internal carotid if the contralateral internal carotid is occluded?**
When the contralateral internal carotid artery is occluded the body will often adjust to maintain the same anterior cerebral perfusion by increasing flow in the internal carotid of interest. This increased flow leads to elevated velocities determined by Doppler. Because these velocities are used to estimate stenosis, the Doppler may artificially predict a tighter stenosis than is in fact present.

VENOUS DISEASE

9. **What noninvasive test is used to diagnose acute DVT?**
   Duplex US has replaced venous occlusion plethysmography as the accepted standard. Color-flow duplex is useful because it helps to identify small veins from the muscle and fascial layers. The US assessment involves the following steps:
   a. Examine the vein for echogenic thrombus.
   b. Compress the vein, using pressure on the US probe, looking for complete collapse. Inability to compress the vein suggests thrombosis. Partial compression suggests partial thrombosis.
   c. A Doppler signal from the vein that is phasic with respiration suggests no proximal occlusive thrombus. A signal that is spontaneously present but nonphasic suggests flow around an occlusion via small collateral veins. Absence of a Doppler signal in the vein suggests absence of flow.

10. **Can duplex US be used for surveillance in patients at high risk for DVT?**
    Diagnosis of DVT in asymptomatic patients presents a dilemma. The sensitivity of duplex US in detection of proximal (above the knee) DVT is reduced from the reported 97% in symptomatic patients to <80% in asymptomatic patients. Furthermore, distal (below the knee) DVT detection is even worse, with metaanalysis pooled sensitivity of 71%. However, serial contrast venography, although more specific, is not a practical surveillance strategy given that several technical issues often lead to inadequate studies.

11. **Which veins are anatomically deep veins, and which veins are superficial veins?**
    Differentiating between superficial and deep veins is important because superficial venous thrombosis carries almost no risk of pulmonary embolism unless first propagating into the deep system. The deep system is identified beneath muscular fascial layers in the body. For greater simplicity, it is often easiest to remember that if a vein runs with a named artery it is considered a deep vein. Thus, the vein that runs with the superficial femoral artery, the femoral vein (formerly called the superficial femoral vein), is a deep vein. There are a few exceptions to this rule, but they are largely limited to muscular calf veins, the gastrocnemius, and soleal veins.

12. **What noninvasive tests are useful for evaluation of venous incompetence?**
    Doppler US can detect venous reflux in the deep veins of the legs and in the greater and lesser saphenous veins. With experience, the test can be done using a simple Doppler (continuous wave versus pulsed Doppler), but duplex US is often used to facilitate identification of the vein segments and valves and to position a pulsed Doppler sample reliably. When a venous valve is incompetent, flow in the vein perpetuates peripherally if pressure is applied in the more central portion of the limb. Differentiating between competent and incompetent venous valves in the superficial and deep system affects options for therapy.

PERIPHERAL ARTERIAL OCCLUSIVE DISEASE

13. **What is the primary test for diagnosis of lower extremity ischemia?**
    The ankle brachial index (ABI) or systolic pressure ratio is normally ≥1.0. Typically, Doppler US is used (instead of a stethoscope) as the flow sensor distal to the pressure cuff, but plethysmographic instruments also may be used. Doppler signals are usually monitored at the posterior tibial artery or dorsalis pedis artery. The ABI is the ratio of the highest systolic blood pressure (SBP) measured at either the dorsalis pedis artery or posterior tibial artery compared to the highest SBP measurement at the brachial artery of either arm. Unfortunately, calcified vessels can prevent compression by pressure cuffs, thus suggesting artificially high SBP. This is most notable in patients who are diabetic who may demonstrate ABI >1.0 despite hemodynamically significant lower extremity stenotic disease.

14. **What is gained by measuring pressures at limb levels other than the ankle?**
    Segmental limb pressure (SLP) measurements, performed at the upper thigh, lower thigh, calf, and ankle, localize the arterial segment(s) involved in peripheral arterial occlusive disease.

15. **What tests are used for assessing peripheral artery disease in patients who are diabetic who may have incompressible arteries caused by medial calcification?**
    Pulse volume recording (PVR) is a pneumoplethysmographic technique that tracks the limb volume changes over the cardiac cycle. It measures the segmental pressure changes with pneumatic cuffs as a function of the limb volume changes. The relative PVR amplitudes identify the presence of peripheral

artery disease and localize the arterial segment involved. The PVR is unaffected by medial calcification. Great toe pressure also may be used to diagnose and assess disease severity in diabetic patients because medial calcification rarely affects the digital arteries.

16. **How should the patient with suspected intermittent claudication be evaluated?**
The patient first should be evaluated by obtaining ABIs or SLPs at rest. The patient with ischemia at rest does not normally need further evaluation. The patient with mild arterial insufficiency at rest or even normal resting pressures should perform an exercise stress test (treadmill walking using either fixed or variable load protocols) followed by ABIs. The distance that the patient is able to walk allows assessment of functional disability, and the postexercise reduction in ankle pressure, or lack thereof, allows assessment of whether the disability is caused by arterial insufficiency rather than musculoskeletal or neurologic pain.

DUPLEX US SURVEILLANCE OF VASCULAR THERAPY

17. **What is the importance of duplex US surveillance of autogenous lower extremity bypass grafts?**
Duplex surveillance of infrainguinal autogenous bypass grafts is critical to the postoperative care in the vascular patient. Occluded autogenous grafts usually do not respond to attempts to regain patency and often require entirely new bypasses. Multiple studies have demonstrated that physical examination (e.g., loss or diminished distal pulse) or return of ischemic symptoms fail to identify new stenoses before occlusion. Early identification of stenosis within or at the periphery of grafts may be treated by minimally invasive open or endovascular techniques before occlusion occurs. Duplex US can easily identify stenoses both within the graft and at the anastomoses by demonstrating significant velocity shifts at these points.

18. **Does duplex US have any role in surveillance of infrainguinal revascularization?**
Infrainguinal revascularization can be categorized by the material used (vein [autogenous versus autologous] or graft bypass) and location of the distal anastomosis (above or below knee bypass). Numerous studies have verified that the patency rate differs depending on which type of conduit is used and the location of the distal anastomosis—vein graft above the knee being best and below knee prosthetic graft being worst in terms of graft failure. It has been documented that early detection of graft failure resulting from significant stenosis and subsequent intervention have a better outcome compared to salvage of an occluded graft. Vein grafts are more likely to develop a progressive stenosis leading to occlusion compared to prosthetic graft, which generally do not stenose before occlusion. Duplex US, therefore, has a role in graft surveillance of vein graft to improve patency. Although prosthetic grafts do not routinely demonstrate intragraft stenosis, they may exhibit progression of atherosclerotic disease of hemodynamically significant narrowing at the anastomoses. If this narrowing is identified and treated, it may be possible to extend prosthetic graft patency as well. Furthermore, current literature tends to support surveillance US for following endovascular stenting and angioplasty in attempts to identify early restenosis to expedite reintervention.

19. **What is the role for surveillance duplex US following carotid endarterectomy (CEA)?**
The rationale for surveillance duplex US following CEA is twofold. Most vascular surgeons will evaluate the repair of the ipsilateral carotid on a 6-month to annual basis. The incidence of recurrent stenosis is rare, but early identification may allow more immediate or minimally invasive intervention before a patient becomes symptomatic. Of potentially greater significance during surveillance duplex US examination is evaluation of the contralateral carotid artery. Up to one-quarter of patients undergoing CEA will demonstrate progression from nonhemodynamically significant disease to significant atherosclerotic disease in the contralateral internal carotid artery over the next 10 years.

CONTROVERSIES

20. **Can CEA be performed on the basis of duplex study alone?**
The argument for elimination of arteriography in selected cases is persuasive because the carotid arteriogram alone has a morbidity rate >1%. To realize the benefit of surgery based on duplex US, the duplex study must have a high positive predictive value (PPV). Fortunately, the PPV is high for severe lesions that meet suitably strict criteria (e.g., peak systolic velocities >290 cm/s and end-diastolic velocities >80 cm/s).

21. **Does duplex US have any role in the preoperative evaluation of peripheral vascular disease?**
Contrast arteriography (CA) is still the gold standard imaging modality in the workup of limb ischemia. However, duplex US is gaining popularity as the preferred modality of choice to image the arterial vasculature to evaluate for potential revascularization. Duplex has several advantages over CA that make it appealing. It can identify areas of thickened or calcified vessels that are still patent and, therefore, would be falsely identified as a potential distal target on contrast imaging or MRA. Volume flow measurements by duplex allow a more objective assessment of hemodynamically significant lesion as compared to a subjective assessment by CA. Other benefits of duplex are the ability to assess the underlying disease of the vessel to determine whether a lesion is a chronic occlusion or an acute embolus with little underlying disease, aneurysms with partial thrombus and no luminal dilation, which would appear normal on CA, and the presence of ulcerated or irregular plaques, which would be a source of embolization. The feasibility and portability of the duplex as a bedside study allows for a more cost-effective and time-efficient study, thus reducing hospital cost and stays. The ability to concurrently evaluate the venous system for potential conduit is also attractive.

22. **What are the potential adverse effects of MRA in patients with renal insufficiency?**
Nephrogenic systemic fibrosis (NSF), first recognized in 1997, is a disease affecting renal failure or dialysis patients. It is characterized by a scleroderma-like dermatosis with thickening of the skin resulting in indurated plaque lesions. It commonly involves extremities, causing contractures, but can also have visceral involvement, which increases morbidity and mortality. Although the actual pathogenesis is currently unknown, there are many associated risk factors including gadolinium-containing contrast media. Because MRA carries the risk of NSF and CTA carries a risk of contrast nephropathy, duplex US may be the diagnostic modality of choice in patients with renal insufficiency.

23. **What are the disadvantages of duplex US?**
Duplex US does have limitations. Factors that limit its visualization are severely calcified vessels, severe lymphedema, dermatitis, ulcer wounds, hyperkeratosis, rest pain, and patient noncompliance. Extremely low-flow states with peak systolic velocity (PSV) <20 cm/s can make duplex interpretations unreliable, as is the case with critically stenotic internal carotid artery (ICA) disease that may be incorrectly interpreted as occluded.

24. **Should D-dimer blood tests be required before patients are evaluated by US for DVT?**
D-dimer is a degradation product of cross-linked fibrin. Blood plasma levels of D-dimer are often elevated in patients with DVT. However, DVT is not the only cause of elevated D-dimers and cannot be used instead of US to diagnose the presence of DVT. Conversely, in selected patient subgroups, a low D-dimer level has a high negative predictive value and can prevent unnecessary US testing. The test should be restricted to nonsurgical patients, patients who are not anticoagulated, patients in the outpatient setting, and patients in whom there is a low clinical suspicion of DVT, such as a painful limb without swelling or bilateral ankle swelling.

25. **Is there a therapeutic component to the noninvasive VDL?**
Duplex US is now being used to localize and guide treatment of many iatrogenic pseudoaneurysms. When a patient develops a pseudoaneurysm after arterial cannulation with a long and narrow neck, treatment can be instituted employing compression at the neck using the US probe. If the flow can be obstructed using the probe (usually requiring 20–30 minutes of pressure), the pseudoaneurysm will often thrombose. Additionally, US can be used to guide thrombin injection into the pseudoaneurysms themselves. Injection is performed only in pseudoaneurysms with long, narrow necks. Cannulation of the aneurysm with a needle is confirmed with US. Color-flow is applied to the aneurysm during thrombin injection to confirm thrombosis. This method, while carrying a small risk of distal embolization, eliminates the discomfort to the patient of extended US compression.

26. **What is the role of duplex US in the treatment and management of abdominal aortic aneurysms (AAA)?**
Conventional US is quite good at identifying AAA but suffers when attempting to determine aneurysm size. This is more significant in large patients or aneurysms containing an abundance of thrombus. Computed tomography (CT) scan remains the test of choice for anatomic delineation of AAA, especially when evaluating for the appropriateness of endovascular AAA repair (EVAR). Duplex US may be valuable in determining success of repair during surveillance after EVAR. Although this application remains controversial, post-EVAR duplex US can identify leaks and evaluate aneurysm sac growth while avoiding the contrast load incumbent to post-EVAR CT scan surveillance.

KEY POINTS: NONINVASIVE VASCULAR DIAGNOSTIC LABORATORY

1. Duplex US has a sensitivity of 99% in detecting carotid artery disease and an accuracy of 95% in correctly classifying carotid stenoses as >70% reduction in diameter.
2. The primary test for diagnosis of lower extremity ischemia is the ABI.
3. The noninvasive test used to diagnose acute DVT is duplex US.
4. Duplex US surveillance of lower extremity revascularization and CEA has become a critical component of the noninvasive VDL.
5. The role of duplex US is rapidly expanding in conjunction with the expansion of minimally invasive vascular therapies. This role includes not only diagnosis but also surveillance and therapy.

WEBSITE

- www.vascular.org

BIBLIOGRAPHY

1. Ascher E, Marks NA. Duplex-guided endovascular treatment for occlusive and stenotic lesions of the femoral-popliteal arterial segment: a comparative study in the first 253 cases. *J Vasc Surg.* 2006;44(6):1230–1237.
2. Baker Jr WF. Diagnosis of deep venous thrombosis and pulmonary embolism. *Med Clin North Am.* 1998;82(3): 459–476.
3. Ballotta E, Da Giau G. Progression of atherosclerosis in asymptomatic carotid arteries after contralateral endarterectomy: a 10-year prospective study. *J Vasc Surg.* 2007;45(3):516–522.
4. Byrnes KR, Ross CB. The current role of carotid duplex ultrasonography in the management of carotid atherosclerosis: foundations and advances. *Int J Vasc Med.* 2012;2012:187872.
5. Carter A, Murphy MO, Halka AT, et al. The natural history of stenoses within lower limb arterial bypass grafts using a graft surveillance program. *Ann Vasc Surg.* 2007;21(6):695–703.
6. Goodacre S, Sampson F. Systematic review and meta-analysis of the diagnostic accuracy of ultrasonography for deep vein thrombosis. *BMC Med Imaging.* 2005;5:6.
7. Hanson JM, Atri M. Ultrasound-guided thrombin injection groin pseudoaneurysm: Doppler features and technical tips. *Br J Radiol.* 2008;81(962):154–163.
8. Jahromi AS, Cinà CS. Sensitivity and specificity of color duplex ultrasound measurement in the estimation of internal carotid artery stenosis: a systematic review and meta-analysis. *J Vasc Surg.* 2005;41(6):962–972.
9. Moneta GL, Edwards JM, Papanicolaou G, et al. Screening for asymptomatic internal carotid artery stenosis: duplex criteria for discriminating 60% to 99% stenosis. *J Vasc Surg.* 1995;21(6):989–994.
10. Roth SM, Bandyk DF. Duplex imaging of lower extremity bypasses, angioplasties, and stents. *Semin Vasc Surg.* 1999;12(4):275–284.
11. Wolf YG, Johnson BL. Duplex ultrasound scanning versus computed tomography angiography for postoperative evaluation of endovascular abdominal aortic aneurysm repair. *J Vasc Surg.* 2003;38(5):1142–1143.
12. McPhee JT, Madenci A. Contemporary comparison of aortofemoral bypass to alternative inflow procedures in the Veteran population. *J Vasc Surg.* 2016;64(6):1660–1666.

VIII
CARDIOTHORACIC SURGERY

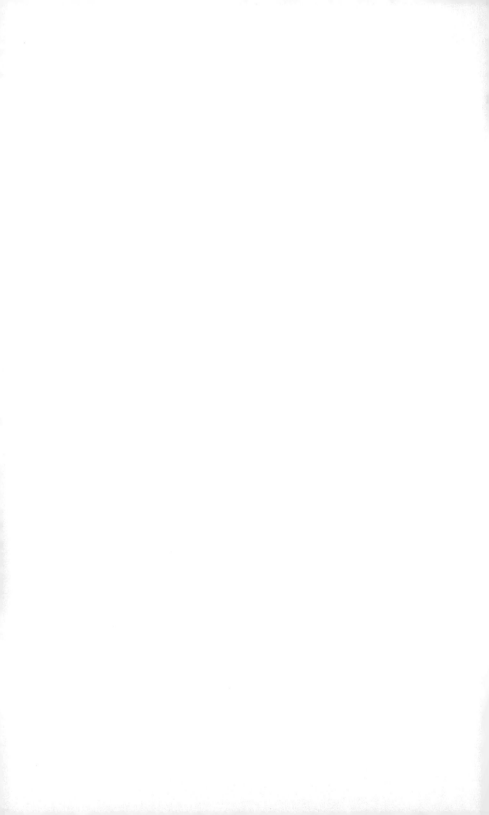

CORONARY ARTERY DISEASE

Joseph C. Cleveland, Jr., MD

CHAPTER 78

1. What is angina, and what causes it?
   Angina pectoris reflects myocardial ischemia. Patients often describe the sensation as pressure, choking, or tightness. Angina typically worsens with exertion or stress and is relieved by rest. Angina is typically produced by an imbalance between myocardial oxygen supply and myocardial oxygen demand. The classic presentation is a man (male/female ratio of 4:1) out shoveling snow on a cold night after a big meal. Alternatively, sometimes (particularly in patients with diabetes mellitus), dyspnea on exertion may also reflect myocardial ischemia. For unclear reasons, patients with diabetes may not complain of chest pain/pressure, but rather dyspnea as their presenting symptom of myocardial ischemia.

2. How is angina treated?
   The treatment options for angina include medical therapy or medical therapy with myocardial revascularization with either percutaneous coronary intervention (PCI) or coronary artery bypass grafting (CABG). Medical treatment is directed toward decreasing myocardial oxygen demand. Strategies include nitrates (nitroglycerin, isosorbide), which dilate coronary arteries minimally but also decrease blood pressure (afterload) and therefore myocardial oxygen demand; β-receptor antagonists, which decrease heart rate, contractility, and afterload; and calcium channel antagonists, which decrease afterload and may prevent coronary vasoconstriction. Antiplatelet therapy (e.g., aspirin, Plavix, prasugrel) is also important. Newer antiplatelet agents such as clopidogrel (Plavix) and eptifibatide (Integrilin) are promoted in the management of acute coronary syndromes. Plavix, however, is a potent, efficacious agent, and operation (i.e., CABG) within 5 days of Plavix exposure increases the risk of postoperative bleeding threefold.

   Once patients are on guideline-directed medical therapy, then revascularization with either PCI or CABG is undertaken if symptoms persist.
   a. What is a heart team? A heart team is composed of an interventional cardiologist and a cardiac surgeon. The heart team endorses a multidisciplinary approach to coronary revascularization and seeks to inform patients about the most appropriate therapy to treat their cardiovascular disease. The use of a heart team is endorsed as a Class I indication by the American Heart Association/American College of Cardiology 2012 Stable Ischemic Heart Disease Guidelines.
   b. What is a syntax score? The SYNTAX trial randomized 1800 patients to receive either a drug-eluting stent (PCI) or CABG for multivessel CAD. In SYNTAX, the degree of CAD was calculated based on a score that was based on the extent, location, and severity of CAD from the coronary angiogram. The cutoff points for syntax scores are as follows: low <22, intermediate 23–32, and high >33. Patients with high syntax scores (>33) and multivessel CAD had improved survival and lower rates of death, myocardial infarction (MI), and repeat reintervention. Thus, this score can aid the heart team in counseling patients regarding revascularization options.

3. What are the indications for coronary artery bypass graft?
   a. Left main coronary artery stenosis: Stenosis >50% involving the left main coronary artery is a robust predictor of poor long-term outcome in patients who are medically treated. A substantial portion of the myocardium is supplied by this artery. Even if the patient is asymptomatic, survival is markedly improved with CABG. Left main disease is a Class I indication for CABG according to the American Heart Association/American College of Cardiology guidelines for CABG surgery.
   b. Three-vessel coronary artery disease (70% stenosis) with depressed left ventricular (LV) function (i.e., <0.50) or two-vessel coronary artery disease (CAD) with proximal left anterior descending (LAD) involvement: In randomized trials, patients with three-vessel disease and depressed LV function showed a survival benefit with CABG compared with medical therapy.
   c. CABG also confers survival benefit in patients with two-vessel CAD with a tight proximal LAD stenosis and an ejection fraction (EF) <0.50 or demonstrable ischemia on noninvasive testing. An important caveat, however, in managing patients with depressed LV function is that operative mortality increases when the EF falls below 30%.

d. Angina despite aggressive medical therapy: Patients who have lifestyle limitations because of CAD are appropriate candidates for CABG, provided surgery can be performed with acceptable risk. Data from the Coronary Artery Surgery Study suggest that patients treated with surgery have less angina, fewer activity limitations, and an objective increase in exercise tolerance compared with medically treated patients.

4. **What is done during a traditional CABG procedure?**
CABG is an arterial bypass procedure that can be done both on bypass and off bypass. The left internal mammary artery (LIMA) is harvested as a pedicled graft, with other conduits including the greater saphenous vein or radial artery procured as well. Cardiopulmonary bypass (CPB) is established by cannulating the ascending aorta and the right atrium, and the heart is arrested with cold blood cardioplegia. Segments of the greater saphenous vein are then reversed and sewn with the proximal (inflow) portion of the bypass graft originating from the ascending aorta and the distal (outflow) portion of the bypass graft anastomosed to the coronary artery distal to the obstructing lesion. The LIMA is typically sewn to the LAD. When the anastomoses are finished, the patient is weaned from CPB, and the chest is closed. Typically, one to six bypass grafts are constructed (hence the terms triple or quadruple bypass).

5. **What is an off-pump CABG (OPCAB)?**
CABG can be performed without CPB and arrest of the heart. When done with the heart beating through a median sternotomy, CABG is then called an OPCAB. The heart is positioned with commercially available stabilization devices, and the vessel to be bypassed is immobilized and snared to provide temporary occlusion. The venous or arterial conduit is then sewn to the immobilized coronary artery, and the occlusion of the vessel is released.

6. **Why would one choose an OPCAB instead of a traditional CABG?**
CABG with CPB remains the gold standard with 80%–85% of CABG procedures reported to the Society of Thoracic Surgeons National Adult Cardiac Database still being performed with CPB. However, CPD is associated with several adverse clinical consequences such as acute lung dysfunction, stroke, renal failure, liver failure, bleeding, and the promotion of a proinflammatory state. It is thought, although not yet well delineated, that performing CABG without CPB may reduce these complications. Patients with comorbidities of lung disease, cerebrovascular disease, renal disease, or severe peripheral vascular disease may have improved outcomes when CABG is performed without the use of CPB. The tradeoff for avoidance of CPB may unfortunately include compromised graft patency because most reports promoting OPCAB do not include graft patency data, and early reports of OPCAB described more early graft occlusions with this technique. To summarize, certain centers have adopted OPCAB. These centers prefer this technique and likely have good outcomes with OPCAB. The majority of CABG is still performed in the United States using cardiopulmonary bypass.

7. **Does CABG improve myocardial function?**
Yes. Hibernating myocardium is improved by CABG. Myocardial hibernation refers to the reversible myocardial contractile function associated with a decrease in coronary flow in the setting of preserved myocardial viability. Some patients with global systolic dysfunction exhibit dramatic improvement in myocardial contractility after CABG.

8. **Is CABG helpful in patients with congestive heart failure (CHF)?**
Possibly. CABG improves CHF symptoms that are related to ischemic myocardial dysfunction. Conversely, if heart failure is secondary to long-standing irreversibly infarcted muscle (i.e., scar), CABG does not prove beneficial. The critical preoperative evaluation must assess the viability of dysfunctional myocardium. A rest-redistribution thallium scan can determine the segments of myocardium that are still viable; however, cardiac magnetic resonance imaging (MRI) is supplanting radionuclide imaging as a better test to detect hibernating myocardium.

9. **Is CABG valuable in preventing ventricular arrhythmias?**
No. Most ventricular arrhythmias in patients with CAD originate from the border of irritable myocardium that surrounds infarcted muscle. Implantation of an automated implantable cardiac defibrillator is indicated for patients with life-threatening ventricular tachyarrhythmias.

10. **What is the difference between PCI and CABG?**
Several randomized, controlled clinical trials have compared PCI with CABG. Although collectively they analyzed data from several thousand patients, the vast majority (>80%) of patients who originally

met inclusion criteria were excluded from participation for a variety of reasons. It is important to understand that although randomized controlled trials are the gold standard for comparison between two therapies, a significant criticism of these CABG versus PCI trials includes the relatively low risk of the populations studied, which may not be reflective of real-world patients who undergo either CABG or PCI (see Controversies).

Several important features emerged from these trials. Overall mortality and adverse cardiac event (MI) rates were no different for CABG and PCI. One study, the Bypass Angioplasty Revascularization Investigation (BARI) study showed a clinically relevant higher survival in type 2 diabetics undergoing CAB than those diabetics who had PCI. This differential survival persisted for 10 years of follow-up.

The major difference between the two treatment strategies was freedom from angina and reintervention. Overall, 40% of patients treated with percutaneous transluminal coronary angioplasty (PTCA) required repeat PTCA or CABG, whereas roughly 5% of patients treated with CABG required reintervention. The patients who underwent CABG also experienced fewer episodes of angina compared with the patients treated with PTCA.

The more recent trials comparing drug-eluting stents (DES) versus CABG do establish a much lower rate of restenosis with DES—roughly 8%–10%. However, DES have been associated with catastrophic thrombosis—occurring suddenly and without antecedent clinical signs—months to even years after placement. The thrombosis of these stents is much more likely to cause sudden death, or a substantial MI than restenosis seen by bare metal stents (BMS). Because of this propensity toward thrombosis with DES, patients are committed to dual antiplatelet therapy (both acetylsalicylic acid and clopidogrel) for a minimum of 1 year, and many patients with DES in place are now being continued on dual antiplatelet therapy indefinitely.

The unavoidable conclusion is that the recommendation of PCI or CABG should be individualized for each patient. The two therapies should not be viewed as exclusionary or competitive; some patients may benefit from a combination of PCI and CABG. CABG results in a more durable revascularization, although with the inherent risk of perioperative complications.

11. **What is the rule of thumb for vessel patency?**
Internal mammary graft: 90% patency at 10 years
Saphenous vein graft: 50% patency at 10 years
PCI with BMS of stenotic vessel: 80% patency at 1 year

12. **What operative and technical problems are associated with CABG?**
The operative complications broadly include technical problems with the bypass graft anastomosis, sternal complications, and incisional complications associated with the saphenous vein harvest incision. Technical problems with the coronary artery anastomosis usually lead to MI. Sternal complications predictably result in sepsis and multiple organ failure. Incisions for saphenous vein harvest also may result in problems with edema, infection, and pain postoperatively.

13. **What are the risks of CABG? Which comorbid factors increase the operative risk for CABG? Why are large databases useful for the reporting of data?**
Estimating operative risk is a critical component of counseling patients before surgical revascularization. The Society of Thoracic Surgeons (STS) and the Veterans' Administration have developed and promoted two large national databases. The STS database now includes outcomes on over 2 million patients and represents the largest cardiothoracic outcomes and quality improvement program in the world. Factors that increase the risk of CABG include depressed left ventricular EF, previous cardiac surgery, priority of operation (emergency versus elective), New York Heart Association Classification, age, peripheral vascular disease, chronic obstructive pulmonary disease, and decompensated heart failure at the time of surgery. These comorbidities figure prominently in outcome. Quite simply, raw mortality data for CABG can be misleading. Different surgeons can perform identical operations but have different raw mortality rates if one surgeon operates on young triathletes with CAD and the other surgeon operates on old couch potatoes who smoke two packs of cigarettes per day. Through assessment of these comorbid factors, a fairer representation of predicted to observed outcome can be determined. In this manner, using observed to expected outcomes with risk-adjusted models represents a more honest comparison of CABG mortality rates. As both the public and payers of healthcare demand transparency in outcomes, the STS database serves as a model for all other specialties to appropriately collect and risk-adjust data for quality improvement.

14. **What steps are taken if a patient cannot be weaned from CPB?**
The surgeon is in fact treating shock. As in hypovolemic shock (e.g., a bullet transecting the aorta), the basic principles include the following:
    - Volume resuscitation until left-sided and right-sided filling pressures are optimized.
    - When filling pressures are adequate, initiation of inotropic support.
    - Push inotropic support to toxicity (usually ventricular tachyarrhythmias) and insert an intraaortic balloon pump. The ultimate extension of CPB includes the placement of an LV or right ventricular assist device (or both). These devices can support the circulation while allowing for myocardial recovery.

CONTROVERSIES

15. **Is there an advantage to surgical revascularization with all arterial conduits?**
Probably; however, the data are much less strong than the data supporting the clear advantage of a LIMA to LAD bypass over a vein graft to LAD bypass. The logical extension of the observation that an internal mammary artery has superior patency to a saphenous vein has sparked an interest in total arterial revascularization. Instead of using saphenous veins as bypass conduits, some surgeons also use the right internal mammary artery, the gastroepiploic artery, and the radial artery as bypass conduits instead of vein. Convincing data suggest a survival benefit and freedom from angina when the LIM artery is used as a conduit. The data supporting total arterial revascularization are much less clear.

16. **What are the options for a patient with continued angina who is deemed not suitable for CABG?**
For patients on optimized medical treatment who are not surgical candidates (because of prohibitive comorbidities or poor quality coronary artery targets for bypass), an alternative is a procedure called transmyocardial revascularization (TMR). TMR uses a laser to burn small holes from the endocardium to the epicardium. Although it was originally believed that the laser brought blood from the endocardial capillary network to the myocardium, it has been repeatedly observed that laser-created channels are filled with thrombus within 24 hours and subsequently occluded. Therefore, it is postulated that the laser energy invokes an inflammatory response with a resultant increase in angiogenic factors (vascular endothelial growth factor, tumor growth factor β, and fibroblast growth factor). Although promising experimental data and clinical trials support TMR as therapeutic, one wonders if a placebo effect is not operative in promoting anginal relief.

17. **What therapy should I offer to a 65-year-old male with diabetes mellitus, stable lifestyle limiting angina, multivessel coronary artery disease (no proximal left anterior descending involvement), and normal ventricular function (EF = 65%)?**
This type of patient explores the debate and interface between three options: (1) continued medical therapy, (2) multivessel PCI, and (3) CABG. A persuasive argument can be made for each therapy, although as surgeons, we would offer this patient a CABG. The key to appropriate decision making for this patient includes a multidisciplinary team of physicians, including cardiologists, and cardiac surgeons to fully inform the patient of his options and the expected benefits, outcomes, and long-term issues with each line of therapy. The decision to undergo multivessel PCI while this patient is on the catheterization table because the problem can be fixed at this moment without a big operation leaves this patient without a fair chance to be adequately counseled and informed of his options. In discussion with this patient, highlight that although CABG represents the most invasive therapy for his CAD, it offers him the most durable long-term treatment of his disease with a small upfront risk of mortality or morbidity and a relatively short (weeks to months) recovery period.

KEY POINTS: CORONARY ARTERY DISEASE

1. Hibernating myocardium is improved by CABG.
2. CABG is not helpful in preventing ventricular arrhythmias.
3. The rule of thumb for vessel patency is 90% patency at 10 years for the internal mammary graft, 50% patency at 10 years for saphenous vein grafts, and 90% patency at 1 year for PCI of stenotic vessel with a BMS.

BIBLIOGRAPHY

1. Cleveland Jr JC, Shroyer AL. Off-pump coronary artery bypass grafting decreases risk-adjusted mortality and morbidity. *Ann Thorac Surg.* 2001;72(4):1282–1288.
2. Fihn SD, Blankenship JC, Alexander KP, et al. 2014 ACC/AHA/AATS/PCNA/SCAI/STS focused update of the guideline for the diagnosis and management of patients with stable ischemic heart disease: a report of the American College of Cardiology/American Heart Association Task Force on Practice Guidelines, and the American Association for Thoracic Surgery, Preventive Cardiovascular Nurses Association, Society for Cardiovascular Angiography and Interventions, and Society of Thoracic Surgeons. *J Am Coll Cardiol.* 2014;64(18):1929–1949.
3. Gundry SR, Romano MA. Seven-year follow-up of coronary artery bypasses performed with and without cardiopulmonary bypass. *J Thorac Cardiovasc Surg.* 1998;115(6):1273–1277.
4. Hannan EL, Racz MJ, Walford G, et al. Long-term outcomes of coronary-artery bypass grafting versus stent implantation. *N Engl J Med.* 2005;352(21):2174–2183.
5. Horvath KA, Aranki SF. Sustained angina relief 5 years after transmyocardial laser revascularization with a CO_2 laser. *Circulation.* 2001;104(12 suppl 1):I81–I84.
6. Taggart DP. Coronary artery bypass grafting is still the best treatment for multivessel and left main disease, but patients need to know. *Ann Thorac Surg.* 2006;82(6):1966–1975.
7. BARI Investigators. The final 10-year follow-up: results from the BARI randomized trial. *J Am Coll Cardiology.* 2007;49(15):1600–1606.
8. Serruys PW, Morice MC, Kappetein AP, et al. Percutaneous coronary intervention versus coronary artery bypass grafting for severe coronary artery disease. *N Engl J Med.* 2009;360(10):961–972.
9. Alexander JH, Smith PK. Coronary artery bypass grafting. *N Engl J Med.* 2016;374(20):1954–1964.

CHAPTER 79

MITRAL STENOSIS

Giorgio Zanotti, MD, John M. Swanson, MD, David A. Fullerton, MD

1. **What is the most common cause of mitral valve stenosis in adults?**
   Rheumatic fever. This usually occurs in early childhood, and many patients do not recall their illness.

2. **Which gender is most commonly affected?**
   Women, by a ratio of 2:1.

3. **What is the main symptom of mitral valve stenosis?**
   Dyspnea on exertion.

4. **What are the physical examination findings associated with mitral valve stenosis?**
   On auscultation, an opening snap and a diastolic murmur best heard at the apex.

5. **How is the diagnosis confirmed?**
   Echocardiography: Transesophageal echocardiography is most accurate (but not always necessary).

6. **What is the normal cross-sectional area of the mitral valve orifice?**
   - Normal is 4–6 cm^2
   - Mild mitral stenosis is <2 cm^2
   - Severe mitral stenosis is <1 cm^2

7. **What is the Gorlin formula?**
   A formula used to calculate the area of a heart valve. In simplified terms:
   Mitral valve area = cardiac output (CO) $\div$ $\sqrt{}$mean pressure gradient across the valve

8. **How is the mitral valve area determined by echocardiogram?**
   By measuring the blood flow velocity across the valve with Doppler ultrasound, and measuring the time required for the flow velocity to decline (referred to as the pressure half-time). In simplified terms:
   Mitral valve area = 220 $\div$ pressure half-time

9. **What is the pathophysiology of mitral stenosis?**
   Mitral valve stenosis occurs when the valve does not open as wide as it should. This creates an increase in left atrial pressure, which is then transmitted retrograde into the pulmonary circulation causing increased pulmonary vein/capillary pressure. This causes dyspnea and, if the pressure is high enough, pulmonary edema.
   Example: To maintain adequate left ventricular filling across a 1.5-cm^2 valve, a pressure gradient of 20 mm Hg is required. With a normal left ventricular end-diastolic pressure of 5 mm Hg, a 20-mm Hg gradient requires a left atrial pressure of 25 mm Hg to allow adequate flow across the narrowed valve. Left atrial pressure rises even further as flow across the valve increases (increased cardiac output during exercise). This high left atrial pressure backs up into the pulmonary veins resulting in pulmonary edema.

10. **What precipitates symptoms in patients with mitral stenosis?**
    The three most common precipitating factors are:
    a. Tachycardia
    b. Atrial fibrillation
    c. Pregnancy
    Blood from the left atrium fills the left ventricle through the mitral valve during diastole. If the valve is narrowed, a longer period of time is required for a given volume of blood to flow through the valve. Likewise, the atrial kick becomes increasingly important to augment flow through the valve. Therefore, anything that shortens diastole (tachycardia) or diminishes the atrial kick (atrial fibrillation) exacerbates symptoms due to inadequate left atrial emptying and left ventricular filling, increased left atrial pressures, and decreased cardiac output.

11. **What complications may result from mitral stenosis?**
    - Hemoptysis, from severe pulmonary venous congestion leading to pulmonary capillary hemorrhage
    - Thromboembolism (stroke, end-organ ischemia) associated with atrial fibrillation
    - Pulmonary hypertension and right-sided heart failure (cor pulmonale)
    - Endocarditis

12. **Why does mitral stenosis cause pulmonary hypertension?**
    - Retrograde transmission of increased left atrial pressure
    - Reflex pulmonary arterial vasoconstriction initiated by left atrial distension (reversible pulmonary hypertension)
    - Hypertrophy of the pulmonary arteries with remodeling of the pulmonary vasculature (this may become irreversible pulmonary hypertension)

13. **What is the medical therapy of mitral valve stenosis?**
    - Diuretics (i.e., furosemide) and dietary salt restriction to improve dyspnea in patients with pulmonary vascular congestion
    - Beta-blockers to slow the heart rate to approximately 60 beats/minute and thereby increase diastolic filling time
    - AV nodal blockers (i.e., digoxin) to slow atrial-ventricular conduction in patients with atrial fibrillation
    - Warfarin (Coumadin) for thromboembolism prophylaxis in patients with atrial fibrillation

14. **Should patients with mitral valve stenosis undergo secondary prevention of rheumatic fever?**
    Yes. Additionally, there should be a low threshold to test and treat these patients for acute group A streptococcal pharyngitis, which may worsen the stenosis.

15. **What is the natural history of mitral valve stenosis?**
    - Progressive congestive heart failure as the valve orifice area decreases.
    - Survival in asymptomatic patients is 80% at 10 years.
    - Survival with moderate mitral stenosis is 50% at 10 years.
    - Survival after symptoms develop is 0%–15% at 10 years.
    - Survival with severe pulmonary hypertension averages <3 years.

16. **What are the interventional options to treat mitral valve stenosis?**
    - Percutaneous mitral balloon valvuloplasty
    - Surgical mitral valve replacement (valve repair is rarely an option because of valve leaflet deformity)
    - Percutaneous mitral valve replacement

17. **What are the indications for intervention in mitral valve stenosis?**
    Since mitral stenosis is a progressively degenerative disorder, its natural history is altered only by interventions including percutaneous balloon valvuloplasty, surgical mitral valve replacement, or percutaneous mitral valve replacements. Indications for specific interventions are as follows:
    - Percutaneous balloon valvuloplasty: (1) Symptomatic patients (NYHA class III-IV) with severe mitral stenosis (valve area <1.5 cm^2) or transvalvular gradient of 5–10 mm Hg; (2) asymptomatic patients with mitral valve area <1 cm^2, transvalvular gradient of >10 mm Hg, or pulmonary artery systolic pressure >50 mm Hg. In any of the above patients, the echo must also demonstrate mobile valve leaflets without evidence of significant mitral valve insufficiency, subvalvular fibrosis, valve thickening, or left atrial thrombus.
    - Surgery (usually mitral valve replacement): Symptomatic patients with severe mitral stenosis who are not at prohibitive risk for surgery, have failed prior percutaneous valvuloplasty, or are not candidates for percutaneous balloon valvuloplasty. Also, patients with severe mitral stenosis undergoing cardiac surgery for other indications.
    - Percutaneous mitral valve replacement: Patients who meet criteria for mitral valve replacement but have prohibitive surgical risk.

18. **What is the initial procedure of choice for mitral stenosis?**
    Percutaneous balloon valvuloplasty if the above criteria are met.

19. What are the results of balloon valvuloplasty?
    - Mortality rate <1%
    - Initial success (mitral valve area >1.5 cm^2 and left atrial pressure <18 mm Hg) can be as high as 95% in properly selected patients, but recurrent stenosis occurs in virtually all patients long term. The need for repeat commissurotomy is 10% at 10 years. The outcomes after repeat procedure may be less favorable than the initial procedure because of increased valve fibrosis and deformity, which ultimately require surgery.

20. Which operations may be done for mitral stenosis?
    - Mitral commissurotomy: Now very rarely done.
    - Mitral valve replacement: Perioperative mortality varies from <5% in young and healthy patients to >10% in older individuals with multiple comorbidities and heart failure. An approximate and individualized risk for perioperative morbidity and mortality may be estimated by calculating the Society of Thoracic Surgeons risk score.

BONUS QUESTION

21. What is the Lutembacher syndrome?
    Mitral stenosis associated with an atrial septal defect. This results in a left-to-right shunt and over-works the right ventricle.

KEY POINTS: MITRAL STENOSIS

1. Rheumatic fever is the leading cause of mitral stenosis.
2. A mitral valve area of <1 cm^2 is considered severe mitral stenosis.
3. The main symptom of mitral stenosis is dyspnea on exertion.
4. Medical management of mitral stenosis is primarily diuretics and beta-blockers.
5. The treatment of choice for symptomatic, severe mitral stenosis is balloon mitral valvuloplasty.

BIBLIOGRAPHY

1. Nishimura RA, Otto CM, Bonow RO, et al. 2014 AHA/ACC Guideline for the management of patients with valvular heart disease: executive summary: a report of the American College of Cardiology/American Heart Association Task Force on Practice Guidelines. *Circulation.* 2014;129(23):2440–2492.
2. Yanagawa B, Butany J. Update on rheumatic heart disease. *Curr Opin Cardiol.* 2016;31(2):162–168.
3. Zeng YI, Sun R. Pathophysiology of valvular heart disease. *Exp Ther Med.* 2016;11(4):1184–1188.
4. Nishimura RA, Vahanian A. Mitral valve disease–current management and future challenges. *Lancet.* 2016;387(10025):1324–1334.

CHAPTER 80

MITRAL REGURGITATION

Giorgio Zanotti, MD, John M. Swanson, MD, David A. Fullerton, MD

1. **What are the causes of mitral regurgitation?**
   a. (Primary) degenerative mitral regurgitation is due to an abnormality of the mitral valve annulus, leaflets, or chordae tendineae. Principal causes include:
      - Mitral valve prolapse
      - Valvular degeneration
      - Annular calcification
      - Rheumatic fever
      - Endocarditis
      - Ruptured chordae tendineae
      - Ruptured papillary muscle
   b. (Secondary) functional mitral regurgitation is due to an abnormality of the left ventricle causing valvular distraction and leak despite structurally intact valve. Principal causes include:
      - Cardiomyopathy
      - Myocardial/papillary muscle ischemia
      - Myocardial infarction

2. **What is the pathophysiology of mitral regurgitation?**
   In a healthy heart, the mitral valve prevents retrograde flow between the left ventricle into the left atrium during systole. However, with mitral regurgitation each ventricular contraction ejects blood via two routes: (1) antegrade, through the aortic valve and (2) retrograde, through the mitral valve. The percentage of each stroke volume inappropriately ejected retrograde into the left atrium is termed the *regurgitant fraction*. The regurgitant fraction joins blood returning from the pulmonary veins causing increased left atrial pressures, which are transmitted back into the left ventricle during diastolic filling. In order to compensate for the regurgitant fraction and maintain cardiac output, the left ventricle must increase the total stroke volume. This produces left ventricular volume overload, dilation, dysfunction, and possibly arrhythmias.

3. **What are the symptoms of mitral regurgitation?**
   Most people are asymptomatic until there is severe regurgitation. When this occurs, people exhibit symptoms of heart failure, including dyspnea on exertion, loss of exercise tolerance, fatigue, and eventually increased peripheral edema.

4. **What murmur is associated with mitral regurgitation?**
   A holosystolic murmur, which is best heard at the precordium with radiation to the left axilla.

5. **What determines left atrial pressure in mitral regurgitation?**
   The compliance of the left atrium.

6. **Why does acute mitral regurgitation cause severe symptoms?**
   With acute mitral regurgitation, the normal-sized left atrium has little time to remodel and increase compliance. Hence, the increase in left atrial volume from the regurgitant fraction causes the left atrial pressure to increases rapidly. This increases the hydrostatic pressure in the pulmonary veins causing pulmonary edema. Conversely, chronic mitral regurgitation is associated with progressive dilation of the left atrium, allowing sufficient time for atrial remodeling and a gradual increase in left atrial compliance. This increased compliance blunts the rise in left atrial pressure.

7. **What hemodynamic conditions exacerbate mitral regurgitation?**
   Increased left ventricular afterload (hypertension). Elevated systemic arterial blood pressure increases the impedance against which the left ventricle must pump. This increases the regurgitant fraction (blood preferentially flows backward into the lower pressure left atrium rather than forward into the high pressure systemic circuit).

8. **What is the best test to confirm the diagnosis and grade the severity of mitral regurgitation?**

By Doppler echocardiography, especially transesophageal echocardiography (TEE) (the esophagus lies directly behind the left atrium, providing excellent echo images of the mitral valve). Echocardiography also allows determination of the cause (degenerative or functional) and severity of mitral regurgitation. It further allows determination of the ability to surgically repair the valve.

9. **What is the medical therapy for mitral regurgitation?**
   - Diuretics (i.e., furosemide) and dietary salt restriction to lower the left ventricular preload and reduce pulmonary vascular congestion
   - ACE inhibitors (i.e., lisinopril) to reduce afterload
   - AV nodal blockers (i.e., digoxin) for ventricular rate control in atrial fibrillation
   - Warfarin (Coumadin) for thromboembolism prophylaxis in patients with atrial fibrillation

10. **What are the indications for surgery in patients with mitral regurgitation?**
   - Symptomatic patients with severe mitral regurgitation and left ventricular ejection fraction (LVEF) >30%
   - Asymptomatic patients with severe mitral regurgitation and LVEF 30%–60% and/or end diastolic left ventricular volume >40 mm
   - Deteriorating left ventricular systolic function. Because mitral regurgitation lowers the total impedance of left ventricular ejection (much of each stroke volume escapes via the low resistance mitral valvular "back door"), the LVEF should be greater than normal in the presence of mitral regurgitation in order to maintain cardiac output. An LVEF <55% in the presence of mitral regurgitation suggests left ventricular dysfunction.
   - Pulmonary hypertension (mean pulmonary artery pressure ≥25) at rest or induced by exercise

11. **How is mitral regurgitation corrected?**

By surgery.
   - Mitral valve repair is the preferred surgical procedure. This preserves the mitral apparatus, maintaining the continuity between the left ventricular muscle and the mitral annulus via the chordae tendineae. Loss of this continuity by resection of the apparatus during mitral valve replacement places the left ventricle at a mechanical disadvantage leading to left ventricular dilatation and dysfunction over time.
   - Surgical mitral valve replacement with a prosthetic valve is performed when repair is not possible. If replacement is necessary, efforts should be made to preserve the posterior leaflet of the mitral valve. In most series, mitral valve replacement is required in <30% of cases.
   - Percutaneous mitral valve repair (using a mitral clip device) is an option in patients with prohibitive surgical risk who have functional mitral regurgitation. Indication for such procedure must be determined by a multidisciplinary heart valve team including cardiologists and cardiac surgeons experienced in the management of valvular heart disease.

12. **Why is it preferable to repair rather than replace the mitral valve?**
   - Lower operative mortality
   - Better long-term left ventricular function
   - Avoids valve-related complications (biologic valve degeneration requiring reoperation, prosthetic valve-related thromboembolism, and prosthetic valve associated endocarditis)

13. **How is the mitral valve surgically repaired?**
   a. The redundant portion(s) of the valve leaflet(s) is resected.
   b. The leaflet is reapproximated.
   c. The mitral annulus is plicated and reinforced with a prosthetic annuloplasty ring.
   d. The annuloplasty ring is sewn around the perimeter of the annulus on the left atrial side of the valve. In so doing, the mitral leaflets are supported by competent chordae tendineae and the circumference of the mitral annulus is decreased, which aids in coaptation. Competency of the repaired valve is assessed intraoperatively using TEE.

14. **What is the operative mortality of mitral valve repair versus mitral valve replacement?**

Repair: 2%
Replacement: 5%

15. How durable are mitral valve repairs?

The risk of requiring another mitral valve operation is approximately 1% per year.

16. What is the role of minimally invasive surgery in patients with mitral regurgitation?

Minimally invasive approaches (i.e., mini-sternotomy, mini-thoracotomy, robotically assisted mitral valve surgery) can be applied to many patients undergoing either mitral valve repair or replacement. These techniques may provide for a decrease in perioperative bleeding and postoperative pain, faster functional recovery, and preserved lung function. Minimally invasive approaches are also advantageous in patients with previous sternotomy, avoiding sternal reentry, and pericardial adhesions. The robotic approach may be particularly useful in facilitating repair of the mitral valve for myxomatous degeneration.

BONUS QUESTION

17. What is systolic anterior motion (SAM) of the mitral valve?

SAM may occur as a consequence of mitral valve repair. After mitral valve repair, the anterior leaflet of the mitral valve may billow into the left ventricular outflow tract during systole, creating two problems: (1) dynamic left ventricular outflow tract obstruction and (2) mitral regurgitation (anterior displacement of the anterior leaflet causes it to be foreshortened). SAM is diagnosed by echocardiography. It is exacerbated by an increased contractile state of the myocardium, so inotropic agents should be avoided. Patients with SAM are treated by volume-loading and beta-blocking agents. If these measures fail, the valve should be replaced. Occurrence of SAM may be predicted preoperatively by echocardiographic assessment and therefore must be prevented by choosing an appropriate repair technique.

Known risk factors for SAM include:
a. Small left ventricle (diameter <45 mm)
b. Large anterior leaflet
c. Anterior/posterior leaflet ratio <1
d. Narrow angle between aortic and mitral valve on two chamber echo view (aorto-mitral angle < 120 degrees)
e. Preoperative SAM

KEY POINTS: MITRAL REGURGITATION

1. The symptoms are dyspnea on exertion and loss of exercise tolerance.
2. The murmur of mitral regurgitation is a holosystolic murmur heard best at the apex with radiation to the left axilla.
3. Mitral regurgitation may be classified as either degenerative or functional.
4. The principal indications for surgery are symptoms despite medical therapy and/or deteriorating left ventricular function (echocardiography).
5. Mitral valve repair is preferable to replacement because of lower operative mortality rates, less risk of thromboembolism, less risk of endocarditis, better long-term left ventricular function, and less need (if any) for chronic anticoagulation.

BIBLIOGRAPHY

1. Nishimura RA, Otto CM, Bonow RO, et al. 2014 AHA/ACC Guideline for the management of patients with valvular heart disease: executive summary: a report of the American College of Cardiology/American Heart Association Task Force on practice guidelines. *Circulation*. 2014;129(23):2440–2492.
2. Yanagawa B, Butany J, Verma S. Update on rheumatic heart disease. *Curr Opin Cardiol*. 2016;31(2):162–168.
3. Zeng YI, Sun R. Pathophysiology of valvular heart disease. *Exp Ther Med*. 2016;11(4):1184–1188.
4. Nishimura RA, Vahanian A. Mitral valve disease-current management and future challenges. *Lancet*. 2016;387(10025):1324–1334.

CHAPTER 81

AORTIC VALVE DISEASE

Elizabeth E. Brown, BA, James M. Brown, MD

1. **What does aortic valve disease mean?**
   Aortic valve disease most often refers to obstruction of the aortic valve, aortic stenosis, or an aortic valve leak known as aortic regurgitation or aortic insufficiency. The vast majority of aortic valve disease is an adult-acquired condition with aortic stenosis predominant. However, because the aortic valve is anatomically integrated with the heart and the sinuses of Valsalva, many conditions including congenital diseases can affect the function of the aortic valve. For example, an aortic aneurysm that stretches the aortic valve attachments can cause aortic valve regurgitation. Hypertrophic muscle below the aortic valve can cause so-called subvalvular aortic stenosis.

2. **What is aortic stenosis?**
   Aortic stenosis is typically an acquired narrowing of the aortic valve from valve leaflet calcification of uncertain etiology. However, the pathobiology mimics atherosclerosis regarding inflammatory cell and mediator activation and occurs with increasing frequency over the age of 70. In people over the age of 80, 4% of the population has moderate to severe aortic stenosis. Furthermore, 2% of the population is born with a bicuspid aortic valve (BAV). BAVs are at higher risk to calcify or become regurgitant. Up to 40% of patients with BAV will develop aortic valve disease with a peak incidence between the ages of 45 and 55. Aortic stenosis accounts for 3% of congenital heart defects. This creates an urgent neonatal health problem when severe.

3. **What are the symptoms of aortic stenosis?**
   In adults, the development of angina, syncope, or dyspnea on exertion, and congestive heart failure portends a poor prognosis unless valve replacement is performed. In the setting of severe aortic stenosis with symptoms, mortality is as high as 80% by 2 years. It is critical to know that up to 50% of patients with severe aortic stenosis underreport their symptoms. If an echocardiogram indicates severe aortic stenosis in patients, more than half may truly be symptomatic when given a stress test using a treadmill. Therefore it is critical to perform a careful history in aortic stenosis patients.

4. **How can a patient with aortic stenosis and normal coronary arteries get angina?**
   Angina occurs because of oxygen supply imbalance in the myocardium. Normally, myocardial blood flow can autoregulate to dramatically increase coronary flow and maintain blood supply.
   In aortic stenosis the myocardium has thickened or hypertrophied. When this occurs, the endocardium becomes more dependent on diastole for blood flow. Add to this the delayed systolic ejection phase of a patient with aortic stenosis, even minor exertion, or an increase in heart rate. This scenario will sacrifice time in diastole and the supply demand balance is broken. The patient will have angina.

5. **What is the expected survival of a patient with untreated aortic stenosis?**
   If the patient has developed symptoms, the mortality from aortic stenosis with medical management is as high as 80% at 2 years. Therefore intervention to replace the valve is usually recommended. Patients with aortic stenosis are at risk for sudden death, often prompted by an increase in heart rate or drop in systemic vascular resistance when, for example, they receive a dose of sedating medicine for a hernia repair when a murmur was not appreciated. Therefore listen for the murmur! It can be lifesaving.

6. **What are the physical findings of aortic stenosis?**
   The murmur of aortic stenosis is a systolic crescendo-decrescendo (diamond shaped) harsh quality murmur radiating to the neck. This can make distinguishing a carotid bruit difficult because the murmur of aortic stenosis is loud. The patient will often have diminished peripheral pulses with a delayed pulse upstroke (call it *pulsus parvus et tardus* if you want to shine on medicine rounds).

7. **For extra credit, what hematologic or bleeding disorders occur in patients with severe aortic stenosis?**
   Impaired platelet function and decreased levels of von Willebrand factor (VWF) occur in patients with severe aortic stenosis. This happens because turbulence of blood passing through the stenotic

valve causes deformation of VWF, causing it to open, and thus makes it vulnerable to metabolism and inactivity. This acquired VWF deficiency or vWD-2A is associated with epistaxis, ecchymoses in 20% of patients, and gastrointestinal bleeding from angiodysplasia in the gastrointestinal track. This is called Hyde's syndrome, which was described in 1958, and occurs in 1% of patients with aortic stenosis. It can be cured by aortic valve replacement.

8. **What are the typical findings of aortic stenosis on chest x-ray (CXR) and electrocardiogram (EKG)?**
   Both chest radiographs and EKG may show normal results even with severe aortic stenosis; thus, these are not good screening tests. On CXR, calcification of the aortic valve and an enlarged cardiac silhouette may be seen. EKG is sensitive in detecting left ventricular hypertrophy and may also reveal conduction defects such as P-R interval prolongation (these occur secondary to extension of valvular calcification into the adjacent conduction tissue). Elderly patients with aortic stenosis are at risk for poor sinus node function and aortic valve node conduction delays.

9. **How is aortic stenosis diagnosed?**
   The mainstays of diagnosis are the history, physical findings, and echocardiogram. Echocardiography is nearly 100% accurate in diagnosing hemodynamically significant aortic stenosis. By measuring the velocity of blood flow and cross-sectional area before and at the aortic valve, the valve area can be calculated using the continuity equation. An aortic valve area of <1 cm^2 is considered severe. Note that a normal aortic valve area is 3–4 cm^2.

Aortic Valve Area

Normal	3–4 cm^2
Severe	<1 cm^2

Velocity measurements can be converted to a gradient using the **Bernoulli equation**, where gradient = $4v^2$. A mean gradient over 40 mm Hg or a velocity of 4 m/s indicates severe aortic stenosis. If there is confusion over the diagnosis after echocardiography then a left heart catheterization can be performed. Pressure transducing catheters can be passed into both the aorta and ventricle and used to assess the gradient and calculate the valve area using the **Gorlin formula:**

$$\frac{\text{Cardiac Output (mL/sec)}}{44.5 \times \sqrt{\text{mean valve gradient}}}$$

10. **Is a cardiac catheterization necessary?**
    Yes, if the patient has a diagnosis of severe or symptomatic aortic stenosis, is over the age of 45, or has risk factors for coronary artery disease. Knowing if there are any coronary artery stenoses of over 50% is important for planning safe valve replacement.

11. **When is aortic valve replacement indicated?**
    Patients with severe aortic stenosis with symptoms should have their aortic valve replaced if they do not have terminal cancer or they are not so frail that their life expectancy is fewer than 2 years. Even between the ages of 90 and 95 the results of aortic valve replacement are good and result in return of survival to normal-for-age and return of quality of life to near normal. Patients who do not report symptoms, but who have either severe calcification or high velocity across the valve by echocardiography likely have diminished survival and an indication for aortic valve replacement. Patients not reporting symptoms, but who have decreased or decreasing ventricular function (ejection fraction <50%) should undergo valve replacement. Furthermore, if the patient is having cardiac surgery for another reason, such as coronary artery disease, then aortic valve replacement is indicated if the aortic valve is moderately or severely stenosed.

12. **What preoperative orders, tests, or procedures are important before valve replacement?**
    As in the preoperative phase of most conditions, the evaluation of the patient should be comprehensive and system based. Left-heart cardiac catheterization, labs including hematologic studies, electrolytes, creatinine, and liver function should be routine. In cases of uncertain aortic anatomy, gated computed axial tomography (CT) scan should be done. The CT scan will be necessary for a patient being considered for transcatheter aortic valve replacement (TAVR). Carotid duplex scanning to

rule out significant carotid stenosis and a peripheral pulse exam to complete the vascular workup are routine. Furthermore, a patient about to receive implantation of a valve prosthesis should be examined by a dentist for the absence of an infected tooth or a tooth at risk for infection. This is because the human mouth harbors dangerous pathogens (e.g., *strep viridans*), which can seed an implanted heart valve and create a life-threatening problem.

13. **What aortic valve types are available to use for replacement?**
    Prosthetic aortic valves are either mechanical or bioprosthetic. Mechanical valves are made of pyrolytic carbon and titanium and require use of daily Coumadin for life. There is an obligate risk of serious anticoagulant-related complications of 1% per patient per year. As such, the majority of aortic valve implants in the last 10 years have been porcine or bovine bioprosthetic valves. These tissues are mounted on a stent mimicking the aortic valves' native anatomy and fixed with a sewing ring to facilitate sutured implantation. A recent development has been TAVR. TAVR valves are bioprosthetic tissue mounted on an expandable stent made of nitinol, cobalt, or steel.

14. **What are the potential approaches for aortic valve replacement?**
    With the advent of TAVR, there is a new option that offers a transcatheter minimally invasive approach. At present, there is enough evidence to suggest that a transcatheter approach can be taken in situations in which the patient is not a candidate for surgical aortic valve replacement or the patient's predicted mortality from surgery is more than 8%. TAVR valves can be delivered via the femoral artery, left ventricular (LV) apex, axillary artery, or directly via the aorta.

    Otherwise, surgical aortic valve replacement can be performed via a standard median sternotomy, a minimally invasive partial sternotomy, or a minimally invasive anterior thoracotomy approach.

15. **What is the mortality rate, complication rate, and benefit for surgical aortic valve replacement?**
    Over the last 15 years, mortality and complication for aortic valve replacement has dropped dramatically. For a healthy 50-year-old, the predicted 30-day mortality risk from the Society of Thoracic Surgeons is 0.5%, and the stroke risk is 0.4%. However, real-world patients are not always completely healthy, so their risk is slightly higher. For example, if the 50-year-old was a smoking hypertensive diabetic with a prior stroke, the risk would be much higher. By contrast, an 85-year-old male with hypertension, mild renal insufficiency, and mild chronic obstructive pulmonary disease would have a mortality risk of 4.3% and a stroke risk of 2.3%. Age and added medical comorbidities make risk of aortic valve replacement higher. Nonetheless, the octogenarian mentioned above would have a full return to predicted life expectancy as well as age-matched quality of life after surgical aortic valve replacement.

16. **What is the mortality rate, the complication rate, and benefit of TAVR?**
    So far the trials comparing TAVR to surgery or TAVR to best medical therapy have shown either:
    a. TAVR noninferiority to surgery or
    b. A survival advantage for TAVR when compared to medical therapy only at 1- and 2-year follow-up
    Mortality from TAVR has ranged from 3.4% to 6%, major stroke rates from 2.9% to 5.0%, vascular complications from 10% to 20%, and major paravalvular leak from 4% to 10%. The presence of stroke or vascular complications increases mortality risk a minimum of threefold in short-term follow up.

    Studies on stroke after TAVR using diffusion-weighted MRI have shown a rate of new brain lesions of 80% compared to less than half that number after open surgery. Clearly, diffusion-weighted MRI is a very sensitive test because a minority of positive findings translate into clinical stroke.

    Recent data from the PARTNER II trial in intermediate-risk patients demonstrate that the newer versions of the transcatheter technology are associated with improved outcomes regarding death, stroke, vascular complications, and perivalvular leak. Strangely, the stroke rate in the surgical group in recent studies has been 6.0%, which is high, compared to historical surgical stroke rates and current national averages.

    Still, the prospective randomized evidence to date suggests noninferiority of TAVR compared to standard surgical treatment. Furthermore, the benefit of TAVR is the rapid mobilization of the patient after the procedure and early discharge from the hospital. Finally, TAVR is a transformative technology. Further trial outcomes comparing TAVR to surgery for low-risk patients are pending.

17. **How common is aortic valve regurgitation?**
    Moderate to severe aortic regurgitation (or aortic insufficiency) affects 1% of the population and males more often than females, reflecting the predominance of males born with BAVs. Of replaced aortic valves, 10% are replaced for aortic regurgitation. Aortic regurgitation of any amount is common in the United States population, with an incidence of 10%.

18. **How deadly is aortic regurgitation?**

    Aortic regurgitation is less deadly than severe aortic stenosis, at least acutely, and here there is a rub, so beware. Once moderate to severe aortic regurgitation with or without symptoms is diagnosed, the 10-year survival can be as low as 50%. A patient's ventricular function can diminish silently. If this happens, the heart function may not recover after aortic valve surgery. Therefore the patient needs careful consistent follow-up with echocardiograms. Aortic regurgitation can cause sudden death, but much less commonly than aortic stenosis.

19. **What causes aortic valve regurgitation?**

    The aortic valve is housed and suspended within the aortic sinuses or aortic root and functions like a suspension bridge. The necessary components for the aortic valve to remain competent are as follows:
    a. The annulus
    b. The sinotubular junction, where the aorta meets the aortic root or sinuses of Valsalva
    c. The valve leaflets

    Any disease that alters any of the above structures can result in aortic insufficiency or aortic regurgitation. For example, any enlargement of the aorta at the sinotubular junction can cause aortic regurgitation. Also, any deficit or surplus of valve leaflet tissue can cause aortic regurgitation. Worldwide, rheumatic heart disease is the leading cause of aortic regurgitation. In the United States, congenital valve anatomy likely accounts for the majority of aortic insufficiency. In the 2% of population born with a BAV, 15% will develop aortic regurgitation. Other causes of aortic regurgitation include infective valvular endocarditis, aortic dissection, connective tissue disease (e.g., Marfan's and Ehlers-Danlos syndromes), aortitis (syphilitic or giant cell), iatrogenic (after aortic balloon valvotomy), and aortic cusp prolapse associated with ventricular septal defects.

20. **How does the pathophysiology of aortic regurgitation differ from aortic stenosis?**

    While aortic stenosis is a pressure overload problem, aortic regurgitation is a volume overload problem. The ventricle responds by eccentric hypertrophy and becomes both thicker and larger. In the compensated state, aortic regurgitation is both a volume and pressure overload stress for the left ventricle. While the hypertrophied heart in aortic stenosis undergoes concentric hypertrophy and maintains size overall, the left ventricle in aortic regurgitation can become extremely large.

21. **What physical findings suggest aortic regurgitation?**

    The physical examination of a patient with aortic regurgitation is a classic part of the history of medicine. The patient's pulse is characterized by a rapid rise and fall of the arterial pulse (a "water-hammer pulse"). The diastolic blood pressure can be low in severe cases, with a widened pulse pressure. These patients exhibit a soft diastolic murmur as opposed to aortic stenosis patients who exhibit a systolic ejection murmur. Maneuvers that increase afterload may accentuate the murmur. Other physical exam findings are listed below:
    - **Quincke sign:** Visible pulsations of the fingernail bed
    - **Corrigan pulse** (water-hammer pulse): Abrupt distention and quick collapse on palpation of the peripheral arterial pulse
    - **Traube sign** ("pistol-shot" pulse): Booming systolic and diastolic sounds auscultated over the femoral artery
    - **de Musset sign:** Bobbing motion of the patient's head with each heartbeat
    - **Hill sign:** Popliteal cuff systolic blood pressure 40 mm Hg higher than brachial cuff systolic blood pressure
    - **Duroziez sign:** Systolic murmur over the femoral artery with proximal compression of the artery and diastolic murmur over the femoral artery with distal compression of the artery
    - **Müller sign:** Systolic pulsations of the uvula
    - **Becker sign:** Systolic pulsations of the retinal arterioles

22. **How is the diagnosis of aortic insufficiency confirmed?**

    As with aortic stenosis following thorough history and physical exam, echocardiography is the test of choice. If size of the regurgitant jet is more than half the size of the ventricular outflow at the annulus then aortic insufficiency is graded as severe. Just as important as the grading of aortic insufficiency is the assessment of ventricular function and ventricular volumes. Reduced ventricular function and enlargement of the heart are key findings on echocardiogram, which should prompt intervention or more careful follow-up. The degree of aortic insufficiency can also be graded during cardiac catheterization with contrast injection of the aortic root.

23. **When is an operation indicated for aortic insufficiency?**
This depends on the cause of the aortic insufficiency and whether it is acute or chronic. Aortic insufficiency caused by an ascending aortic dissection is a surgical emergency. Aortic insufficiency secondary to infective endocarditis may also require surgery emergently. Patients with chronic (mild to moderate) aortic insufficiency that does not progress enjoy a near-normal life expectancy. Patients with severe aortic insufficiency require valve surgery before they develop irreversible LV dysfunction. Aortic valve repair or replacement is indicated for a symptomatic patient irrespective of LV function. For asymptomatic patients, aortic valve repair or replacement is indicated in the setting of the following:
    a.   Reduced ventricular function (ejection fraction <50%)
    b.   Increasing ventricular systolic or diastolic volumes (end diastolic dimension >75 mm)
    c.   The need for open heart surgery unrelated to the aortic valve regurgitation

24. **What are the surgical options for aortic valve regurgitation?**
The surgical therapy needs to be directed at the causal pathophysiology. As before, a regurgitant valve can be replaced with either a mechanical or a tissue valve, the tissue option being favored currently. In the setting of pliable noncalcified leaflet aortic valve, repair can be attempted with good success and lower long-term valve-related complications (thromboemboli, stroke, transient ischemic events, or infection) than valve replacement. Furthermore, if a dilated ascending aorta is the cause of aortic insufficiency, then the aorta can be replaced, often with sparing of the native valve and a competent aortic valve created.

KEY POINTS: AORTIC VALVE DISEASE

1. The most common causes of aortic stenosis in adults are calcific (degenerative) disease and a degenerated calcified congenitally BAV.
2. Severe symptomatic aortic stenosis is a lethal disease that can be cured with valve replacement.
3. Aortic stenosis is associated with a harsh, easy to hear systolic ejection murmur, whereas aortic insufficiency is associated with a soft diastolic murmur.
4. Aortic stenosis is prevalent and will become epidemic as the baby-boomer population ages.
5. There are now numerous options for aortic valve replacement including surgical sewn, surgical stented valves performed minimally invasively as well as transcatheter valves placed from the femoral arteries, apex of the heart, the axillary arteries, or directly into the aorta.
6. Patients with aortic stenosis should receive antibiotic prophylaxis before noncardiac surgeries.

WEBSITES

- www.ctsnet.org/
- http://www.sts.org/quality-research-patient-safety/quality/risk-calculator-and-models/risk-calculator
- http://circ.ahajournals.org/content/circulationaha/early/2014/02/27/CIR.0000000000000029.full.pdf
- http://professional.heart.org/professional/GuidelinesStatements/UCM_316885_Guidelines-Statements.jsp
- http://tools.acc.org/TAVRRisk/#!/content/evaluate/
- riskcalc.sts.org

BIBLIOGRAPHY

1. Nishimura RA, Otto CM, Bonow RO, et al. AHA/ACC Guideline for the management of patients with valvular heart disease: executive summary: a report of the American College of Cardiology/American Heart Association Task Force on practice guidelines. *J Am Coll Cardiol*. 2014;63(22):e57–e185.
2. Lindman BR, Bonow RO. Current management of calcific aortic stenosis. *Circ Res*. 2013;113(2):223–237.
3. Carabello BA. Aortic stenosis. *New Engl J Med*. 2002;346(9):677–682.
4. Heyde EC. Gastrointestinal bleeding in aortic stenosis (letter). *N Engl J of Med*. 1958;259(4):196–196.
5. Brown JM, O'Brien SM. Isolated aortic valve replacement in North America comprising 108,687 patients in 10 years: changes in risks, valve types, and outcomes in the Society of Thoracic Surgeons National Database. *J Thorac Cardiovasc Surg*. 2009;137(1):82–90.

6. Bonacchi M, Prifti E. Does ministernotomy improve postoperative outcome in aortic valve operation? A prospective randomized study. *Ann Thorac Surg.* 2002;73(2):460–465.
7. Svensson LG, Adams DH, Bonow RO, et al. Aortic valve and ascending aorta guidelines for management and quality measures: executive 8. Borer JS. Aortic valve replacement for the asymptomatic patient with aortic regurgitation: a new piece of the strategic puzzle. *Circulation.* 2002;106(1):2637–2639.
8. Chaliki HP, Mohty D, Avierinos JF, et al. Outcomes after aortic valve replacement in patients with severe aortic regurgitation and markedly reduced left ventricular function. *Circulation.* 2002;106(21):2687–2693.
9. Lamb HJ, Beyerbacht HP, de Roos A, et al. Left ventricular remodeling early after aortic valve replacement: differential effects on diastolic function in aortic valve stenosis and aortic regurgitation. *J Am Coll Cardiol.* 2002;40(12): 2182–2188.
10. Akins CW, Hilgenberg AD. Results of bioprosthetic versus mechanical aortic valve replacement performed with concomitant coronary artery bypass grafting. *Ann Thorac Surg.* 2002;74(4):1098–1106.
11. Lichtenstein SV, Cheung A, Ye J, et al. Transapical transcatheter aortic valve implantation in humans: initial clinical experience. *Circulation.* 2006;114(6):591–596.
12. Mihaljevic T, Cohn LH. One thousand minimally invasive valve operations: early and late results. *Ann Surg.* 2004;240(3):529–534.
13. McCrindle BW, Blackstone EH, Williams WG, et al. Are outcomes of surgical versus transcatheter balloon valvotomy equivalent in neonatal critical aortic stenosis? *Circulation.* 2001;104(12 suppl 1):I152–I158.
14. Paparella D, David TE. Mid-term results of the Ross procedure. *J Card Surg.* 2001;16(4):338–343.
15. Rankin JS, Hammill MS, Ferguson TB, et al. Determinants of operative mortality in valvular heart surgery. *J Thorac Cardiovasc Surg.* 2006;131(3):547–557.
16. Russo CF, Mazzetti S, Garatti A, et al. Aortic complications after bicuspid aortic valve replacement: long-term results. *Ann Thorac Surg.* 2002;74(5):S1773–S1776.
17. Leon MB, Smith CR, Mack M, et al. Transcatheter aortic-valve implantation for aortic stenosis in patients who cannot undergo surgery. *N Engl J Med.* 2010;363(17):1597–1607.
18. Thourani VH, Kodali S, Makkar RR, et al. Transcatheter aortic valve replacement versus surgical valve replacement in intermediate-risk patients: a propensity score analysis. *Lancet.* 2016;387(10034):2218–2225.
19. Leon MB, Smith CR, Mack MJ, et al. Transcatheter or surgical aortic-valve replacement in intermediate-risk patients. *N Engl J Med.* 2016;374(17):1609–1620.
20. Adams DH, Popma JJ, Reardon MJ, et al. Transcatheter aortic-valve replacement with a self-expanding prosthesis. *N Engl J Med.* 2014;371(10):967–968.
21. Walther T, Simon P, Dewey T, et al. Transapical minimally invasive aortic valve implantation. *Circulation.* 2007;116(suppl 11):I240–I245.
22. Webb JG, Chandavimol M, Thompson C, et al. Percutaneous aortic valve implantation retrograde from the femoral artery. *Circulation.* 2006;113(6):842–850.
23. Webb JG, Pasupati S, Humphries K, et al. Percutaneous transarterial aortic valve replacement in selected high-risk patients with aortic stenosis. *Circulation.* 2007;116(7):755–763.
24. Yener N, Oktar GL. Bicuspid aortic valve. *Ann Thorac Cardiovasc Surg.* 2002;8(5):264–267.

CHAPTER 82

THORACIC SURGERY FOR NONNEOPLASTIC DISEASE

Laurence H. Brinckerhoff, MD

PLEURAL EFFUSION

1. **What is a pleural effusion?**

   Pleural fluid is generated in normal adults at a rate of 5–10 L per 24 hours in the combined hemithoraces, but normal adults have only 20 mL of pleural fluid present at any time. Pleural effusions develop when there is either increased production or decreased resorption. Pathologic conditions leading to effusions include increased capillary permeability (inflammation, tumor), increased hydrostatic pressure (e.g., in congestive heart failure [CHF]), decreased lymphatic drainage (tumor, radiation fibrosis), decreased oncotic pressure (hypoalbuminemia), or combinations of these.

2. **How does one determine the cause of a pleural effusion?**

   History and physical examination, chest radiograph (upright and decubitus), chest computed tomography (CT) scans, and thoracentesis are used. Thoracentesis should be used to evaluate the pleural fluid. Bloody fluid is typical of trauma, pulmonary embolism, or malignancy. Milky fluid can be evidence of a chylothorax (triglyceride >110), and purulent fluid evidence of an empyema. Fluid should be checked for cell count; cytology; acid-base balance (pH); Gram stain; culture; and glucose, protein, lactate dehydrogenase (LDH), amylase, and triglyceride level. Exudates have a protein ratio >0.5 and an LDH ratio >0.6. The most common cause of transudate is CHF; the most common cause of exudate is malignancy. Glucose <60 mg/dL is seen in parapneumonic effusions, rheumatoid effusion, tuberculous pleuritis, and malignancy.

3. **What is the management of a pleural effusion?**

   Treatment for effusions differs based on the kind of effusion: transudative or exudative. Thoracentesis or a tube thoracostomy should be used to evacuate the effusion and determine the type. If the effusion is transudative, one should correct the underlying problem (e.g., CHF). If the effusion is exudative, one needs to consider operative intervention (e.g., pleurodesis or decortication). A decortication is the removal of an infective rind from the lung surface, allowing for full expansion of the lung tissue, thus filling an infected pleural space. A pleurodesis is used to treat a malignant effusion. A pleurodesis (stick the parietal and visceral pleurae together) can be performed with sclerosants (talc) or mechanical abrasion. Pleural symphysis (stuck pleura) results in decreased surface area for production, eliminates the pleural space for accumulation, and prevents lung collapse and compression. Chest tubes are generally removed when output is <150 mL per 24 hours.

4. **What does an air-fluid level on an initial chest radiograph indicate?**

   An air-fluid level before any drainage procedure may represent a bronchopleural fistula. These fistulas may resolve with chest tube drainage or require open thoracotomy for definitive repair.

EMPYEMA

5. **What is an empyema, and what causes it?**

   An empyema is a purulent (infected) effusion. Fluid or blood in the pleural space can be directly inoculated with bacteria during surgery or trauma (33%) or by contamination from contiguous sites (50%) such as bronchopulmonary infection (most common). Most empyemas are parapneumonic, and the most commonly involved organisms are *Staphylococcus aureus*, enteric gram-negative bacilli, and anaerobes. Many times, infections are polymicrobial. Often there is no growth of an empyema culture because of effective antibiotic therapy or inadequate culture techniques, particularly with anaerobes.

6. **What are the three stages of empyema development?**

   They are the exudative stage (low viscosity fluid), fibrinopurulent stage (transitional phase with heavy fibrinous deposits and turbid fluid), and organizing stage (capillary ingrowth with lung trapping by collagen). This process usually evolves over 6 weeks.

7. **How is an empyema diagnosed?**

   Characteristic clinical and radiographic findings are used. CT scans are helpful in defining loculations. Thoracentesis may reveal frank pus. Gram stain may show many white blood cells (WBCs) and organisms. Biochemical analysis varies, but it is generally an exudate with a low pH (<7), high LDH (>1000 IU/L), and low glucose (<50 mg/dL).

8. **How should an empyema be treated?**

   Antibiotic therapy directed by Gram stain and culture. If early in the disease process, tube thoracostomy may be curative. Instillation of fibrinolytic enzymes (e.g., DNase and tissue plasminogen activator) is often used as a first treatment method for an early empyema. An infected loculated (many discontinuous cystic pockets) effusion <14 days old or an effusion that fails to resolve after a trial of lytic therapy should undergo video-assisted thoracoscopic surgery decortication (i.e., resection of the thickened, adherent peel). The probability of conversion to open thoracotomy increases with the age of the effusion or empyema.

9. **What is a decortication?**

   The cortex is the outside wall or peel of the empyema (like an orange). Thus, decortication is the surgical release of the lung and removal of the abscess cavity walls. Successful decortication allows the lung to expand and fill the entire pleural space; if complete expansion does not occur, then the effusion may recur, and continued lung trapping is likely. There are two indications for decortication: (1) ongoing signs of infection (fever, sepsis high WBC) after drainage and (2) a significant rind on the lung resulting in a trapped lung and a pleural effusion.

10. **What are the complications of an empyema if left untreated?**

    The most common is pulmonary fibrosis with lung trapping and resultant dyspnea. Others include contraction and deformity of the chest wall, spontaneous drainage through the chest wall (empyema necessities), bronchopleural fistula, osteomyelitis, pericarditis, mediastinal or subphrenic abscess, sepsis, and death. None of these outcomes is particularly appealing, so in the absence of overwhelming contraindications, all empyemas warrant therapy.

INFECTIONS AND TUBERCULOSIS

11. **What is a lung abscess, and how is it treated?**

    A lung abscess is a localized site of infection located within the lung tissue with associated tissue necrosis. There are many potential lung infections that can produce lung abscesses, but anaerobic infections remain the most frequent types of pathogens. Unlike abscesses in other areas of the body, most lung abscesses do not require drainage and can be treated with systemic antibiotic therapy. This is because most lung abscesses are essentially drained by the airway. Surgery is only considered when medical therapy has failed.

12. **What are the clinical manifestations of pulmonary tuberculosis (TB)?**

    They can be almost anything or nothing (it has been stated that if you know TB, you know all of medicine), but the most common signs and symptoms are chronic fever; weight loss; night sweats; and cough, sometimes with hemoptysis. A chest radiograph typically shows upper lobe infiltrates, with or without cavitation, and can be misdiagnosed as a neoplastic process. Patients who are human immunodeficiency virus (HIV) positive and who are immunocompromised usually have mediastinal adenopathy, pleural effusions, and a miliary pattern.

13. **How is the diagnosis of pulmonary TB made?**

    Positive acid-fast bacilli ("red snappers") smear in sputum sample; sensitivity improves with bronchoalveolar lavage specimens. Culture growth will identify specific organisms (i.e., atypicals) and drug sensitivity (watch out for multidrug resistance [MDR]).

14. **What is the current medical treatment for active TB?**

    Initial therapy consists of a 6-month regimen with isoniazid, rifampin, and pyrazinamide for the first 2 months and then isoniazid and rifampin for another 4 months. With this schedule, 95% of patients have TB-negative sputum at the end of therapy. Partial responders should receive therapy for longer than 6 months, and those with MDR-TB may receive ethambutol or streptomycin.

15. **What are the indications for surgery in patients with TB?**
Surgery is indicated for complications of the disease. The most common surgical indication in the United States is MDR-TB with destroyed lung and persistent cavitary disease. This lung tissue is resistant to drug penetration and can "spill" organisms into healthy lung tissue. Other indications include hemoptysis, exclusion of lung cancer, bronchial stenosis, bronchopleural fistula, middle lobe syndrome, or mycobacterium other than tubercle bacilli (MOTT).

16. **What is MOTT, and what is the role of surgery with this disease?**
Atypical mycobacterial infections, non-TB mycobacterial infections, infection with mycobacteria other than TB and environmental mycobacteria are synonyms. The most common of these organisms is the *Mycobacterium avium* complex (MAC). Others include *M. chelonae* and abscesses, *M. kansaii, M. fortuitum,* and *M. xenopi.* MAC typically produces fibrocavitary disease of the upper lobes or the middle lobe or lingula of thin, white women. Surgery is indicated for localized disease, and in combination with drug therapy, it results in sputum conversion in 95% of patients with relapse rates of <5%. Other indications for surgery are the same as for regular TB.

KEY POINTS: THORACIC SURGERY FOR NONNEOPLASTIC DISEASE

1. An empyema is a purulent (infected) effusion. The primary treatment is drainage.
2. The three stages of empyema are the exudative stage (low viscosity fluid), fibrinopurulent stage (transitional phase with heavy fibrinous deposits and turbid fluid), and organizing stage (capillary ingrowth with lung trapping by collagen).
3. Surgery is indicated for complications of TB, with the most common indication in the United States being MDR-TB with destroyed lung and persistent cavitary disease.

WEBSITE

• www.sts.org

BIBLIOGRAPHY

1. Colice GL, Curtis A, Deslauriers J, et al. Medical and surgical treatment of parapneumonic effusions: an evidence-based guideline. *Chest.* 2000;200;118(4):1158–1171.
2. Rahman NM, Maskell NA, West A, et al. Intrapleural use of tissue plasminogen activator and DNase in pleural infection. *N Engl J Med.* 2011;365(6):518–526.
3. Raymond D. Surgical intervention for thoracic infections. *Surg Clin North Am.* 2014;94(6):1283–1303.
4. Psallidas I, Corcoran JP, Rahman NM. Management of parapneumonic effusions and empyema [Review]. *Semin Respir Crit Care Med.* 2014;35(6):715–722.
5. Molnar TF. Current surgical treatment of thoracic empyema in adults [Review]. *Eur J Cardiothorac Surg.* 2007;32(3):422–430.
6. Shiraishi Y. Surgical treatment of nontuberculous mycobacterial lung disease. *Gen Thorac Cardiovasc Surg.* 2014;62(8):475–480.
7. Takeda S, Maeda H, Hayakawa M, et al. Current surgical intervention for pulmonary tuberculosis. *Ann Thorac Surg.* 2005;79(3):959–963.

CHAPTER 83

LUNG CANCER

James M. Brown, MD

1. **Is lung cancer a single disease?**
   Traditionally, lung cancer has been stratified histologically as squamous/epidermoid, adenocarcinoma, and small/large cell lung cancers. Our current ability to profile cancers at the molecular level appears to have both prognostic and therapeutic value.

2. **What are the major histologic types of lung cancer?**
   The most important distinction is between small cell and non–small cell carcinoma because of fundamental differences in tumor biology and clinical behavior (Table 83.1). Patients with small cell lung cancer are classified as having either limited or extensive disease. **Limited** means that all known disease is confined to one hemithorax and regional lymph nodes, including mediastinal, contralateral hilar, and ipsilateral supraclavicular nodes. **Extensive** describes disease beyond these limits, including brain, bone marrow, and intraabdominal metastases.

   With small cell or neuroendocrine carcinoma, the small cell type is usually extensive at presentation, and 5-year survival is 5%. Neuroendocrine carcinoma, which is well differentiated, is known as atypical carcinoid and has a good prognosis but is not benign.

Table 83.1 Major Histologic Types of Lung Cancer		
TYPE	**INCIDENCE**	**COMMENTS**
Non–small cell carcinomas	80%	
Adenocarcinoma	40%	Has increased in nonsmokers
Squamous cell carcinoma	40%	Referred to as epidermoid, is associated histologically with keratin pearls, and is promoted by smoking and other inhaled irritants
Large cell carcinoma	15%	
Bronchoalveolar carcinoma	5%	Single nodule, multiple nodules, or nonresolving infiltrate on chest radiography
Small cell carcinoma	20%	Very poor prognosis

3. **Do genes and heredity play a role in lung cancer?**
   Yes. A family history of lung cancer probably increases the risk of getting lung cancer. Furthermore, a large array of important biomarkers that influence prognosis have been identified in lung cancer cells and lung cancer tissue.
   Past:
   - Light microscopic evidence of vascular invasion
   - Lymphatic invasion
   - Cellular pleomorphism and mitotic figures

   Present:
   - Proto-oncogenes, growth factors, growth factor receptors
   - Insulin-like growth factor
   - Epidermal growth factor receptor (EGFR)
   - K-*ras* mutation (cell growth regulation)
   - C-*myc* overexpression (cell growth)
   - *bcl*-2 underexpression (loss of apoptosis regulation)
   - Loss of tumor suppressor genes

- p53
- Retinoblastoma (RB gene)
- Chromosomal allele loss
- Fragile histidine triad gene
- Retinoic acid receptor a
- Overactivation of angiogenesis
- Platelet-derived growth factor
- Vascular endothelial-derived growth factor

Future:
- Gene therapy directed at those listed in present
- Antiangiogenesis therapy
- Immunopotentiation
- Adoptive immunotherapy: Isolation, expansion, and reinfusion of tumor-infiltrating lymphocytes
- Nonspecific immunostimulation
- Tumor vaccines
- No single marker yet has a clear meaning with respect to prognosis in a given patient

4. **What risk factors are thought to be important in the development of lung cancer?**
   - Ninety percent of patients have a smoking history
   - Chemicals (aromatic hydrocarbons, vinyl chloride)
   - Radiation (radon gas and uranium)
   - Asbestos
   - Metals (chromium, nickel, lead, and arsenic)
   - Environmental factors (air pollution, coal tar, petroleum products)

5. **Have culprit genes been identified?**
   EGFR-activating mutations are associated with increased frequency of stage IV disease and decreased overall survival.

6. **Is lung cancer screening effective?**
   Old dogma: No.
   Current thinking: Maybe.
   The thinking is as follows: Lung cancer accounts for more cancer deaths than other cancers. Eighty-five percent of patients present with advanced incurable lung cancer. We have not changed survival for lung cancer. Early-stage cancers that are asymptomatic can be found by chest radiograph and helical computed tomography (CT). Unfortunately, CT also detects many false positives. Also, public health policy does not endorse screening for lung cancer.

7. **How do patients with lung cancer present?**
   - Cough: 70%
   - Weight loss: 10%
   - Bone pain: 30%
   - Paraneoplastic syndrome: 10%
   - Asymptomatic: 10%

8. **What is a paraneoplastic syndrome?**
   Paraneoplastic syndromes of lung cancer may be metabolic (e.g., hypercalcemia, Cushing's syndrome), neurologic (e.g., peripheral neuropathy; polymyositis; or Lambert-Eaton syndrome, which is similar to myasthenia gravis), skeletal (e.g., clubbing, hypertrophic osteoarthropathy), hematologic (e.g., anemia, thrombocytosis, disseminated intravascular coagulation [DIC]), or cutaneous (e.g., hyperkeratosis, acanthosis nigricans, dermatomyositis). Of interest, the presence of a paraneoplastic syndrome does not influence the ultimate curability of the lung cancer.

9. **Does the staging system for lung cancer have prognostic and therapeutic importance?**
   Yes. The patient's survival is related to the stage at presentation (Table 83.2).

Table 83.2 Staging of Lung Cancer

STAGE	SUBSET	DESCRIPTION
I	Ia	Intraparenchymal tumor with or without extension to the visceral pleura, 2 cm from the carina, and no lymph node metastases spread
	Ib	Tumor >3 cm or through parietal pleura, no positive nodes
II	IIa	Primary tumor is similar to that of stage I with extension to interbronchial lymph nodes (N_1)
	IIb	Tumor invades chest wall without nodal involvement (T_3N_0)
III	IIIa	Extension of tumor into hilar or mediastinal lymph nodes (N_2) or chest wall with N_1 nodes
	IIIb	All elements of IIIa plus extension of tumor to mediastinal structures (heart or great vessels) or contralateral hilar, paratracheal, or supraclavicular lymph nodes (N_3)
IV		Malignant pleural effusion or metastatic disease (M_1)

10. **Describe the workup of a patient with a mass on chest radiograph.**
    The workup should be directed toward diagnosis, staging, and risk assessment.
    a. Diagnosis
       - Prior radiographs are invaluable
       - CT and positron emission tomography (PET): Defines size, mets, nodes, and malignancy risk
       - Sputum cytology: Low diagnostic yield
       - Bronchoscopy: Low diagnostic yield if tumor not visible
       - CT-guided fine-needle aspiration
       - Thoracoscopy and biopsy: Wedge excision
    b. Staging
       - CT scan (chest): Tumor, mediastinal lymph node assessment
       - PET: 90% sensitive and 80% specific for nodes, mets
       - Bronchoscopy: Endobronchial invasion
       - Thoracoscopy: Lymph node sampling
       - Mediastinoscopy: Sample N2 and N3 nodes
    c. Risk assessment
       i. Pulmonary
          - Spirometry: Ventilation/perfusion screening; if borderline, must leave patient with approximately 800 mL forced expiratory volume after resection
          - Arterial blood gas analysis
       ii. Cardiac
          - Electrocardiogram
          - History of myocardial infarction, prior intervention
       iii. Cardiopulmonary
          - Able to walk a flight of stairs; if yes, will tolerate lobectomy
          - Maximal oxygen consumption <15 mL/kg per minute

11. **How are patients with lung cancer treated?**
    The most effective treatment for lung cancer is surgical resection. Unfortunately, 75% of patients present with advanced disease and are not candidates for resection. Fortunately, preoperative chemotherapy with a cisplatinum-containing regimen has increased the number of patients with stage III who are candidates for resection. This recent innovative therapy may translate into improved survival rates. For stage III lung cancer, several clinical trials have shown an advantage to preoperative chemotherapy and radiation treatment called neoadjuvant therapy. Even lower-stage disease or tumors at high risk of recurrence may benefit from newer chemotherapeutic regimens.

12. **Do chemotherapy and radiation therapy have a place in the therapy of lung cancer?**
    Radiation therapy is effective palliative, but not curative, therapy for lung cancer. Specifically, patients who present with a superior vena cava syndrome or a blocked bronchus with distal pneumonia

frequently can be "opened up" with radiation therapy. Radiation is also excellent for the palliation of pathologic bone pain. Some—but not all—clinical trials have shown some benefit from preoperative chemoradiation treatment in advanced-stage lung cancer. There is evidence to suggest that patients with stage Ib, IIa, or IIb lung cancer benefit from induction chemotherapy. The treatment of stage III disease based on the presence of mediastinal lymph nodes is still controversial, despite much attention and many trials over the last 10 years. For now, most patients with stage III disease have only a 20% survival at best. Most should be offered induction preoperative chemotherapy.

13. **What is the survival rate of patients treated for non-small cell lung cancer at 5 years?**
Stage I:
    Ia 65% (up to 84% with no nodes or N1)
    Ib 55%
Stage II:
    IIa 55%
    IIb 40%
Stage III:
    IIIa 20%
    IIIb 10%
Stage IV: 2%
Note that for chest wall invasion with no lymph nodes, survival is 50% at 5 years, although this is still called stage IIb. Also, if stage Ia (small tumor, no positive nodes) cancer is not resected, survival decreases from 70% to 7%.

14. **What is mediastinoscopy?**
Mediastinoscopy is a staging procedure in which the paratracheal, subcarinal, and proximal peribronchial lymph nodes are sampled from a small incision made in the suprasternal notch.

15. **What are the indications for mediastinoscopy?**
Mediastinal staging is indicated in patients with either apparent or documented lung cancer who have:
- Known lung cancer with mediastinal lymph nodes >1 cm accessible by cervical mediastinal exploration, as assessed by CT scan
- Adenocarcinoma of the lung and multiple mediastinal lymph nodes <1 cm
- Central or large (>5 cm) lung cancers with mediastinal lymph nodes <1 cm
- Lung cancer when the patient is at high risk of thoracotomy and lung resection
- Highly suggestive PET scan for mediastinal nodal mets

If the mediastinoscopy has negative results, the surgeon should proceed with minimally invasive thoracotomy, biopsy, and curative lung resection.

16. **Is malignant pleural effusion or recurrent nerve involvement with tumor an absolute contraindication to surgical resection for lung cancer?**
A malignant pleural effusion defines the tumor—T as T4 and the stage is at least IIIb. Most such patients will have metastatic disease after evaluation. Rarely, a small malignant pleural effusion will occur in the presence of a pleurally based but resectable primary tumor. Conversely, both King George V and Arthur Godfrey had successful surgical resections in the face of recurrent nerve involvement with tumor.

KEY POINTS: LUNG CANCER

1. The overall survival rate for patients with lung cancer is 10%.
2. Ninety percent of patients have a smoking history.
3. The most effective treatment for lung cancer is surgical resection.

WEBSITE

- https://www.cancer.gov/types/lung/hp/non-small-cell-lung-treatment-pdq

BIBLIOGRAPHY

1. Alegre E, Fusco JP, Restituto P, et al. Total and mutated EGFR quantification in cell-free DNA from non-small cell lung cancer patients detects tumor heterogeneity and presents prognostic value. *Tumour Biol.* 2016;37(10):13687–13694.
2. Arriagada R, Bergman B, Dunant A, et al. Cisplatin-based adjuvant chemotherapy in patients with completely resected non-small-cell carcinoma. *N Engl J Med.* 2004;350(4):351–360.
3. Ginsberg RJ, Ruckdeschel JC, eds. *Lung cancer: past, present, and future. Part I. Chest surgery clinics of North America.* Philadelphia: W.B. Saunders; 2000.
4. Sonett JR, Krasna MJ, Suntharalingam M, et al. Safe pulmonary resection after chemotherapy and high-dose thoracic radiation. *Ann Thorac Surg.* 1999;68(2):316–320.
5. Strauss GM. Prognostic markers in resectable non-small-cell lung cancer. *Hematol Oncol Clin North Am.* 1997;11(3):409–434.
6. Toloza EM, Harpole L. Invasive staging of non small cell lung cancer. *Chest.* 2003;123(suppl 1):157S–166S.

CHAPTER 84

SOLITARY PULMONARY NODULE

James M. Brown, MD

1. **Does lung cancer screening save lives?**

   The United States National Lung Screening Trial (NLST) reported a reduction in lung cancer mortality of 20%, and a 6.7% decrease in all-cause mortality. Low-dose computed tomography (CT) scans may prove beneficial in high-risk patients. Multiple other screening trials have not proven to be so optimistic; lung screening remains controversial.

2. **What is a solitary pulmonary nodule?**

   A solitary pulmonary nodule or "coin lesion" is found on chest radiograph, or CT, and is <3 cm. It is completely surrounded by lung parenchyma.

3. **What causes a solitary pulmonary nodule?**

   The most common causes of a pulmonary nodule are either neoplastic (carcinoma, 60%–70% of resected nodules) or infectious (granuloma). Pulmonary nodules may also represent lung abscess, pulmonary infarction, arteriovenous malformations, resolving pneumonia, pulmonary sequestration, and hamartoma. As a general rule of thumb, likelihood of malignancy is proportionate to the nodule's size, the patient's age, and history of smoking. Thus, whereas lung cancer is rare (although it does occur) in 30-year-old individuals, in 50-year-old smokers the chance that a solitary pulmonary nodule represents malignancy is 50%–60%. In a 70-year-old person with a smoking history and a 2.9-cm pulmonary nodule the malignancy risk is 75%.

4. **How does a solitary pulmonary nodule present?**

   Typically, a solitary nodule presents incidentally as a finding on routine chest radiograph. In several large series, more than 75% of lesions were surprise findings on routine chest radiograph. Fewer than 25% of patients had symptoms referable to the lung. Solitary nodules are now seen on other sensitive imaging tests such as helical CT.

5. **How frequently does a solitary pulmonary nodule represent metastatic disease?**

   Fewer than 10% of solitary nodules represent metastatic disease. Accordingly, an extensive workup for a primary site of cancer other than the lung is not indicated.

6. **Can a tissue sample be obtained by fluoroscopic or CT-guided needle biopsy?**

   Yes, but the results do not change the treatment. If the needle biopsy tissue indicates cancer, the nodule must be removed. If the needle biopsy is negative for cancer, the nodule must still be removed. Positron emission tomography (PET) is 90% sensitive in identifying malignant tumors. Nodule characteristics on CT scanning combined with PET may be 90% accurate in ruling out malignancy. But most patients are not satisfied with 90% accuracy. They want 100%.

7. **Are radiographic findings important?**

   Only relatively. The resolution of CT scanners allows the best identification of characteristics that suggest cancer.

   a. Indistinct or irregular spiculated borders of the nodule.

   b. The larger the nodule, the more likely it is to be malignant.

   c. Calcification in the nodule generally is associated with benign disease (the opposite of breast cancer). Specifically, whereas central, diffuse, or laminated calcifications are typical of a granuloma, calcifications with more dense and irregular "popcorn" patterns are associated with hamartomas. Unfortunately, eccentric foci of calcium or small flecks of calcium may be found in malignant lesions.

   d. Nodules can be studied using a CT scanner by measuring their change in relative radiodensity after injection of contrast. This is called Hounsfield attenuation and improves the accuracy of predicting the presence of malignancy.

8. **What social or clinical findings suggest that a nodule is malignant rather than benign?**
Unfortunately, none of these findings is sufficiently sensitive or specific to influence the workup. Both increasing age and a long smoking history predispose patients to lung cancer. Winston Churchill should have had lung cancer and cirrhosis, but he did not. Thus, the fact that the patient is the president of the spelunking club (histoplasmosis), has a sister who raises pigeons (cryptococcosis), grew up in the Ohio River Valley (histoplasmosis), works as sexton for a dog cemetery (blastomycosis), or just took a hiking trip through the San Joaquin Valley (coccidioidomycosis) is interesting associated history but does not affect the workup of a solitary pulmonary nodule.

9. **What is the most valuable bit of historic data?**
The patient's age and smoking history. Beyond the obvious, the most valuable data piece is an old chest radiograph. If the nodule is new, it is more likely to be malignant, whereas if the nodule has not changed in the past 2 years, it is less likely to be malignant. Unfortunately, even this observation is not absolute.

10. **If a patient presents with a treated prior malignancy and a new solitary pulmonary nodule, is it safe to assume that the new nodule represents metastatic disease?**
No. Even in patients with known prior malignancies, <50% of new pulmonary nodules are metastatic. Thus, the workup should proceed exactly as for any other patient with a new solitary pulmonary nodule.

11. **How should a solitary pulmonary nodule be evaluated?**
A complete travel and occupational history is interesting but does not affect the evaluation. Because of the peripheral location of most nodules, bronchoscopy has a diagnostic yield of <50%. Even in the best hands, sputum cytology has a low yield. CT scanning is recommended because it can define to a degree the nodule (size, calcification, density, etc.), identify other potentially metastatic nodules, and delineate the status of mediastinal lymph nodes. As indicated previously, percutaneous needle biopsy has a diagnostic yield of approximately 80% but rarely alters the subsequent management. PET scanning may suggest cancer with accuracy. More importantly, PET scanning may suggest the presence of extramediastinal or covert mediastinal disease with more sensitivity than CT scanning.
   The mainstay of management in patients who can tolerate surgery is resection of the nodule, usually by minimally invasive thoracoscopic lobectomy if cancer is suspected. Decisions to observe pulmonary nodules should be made selectively (e.g., old patient, poor candidate for surgery) and with a careful follow-up plan.

12. **If the lesion proves to be cancer, what is the appropriate surgical therapy?**
Like all clinical decision making, that would depend. Although several series have suggested that wedge excision of the nodule is sufficient, an anatomic lobectomy remains the procedure of choice for a known cancer of the lung. This can typically be accomplished by a video-assisted approach. A solitary node that turns out to be metastatic cancer should be wedged out with likely benefit. Unfortunately, the recurrence rate even for stage I tumors or a small nodule is 30% over 5 years. Recurrences are split between local and distant.

KEY POINTS: SOLITARY PULMONARY NODULE

1. A solitary pulmonary nodule or coin lesion is <3 cm and is discrete on chest radiograph.
2. The most common causes of a pulmonary nodule are either neoplastic or infectious.
3. If the lesion proves to be cancer, anatomic lobectomy is the procedure of choice.

WEBSITE

- https://www.thoracic.org/professionals/career-development/residents-medical-students/ats-reading-list/lung-cancersolitary-pulmonary-nodule.php

BIBLIOGRAPHY

1. Park YS. Lung cancer screening: subsequent evidences of national lung screening trial. *Tuberc Respir Dis (Seoul).* 2014;77(2):55–59.
2. Birim O, Kappetein PA, Stijnen T, et al. Meta-analysis of positron emission tomographic and computed tomographic imaging in detecting mediastinal lymph node metastases in nonsmall cell lung cancer. *Ann Thoracic Surgery.* 2005;79(1):375–382.
3. Davies B. Ghosh S. Solitary pulmonary nodules: pathological outcome of 150 consecutively resected lesions. *Interact Cardiovas Thorac Surg.* 2005;4(1):18–20.
4. Dewey TM, Mack MJ. Lung cancer: surgical approaches and incisions. *Chest Surg Clin North Am.* 2000;10(4):803–820.
5. Ginsberg RJ, Rubinstein LV. Randomized trial of lobectomy versus limited resection for T1 N0 non-small cell lung cancer. Lung Cancer Study Group. *Ann Thorac Surg.* 1995;60(3):615–622.
6. Khouri NF, Meziane MA. The solitary pulmonary nodule: assessment, diagnosis, and management. *Chest.* 1987;91(1):128–133.
7. Miller DL, Rowland CM. Surgical treatment of non-small cell lung cancer 1 cm or less in diameter. *Ann Thorac Surg.* 2002;73(5):1541–1545.
8. Nesbitt J, Putnam JB. Survival in early stage non-small cell lung cancer. *Ann Thorac Surg.* 1995;60(2):466–472.
9. Varoli F, Vergani C, Caminiti R, et al. Management of the solitary pulmonary nodule. *Eur J Cardiothorac Surg.* 2008;33(3):461–465.
10. Walsh GL, Pisters KM. Treatment of stage I lung cancer. *Chest Surg Clin North Am.* 2001;11(1):17–38.

DISSECTING AORTIC ANEURYSM

Richard-Tien V. Ha, MD

CHAPTER 85

1. **Why is the term *dissecting aortic aneurysm* really incorrect?**
   The correct term should be *dissecting aortic hematoma* because the lesion is not an aneurysm. Blood passes into the media, creating a hematoma that separates the intima from the media or adventitia. It is unclear whether the inciting event is the intimal tear or blood from the media tearing through the intima. Hence, an intimal tear is not a prerequisite because 5%–13% of patients do not have one.

2. **When should the diagnosis be entertained?**
   Suspicion is the most important factor because no one feature is common to patients presenting with aortic dissections. In any patient who presents with severe knifelike, ripping chest and back pain, the diagnosis of aortic dissection should be considered. Other symptoms include syncope and neurologic symptoms.

3. **After the diagnosis is entertained, how should the patient be managed?**
   Two-thirds of patients are hypertensive, so blood pressure (BP) must be controlled to a systolic BP of <100 mm Hg. Pain must also be managed to reduce catecholamine surge. The other diagnosis to be strongly considered is acute myocardial infarction (MI). An electrocardiogram often rules out MI, but some aortic dissections tear off a coronary artery; thus, both acute infarction and aortic dissection occur concurrently (this patient group has a higher mortality).

4. **What is the most significant diagnostic clue on physical examination?**
   A new aortic valvular diastolic murmur, indicating aortic valvular regurgitation caused by distortion of the valve structure by the mural hematoma. In addition, the dissecting hematoma can encircle the lumen or actually cleave the takeoff of the subclavian or femoral vessels, resulting in the loss of pulses or systolic variation between arms. Neurologic findings, including paraplegia and hemiplegia, may also be present because of similar flap occlusion of the great vessels.

5. **Which chest radiograph findings are helpful in diagnosis?**
   Widened mediastinum and loss of aortic knob silhouette—a hematoma surrounding the aorta makes the aortic outline blurry—are helpful findings. In 15%–25% of patients, a left-sided pleural effusion is present.

6. **How is the diagnosis confirmed? What are the best diagnostic studies?**
   The literature reports the high accuracy of transesophageal echocardiography (TEE) and spiral computed tomography angiography (CTA) in the diagnosis of aortic dissections. On the other hand, unlike these modalities, angiography allows for visualization of the coronary arteries or estimation of aortic valvular insufficiency. The decision to use one modality over the other lies in the stability of the patient and the modalities available at a given institution. TEE should be the first modality if available in unstable patients, followed by CTA. Angiography may be used in stable patients to define the coronary anatomy and valvular architecture, although studies show that in-house mortality is not improved with coronary angiography.

7. **What are the types of dissection?**
   There are two classification schemes: DeBakey and Stanford. DeBakey type I involves the ascending aorta and propagates to at least the aortic arch. Type II involves only the ascending aorta. Type III involves the descending aorta.
   The Stanford classification has both therapeutic and prognostic value:
   - Ascending (type A) involves only the ascending or both the ascending and descending aorta.
   - Descending (type B) involves only the descending aorta. Ascending dissections are twice as common as descending dissections and often begin at the right lateral wall and involve the aortic arch in 30%.

8. **Who cares whether a dissection involves the ascending (type A) or descending (type B) aorta?**
Ascending dissections require early surgical correction to avoid extension into the coronary or carotid arteries, rupture into the pericardium (tamponade), or both. Descending dissections do not involve the ascending aorta and currently are managed with a stent graft as the primary solution. If stent grafting is not possible, open repair is the next option.

9. **What is the key to medical management?**
The BP should be lowered to 100 mm Hg (systolic) with a combination of sodium nitroprusside and propranolol. Propranolol or labetalol is particularly important because it decreases the contractility of the myocardium (dp/dt), thereby decreasing the shearing force that prevents propagation of the dissection down the aorta. Conceptually, the BP should be lowered as much as possible, but the patient must continue to perfuse the end organs (i.e., make urine). Sodium nitroprusside may be added for further BP control.

10. **What are the principles and advantages of surgical management of acute aortic dissection?**
Ascending dissection:
a. To close off the hematoma by obliterating the most proximal intimal tear
b. To restore competency of the aortic valve
c. To restore flow to any branches of the aorta that have been sheared off and receive blood flow from a false lumen
d. To protect the heart during these maneuvers and to restore coronary blood flow if a coronary artery has been sheared off
e. To look for tears in the transverse aortic arch
Technique: Use of deep hypothermia circulatory arrest with or without retrograde cerebral perfusion is in vogue at present. This technique allows the arch to be inspected and the distal anastomosis of the Dacron graft to be sewn accurately to the distal ascending aorta in an open fashion. Whether to replace or repair the aortic valve is controversial.
Descending dissection:
a. To close off the hematoma by obliterating the most proximal intimal tear
b. To restore blood flow to branches of the aorta fed by the false channel
Technique: Surgery is performed using partial cardiopulmonary bypass, or the clamp and run technique, in which the aorta is crossclamped and the graft is sewn in as fast as possible (see Controversies). Endovascular repair with stents is gaining popularity, and in some clinical situations may be the better choice (see Controversies).

11. **What are the operative complications?**
- Hemorrhage (20%): Quite common because of the use of heparin and the poor quality of aortic tissue (like wet Kleenex)
- Renal failure (20%)
- Pulmonary insufficiency (30% higher in repair of descending dissections)
- Paraplegia: Often presents before operation; as a surgical complication, it usually occurs only with descending dissections (11%)
- Acute MI or low cardiac output (30%)
- Bowel infarction (5%)
- Death (15%): Higher for acute than chronic dissections and higher for repair of ascending dissections

12. **What are the long-term results?**
Of patients who survive the operation, two-thirds die within 7 years because of comorbid cardiac and cerebrovascular disease.

CONTROVERSIES

13. **Which is preferred, surgical or medical management of descending dissections?**
Initial surgical management:
- Approximately 25% of patients initially treated medically need an operation eventually.
- Operative mortality is much lower today (20%–30%) than in the past.
- Stent graft repair is showing promise as an early and less morbid treatment.
Initial medical management:
- Medical management has a lower in-hospital mortality rate (10%–15%).
- This avoids unnecessary operation and its attendant cost and complication rate.

14. **What is the preferred management of aortic insufficiency in ascending dissections?**
    Replacement of aortic valve:
    - Easy (valved conduits now available)
    - Eliminates aortic insufficiency completely
    - Should be done in patients with Marfan's syndrome

    Repair of aortic valve:
    - With native valve reconstruction, when done correctly, the need to replace the valve at a later time is only 10%.
    - Avoids need for anticoagulation, which is necessary when a mechanical valve is used to replace the aortic valve.

15. **What is the preferred repair of descending dissections?**
    a. Partial left atrial-to-femoral artery bypass
       For:
       - Allows unloading of the heart
       - Allows distal perfusion to avoid visceral ischemia
       - Allows as much time as needed to complete anastomosis

       Against:
       - Requires heparinization
    b. Simple aortic crossclamping
       For:
       - Fast

       Against:
       - Placement of the graft has to be done in <30 minutes or the complication rate, particularly paraplegia, increases significantly
    c. Placement of a stent graft across the intimal tear
       For:
       - Decreased in-hospital mortality (10%) compared to surgery
       - Decreased hospital stay, faster recovery, and decreased postprocedure pain
       - Allows reexpansion of compressed true lumen
       - Decreased risk of paraplegia

       Against:
       - May occlude previously normal branch arteries
       - Effectiveness in stable type B dissections under investigation
       - Long-term results are not known at this time

KEY POINTS: DISSECTING AORTIC ANEURYSM

1. The correct term should be *dissecting aortic hematoma* because the lesion is not an aneurysm.
2. A new aortic valvular diastolic murmur, indicating aortic valvular regurgitation caused by distortion of the valve structure by the mural hematoma.
3. Ascending dissections require early surgical correction to avoid extension into the coronary or carotid arteries, rupture into the pericardium, or both.
4. Descending dissections may be managed medically; however, even surgical patients should have BP lowered to between 100 and 110 mm Hg with a combination of sodium nitroprusside and propranolol/labetalol.

BIBLIOGRAPHY

1. Barron DJ, Livesey SA. Twenty-year follow-up of acute type a dissection: the incidence and extent of distal aortic disease using magnetic resonance imaging. *J Card Surg.* 1997;12(3):147–159.
2. Glower DD, Fann JI, Speier RH. Comparison of medical and surgical therapy for uncomplicated descending aortic dissection. *Circulation.* 1990;82(suppl 5):IV39–IV46.
3. Khan IA, Nair CK. Clinical, diagnostic, and management perspectives of aortic dissection. *Chest.* 2002;122(1):311–328.
4. Okita Y, Takamoto S. Mortality and cerebral outcome in patients who underwent aortic arch operations using deep hypothermic circulatory arrest with retrograde cerebral perfusion: no relation of early death, stroke, and delirium to the duration of circulatory arrest. *J Thorac Cardiovasc Surg.* 1998;115(1):129–138.

5. Nienaber CA, Eagle KA. Aortic dissection: new frontiers in diagnosis and management. Part I: from etiology to diagnostic strategies. *Circulation.* 2003;108(5):628–635.
6. Nienaber CA, Eagle KA. Aortic dissection: new frontiers in diagnosis and management. Part II: therapeutic management and follow-up. *Circulation.* 2003;108(6):772–778.
7. Ince H, Nienaber CA. Diagnosis and management of patients with acute aortic dissection. *Heart.* 2007;93(2):266–270.
8. Divchev D, Aboukoura M, Weinrich M. Risk evaluation of type B aortic dissection: importance for treatment of acute aortic syndrome. *Chirurg.* 2014;85(9):774, 776–781.
9. Mussa FF, Horton JD. Acute aortic dissection and intramural hematoma: a systematic review. *JAMA.* 2016;316(7): 754–763.

IX
PEDIATRIC SURGERY

HYPERTROPHIC PYLORIC STENOSIS

Ann M. Kulungowski, MD

CHAPTER 86

1. **What is hypertrophic pyloric stenosis (HPS)?**
   HPS is the most common cause of gastric outlet obstruction in infants resulting in nonbilious vomiting. The pathogenesis of HPS is unknown; it is not thought to be a developmental defect. Hypotheses include nitric oxide deficiency, decreased neurotrophins, and alterations in growth factors and gastrointestinal peptides. It is more common in boys than girls (2:1). Offspring of an affected parent have an increased risk of HPS (10%); the highest rate (20%) occurs in boys born to affected mothers. The pylorus muscle grossly and histologically appears thickened and hypertrophied.

2. **Describe the typical presentation of an infant with HPS.**
   Typically, an otherwise healthy infant who was feeding without issue develops nonbilious emesis at 2–8 weeks of age. Initially, the emesis is not frequent or forceful. Over a period of days, the infant develops projectile vomiting with most feeds. The emesis may have a coffee-ground appearance as a result of gastritis or esophagitis. The infant remains hungry after emesis. In premature infants, the diagnosis often presents 2 weeks later. As HPS goes unrecognized, the infant becomes dehydrated.

3. **What are the physical findings?**
   The infant may appear normal, especially if the diagnosis is made early. Some infants are dehydrated, malnourished, or lethargic. The abdomen is nondistended and soft. A palpable "olive" confirms the diagnosis. The pylorus can be palpated in a relaxed infant in the epigastrium. This is becoming a lost skill in the era of ultrasonography.

4. **Why do some infants with HPS appear jaundiced?**
   Approximately 5% of infants have mild jaundice from indirect hyperbilirubinemia related to glucuronyl transferase deficiency.

5. **How is the diagnosis confirmed?**
   Ultrasonography is the imaging test of choice. Ultrasonographic criteria include a pyloric muscle thickness of ≥3.5 mm, pyloric channel length of ≥15 mm, and pyloric diameter ≥14 mm. Muscle thickness of ≥3 mm is considered positive for infants younger than 30 days of age. If ultrasonography is not available or nondiagnostic, an upper gastrointestinal (UGI) contrast examination can assist with diagnosis or provides alternative causes of nonbilious vomiting (e.g., gastroesophageal reflux, malrotation, duodenal stenosis).

6. **Describe the likely electrolyte abnormalities.**
   Electrolytes are often normal because of earlier consideration of the diagnosis. In the case of long-standing vomiting, a hypokalemic, hypochloremic metabolic alkalosis results because of the loss of gastric acid (HCl). Dehydration is corrected with 0.9% sodium chloride (NaCl) with 20 mEq/L of potassium chloride (KCl). Withholding KCl while awaiting urine output delays appropriate replacement. The rare exception is acute renal compromise or preexisting renal impairment. Once the infant is resuscitated and electrolytes corrected, pyloromyotomy is performed. The serum bicarbonate level should be <30 mEq/L to avoid respiratory depression and prolonged postoperative intubation.

7. **What procedure is performed to treat HPS?**
   The operative procedure of choice remains the Ramstedt pyloromyotomy. A superficial incision is made longitudinally over the pyloric muscle in an avascular area. The muscle's fibers are fractured bluntly with either the back of a scalpel or a pyloric spreading clamp. A few pyloric muscle fibers are left intact on the duodenal end to reduce the risk of perforation. At conclusion of the pyloromyotomy, the gastric mucosa should bulge upward into the cleft. The pyloric muscle walls should move

independently. Air is injected into the stomach via the nasogastric tube to identify mucosal perforation. Pyloromyotomy can be performed open (transverse right upper quadrant or supraumbilical incision) or laparoscopically (three small incisions).

8. **What are the complications of pyloromyotomy?**
Incomplete pyloromyotomy, mucosal perforation, wound infection, and abdominal wall hernias are some of the potential complications. Most incomplete pyloromyotomies are a result of failure to extend it far enough on the proximal antrum. Laparoscopic pyloromyotomy benefits include faster recovery and advancement to full feeds, decreased pain, and improved cosmesis. Incomplete pyloromyotomy risk is slightly higher with the laparoscopic approach (1%) compared to the open approach (0.3%); mucosal perforation rates are equivalent.

9. **What should be done if a mucosal perforation is identified?**
Mucosal perforation is a rare event (0.5%). The submucosa should be approximated with interrupted fine absorbable suture and covered with an omental patch. An infrequently needed alternative is closure of the original myotomy and a second, parallel myotomy made 180 degrees on the opposite side of the pylorus.

10. **When can postoperative feeding begin?**
Small-volume feedings are started after the infant has recovered from anesthesia (2–3 hours). The feeds are advanced to goal. Small-volume emesis is common (20%), but most infants achieve full feeds 24 hours postoperatively. An incomplete pyloromyotomy is considered when symptoms of gastric outlet obstruction persist for 7 days postoperatively.

KEY POINTS: HYPERTROPHIC PYLORIC STENOSIS

1. Infants with HPS present with nonbilious, projectile vomiting. A hypokalemic, hypochloremic metabolic alkalosis can develop with long-standing emesis.
2. Ultrasonography is the diagnostic test of choice to confirm HPS; a positive study shows a muscle thickness of ≥ 3.5 mm and pyloric channel length of ≥ 15 mm.
3. After resuscitation and correction of electrolyte abnormalities, pyloromyotomy, laparoscopic or open, is performed. Complications of the pyloromyotomy include mucosal perforation and incomplete pyloromyotomy.

BIBLIOGRAPHY

1. Adibe OO, Iqbal CW, Sharp SW, et al. Protocol versus ad libitum feeds after laparoscopic pyloromyotomy: a prospective randomized trial. *J Pediatr Surg.* 2014;49(1):129–132. discussion 132.
2. Hall NJ, Eaton S, Seims A, et al. Risk of incomplete pyloromyotomy and mucosal perforation in open and laparoscopic pyloromyotomy. *J Pediatr Surg.* 2014;49(7):1083–1086.
3. Acker SN, Garcia AJ. Current trends in the diagnosis and treatment of pyloric stenosis. *Pediatr Surg Int.* 2015;31(4):363–366.

INTESTINAL OBSTRUCTION OF NEONATES AND INFANTS

Stig Sømme, MD, MPH, Ann M. Kulungowski, MD

1. **What signs and symptoms suggest intestinal obstruction in the neonate?**

   Signs and symptoms vary according to the location of the obstruction. Proximal intestinal obstruction leads to early bilious vomiting, typically with minimal distention. Neonates with distal intestinal obstruction often present after the first day of life with distention and bilious emesis. Bilious emesis in infants and children deserves immediate investigation. An upper gastrointestinal (UGI) contrast study will identify a surgical cause in about one-third of cases. In particular, malrotation with midgut volvulus should always be ruled out as this condition requires prompt surgical intervention.

2. **What is the differential diagnosis of intestinal obstruction in neonates?**

   Rule out proximal and distal anatomical abnormalities—esophageal atresia and anorectal malformation. Perform a rectal examination. Evacuation of stool during rectal examination suggests Hirschsprung disease. Next, obtain a two-view abdominal x-ray. The extent of gaseous distention of the bowel helps differentiate proximal versus distal bowel obstruction.

   Proximal (minimal bowel gas)
   Duodenal atresia, stenosis (commonly double bubble)
   Malrotation with midgut volvulus
   Jejunal atresia (sometimes triple bubble)
   Distal (bowel gas in multiple loops and distention)
   Ileal atresia
   Meconium ileus or plug
   Small left colon syndrome
   Hirschsprung disease

3. **When are contrast studies of the gastrointestinal tract indicated?**

   Immediate abdominal exploration is indicated if there is peritonitis or pneumoperitoneum. Malrotation with midgut volvulus must be distinguished from other causes of congenital duodenal obstruction (duodenal atresia/stenosis). In malrotation with midgut volvulus, the UGI demonstrates a distended duodenum, failure of the duodenal-jejunal junction to cross the midline, corkscrewing of the distal duodenum, and minimal or no passage of contrast into the jejunum. Duodenal atresia often presents with a double bubble (first bubble stomach and second bubble duodenum) on plain x-ray at the time of birth. A contrast study may be helpful for the diagnosis of duodenal stenosis. Contrast enema is indicated for distal intestinal obstruction.

Disorder	Findings on Contrast Enema
Ileal atresia	Microcolon; no reflux into terminal ileum
Meconium ileus	Microcolon; reflux into terminal ileum with filling defects (can be therapeutic)
Meconium plug	Normal colon: large filling defects of left colon
Hirschsprung disease	Narrow rectosigmoid, proximal dilation

4. **Describe intestinal atresia.**

   Intestinal atresia can occur anywhere in the GI tract—duodenal (50%), jejunoileal (45%), or colonic (5%). Duodenal atresia is due to failure of recanalization in the first trimester. Jejunoileal and colonic atresias are caused by an in utero mesenteric vascular accident.

5. **Distinguish duodenal atresia from other forms of intestinal atresia.**

   - Duodenal atresia is characterized by early feeding intolerance and bilious vomiting (85% of atresia distal to ampulla of vater). A double bubble gas pattern without distal gas (atresia) or with distal gas (stenosis) is observed on plain abdominal radiograph. The abdomen is scaphoid and not distended. Approximately 25% of infants with duodenal atresia have trisomy 21. Surgical correction involves creating a duodenoduodenostomy.

- Jejunoileal atresia presents early (<24 h) if the obstruction is in the proximal jejunum or later (>24 h) with more abdominal distention if the obstruction is in the ileum. Associated anomalies are uncommon. Plain abdominal radiographs may show dilated loops of bowel with air-fluid levels. A contrast enema demonstrates a microcolon with no contrast refluxing into dilated intestine. Surgical correction involves limited intestinal resection and end-to-end anastomosis.
- Colonic atresia presents similar to other distal bowel obstructions. A contrast enema is usually diagnostic and demonstrates a distal microcolon without reflux of contrast into dilated proximal intestine. Associated anomalies of the heart, musculoskeletal system, and abdominal wall are identified in 20% of infants. Surgical correction involves limited colonic resection and intestinal anastomosis.

6. **Describe malrotation with midgut volvulus.**

During the sixth to twelfth week of gestation, the intestine develops outside the abdominal cavity, returns to the abdomen, rotates counterclockwise, and becomes fixed. Malrotation is an error in rotation and fixation. The result is a narrow-based mesentery supplying the midgut, which is prone to twisting causing intestinal ischemia. Midgut volvulus results in proximal obstruction (at the level of third portion of duodenum), bilious emesis, and intestinal ischemia.

Malrotation with volvulus is rarely present at birth. An infant with volvulus goes from doing well to suddenly developing feeding intolerance and bilious emesis. An acutely ill infant undergoes immediate abdominal exploration. A UGI can be performed in a stable infant. The operation for malrotation with volvulus consists of (1) counterclockwise (from the surgeon's perspective) detorsion of the bowel, (2) division of abnormal peritoneal bands, (3) broadening the base of the mesentery, (4) appendectomy (to avoid confusion because cecum will be located in the left upper quadrant), and (5) placement of the small intestine to the right and colon to the left of midline.

7. **What is meconium ileus (MI)?**

MI is obstruction of the terminal ileum by viscid, tenacious meconium. MI is a complication of cystic fibrosis related to pancreatic insufficiency and abnormal intestinal glands producing hyperviscous mucous. Fifteen percent of neonates with cystic fibrosis present with MI. Infants present in the first few days of life with distention and bilious emesis. The obstruction is demonstrated with a water-soluble contrast enema (Gastrografin). The hyperosmolar contrast enema can break up the impacted meconium. The enemas can be repeated until the meconium is cleared. In about 40% of cases, surgery is necessary to relieve the obstruction. The objective of surgery is removal of the obstruction by limited resection or enterostomy with evacuation of the meconium and distal intestinal irrigation.

8. **What is Hirschsprung disease?**

Ganglion cells in the smooth muscle of the intestine wall facilitate peristalsis. When ganglion cells are absent, the intestine remains contracted and produces a functional obstruction. Typical presenting symptoms of Hirschsprung disease include failure to pass meconium within 24 hours of birth, distention, feeding intolerance, and bilious emesis. The disease begins just proximal to the dentate line and extends proximally. The majority of patients (approximately 85%) have involvement of the rectosigmoid colon. The remaining patients have varying degrees of proximal extension into the colon and small intestine. The condition is more common in boys (4:1). Contrast enema can show a contracted rectum with proximally dilated bowel; it is helpful for surgical planning. Definitive diagnosis of Hirschsprung disease is based on histologic evaluation of a distal rectal biopsy (usually suction rectal biopsy) showing the absence of ganglion cells, nerve hypertrophy, and lack of calretinin staining. Surgical correction consists of excision of the aganglionic intestine with a coloanal anastomosis, most commonly performed transanally.

9. **What is intussusception? What are the therapeutic options?**

Intussusception is the invagination of the proximal bowel (intussusceptum) into the distal bowel (intussuscipien). This results in intestinal obstruction and can lead to bowel ischemia. Lymphoid hyperplasia in the terminal ileum due to a viral infection is theorized to be the cause, resulting in the most common type of intussusception, ileocolic. Typical presenting symptoms of ileocolic intussusception include a previously healthy infant or toddler (3 months to 3 years of age) with intermittent crampy abdominal pain and bloody stools.

Ultrasonography showing a target or doughnut sign is confirmatory. A stable patient can undergo pneumatic air or hydrostatic barium enema reduction under fluoroscopic or ultrasonographic guidance. If there is concern for intestinal ischemia, perforation, or the enema is unsuccessful, laparoscopic or open reduction of the intussusception should be performed. The risk of recurrent intussusception is 10% with radiographic reduction and <7% with surgical reduction.

10. **What examples of neonatal obstruction can escape early detection and present later in life?**
   - Duodenal stenosis: This can escape early detection because the infant consumes a liquid or pureed diet. As solids are introduced, food may get stuck at the stenotic area. An UGI study will be diagnostic.
   - Malrotation: One-third of patients with malrotation are diagnosed after the first month of life. Malrotation with midgut volvulus should be suspected in any child who presents with bilious vomiting, signs of intestinal obstruction, and no history of abdominal surgery. Surgical correction of asymptomatic malrotation is controversial.
   - Hirschsprung disease: One-third of patients are diagnosed after 1 year of age. Older patients often present with chronic constipation, distention, and failure to thrive. A long history of constipation refractory to standard treatment mandates a rectal biopsy, especially in patients with trisomy 21.
   - Intussusception: A pathologic lead point (i.e., tumor, polyp, or Meckel's diverticulum) is present in one-third of older patients.

KEY POINTS: INTESTINAL OBSTRUCTION OF NEONATES AND INFANTS

1. Bilious emesis in an infant or child is an emergency and warrants immediate evaluation for malrotation with midgut volvulus. A UGI contrast study can be performed in a stable patient for diagnostic purposes. Surgical correction of malrotation with volvulus consists of detorsion of the intestine, lysis of abnormal peritoneal bands, widening of the mesentery, appendectomy, and placement of small intestine to the right and colon to the left of midline.
2. Intestinal atresia can occur anywhere along the GI tract. Duodenal atresia is most common (50%), followed by jejunoileal (45%) and colonic (5%) atresias. Contrast enema is useful for evaluation of distal intestinal obstruction.
3. Hirschsprung disease is due to absence of ganglion cells and typically affects the rectosigmoid colon.

BIBLIOGRAPHY

1. Langer JC. Hirschsprung disease. *Curr Opin Pediatr.* 2013;25(3):368–374.
2. Graziano K, Islam S, Dasgupta R, et al. Asymptomatic malrotation: diagnosis and surgical management: an American Pediatric Surgical Association outcomes and evidence based practice committee systematic review. *J Pediatr Surg.* 2015;50(10):1783–1790.
3. Escobar MA, Ladd AP, Grosfeld JL, et al. Duodenal atresia and stenosis: long-term follow-up over 30 years. *J Pediatr Surg.* 2004;39(6):867–871.
4. Somme S, To T. Factors determining the need for operative reduction in children with intussusception: a population-based study. *J Pediatr Surg.* 2006;41(5):1014–1019.
5. Stewart CL, Kulungowski AM. Rectal biopsies for Hirschsprung disease: patient characteristics by diagnosis and attending specialty. *J Pediatr Surg.* 2016;51(4):573–576.
6. Rattan KN, Singh J. Neonatal duodenal obstruction: a 15-year experience. *J Neonatal Surg.* 2016;5(2):13.

CHAPTER 88

ANORECTAL MALFORMATION

Alberto Peña, MD, FAAP, FACS, FRCS, Andrea Bischoff, MD

1. **What is an anorectal malformation?**
   Anorectal malformation is a term used to designate a series of congenital defects characterized by the absence of an anal opening. However, most of the time, the rectum is abnormally connected to the perineum or to the urogenital tract. Actually, only 5% of all cases suffer from a real blind rectum and half of that particular group suffers from Down syndrome.

   Fifty percent of the cases have a urologic abnormality, 30% a vertebral one, 25% a spinal cord anomaly, 10% a cardiac condition that requires treatment, and 8% esophageal atresia.

2. **How do you determine the severity of the defects?**
   The malformation occurs in the form of a spectrum. On the good side of the spectrum are malformations relatively easy to repair, with an excellent functional prognosis. On the bad side of the spectrum, we see complex defects, such as cloacas and cloacal exstrophies, that require a specialized team of surgeons to repair; and the patients suffer from very serious functional sequelae, mainly related to bowel and urinary control as well as sexual and fertility problems.

   Important prognostic factors include (1) characteristics of the sacrum, (2) presence or absence of tethered cord, and (3) specific type of malformation.

   The functional prognosis in patients who receive an adequate repair and have normal sacrum and no tethered cord is:
   In males:
   - Perineal fistula: 100% chances of bowel control
   - Anorectal malformation without fistula: 90%
   - Rectourethral bulbar fistula: 85%
   - Rectourethral prostatic fistula: 60%
   - Rectobladder neck fistula: 15%

   In females:
   - Perineal fistula: 100% chances of bowel control
   - Vestibular fistula: 93%
   - Cloaca with short common channel (<3 cm common channel)
     70% chances of bowel control
     80% chances of urinary control
   - Cloaca with a long common channel (>3 cm common channel)
     50% chances of bowel control
     20% chances of urinary control

   (Real rectovaginal fistulae cases are extremely rare.)

3. **What are the external signs that help to suspect and differentiate a malformation with good functional prognosis from a one with bad prognosis?**
   Signs of good functional prognosis:
   - Anal orifice in the perineum or the presence of subepithelial meconium
   - Good midline intergluteal groove (well-formed buttocks)
   - Prominent anal dimple
   - In females, the presence of three identifiable orifices (urethra, vagina, and anus)

   Signs of bad functional prognosis:
   - Flat bottom (absence of midline groove and anal dimple)
   - In females, presence of single perineal orifice (cloaca)

4. **What are the diagnostic and therapeutic priorities in the management of a newborn with anorectal malformation?**
First 24 hours:
- Do not operate; rule out important associated malformations
- ECHO cardiogram, babygram (esophageal atresia? Duodenal atresia? Spinal abnormalities? Sacral anomalies?)
- Kidney ultrasound: Renal anomalies, absent kidney
- Pelvic ultrasound (females with cloaca): Rule out hydrocolpos

After 24 hours:
- Make a decision to operate (colostomy or anoplasty). Depending on the experience of the surgeon: Colostomy to be done in the majority of malformations. Anoplasty in cases of perineal fistulae, in some cases of vestibular fistula

5. **What type of colostomy is indicated in cases of anorectal malformations?**
- Totally diverting colostomy (separated stomas) to avoid passing of stool distally and contaminate the urinary tract
- Located in the descending colon to leave enough distal colon to facilitate the pull-through
- Patients with cloaca associated with hydrocolpos require a colostomy and a permanent drainage of the hydrocolpos with a transabdominal catheter

6. **After the colostomy is done, when is the main repair performed?**
Depending on the experience of the surgeons and the general condition of the patient, the main repair can be done as soon as the patient shows normal growth and development.

7. **What type of operations are used to repair anorectal malformations?**
The most common type of repair is called posterior sagittal anorectoplasty (PSARP). It consists of approaching the defect through a midsagittal, posterior incision in between both buttocks. To identify the sphincter mechanism with an electrical stimulator, to separate the rectum form the urogenital tract under direct vision, mobilize the rectum, and place it in the center of the sphincter mechanism.

In cases of perineal fistula, the procedure follows the same principles but is done with a small incision.

An abdominal approach (laparotomy or laparoscopy) is indicated to find and mobilize an extremely highly located rectum in 10% of the male cases and 35% of the patients with cloacas.

8. **What are the indications of a laparoscopic approach in cases of anorectal malformations?**
The ideal indication is in those cases that require a laparotomy. Depending on the experience of the surgeon, some cases of rectoprostatic fistula can also be repaired via laparoscopy.

Some surgeons have tried to repair cloacas laparoscopically. They have actually repaired only the rectal component of the malformation.

KEY POINTS: ANORECTAL MALFORMATIONS

1. *Anorectal malformation* is a term used to designate a series of congenital anomalies of the anus and rectum, characterized by the absence of an external anal opening. The rectum is connected to the perineum or to the urogenital tract in 95% of the cases.
2. These malformations present in the form of a spectrum, including benign defects in one extreme and very severe and complex in the other.
3. The majority of cases require a colostomy at birth, and later on, a procedure called PSARP. Ten percent of the male cases and 35% of the cloacas in females need, in addition, a laparotomy or laparoscopy. Benign malformations can be treated with an anoplasty at birth.
4. Patients with anorectal malformations do not die from the anorectal defect, but rather from one of the associated conditions (cardiac and/or urologic).

BIBLIOGRAPHY

1. Peña A, Bischoff A. *The Surgical Treatment of Colorectal Problems in Children.* Gewerbestrasse: Springer International Publishing; 2015.
2. Bischoff A, Levitt MA. Update on the management of anorectal malformations. *Pediatr Surg Int.* 2013;29(9):899–904.
3. Bischoff A, Frischer J. Anorectal malformation without fistula: a defect with unique characteristics. *Pediatric Surg Int.* 2014;30(8):763–766.
4. Fernandez E, Bischoff A. Esophageal atresia in patients with anorectal malformations. *Pediatr Surg Int.* 2014;30(8):767–771.
5. Bischoff A, Martinez-Leo B. Laparoscopic approach in the management of anorectal malformation. *Pediatr Surg Int.* 2015;31(5):431–437.

CHAPTER 89

TRACHEOESOPHAGEAL MALFORMATIONS

Ann M. Kulungowski, MD

1. **What are tracheoesophageal fistula and esophageal atresia?**
   The pathogenesis for the development of esophageal atresia, with and without fistula, is still unknown. Theories include imperfect separation of the tracheoesophageal septum or defective pharyngeal arch development. More than 50% of cases of esophageal atresia with tracheoesophageal atresia are associated with other anomalies; 10% are found in specific chromosomal or single gene disorders.

2. **Describe the three most common anatomic patterns of tracheoesophageal disorders and their relative incidence.**
   The overall incidence of esophageal atresia, with or without tracheoesophageal fistula, is 1:3500 live-born infants.
   - Proximal esophageal atresia with distal tracheoesophageal fistula: 85% (type C, proximal pouch with distal fistula)
   - Pure esophageal atresia: 10% (type A)
   - Tracheoesophageal fistula without atresia: 5% (type E, H fistula)

3. **What are the other common anomalies that occur with tracheoesophageal malformations?**
   Tracheoesophageal fistula and esophageal atresia occur as early disturbances in organogenesis during weeks 3–8 of development. Approximately 70% of affected infants have at least one associated congenital malformation. The most common anomalies include cardiovascular (35%), genitourinary (25%), gastrointestinal (25%), musculoskeletal (15%), and central nervous system (7%). The incidence of VACTERL association, which incudes vertebral, anorectal, cardiac, tracheoesophageal, renal, and limb anomalies, in the esophageal atresia population is 20%.

4. **What are additional prognostic factors to consider when evaluating an infant with esophageal atresia with and without tracheoesophageal fistula?**
   Infants weighing 2 kg or more without cardiac anomalies have a better prognosis than those weighing <2 kg with heart defects. Infants without major additional anomalies generally undergo early repair with near 100% survival. Severely premature infants or those with life-threatening anomalies may benefit from delayed repair. Infants with chromosomal anomalies tend to have poorer outcomes.

5. **Describe the clinical presentation, diagnosis, and preoperative management of esophageal atresia with distal tracheoesophageal fistula.**
   The earliest clinical signs of esophageal atresia with distal tracheoesophageal fistula include excessive salivation and pooling of secretions in the pharynx. The first feeding results in choking, regurgitation, and coughing. Respiratory distress develops because of aspiration of secretions or feeds from the proximal pouch. Reflux of gastric acid into the airways and lungs via the distal tracheoesophageal fistula contributes to respiratory distress. A nasogastric tube cannot be advanced into the stomach. Radiographs demonstrate a blind-ending proximal esophageal pouch. An air-filled stomach and normal bowel gas pattern are present because of the anomalous connection of the distal esophagus (fistula) to the airway. The infant is maintained in the semi-upright position with sump catheter drainage of the proximal esophageal pouch to minimize lung contamination. Associated anomalies should be identified. An echocardiogram should be obtained before proceeding to the operating room.

6. **Describe the clinical presentation, diagnosis, and preoperative management of isolated esophageal atresia.**
   Isolated esophageal atresia is associated with excessive secretions, choking, and regurgitation of feeds. A nasogastric tube cannot be placed. The radiograph demonstrates a gasless abdomen. A sump catheter is placed in the proximal pouch to minimize aspiration. Gastrostomy is generally performed

within the first 48 hours of life for enteral nutrition. Gap length is determined between the proximal and distal esophageal pouches. The esophagus is either placed on traction (Foker technique) or allowed to grow to reduce gap distance for eventual anastomosis.

7. **Describe the clinical presentation, diagnosis, and preoperative management of tracheoesophageal fistula without esophageal atresia.**
These infants frequently choke or have cyanotic spells with feeds due to reflux from the esophagus into the lungs via the anomalous connection between esophagus and airway. The diagnosis is often delayed. Older infants and children may have recurrent pneumonias or reactive airway disease. Prone pull-back contrast esophagram can be diagnostic; bronchoscopy and esophagoscopy are confirmatory.

8. **How are tracheoesophageal malformations surgically corrected?**
The surgical goals are separating the pathologic connection of the esophagus to the trachea, eliminating contamination of the airway, and establishing esophageal continuity for feeding. Correction of esophageal atresia with distal tracheoesophageal fistula can be performed open via a thoracotomy or thoracoscopically. The first goal is ligation of the tracheoesophageal fistula followed by an end-to-end esophageal anastomosis when possible. An esophagram is obtained five to seven days postoperatively. If no leak is present, oral feedings are commenced. The pleural drain is removed.

In infants with pure esophageal atresia, an anastomosis between the proximal and distal esophagus is usually attempted after a period of waiting or traction. If the distance between the two ends is too long, the stomach can be used as a conduit to allow for a connection between the proximal esophagus and the bowel.

9. **What are the pros and cons of open versus thoracoscopic repairs for tracheoesophageal fistula with esophageal atresia?**
The open approach is the gold standard approach for repairing the anomaly. It avoids hypercapnia and allows for an extrapleural repair. Ventilator and hospital days are equivalent between the two approaches. Scoliosis and scapula alata occur more commonly in patients who have undergone open repairs versus thoracoscopic repair. The major advantage of the thoracoscopic approach is avoidance of an open thoracotomy and scar. Thoracoscopic repair is associated with a higher rate of vocal cord paresis/paralysis due to dissection of the esophagus high into the thoracic inlet. It appears that there is no difference between the approaches with regard to anastomotic stricture, leak, or tracheomalacia.

10. **What are the early and late complications of surgical repair?**
Early complications
    Anastomotic disruption: 5%
    Recurrent TEF: 5%
    Anastomotic leak: 15%
    Tracheomalacia: 15%
Early complications are related to basic aspects of wound healing, which includes blood supply and tension.

Late complications
    Anastomotic stricture: 25%
    Gastroesophageal reflux: 50%
    Esophageal dysmotility: 100%

11. **How are esophageal strictures managed?**
Many esophageal strictures occur in the first weeks to months after the repair. The presentation of an infant with a stricture is variable. Symptoms include drooling, pooling of secretions, choking, need for prolonged and frequent feeds, and emesis. Most strictures respond to one to three dilations performed in the first 6 months of life. Refractory strictures can be related to gastroesophageal reflux. Medical treatment of gastroesophageal reflux is important in all patients. In general, the longer the gap, the more gastroesophageal reflux.

KEY POINTS: TRACHEOESOPHAGEAL MALFORMATIONS

1. The three most common variants are proximal esophageal atresia with distal tracheoesophageal fistula, isolated esophageal atresia, and tracheoesophageal fistula without esophageal atresia.
2. Surgical treatment includes separation of the pathologic connection between the esophagus and airway and establishment of esophageal continuity.
3. Common complications of repair of tracheoesophageal malformations include leak, stricture, and gastroesophageal reflux.

BIBLIOGRAPHY

1. Davenport M, Rothenberg SS. The great debate: open or thoracoscopic repair for oesophageal atresia or diaphragmatic hernia. *J Pediatr Surg.* 2015;50(2):240–246.
2. Pierro A. Hypercapnia and acidosis during the thoracoscopic repair of oesophageal atresia and congenital diaphragmatic hernia. *J Pediatr Surg.* 2015;50(2):247–249.
3. Bairdain S, Hamilton TE, Smithers CJ, et al. Foker process for the correction of long gap esophageal atresia: primary treatment versus secondary treatment after prior esophageal surgery. *J Pediatr Surg.* 2015;50(6):933–937.
4. Woo S, Lau S, Yoo E. Thoracoscopic versus open repair of tracheoesophageal fistulas and rates of vocal cord paresis. *J Pediatr Surg.* 2015;50(12):2016–2018.

CHAPTER 90

CONGENITAL DIAPHRAGMATIC HERNIA

Shannon N. Acker, MD, Timothy M. Crombleholme, MD

1. **What is the most common type of congenital diaphragmatic hernia (CDH)?**
   Congenital abnormalities of the diaphragm include a posterolateral defect (Bochdalek hernia), an anteromedial defect (Morgagni hernia), or the eventration (central weakening) of the diaphragm. The Bochdalek hernia is the most common variant and accounts for approximately 80% of CDH cases. This defect is most common on the left (80%), 20% are right-sided lesions, and <1% are bilateral.

2. **How is CDH Diagnosed?**
   CDH is usually diagnosed based on prenatal ultrasound (US) when the stomach is detected in the fetal thorax or at the same cross-sectional level as the heart. US may be obtained as a part of a normal prenatal screening examination or to evaluate a finding of polyhydramnios. Mean age at diagnosis is 24 weeks. Occasionally, the diagnosis of CDH is not made prenatally but may present soon after birth. Neonatal respiratory distress is the most common manifestation of CDH. At birth or shortly thereafter, the infant can develop severe dyspnea, retractions, and cyanosis. On physical examination, breath sounds are diminished on the ipsilateral side. Heart sounds can be heard more easily in the contralateral chest, and the abdomen is scaphoid because of the herniation of abdominal viscera into the chest.

3. **How is the diagnosis confirmed?**
   A chest radiograph can be obtained at birth to confirm the diagnosis. The radiograph demonstrates multiple loops of air-filled intestine or stomach in the ipsilateral thorax. If a chest radiograph is obtained before entry of significant amounts of air into the bowel, a confusing pattern of mediastinal shift, cardiac displacement, and opacification of the hemithorax may be observed. Insertion of a nasogastric (NG) tube followed by repeat chest radiograph often demonstrates the tube (i.e., stomach) in the chest and confirms the diagnosis.

4. **Are other anomalies associated with CDH?**
   The incidence of associated congenital anomalies among infants with CDH ranges from 10% to 50%. Fewer than 10% of patients with multiple major concurrent anomalies survive. Excluding intestinal malrotation and pulmonary hypoplasia, cardiac anomalies (24%–63%) are the most frequent, followed by skeletal defects (32%), genitourinary (23%), gastrointestinal (17%), central nervous system (14%), and other pulmonary (5%) anomalies.

5. **What therapeutic measures should be initiated to stabilize an infant with CDH and respiratory distress at birth?**
   If a prenatal diagnosis of CDH is made, the fetus and mother should be referred to a tertiary care center, preferably with expertise in CDH management. After birth, resuscitation should begin with endotracheal intubation and NG tube insertion. Bag-mask ventilation should be avoided to prevent gastric distention. Arterial and venous access should be obtained via the umbilicus. It is important to maintain temperature, glucose, and volume homeostasis. Goals of mechanical ventilation include maintaining a preductal PO_2 >60 mm Hg and PCO_2 <60 mm Hg. If conventional ventilator settings fail to achieve these goals, high-frequency oscillatory ventilation can be used to stabilize the infant.

6. **When should operative repair occur?**
   The optimal timing of operative repair is still unclear. Previously, infants were taken emergently to the operating room for reduction of the intraabdominal contents and repair of the hernia soon after birth. More recent data suggest that operative repair should be delayed until pulmonary hypertension and the infant's hemodynamics have stabilized. The length of preoperative stabilization is highly variable, ranging from days to weeks.

7. **What operative approach is used to repair a diaphragmatic defect?**
There is no single best approach to CDH repair. The operation can be performed from either the abdomen (laparotomy or laparoscopy) or the chest (thoracotomy or thoracoscopy). Thoracoscopic repair may be associated with higher rates of recurrence and unacceptably high levels of acidosis due to CO_2 insufflation and is generally reserved for stable infants or older children with delayed diagnosis of CDH. The choice of approach is dependent on the surgeon's preference. Principles of repair are the same whether approached from the chest or the abdomen—reduce the abdominal contents; assess the amount of diaphragmatic tissue available for repair; and decide whether to repair the defect primarily, using prosthetic tissue, or with the patient's own tissue. Recent data suggest an abdominal wall muscle flap is safe, even in the setting of extracorporeal membrane oxygenation (ECMO) with an acceptably low rate of recurrence.

8. **What factors predict morbidity and mortality in infants with CDH?**
The degree of pulmonary hypoplasia and severity of pulmonary hypertension are the biggest predictors of morbidity and mortality among infants with CDH. In infants with CDH, the lungs exhibit decreased alveolarization with decreased surface area available for gas exchange as well as immaturity of pulmonary vasculature with hyperplasia of the pulmonary arteries. These histologic changes contribute to elevated pulmonary vascular resistance and pulmonary arterial hypertension. This then leads to right-to-left shunting of deoxygenated blood to the systemic circulation through the patent ductus arteriosus and patent foramen ovale then causing hypoxemia, acidosis, and shock.

9. **What strategies can be used to treat pulmonary hypertension among infants with CDH?**
    a. Monitoring: Oximetry or arterial sampling (preductal in the right upper extremity; postductal in the lower extremity) permits early detection of shunting of deoxygenated blood to the systemic circulation.
    b. Ventilation: Hypercarbia is corrected by mechanical ventilation with adequate sedation.
    c. Oxygenation: Hypoxemia is corrected by adequate ventilation and high concentrations of inspired oxygen (generally, fraction of inspired oxygen = 100%).
    d. Resuscitation: Metabolic acidosis is managed by restoring adequate tissue perfusion (intravenous fluids or blood, inotropes, and sodium bicarbonate).
    e. Rescue: Salvage therapies include administration of pulmonary vasodilators via the ventilatory circuit (nitric oxide) or systemic circulation (Priscoline, prostaglandin E2), high-frequency ventilation, and ECMO.

10. **What is the survival rate for patients with CDH?**
The overall survival rate is 60%–90%. The major determinants of survival are the degree of pulmonary hypoplasia, severity of pulmonary hypertension, and associated major congenital anomalies. Late deaths occur in approximately 10% of children, secondary to persistent pulmonary hypertension.

11. **Does in utero intervention have a role in the treatment of patients with CDH?**
Fetal intervention for CDH is becoming more common. Early trials failed to demonstrate a benefit with in utero repair of the defect. However, current research has focused on the role of tracheal occlusion during the fetal period as a means to promote lung growth. Techniques of in-utero fetoscopic endoluminal tracheal occlusion (FETO) promoting lung growth and development followed by postnatal repair of the diaphragmatic hernia are currently being investigated. Early trials of FETO suggest a potential survival advantage compared to control groups with similar disease severity.

KEY POINTS: CONGENITAL DIAPHRAGMATIC HERNIA

1. CDH is usually diagnosed in the prenatal period based on routine ultrasonography.
2. Infants with CDH usually develop respiratory distress at birth.
3. CDH should be repaired when the baby is stable from a pulmonary hypertension and hemodynamic standpoint.
4. Morbidity and mortality in CDH are determined by the severity of pulmonary hypertension and degree of pulmonary hypoplasia.

BIBLIOGRAPHY

1. Chiu PP, Sauer C, Mihailovic A, et al. The price of success in the management of congenital diaphragmatic hernia: is improved survival accompanied by an increase in long-term morbidity? *J Pediatr Surg*. 2006;41(5):888–892.
2. Clugston RD, Greer JJ. Diaphragm development and congenital diaphragmatic hernia. *Semin Pediatr Surg*. 2007;16(2):94–100.
3. Kinsella JP, Ivy DD. Pulmonary vasodilator therapy in congenital diaphragmatic hernia: acute, late, and chronic pulmonary hypertension. *Semin Perinatol*. 2005;29(2):123–128.
4. Kitano Y. Prenatal intervention for congenital diaphragmatic hernia. *Semin Pediatr Surg*. 2007;16(2):101–108.
5. Lally KP, Lally PA, Lasky RE, et al. Defect size determines survival in infants with congenital diaphragmatic hernia. *Pediatrics*. 2007;120(3):e651–e657.
6. Logan JW, Rice HE. Congenital diaphragmatic hernia: a systematic review and summary of best-evidence practice strategies. *J Perinatol*. 2007;27(9):535–549.
7. Migliazza L, Bellan C. Retrospective study of 111 cases of congenital diaphragmatic hernia treated with early high-frequency oscillatory ventilation and presurgical stabilization. *J Pediatr Surg*. 2007;42(9):1526–1532.
8. Rozmiarek AJ, Qureshi FG. Factors influencing survival in newborns with congenital diaphragmatic hernia: the relative role of timing of surgery. *J Pediatr Surg*. 2004;39(6):821–824.
9. Stolar CJH, Dillon PW. Congenital diaphragmatic hernia and eventration. In: Coran AG, Caldamone A, eds. *Pediatric Surgery*. 7th ed. Philadelphia, PA: Elsevier, 2012;809–824.
10. Gander JW, Fisher JC, Gross ER, et al. Early recurrence of congenital diaphragmatic hernia is higher after thoracoscopic than open repair: a single institutional study. *J Pediatr Surg*. 2011;46(7):1303–1308.
11. Barnhart DC, Jacques E, Scaife ER, et al. Split abdominal wall muscle flap repair vs patch repair of large congenital diaphragmatic hernias. *J Pediatr Surg*. 2012;47(1):81–86.
12. Al-Maary J, Eastwood MP. Fetal tracheal occlusion for severe pulmonary hypoplasia in isolated congenital diaphragmatic hernia: a systematic review and meta-analysis of survival. *Ann Surg*. 2016;264(6):929–933.
13. Wynn J, Krishnan U, Aspelund G, et al. Outcomes of congenital diaphragmatic hernia in the modern era of management. *J Pediatr*. 2013;163(1):114–119.

CHAPTER 91

ABDOMINAL TUMORS

Ann M. Kulungowski, MD, Jennifer L. Bruny, MD, FACS

1. **What are the most common malignant solid abdominal tumors in children?**
   a. Neuroblastomas are derived from neural crest tissue. In the abdomen, they originate from the adrenal glands and parasympathetic ganglia.
   b. Wilms' tumors, nephroblastomas, are derived from the kidney. The classic Wilms' tumor consists of three elements—blastemal, stromal, and epithelial.
   c. Hepatoblastomas originate in the liver.

2. **How does the presentation of neuroblastoma differ from Wilms' tumor?**

Table 91.1 Differences Between Wilms' Tumor And Neuroblastoma

	WILMS' TUMOR	NEUROBLASTOMA
Age at presentation	3–4 y	1–2 y
Crosses midline	Rare	Common
Surface on palpation	Smooth	Knobbly
X-ray calcifications	No	Yes

3. **How are Wilms' tumors and neuroblastomas treated?**

Table 91.2 Treatment Of Wilms' Tumors And Neuroblastomas

TREATMENT	WILMS' TUMOR	NEUROBLASTOMA
Primary surgical excision	Important	Important (less likely)
Chemotherapy	Enormous impact	Less responsive

4. **What are the major prognostic factors in Wilms' tumor?**
   The current prognostic factors include histology, stage, age, tumor weight, response to therapy, and loss of heterozygosity (LOH). Histology and stage are the most important. Favorable histology tumors comprise 90% of the unilateral and bilateral tumors. Anaplastic histology is unfavorable histology and indicates a tumor's resistance to chemotherapy and not its aggressiveness. LOH on chromosomes at 1p and 16q portends a worse prognosis.

5. **What are the major prognostic factors in neuroblastoma?**
   Age at diagnosis is the best predictor of outcome. Infants <18 months of age have survival rates of approximately 75%; survival in children >18 months of age declines to 30%. Tumors with favorable histology (stroma rich) have improved survival compared to unfavorable histology (stroma poor). Tumors with amplification of the *MYCN* oncogene (>10 copies), allelic loss on chromosome 1p (1p36), diploidy, and a high mitotic karyorrhexis index are associated with poorer outcomes.

6. What are the differences between hepatoblastoma and hepatocellular carcinomas? How are the tumors treated?

Table 91.3 Differences Between Hepatoblastoma And Hepatocellular Carcinoma

	HEPATOBLASTOMA	HEPATOCELLULAR CARCINOMA
Age at presentation	6 m–3 y	>10 y
Alpha-fetoprotein	Elevated in 90%	Elevated in 50%
Risk factors	Prematurity Very low birth weight	Hepatitis B Cirrhosis
Location of tumor	Solitary (80%) Right hepatic lobe (60%)	Solitary and multifocal
Treatment	Surgical resection (transplant) and adjuvant chemotherapy	Surgical resection and transplant Chemoresistant

KEY POINTS: ABDOMINAL TUMORS

1. Neuroblastoma, Wilms' tumor, and hepatoblastoma are the three most common solid intraabdominal malignancies of childhood.
2. Age is the most important prognostic factor for patients with neuroblastoma (<18 months have a better prognosis).
3. Hepatoblastomas occur in infants and younger children. Hepatocellular carcinoma occurs in school age children (>10 years of age).

BIBLIOGRAPHY

1. Englum BR, Rialon KL, Speicher PJ, et al. Value of surgical resection in children with high-risk neuroblastoma. *Pediatr Blood Cancer.* 2015;62(9):1529–1535.
2. Dome JS, Graf N, Geller JI, et al. Advances in Wilms tumor treatment and biology: progress through international collaboration. *J Clin Oncol.* 2015;33(27):2999–3007.
3. Czauderna P, Haeberle B, Hiyama E, et al. The Children's Hepatic tumors International Collaboration (CHIC): Novel global rare tumor database yields new prognostic factors in hepatoblastoma and becomes a research model. *Eur J Cancer.* 2016;52:92–101.

CHAPTER 92

CONGENITAL CYSTS AND SINUSES OF THE NECK

Ann M. Kulungowski, MD

1. **What are branchial cleft anomalies?**

   They can occur as cysts, sinuses, and fistulas found in the head and neck related to incomplete obliteration of the first, second, third, or fourth (extremely rare) branchial clefts during early fetal development. Cysts have mucosal or epithelial lining but no external openings. Sinuses may communicate either externally with the skin or internally with the pharynx. Fistulae, however, connect to both.

2. **How do patients with branchial cleft anomalies present?**

   A complete fistula or sinus presents with intermittent drainage of a mucoid fluid on the neck. A cyst typically presents later with a mass (sterile or infected). Complete excision is the goal because of the risks of infection, enlargement, or malignancy. Elective excision is recommended beyond 3–6 months of age. An infected branchial cleft remnant is preferably treated with systemic antibiotics and aspiration; resection is performed after infection resolution.

3. **Which branchial cleft anomaly is the most common?**

   Second branchial cleft anomalies are by far the most common. The typical presentation is a small draining cutaneous pit along the anterior border of the lower sternocleidomastoid muscle. The sinus tract travels through the carotid bifurcation, over the glossopharyngeal and hypoglossal nerves, and enters the tonsillar fossa of the pharynx.

Table 92.1 Branchial Cleft Anomalies

BRANCHIAL CLEFT	INTERNAL OPENING	EXTERIOR OPENING	FREQUENCY
First	External auditory canal	Angle of the jaw	8%
Second	Tonsillar fossa	Anterior border of SCM	90%
Third	Piriform sinus	Suprasternal notch	<1%

4. **What are the operative hazards of first and third branchial cleft remnant excisions?**

   The first branchial cleft anomalies are closely associated with the parotid gland and facial nerve. They are commonly in the preauricular region. Third branchial cleft anomalies are near the superior laryngeal and recurrent laryngeal nerves.

5. **What is a dermoid cyst?**

   Dermoid cysts are thought to arise from elements trapped during fusion of the anterior branchial arches. They are composed of ectodermal and mesodermal elements. Dermoids are typically well circumscribed, lined by a squamous epithelium, and contain sebaceous debris. The overlying skin can be adherent; a small pit may be visible. They can become infected. Complete excision is appropriate.

6. **What is a thyroglossal duct cyst?**

   Thyroglossal duct cysts are a common midline congenital cervical anomaly. They occur along the path of thyroid descent from the foramen cecum at the base of the tongue to the lower neck. They are caused by failure of this path to obliterate. The thyroid descends before formation of the hyoid cartilage; the tract may pass through the hyoid.

7. **How do thyroglossal duct cysts present?**
They present as a paramidline/midline mass in the upper neck and are intimately associated with the hyoid bone. The cysts often move cephalad with swallowing or tongue protrusion. When infected, the patient may present with fever, tenderness, and erythema.

8. **How are thyroglossal duct cysts treated?**
Surgical resection is indicated to avoid infection and malignancy. The goal is complete resection of the cyst, its tract up to the base of the tongue, and the central portion of the hyoid bone (i.e., the Sistrunk procedure). Recurrences are due to incomplete excision of the tract or infection.

9. **What is a lymphatic malformation?**
Lymphatic malformations arise because of errors in vasculogenesis and are slow-flow lesions. They are not vascular tumors. Lymphatic malformations may involve any location but are common in the head and neck. Cervical lymphatic malformations can extend into the mediastinum. They can present as a bulky mass with a bluish hue visualized through the skin. Intralesional bleeding and infection are the most common complications.

10. **How are cystic lymphatic malformations classified and treated?**
There are three morphologic types of cystic lymphatic malformations—macrocystic, microcystic, or mixed macrocystic and microcystic. The type is designated by whether or not the cystic cavity can be aspirated to achieve visible decompression. Sclerotherapy is the often-preferred primary treatment for lymphatic malformations. The only potential curative therapy for lymphatic malformations is surgical resection. This can be tedious in the head and neck. Neurovascular structures should be preserved.

KEY POINTS: CONGENITAL CYSTS AND SINUSES OF THE NECK

1. Second branchial cleft anomalies found along the anterior border of the sternocleidomastoid are the most common branchial cleft anomalies.
2. Thyroglossal duct cyst is treated by complete surgical excision of the cyst, its tract, and central portion of the hyoid bone.
3. Lymphatic malformations in the head and neck can be macro-, micro-, or mixed lesions.

BIBLIOGRAPHY

1. LaRiviere CA, Waldhausen JH. Congenital cervical cysts, sinuses, and fistulae in pediatric surgery. *Surg Clin North Am.* 2012;92(3):583–597, viii.
2. Gaddikeri S, Vattoth S, Gaddikeri RS, et al. Congenital cystic neck masses: embryology and imaging appearances, with clinicopathological correlation. *Curr Probl Diagn Radiol.* 2014;43(2):55–67.
3. Oomen KP, Modi VK, Maddalozzo J. Thyroglossal duct cyst and ectopic thyroid: surgical management. *Otolaryngol Clin North Am.* 2015;48(1):15–27.
4. Foley LS, Kulungowski AM. Vascular Anomalies in Pediatrics. *Adv Pediatr.* 2015;62(1):227–255.

X
TRANSPLANTATION

CHAPTER 93

LIVER TRANSPLANTATION

Megan Adams, MD, Thomas Bak, MD

1. **When and where was the first liver transplant performed?**
   Dr. Thomas Starzl performed the first liver transplant at the University of Colorado in Denver in March of 1963. Early results were dismal but laid the foundation for the future of transplantation.

2. **Is liver transplantation a safe and effective operation?**
   Liver transplant is still a relatively new procedure. As recently as 30 years ago, it was still considered experimental and not universally approved by insurance companies. It has evolved into the standard of care for end-stage liver disease, with survival rates well over 90% expected at 1 year.

3. **What are the most common indications for liver transplantation in the United States?**
   Indication for liver transplant come in a wide variety of acute and chronic disease processes. Viral hepatitis (B and C), alcoholic liver disease (Laennec's), and nonalcoholic steatohepatitis (NASH) remain the most common diagnoses. Primary biliary cirrhosis and primary sclerosing cholangitis are the most common cholestatic diseases. Budd-Chiari syndrome, autoimmune hepatitis, malignant neoplasms, fulminant hepatic failure, and metabolic disorders also are indications.

4. **Has the recipient diagnosis shifted over the years?**
   Yes. Initial liver transplants were performed for tumors and alcoholic cirrhosis. The past 2 decades have seen viral hepatitis as the most common diagnosis. With the improved treatment options for viral disease and the continued increase in our population obesity levels, NASH will be the most common transplant diagnosis within the next 10 years.

5. **What factors control allocation of livers?**
   A standardized nationwide scoring system is utilized to stratify patients on the waiting list. This scoring system is named MELD (Model for End-Stage Liver Disease) and is a logarithmic equation utilizing serum bilirubin, creatinine, and international normalized ratio. This numeric value ranks patients based on their illness severity and projected mortality rates. Upgraded point totals may be petitioned for when certain criteria are met. Length of time on the list is a minimal factor in getting a liver transplant.

6. **Has the severity of illness in patients requiring transplant shifted?**
   Patients on the waiting list are much more ill than previously. Greater than 40% of patients on the list have a MELD >30, with 26% having MELD >35.

7. **What are some common postoperative complications?**
   Postoperative bleeding due to coagulopathy is the most common postoperative complication. Others include infection, biliary leaks/strictures, vascular thrombosis/stenosis, and rejection. Primary non-function of the graft is rare (1%–2%), but is life threatening and requires emergent retransplant.

8. **What is the piggy-back technique?**
   It is a surgical technique in which the recipient's native liver is carefully dissected free from the vena cava and the donor liver is sewn to a common cuff of the recipient's hepatic veins. Using this method, it is possible to do the entire liver transplant without occluding the vena cava blood flow.

9. **Are living-donor liver transplants available?**
   Yes. Initially utilized in the pediatric population, live-donor liver transplantation has become an important addition to the field. Both right and left lobe adult-to-adult liver transplants are being performed successfully. Both donor and recipient lobes regenerate to near normal size quickly after the operation. This is a valuable option for people sick enough to need transplant but with insufficiently high MELD scores to get a cadaver graft.

10. **Are recent advances in medical therapy for hepatitis C changing liver transplant practices?**
    Over the past year, new therapies for all genotypes of hepatitis C have been introduced, with minimal side effects and near 100% response rates. In the past, the transplanted liver would be reinfected

with hepatitis C, resulting in lower long-term survival rates in this patient population. Now most patients can be treated and be viral negative at time of transplant and, in effect, be cured of the disease.

11. **Can a liver cancer patient be transplanted?**
If a patient has a primary hepatic tumor that is not resectable and within certain criteria, they can still be eligible for transplant. Even with a MELD upgrade, typical wait times are well over a year. Bridging techniques such as chemoembolization or ablation are used. Live donor transplant is also a good option in these cases.

12. **What are some indications that used to be absolute contraindications for liver transplant?**
Cholangiocarcinoma patients and patients with HIV are both potential transplant candidates when specific criteria are met.

13. **Should non-heart beating donors be used for transplant?**
Non-heart beating donors or donation after cardiac death (DCD) livers are being used more commonly. The donor must die quickly after extubation to limit warm ischemia time to the liver. When selected properly, DCD livers are able to be used successfully. There is a higher biliary complication rate and retransplant rate in these livers, but we continue to use them because of the severe cadaveric organ shortage.

14. **Should organ donors be compensated?**
There has been much debate over this issue here and across the world. Organ tourism exists where recipients travel to other areas of the world and buy live-donor organs. Compensation or other incentives for either live donation or cadaver donation would increase the number of organs available for transplant. Ethicists argue that this would be socially biased against disadvantaged people. Presumed donor consent (organ donor unless specifically opts out) is another controversial way to increase available organs.

15. **Should liver transplants be performed in individuals with alcoholic liver disease?**
Transplant centers have strict criteria that they must abide by when listing a patient with a history of alcoholism. Extensive social-worker interaction, psychologic counseling, and documented abstinence are all essential. Acute alcoholic decompensation in young, otherwise healthy people who will die without urgent liver transplant remains a center-specific decision. These cases have the potential for most useful life-year use of livers but also have higher recidivism rates.

KEY POINTS: LIVER TRANSPLANTATION

1. The most common indication for liver transplantation in the United States is noncholestatic cirrhosis, usually for viral disease.
2. Optimal cold ischemia time for the liver is <12 hours.
3. A transjugular intrahepatic portosystemic shunt can be used in potential transplant recipients as a bridge to transplantation.

BIBLIOGRAPHY

1. Trotter JF, Wachs M. Adult-to-adult transplantation of the right hepatic lobe from a living donor. *N Engl J Med.* 2002;346(14):1074–1082.
2. Townsend CM, Beauchamp RD. *Sabiston Textbook of Surgery: The Biological Basis of Modern Surgical Practice.* 19th ed. Philadelphia: Elsevier; 2012:655–665.

CHAPTER 94

KIDNEY TRANSPLANTATION

Thomas Pshak, MD, Thomas Bak, MD

1. **When was the first successful kidney transplant performed?**
   In 1954, Dr. Joseph Murray successfully transplanted a kidney between identical twins at the Brigham Hospital in Boston.

2. **What are the most common causes for end-stage renal disease (ESRD) in the United States?**
   In adults, hypertension and diabetes are now the most common cause of ESRD, whereas glomerular disease, which used to be the most prevalent, now accounts for only 21%. Other causes are interstitial and cystic diseases. In children, the most common cause is congenital anomalies of the kidney and urinary tract, accounting for approximately 50%.

3. **Why is kidney transplantation considered a better option than dialysis?**
   Kidney transplantation offers patients better long-term outcomes. Quality of life is improved and overall survival is projected to be 10 years longer than if the patient remained on dialysis.

4. **In general, how long is kidney graft survival (Table 94.1)?**
   This largely depends on the type of donor, namely donation after cardiac death (DCD), standard criteria donor (SCD), extended criteria donor (ECD), or living donor. In general, DCD kidneys have higher rates of delayed graft function but nearly equivalent overall graft survival rates compared to SCD grafts.

Table 94.1 Graft Survival

DONOR TYPE	Graft Survival (%)		
	1 Y	5 Y	10 Y
DCD & SCD	91.7	70.4	43.7
ECD	84.8	54.8	26.3
Living	95.7	80.8	57.9

5. **How long can be kidneys be kept on ice?**
   Kidneys are more resilient than other organs and can maintain function for up to 72 hours. However, delayed graft function significantly increases at 24 hours. Most centers aim to transplant under 36 hours. Perfusion pumps can be used if long cold ischemia time is anticipated.

6. **What location is a kidney transplant placed?**
   The kidney can be placed in the left or right iliac fossa, most commonly the right. A Gibson incision is used, and the retroperitoneal space is entered to expose the external iliac vessels and bladder. An end-to-side vascular anastomosis is performed, followed by a ureteral implant into the bladder. For third or more transplants, an intraabdominal location is usually used.

7. **Are the native kidneys removed at the time of transplant?**
   This is rarely done nowadays. The indications for this are chronic infection (pyelonephritis), symptomatic polycystic kidneys, intractable hypertension, heavy proteinuria, or tumor.

8. **What are the contraindications to living kidney donation?**
   The general contraindications to living kidney donation are BMI >40, age >70, diabetes, active malignancy, glomerular filtration rate (GFR) <70, recurrent nephrolithiasis, and hypertension requiring more than one medication.

9. **What are the indications for pancreas transplantation?**
   In general, all type I diabetics with ESRD who have had or plan to undergo kidney transplant should be considered for a pancreas transplant, as long as they have acceptable surgical risks. The addition of a pancreas transplant does not jeopardize overall patient survival but may improve kidney graft survival and restore normal glycemia. Overall, there are three types of pancreas transplants. A simultaneous kidney-pancreas (SKP) is the most common, but patients may opt for a pancreas after kidney (PAK) transplant or a pancreas transplant alone (PTA).

10. **What is the general 1-year pancreas graft survival for a SKP?**
    This has greatly improved since the first pancreas transplant in 1966, which had a 25% 1-year survival rate. Nowadays, the reported 1-year survival for SKP transplant is 86%–95%, largely attributed to better surgical technique and immunosuppression. The overall 5-year survival is estimated at 69%.

11. **How can a patient with type I diabetes and no ESRD qualify for a PTA?**
    The indications for a PTA are significant hypoglycemic unawareness/events as well as stable renal function. Because these patients will require calcineurin inhibitors (CNI) post transplant, most centers require a GFR >70 and <1 g of proteinuria at the time of PTA. As a result of the necessity of CNI, PTA has been shown to be an independent risk factor in the development of renal failure.

12. **In general, why do SKP have better overall survivals than PAK or PTA?**
    Having the kidney and pancreas come from the same donor offers the transplant physicians the ability to monitor rejection of the pancreas through the kidney.

13. **How is the pancreas transplanted?**
    Typically, this occurs at the same time as the kidney transplant through a lower midline incision. The kidney is placed on one side and the pancreas on the other. The pancreas is procured with a duodenal cuff, which drains the digestive enzymes of the new graft. The duodenal cuff used to be routinely anastomosed to the bladder but nowadays is typically anastomosed to the distal ileum. Even more recently, some centers have begun using exocrine drainage directly into the portal system via the superior mesenteric vein.

14. **Does pancreas transplantation halt the progression of diabetic disease?**
    Intuitively, this would seem to be the case; however, it is largely unproven. Several reports of regression of neuropathy, nephropathy, and eye disease certainly exist. However, it appears that the only proven benefits to date are quality of life without insulin and prolonged kidney graft survival.

15. **Are islet cell transplants the future?**
    The more recent results of this are promising, compared to the 1970s. Theoretically, if this could be perfected, the potential surgical morbidity of pancreas transplant could be avoided altogether. However, there are still several limitations to this. First, the amount of islet cells (6000 equivalents/kg) requires multiple injections and, typically, multiple donors. The site of injection is the portal vein, and there are potentially dangerous complications with this such as portal thrombosis, portal hypertension, hepatic infarct, etc. In addition, the latest survival data pales in comparison to pancreas transplant, with only 70% euglycemic at 1 year and 35% euglycemic at 3 years.

KEY POINTS: KIDNEY AND PANCREAS TRANSPLANT

1. The most common indication for kidney transplantation is ESRD caused by hypertension, diabetes, glomerulonephritis, and polycystic kidney disease.
2. Cadaveric kidney transplant survival rates have steadily improved over the years, with current 1-year graft survival rates of 90% and a 10-year graft survival rate of >50%.
3. Kidney transplants from live donors have a significantly higher graft survival rate than cadaveric kidneys.
4. In general, all type 1 diabetics with poorly controlled diabetes despite optimal medical management should be considered for kidney-pancreas transplantation as long as they are acceptable surgical risks. SKP have a higher pancreatic graft survival at 5 years than PTA and PAK. There is significant debate currently whether the risk of PAK is warranted.

BIBLIOGRAPHY

1. Wolfe RA, Ashby VB, Milford EL, et al. Comparison of mortality in all patients on dialysis, patients on dialysis awaiting transplantation, and recipients of a first cadaveric transplant. *N Engl J Med.* 1999;341(23):1725–1730.
2. Abecassis M, Bartlett ST, Collins AJ, et al. Kidney transplantation as primary therapy for end-stage renal disease: a National Kidney Foundation/Kidney Disease Outcomes Quality Initiative conference. *Clin J Am Soc Nephrol.* 2008;3(2): 471–480.
3. Lipshutz GS, Wilkinson AH. Pancreas-kidney and pancreas transplantation for the treatment of diabetes mellitus. *Endocrinol Metab Clin North Am.* 2007;36(4):1015–1038.
4. Shapiro AM, Lakey JR, Ryan EA, et al. Islet transplantation in seven patients with type 1 diabetes mellitus using a glucocorticoid-free immunosuppressive regimen. *N Engl J Med.* 2000;343(4):230–238.

CHAPTER 95

HEART TRANSPLANTATION

Chun W. Choi, MD, Richard-Tien V. Ha, MD

1. **What is the gold standard therapy for end-stage heart disease?**
   Heart transplantation remains the gold standard therapy for end-stage heart failure. The most common technique is to place the heart in its anatomical or orthotopic position. Ventricular assist devices (VADs) have become more popular either as a bridge-to-transplant or as a destination-therapy for those who are not transplant candidates, with promising results.

2. **Who were the pioneers in developing heart transplantation?**
   In 1905, Alexis Carrel and Charles Guthrie performed a heart transplant heterotopically. Vladmir Demikhov was successful in transplanting hearts both heterotopically and orthotopically.
   In the 1960s, Norman Shumway and Richard Lower refined the techniques of orthotopic heart transplantation, which have served as the basis for modern clinical operative techniques.

3. **Who performed the first human-to-human heart transplant? When?**
   Christian Barnard performed the first human-to-human heart transplantation in December 1967 (in Cape Town, South Africa). In 1968, Norman Shumway performed the first successful human-to-human heart transplantation in the United States.

4. **Who performed the first successful heart-lung transplant? When?**
   In 1981, Bruce Reitz at Stanford performed the first successful heart-lung transplantation in a human. The patient was a 21-year-old woman with pulmonary hypertension secondary to an atrial septal defect.

5. **How many heart transplants are performed annually? Is the number increasing or decreasing?**
   According to the most recent International Society for Heart and Lung Transplantation Registry in 2015, a total of 4477 heart transplants (3817 adult) were performed at 252 centers worldwide. The number has remained relatively stable for several years, with subtle fluctuations, despite the increase in the number of patients on the waitlist. The limiting factor is the number of donors.

6. **What are the anastomoses required to perform a heart transplant?**
   Aorta, pulmonary artery, left atrium, and either right atrium or vena cavae (superior vena cava [SVC] and inferior vena cava [IVC]). The preferred method at most centers is the bicaval technique, in which SVC and IVC are anastomosed separately, rather than anastomosing the right atrium to right atrium (biatrial technique). It is thought that the incidence of postoperatively tricuspid regurgitation and atrial arrhythmias are less with the bicaval technique.

7. **What are the indications and contraindications for heart transplant?**
   Indications:
   - New York Heart Association class III or IV heart failure refractory to medical therapy with expected 2-year survival <60%
   - Debilitating angina with no interventional or surgical options
   - Ventricular arrhythmias refractory to medical treatment, implantable cardioverter-defibrillator, or surgical therapy
   - VO_2 max up to 14 mL/kg/min

   Contraindications:
   - Irreversible pulmonary hypertension (PVR <6 Wood units)
   - Severe obstructive or restrictive lung disease
   - Advanced age (generally older than 70 years)
   - Obesity
   - Unresolved recent malignancy
   - Active infection
   - Significant systemic disease or end-organ dysfunction (e.g., end-stage liver failure, end-stage renal failure, severe peripheral vascular disease)
   - Lack of psychosocial well-being or support, including active substance abuse
   - Medical noncompliance

8. What are acceptable donor selection criteria?
   - Age <55 years
   - No history of chest trauma or cardiac disease
   - No prolonged hypotension or hypoxemia
   - Normal electrocardiogram, echo, and/or coronary angiogram
   - Negative hepatitis B and C serology
   - Negative HIV serology

9. How are the organs allocated?
   Donor organ allocation, including hearts, is managed by United Network for Organ Sharing. The heart allocation algorithm takes into account severity of illness of the potential recipient, time on the waiting list, and ABO type. The recipient status is categorized as 1A, 1B, 2, or 7 (inactive).
   The organs are allocated by geographical regions, with priority given to local recipients.

10. What is the survival rate of heart transplant recipients?
    Results from cumulative data between 1982 and June 2013 show 1-year survival of 82% and 5-year survival of 69%. Median survival was 11 years, with 13 years for those surviving the first year.

11. What are the leading causes of death among heart transplant recipients?
    - Graft failure, infection, and multisystem organ failure
    - Nonspecific graft failure (days to weeks)
    - Noncytomegalovirus infection (months)
    - Acute rejection (months)
    - Cardiac allograft vasculopathy (CAV) (years)

12. What are other surgical options for end-stage heart failure patients besides heart transplant?
    Left VAD has become more common in the surgical treatment of advanced heart failure. For those with right-sided heart failure, right VAD can be implanted either alone or in the setting of left-sided mechanical support. For more acute and emergent cases, extracorporeal membranous oxygenation has gained increased utilization as salvage or bridge-to-decision therapy.

13. What is an acceptable donor heart ischemic time?
    Most centers aim to maintain donor heart ischemic time (form the time of aortic cross clamp of the donor heart to implantation into the recipient and coronary reperfusion) <4 hours. In general, ischemic time of 6 hours is the limit. Within ischemic time of 4–5 hours, many studies have shown no significant difference in survival.

14. When is prolonged donor ischemic time appropriate?
    A center may accept an organ from a greater distance and accept a prolonged ischemic time (>6 hours) under extenuating circumstances, for recipients whose conditions are deteriorating and are less likely to find a suitable donor from the usual allocation locale and have no good options for mechanical circulatory support. Donor hearts with prolonged ischemic time tend to have greater incidence of graft dysfunction with poor cardiac output. Often, temporary mechanical circulatory support is utilized in these cases during the initial recovery period.
    In pediatric cases, most centers accept an ischemic time up to 8–9 hours. Pediatric donor hearts tend to tolerate longer ischemic time.

15. What is the typical infection pattern for a patient after transplant?
    - First postoperative month: Usual bacterial pathogens encountered in most surgical patients
    - 1–4 months: Opportunistic pathogens, especially CVM
    - >4 months: Both conventional and opportunistic infections

16. How is cardiac allograft rejection prevented?
    Host immune system immediately recognizes the donor allograft as foreign. ABO and human leukocyte antigen (HLA) typing aids in preventing hyperacute and acute rejection. To prevent chronic or antibody mediated rejection, pharmacologic agents that render the host immunosuppressed are used. Immunosuppression consists of preoperative induction therapy or postoperative maintenance therapy. Induction therapy is primarily either interleukin-2 receptor (CD52) antibodies or antithymocyte globulin (ATG). OKT3 is no longer recommended for induction because of a higher incidence of pulmonary edema, hypotension, and high fevers. Maintenance therapy usually consists of a calcineurin inhibitor (tacrolimus >> cyclosporine), an antiproliferative agent (mycophenolate mofetil >> rapamycin), and prednisone.

17. **What are the mechanisms of these therapies?**
Induction agents are antibodies that bind directly to receptors on B and T cells and inhibit their function. These aim to prevent downstream cell and antibody recognition of the allograft as foreign.

Tacrolimus and cyclosporine are calcineurin inhibitors that prevent IL-2 production in T cells, thereby suppressing proliferation. Mycophenolic acid is a cell-cycle inhibitor. It inhibits de novo synthesis of guanine nucleotides. Therefore, it suppresses proliferative responses of B and T cells as well as inhibiting antibody production by B cells.

Prednisone is a steroid, an intranuclear binding agent that directly inhibits DNA synthesis that affects downstream production of IL-2.

18. **How is cardiac allograft rejection diagnosed?**
Clinical suspicion is raised by new-onset cardiac arrhythmia, fever, or hypotension. Diagnosis depends on endomyocardial biopsy, which is performed at regular intervals to detect histologic evidence of rejection before signs or symptoms occur. Gene expression profiling of peripheral blood lymphocytes is a novel and increasingly accepted noninvasive tool for diagnosis of rejection. Its negative predictive value is >99%, avoiding the need for biopsy in certain settings.

19. **How is allograft rejection treated?**
Patients can develop significant hemodynamic compromise from rejection. These patients should be treated for their cardiogenic shock with intensive and/or invasive monitoring and inotropic support.

Acute cellular rejection is treated with antithymocyte globulin or pulse corticosteroids.

Antibody-mediated rejection is treated with plasmapheresis, intravenous immunoglobulin, pulse steroids, ATG, and rituximab in variety of combinations.

20. **What are some complications of transvenous endomyocardial biopsy?**
Cardiac perforation occurs in <1%. But when it happens, it can result in acute hemopericardium and cardiac tamponade. Tricuspid regurgitation from trauma of the biopsy catheters has been reported to be about 5%–10%. In severe cases of tricuspid regurgitation from biopsy, a tricuspid valve replacement is warranted.

21. **What is the incidence of CAV? What are the risk factors?**
CAV (also known as transplant vasculopathy, transplant CAD, or accelerated graft arteriosclerosis) occurs in more than 50% of patients by 5 years after transplant and is the main factor limiting long-term survival. Risk factors for CAV include male gender of the donor or recipient, older donor age, donor hypertension, recipient pretransplant coronary artery disease (CAD), and HLA-DR mismatches.

22. **What is the difference between nontransplant CAD or atherosclerosis and CAV?**
Unlike nontransplant CAD, CAV is a diffuse, concentric process involving large- and medium-sized vessels. Preservation injury, alloimmune responses (cellular and humoral), and possibly chronic CMV infection may contribute to its pathogenesis.

23. **How is CAV diagnosed and treated?**
CAV is diagnosed predominantly by angiogram and more recently by intravascular ultrasound. Statin therapy ± diltiazem decreases the incidence of developing CAV. In patients with established CAV, rapamycin may reduce subsequent cardiac events. Otherwise, treatment has been disappointing. Retransplantation is controversial because of only a 55% 1-year survival rate and a 46% incidence of recurrent CAV. Coronary angioplasty ± stenting has been primarily palliative as a result of the diffuse nature of CAV.

24. **What work remains to be done in heart transplantation?**
Xenograft transplantation is a concept that has gained increasing interest with advances in immunology. Animal models have been successful, and human trials in other organs are on the horizon. It is not inconceivable that heart transplantation from a host animal to a human may be a possibility in the future.

Another area of clinical research is the use of ex vivo platforms to recover donor hearts before transplantation. This technology may allow us to expand donor organ utilization by procuring hearts that may be marginal in function and resuscitate them to acceptable quality for transplantation.

KEY POINTS: HEART TRANSPLANTATION

1. Heart transplantation is the gold-standard therapy for end-stage heart failure.
2. Indications for heart transplantation are advanced heart failure that is refractory to medical therapy with limited expected survival.
3. Contraindications for heart transplantation include severe lung disease, active malignancy, and medical noncompliance.
4. For patients who are not transplant candidates or cannot wait for a suitable donor, ventricular assist device has proven to be effective.
5. Various immunosuppressive agents are used to prevent and treat rejection.

BIBLIOGRAPHY

1. Al-khaldi A, Robbins RC. New directions in cardiac transplantation. *Annu Rev Med.* 2006;57:455–471.
2. Canter CE, Shaddy RE, Bernstein D, et al. Indications for heart transplantation in pediatric heart disease: a scientific statement from the American Heart Association Council on Cardiovascular Disease in the Young; the Councils on Clinical Cardiology, Cardiovascular Nursing, and Cardiovascular Surgery and Anesthesia; and the Quality of Care and Outcomes Research Interdisciplinary Working Group. *Circulation.* 2007;115(5):658–676.
3. Crisostomo PR, Wang M, Markel TA, et al. Stem cell mechanisms and paracrine effects: potential in cardiac surgery. *Shock.* 2007;28(4):375–383.
4. Rahmani M, Cruz RP. Allograft vasculopathy versus atherosclerosis. *Circ Res.* 2006;99(8):801–815.
5. Scheule AM, Zimmerman GJ. Duration of graft cold ischemia does not affect outcomes in pediatric heart transplant recipients. *Circulation.* 2002;106(12 suppl 1):I163–I167.
6. Steinman TI, Becker BN, Frost AE, et al. Guidelines for the referral and management of patients eligible for solid organ transplantation. *Transplantation.* 2001;71(9):1189–1204.
7. Taylor DO, Edwards LB, Boucek MM, et al. Registry of the International Society for Heart and Lung Transplantation: twenty-fourth official adult heart transplant report—2007. *J Heart Lung Transplant.* 2007;26(8):769–781.
8. Uber PA, Mehra MR. Induction therapy in heart transplantation: is there a role? *J Heart Lung Transplant.* 2007;26(3):205–209.
9. Wang M, Tsai BM. Tumor necrosis factor receptor 1 signaling resistance in female myocardium during ischemia. *Circulation.* 2006;114(suppl 1):I282–I289.
10. West LJ, Pollock-Barziv SM, Dipchand AI, et al. ABO-incompatible heart transplantation in infants. *N Engl J Med.* 2001;344(11):793–800.
11. Zaroff JG, Rosengard BR, Armstrong WF, et al. Consensus conference report: maximizing use of organs recovered from the cadaver donor: cardiac recommendations, March 28-29, 2001, Crystal City, Va. *Circulation.* 2002;106(7):836–841.
12. Deckers JW, Hare JM. Complications of transvenous right ventricular endomyocardial biopsy in adult patients with cardiomyopathy: a seven-year survey of 546 consecutive diagnostic procedures in a tertiary referral center. *J Am Coll Cardiol.* 1992;19(1):43–47.
13. Del Rizzo DF, Menkis AH, Pflugfelder PW, et al. The role of donor age and ischemic time on survival following orthotopic heart transplantation. *J Heart Lung Transplant.* 1999;18(4):310–319.
14. Russo MJ, Chen JM, Sorabella RA, et al. The effect of ischemic time on survival after heart transplantation varies by donor age: an analysis of the United Network for Organ Sharing database. *J Thorac Cardiovasc Surg.* 2007;133(2):554–559.
15. Williams MJ, Lee MY, DiSalvo TG, et al. Biopsy-induced flail tricuspid leaflet and tricuspid regurgitation following orthotopic cardiac transplantation. *Am J Cardiol.* 1996;77(15):1339–1344.

CHAPTER 96

MECHANICAL CIRCULATORY SUPPORT

T. Brett Reece, MD, Joseph C. Cleveland, Jr., MD

1. **What are the indications for ventricular assist device (VAD)?**
   - Bridge to transplant: Patients are in need of and are eligible for transplant, but their clinical course is such that they will not survive until a donor organ is available. Thus, mechanical circulatory support (MCS) is required to "bridge" the gap until an organ is available. The ultimate goal for these patients is heart transplantation, and they must be listed for transplant before VAD placement.
   - Destination therapy: Patients are those with end-stage heart disease who are not eligible or candidates for heart transplantation. Although they are not candidates for transplantation at the time of device implantation, these patients can evolve into heart transplant candidates in some cases where the ventricular unloading leads to other hemodynamic changes; for instance, improvement in pulmonary hypertension. Goals of destination therapy are to prolong life, reduce hospitalizations, and improve quality of life. Destination therapy is an alternative to medical management for those who have class III–IV heart failure. To qualify for destination therapy, patients should receive optimal medical management (OMM) for at least 60 out of the last 90 days. Destination therapy is also known as durable long-term support.
   - Recovery: Patients with acute situations that may improve fall into this category. Most commonly, this involves postinfarct cardiogenic shock or failure to separate from cardiopulmonary bypass (CPB). Shorter-term devices can allow for recovery or further workup for longer-term devices or transplantation. Some recovery devices use the same cannulas as in CPB, facilitating their implantation.

2. **What are contraindications for VAD?**
   - Lack of social support
   - Cognitive: Inability to learn/adapt to dependency on a device
   - Infection
   - Severity of disease: For example, too debilitated to receive benefit
   - Comorbid conditions other than heart failure that are likely to interfere with survival on VAD

3. **What workup needs to be done prior to VAD placement?**
   - Cultures need to be sent. Remember that these patients tend to have central lines, Foleys, etc., so infection remains a huge problem for them.
   - Echocardiogram (ECHO) looking for clot in the ventricles. Thrombus may not exclude the patient alone but may make stroke more of a risk. ECHO should also evaluate status of valves if repair or replacement is needed and can be done concurrently with VAD placement. If mechanical valve is in place, it should be changed out for bioprosthetic valve at time of implant.
   - Optimize nutrition because this is a huge indicator of long-term and short-term outcome.
   - Left ventricular assist device (LVAD): The right ventricle needs to be evaluated closely because some right ventricular (RV) failure may be secondary to left ventricular (LV) failure. However, the right ventricle may not be able to tolerate the VAD placement either. Unfortunately, predictors of RV failure do not rule out the need for biventricular support.
   - Right ventricular assist device (RVAD): Pulmonary hypertension may be the most important issue to be defined in RV support. If the ventricular issues arise from the pulmonary vasculature, the VAD may not be able to overcome the resistance, or it wears out prematurely.

4. **What is OMM prior to VAD placement?**
   Optimizing heart failure management with β-blocker, angiotensin-converting-enzyme inhibitor, hydralazine, diureses, and possibly digoxin as indicated.

5. **What predicts outcomes with VAD placement?**

   Preoperative renal function, nutritional status, mechanical ventilation, redo sternotomy, elevated central venous pressure, and prothrombin time and international normalized ratio have all demonstrated correlation with poor outcomes. Several risk scores have been developed to try to predict outcomes that use multiple preoperative factors.

6. **How long do the devices last?**

   Durability is device dependent. The short-term devices should probably be either removed or changed to a longer-term device within 1–2 weeks because of increased risk of infection and thromboembolism. The long-term devices should last potentially several years. Four-year survival on LVADs is now 48% (half of the patients are still alive at 4 years). Short-term devices that are intended for recovery actually can be in for a number of weeks depending on the device. A paracorporeal ventricular assist device (PVAD)—not to be confused with a percutaneous ventricular assist device (pVAD)—can be in for weeks to months (i.e., Thoratec PVAD, Abiomed Ventricle). Extracorporeal VADs (i.e., CentriMag) are really only approved by the Food and Drug Administration for hours, but most are left in for days to weeks.

7. **How does the presence of a VAD affect transplantation?**

   Despite the complexity of the dissection in the removal of the devices, the transplant outcomes are not compromised. This is thought to be secondary to many of the patients with a VAD being better stabilized than their heart-failure counterparts. However, the explanting surgeon must be wary of the outflow tracts, whether they are to the pulmonary artery or aorta.

8. **What are the general classes of devices used today, and what are their advantages and disadvantages?**

   Internal:
   - Advantage: The device is protected within the abdomen and thorax.
   - Disadvantage: The drive line remains an issue for both wound healing and infection. Further, the size of the devices can limit utilization in smaller patients.

   External:
   - Advantage: Size of the device does not exclude smaller patients.
   - Disadvantage: The inflow and outflow of the device traverse the skin, which can be more difficult to prevent infection. Further, the external devices may not allow for the patient to actually leave the hospital.

   Axial/centrifugal flow:
   - Advantage: In general the devices are much smaller.
   - Disadvantage: Loss of pulsatility creates an abnormal environment for the systemic vascular bed. Also, the medical staff needs further education on how to take and evaluate the vitals of patients with these devices.

   Percutaneous:
   - Advantage: They are small, can be placed in the catheter lab through peripheral vessels, and do not need to be placed on CPB for implantation. May be best suited for short-term recovery.
   - Disadvantage: Their durability is still being evaluated. They are not long-term devices. Their implantation may not prevent infection in the long term. These devices do not augment flow as well as the other devices.

9. **What are the perioperative issues that must be observed or addressed?**
   - Coagulopathy: Notorious procedures for postoperative bleeding
   - Volume status: Related to bleeding but also to preoperative volume status
   - Afterload: Directly affects pump output; most important in axial flow devices
   - Other ventricle: Most difficult to deal with
   - Thrombosis or embolism

10. **What needs to be done for anticoagulation for these devices?**

    Anticoagulation is device specific. For the most part, all patients with VAD need to be anticoagulated with coumadin and aspirin.

11. **What long-term management issues must be addressed?**
    - Teaching the patient, family, and local medical services how to deal with the VAD
    - Nutrition
    - Drive line healing closely related to nutrition

- Anticoagulation (which is device specific)
- Follow-up echocardiography: Evaluate for ventricular function, valve opening, inflow and outflow orientation, and any indication of device dysfunction including thrombus formation or valve degeneration
- Emergency procedures with community education because these issues may not arise near the implantation institution

12. **When to transplant the bridges?**
    The patient needs to recover from the VAD placement. This is an opportunity to address overall body volume issues, improve the patient's nutrition, and improve activity status. Although transplants are done shortly after device placement, the decision to list takes many different factors into account that might improve the transplant outcome. This is not a patient to place a marginal donor organ into because of fear of deterioration. On the other hand, device complications may accelerate the need for transplantation.

13. **What must be evaluated before explantation?**
    Explantation can be a difficult call to make. The heart function can be temporarily lessened by explantation process, so some reserve must be present to tolerate removal in the perioperative period. Pathology can play a significant role, especially if the recovery of the myocardium is possible. ECHO plays a real role as the assist device can be turned down to evaluate the underlying ventricular function. Finally, the decision for assist device explantation must be multidisciplinary, including the patient in these discussions.

KEY POINTS: MECHANICAL CIRCULATORY SUPPORT

1. Durable MCS now provides 2-year survival of 80%, while medical therapy for these New York Heart Association Class IV individuals is <10% at 2 years.
2. Prompt evaluation and institution of MCS before irreversible end-organ dysfunction occurs yields optimal outcomes.
3. Continuous flow devices have replaced pulsatile devices.
4. Bleeding, infection, and stroke remain the most common complications following MCS.
5. All MCS devices require anticoagulation with heparin or warfarin plus aspirin.

BIBLIOGRAPHY

1. Birks EJ, Tansley PD, Hardy J, et al. Left ventricular assist device and drug therapy for the reversal of heart failure. *N Engl J Med.* 2006;355(18):1873–1874.
2. Lietz K, Long JW, Kfoury AG, et al. Outcomes of left ventricular assist device implantation as destination therapy in the post-REMATCH era: implications for patient selection. *Circulation.* 2007;116(5):497–505.
3. Rao V, Oz MC, Flannery MA, et al. Changing trends in mechanical circulatory assistance. *J Card Surg.* 2004;19(4): 361–366.
4. Rose EA, Gelijns AC, Moskowitz AJ, et al. Long-term mechanical left ventricular assistance for end-stage heart failure. *N Engl J Med.* 2001;345(20):1435–1443.
5. Kirklin JK, Naftel DC, Pagani FD, et al. Seventh INTERMACS annual report: 15,000 patients and counting. *J Heart Lung Transplant.* 2015;34(12):1495–1504.

CHAPTER 97

LUNG TRANSPLANTATION

Daniel R. Meldrum, MD, FACS, FAHA, Joseph C. Cleveland, Jr., MD

1. **Which human organ transplant was performed first, the heart or the lung?**
   Although heart transplantation has progressed more rapidly, the first human lung transplant preceded the first heart transplant.

2. **Who performed the first human lung transplant? When?**
   James Hardy performed the first human lung transplant in 1963; however, more than 20 years passed before lung transplantation was performed routinely in clinical practice (during that 20-year period, only one patient did well enough to leave the hospital). This delay was caused by initial graft failure secondary to inadequate organ preservation, long ischemic times, lack of good immunosuppressive agents, and technical difficulties (primarily with the bronchial—not the vascular—anastomoses).

3. **What are the general types of lung transplants?**
   Single, double (bilateral), and heart-lung.

4. **How many lung transplants are performed annually? Is the number increasing or decreasing?**
   Although first performed in 1963, significant numbers were not performed until the late 1980s (in 1986, one lung transplant; in 1989, 132 lung transplants). Since 1994, the number of single lung transplants performed annually has remained stable (around 700). However, bilateral lung transplantations have rapidly increased from approximately 100 in 1994 to more than 1400 in 2005 and continue to increase worldwide.

5. **Why is the number of combined heart-lung transplants performed annually decreasing?**
   Approximately 250 heart-lung transplants were performed in 1990; the number has decreased to approximately 75 in 2005. As the results of single lung and double lung transplants have improved, the need to perform heart-lung transplants in patients with isolated pulmonary disease has been obviated.

6. **Who is a candidate for a lung transplant?**
   Candidates include patients with no other medical or surgical alternative who are likely to die of pulmonary disease within 2–3 years, are younger than 65 years, are not ventilator dependent, and do not have a history of malignancy. Psychologic stability in the recipient is also important.

7. **What are the most common indications for single lung transplant?**
   - Emphysema (50%)
   - Idiopathic pulmonary fibrosis (25%)
   - α-1 antitrypsin deficiency (7.5%)
   - Cystic fibrosis (CF; 2%)
   - Sarcoidosis (2%)

8. **What are the most common indications for a double lung transplant?**
   - CF (30%)
   - Emphysema (25%)
   - Idiopathic pulmonary fibrosis (13%)
   - α-1 antitrypsin deficiency (8.5%)
   - Primary pulmonary hypertension and pulmonary hypertension secondary to correctable congenital heart disease (6%)

9. **What are the most common indications for heart-lung transplant?**
   Primary pulmonary hypertension (25%) and CF (15%) are instances in which bad lungs have ruined a good heart. Conversely, with congenital heart disease (34%), a bad heart has destroyed good lungs.

10. **What is sewn to what during a single lung transplant? A double lung transplant?**
During a single lung transplant, recipient-to-graft bronchial, pulmonary artery, and pulmonary vein (atrial cuff) anastomoses are required. Anastomoses for double transplant are the same; however, cardiopulmonary bypass (CPB) is required more often during double lung transplant. During implantation of the second lung, diversion of the entire cardiac output to the freshly ischemic lung often results in reperfusion lung edema and hypoxemia.

11. **Which diagnoses carry the best results for single lung transplants?**
Patients with emphysema, α-1 antitrypsin deficiency, and CF do significantly better, with 1-year survival rates of approximately 75%. However, patients with CF or idiopathic pulmonary fibrosis may derive more of a survival benefit from lung transplantation than patients with chronic obstructive pulmonary disorder because mortality without transplantation is higher.

12. **Are the survival rates different for single lung and double lung transplants?**
Yes. Although survival rates for single and bilateral transplant recipients are similar for the first year, in subsequent years, bilateral lung transplants (half-life = 5.9 years) have significantly improved survival compared to single lung transplants (half-life = 4.4 years).

13. **What are the most common complications after lung transplant?**
- Hypertension (85%)
- Renal dysfunction (38%)
- Hyperlipidemia (52%)
- Diabetes (33%)
- Bronchiolitis obliterans (33%)

14. **What are the major causes of death after lung transplantation?**
- Primary graft dysfunction (PGD; days)
- Non-cytomegalovirus (CMV) infection (weeks to years)
- Bronchiolitis obliterans (months to years)

15. **What is PGD? How is it treated?**
PGD is a form of acute lung injury resulting from ischemia or reperfusion injury, edema, preservation, surgical technique, and recipient or donor risk factors. It manifests clinically as poor oxygenation, compliance, and edema. Treatment consists of increased ventilatory support, diuretics, pulmonary vasodilation (prostaglandins and inhaled nitric oxide), surfactant replacement (nebulized synthetic), extracorporeal membrane oxygenation, and retransplantation.

16. **What is the most common nonbacterial cause of pneumonia in lung transplant patients?**
CMV, usually occurring 4–8 weeks postoperatively. Primary CMV infection usually results in more serious illness than reactivation disease. CMV-seronegative recipients should receive only blood products that are serologically negative.

17. **In addition to immune suppressive therapy, what other factors put transplanted lungs at risk for infection?**
Lung denervation, interruption of lymphatic clearance and bronchial circulation, and impaired mucociliary clearance.

18. **What is bronchiolitis obliterans?**
Bronchiolitis obliterans, a major cause of long-term morbidity after lung transplantation, is a chronic irreversible scarring process that results in progressive obliteration of the small airways of the lung allograft and resultant obstructive lung disease. Clinically, it is characterized by dyspnea and airflow obstruction.

19. **How does bronchiolitis obliterans develop?**
Lymphocytes infiltrate the bronchiole submucosa and migrate through the basement membrane to the airway mucosa. Cytotoxic alloreactive injury and epithelial necrosis follow. In response to ulceration, fibropurulent exudate forms within the airway and is accompanied by proliferation of fibroblasts, endothelial cells, and lymphocytes. This myxoid tissue partially or completely can occlude the airway.

20. **What are the risk factors for the development of bronchiolitis obliterans after lung transplant?**
Episodes of acute allograft rejection are undoubtedly the most important risk factor. CMV infection, noncompliance with immunosuppressive medications, and lymphocytic bronchitis are also important risk factors.

21. **How is lung allograft rejection prevented?**

Immunosuppressive practices for lung transplantation have generally paralleled those for heart transplantation. Less than half receive induction therapy (interleukin-2 receptor [CD25] antibodies > antithrombocyte globulin). Maintenance therapy usually consists of a calcineurin inhibitor (tacrolimus > cyclosporine), an antiproliferative agent (mycophenolate mofetil > rapamycin), and prednisone.

22. **What is the incidence of acute rejection? How is lung transplant rejection diagnosed?**

Almost 50% of recipients are treated for acute rejection during the first year after transplant. Unlike heart transplants, the diagnosis of rejection in transplanted lungs is imprecise and can be difficult to distinguish from infection. Transbronchial biopsy remains the gold standard but often requires three or several more "good" biopsies. Bronchoscopy with bronchoalveolar lavage and clinical assessment are also necessary for diagnosis.

23. **What additional tests can help distinguish between acute rejection and infection?**

Polymerase chain reaction (PCR) assays for CMV or *Aspergillus* and *Pneumocystis jirovecii* pneumonia, as well as multiplex PCR for multiple community-acquired and opportunistic infective agents, can supplement standard transbronchial biopsy staining and may facilitate discrimination of occult infection from acute rejection.

24. **Describe the phenomenon of chimerism in transplantation.**

Transplant-mixed chimerism is a condition in which cells from the recipient engraft into the donor transplant so that the allograft becomes a genetic composite of both the donor and recipient. Chimerism enhances the host's tolerance of the graft because the recipient does not recognize the donor organ as foreign.

25. **Does chimerism develop in the heart and the lungs?**

Yes. The first evidence of heart transplant chimerism was observed in 2002 by Quaini and colleagues in male patients who received hearts from female donors. In 2003, Kleeberger and colleagues also demonstrated evidence of lung transplant chimerism in lung epithelium, type II pneumocytes, and seromucous glands.

26. **Why is chimerism exciting?**

Nature is trying to teach us how to perform transplantation without the use of immunosuppression. Our job is to learn why chimerism is induced in some recipients and not in others. That is, we should dissect the mechanisms of chimerism induction so that we may therapeutically induce chimerism in all recipients.

27. **What are the major types of preservation solutions for heart and lung grafts?**

For nearly 2 decades, Euro-Collins (EC) solution or University of Wisconsin (UW) were considered the gold standard for lung transplant. Perfadex is increasingly accepted for lung transplant and improves posttransplant lung function and decreases PGD in comparison to other solutions.

The gold standard for heart transplant is crystalloid cardioplegia (arrest) and UW solution (preservation). Celsior is a novel combination arrest and preservation solution for heart transplants that requires further study.

28. **What are the main differences in composition between EC and UW solutions and Perfadex and Celsior?**

EC and UW are high potassium intracellular preservation solutions originally developed for kidney transplant. In lung transplant, they cause severe vasoconstriction. Perfadex is a low potassium extracellular dextran plus glucose solution that demonstrates less vasoconstriction and decreased interstitial edema formation. Celsior is also extracellular.

29. **What percentage of pulmonary blood flow goes to the transplanted lung after single lung transplant?**

Predictably, almost all of the pulmonary blood flow passes through the lower resistance circuit of the transplanted lung (depending on the pulmonary vascular resistance of the contralateral native; i.e., sick lung). If a preoperative perfusion scan exists, other factors being equal, the lung with the best perfusion is preserved and the bad lung is replaced.

KEY POINTS: LUNG TRANSPLANTATION

1. The most common indication for single lung transplant is emphysema.
2. The most common indication for double lung transplant is CF.
3. Chimerism is a condition in which cells from the recipient engraft into the donor transplant so that the allograft becomes a genetic composite of both donor and recipient.
4. Bronchiolitis obliterans, a major cause of long-term morbidity after lung transplantation, is a chronic irreversible scarring process that results in progressive obliteration of the small airways of the lung allograft and resultant obstructive lung disease.
5. EVLP offers promise to increase lung utilization for transplantation.

30. **Is cardiopulmonary bypass required for lung transplantation?**
No. However, for patients with pulmonary hypertension (primary or secondary), CPB is routinely used before removal of the recipient's lung. CPB is always on standby. This is tricky anesthesia. One lung is transiently excised from a patient who is living (barely) on two bad lungs.

31. **Is living-related lung transplant possible?**
Yes. Living-related lung transplants are an innovative approach to increasing the donor pool. Typically, one lobe from each of two to three donors is used to replace a whole lung in the recipient.

32. **How can stem cells improve pulmonary function before and after lung transplantation?**
Recent studies show that stem cells have acute paracrine effects that result in repair and protection of injured tissue. Specifically, stem cells transplanted to the lung produce antiinflammatory factors, such as interleukin 10 and transforming growth factor beta. These antiinflammatory factors and other angiogenic and antiapoptotic factors may improve pulmonary function after acute lung injury and transplantation.

33. **What is lung volume reduction surgery? How may it be important to patients on the lung transplant waiting list?**
Lung volume reduction surgery offers a therapeutic option for patients who are either not candidates to receive a lung transplant or on a long waiting list. Lung volume reduction surgery removes nonfunctional or destroyed lung. Removal of defunctionalized lung makes more room for airflow in the functional lung, resulting in decreased mortality and increased function.

34. **Who is the best candidate for lung volume reduction surgery?**
The National Emphysema Treatment Trial suggests that the best candidates (lowest mortality) are patients with an obvious upper lobe apical target, marked thoracic distention, forced expiratory volume (FEV_1) >20%, diffusing capacity of the lung for carbon monoxide >20%, and age <70.

35. **What are the contraindications to lung reduction surgery?**
- Pulmonary hypertension (mean pulmonary artery pressure [PAP] >35 mm Hg or systolic PAP >45 mm Hg)
- Clinically significant heart disease
- Previous thoracotomy or pleurodesis (visceral and parietal pleural fusion)
- Diffuse disease without target
- FEV_1 <20%
- Hypercarbia, partial pressure of carbon dioxide >55

36. **What are the 1-year, 3-year, and 5-year actuarial survival rates for single lung retransplants?**
Actuarial survival rates are 60%, 50%, and 45%, respectively. Predictably, such patients do significantly worse. These poor results and the donor shortage make retransplantation of the lung an ethical dilemma.

37. **Is a simultaneous lung and pancreas transplant possible?**
Yes. In 2006, the first simultaneous double lung and pancreas transplant was performed in a patient with CF at Methodist Hospital, Indiana.

38. What is EVLP? How can EVLP alter lung transplantation?

Ex vivo lung perfusion is a technique whereby donor lungs can be preserved and even potentially improved/repaired for transplantation. The technique has evolved as lungs are often injured during the brain death process. If one could repair them with a reliable perfusion technique, then more lungs would be available for the ever increasing number of potential recipients. While EVLP seeks to repair lungs, the Toronto group has attempted to deliver genes into the airways to perhaps modulate rejection and organ tolerance. Such a development would be revolutionary in thoracic organ transplantation.

WEBSITE

- www.ishlt.org

BIBLIOGRAPHY

1. Boku N, Tanoue Y. A comparative study of cardiac preservation with Celsior or University of Wisconsin solution with or without prior administration of cardioplegia. *J Heart Lung Transplant.* 2006;25(2):219–225.
2. Crisostomo PR, Markel TA. In the adult mesenchymal stem cell population, source gender is a biologically relevant aspect of protective power. *Surgery.* 2007;142(2):215–221.
3. Crisostomo PR, Meldrum DR. Stem cell delivery to the heart: clarifying methodology and mechanism. *Crit Care Med.* 2007;35(11):2654–2655.
4. Fishman A, Martinez F, Naunheim K, et al. A randomized trial comparing lung-volume-reduction surgery with medical therapy for severe emphysema. *N Engl J Med.* 2003;348(21):2059–2073.
5. Kawut SM, Lederer DJ, Keshavjee S, et al. Outcomes after lung retransplantation in the modern era. *Am J Respir Crit Care Med.* 2008;177(1):114–120.
6. Kleeberger W, Versmold A, Rothamel T, et al. Increased chimerism of bronchial and alveolar epithelium in human lung allografts undergoing chronic injury. *Am J Pathol.* 2003;162(5):1487–1494.
7. Oto T, Griffiths AP. Early outcomes comparing Perfadex, Euro-Collins, and Papworth solutions in lung transplantation. *Ann Thorac Surg.* 2006;82(2):1842–1848.
8. Quaini F, Urbanek K, Beltrami AP, et al. Chimerism of the transplanted heart. *N Engl J Med.* 2002;346(1):5–15.
9. Snell GI, Boehler A, Glanville AR, et al. Eleven years on: a clinical update of key areas of the 1996 lung allograft rejection working formulation. *J Heart Lung Transplant.* 2007;26(5):423–430.
10. Trulock EP, Christie JD, Edwards LB, et al. Registry of the International Society for Heart and Lung Transplantation: twenty-fourth official adult lung and heart-lung transplantation report—2007. *J Heart Lung Transplant.* 2007;26(8):782–795.
11. Wilkes DS, Egan TM. Lung transplantation: opportunities for research and clinical advancement. *Am J Respir Crit Care Med.* 2005;172(8):944–955.
12. Machuca TN, Cypel M. Ex vivo lung perfusion. *J Thorac Dis.* 2014;6(8):1054–1062.

CHAPTER 98

PENILE AND SCROTAL UROLOGIC EMERGENCIES

Timothy K. Ito, MD, Yuka Yamaguchi, MD, Sarah D. Blaschko, MD

1. **What is priapism?**
   A prolonged erection lasting for more than 4 hours, beyond or unrelated to sexual activity or stimulation.

2. **Why is priapism an emergency?**
   Prolonged ischemia to the penis results in corporal body fibrosis and future erectile dysfunction.

3. **What are the three types of priapism?**
   Ischemic (low flow), nonischemic (high flow), and stuttering (intermittent). In ischemic priapism the corpora cavernosa are typically fully rigid and painful. In contrast, the penis is not typically fully rigid or painful in nonischemic priapism. Patients with nonischemic priapism may relay a history of prior perineal trauma. Stuttering priapism is associated typically with hematologic malignancies and sickle cell disease.

4. **What laboratory tests should be obtained for a priapism patient?**
   a. Corpus cavernosum blood gas testing: Ischemic priapism has dark hypoxic blood typically with a pO_2 <30 mm Hg, pCO_2 >60 mm Hg, and pH <7.25. Nonischemic priapism has oxygenated red blood with blood gas similar to serum.
   b. Complete blood count (CBC): Sickle cell anemia, platelet dysfunction, and leukemia may all result in priapism and can be identified by CBC.
   c. Consider a urine toxicology test: Illegal and psychoactive drugs may result in priapism.
   d. Hemoglobin electrophoresis testing for sickle cell or reticulocyte count may be considered in the appropriate clinical situation.

5. **What is the treatment of ischemic priapism?**
   Injection of phenylephrine and irrigation and evacuation of corporal body blood. If this fails to work, surgical shunting is required.

6. **What is the treatment of nonischemic priapism?**
   Observation. Many cases will spontaneously resolve. Embolization may be performed in cases that do not spontaneously resolve, with surgery typically reserved as a last resort.

7. **What is the difference between phimosis and paraphimosis?**
   Phimosis is the inability to retract the foreskin of the penis over the glans penis due to a narrowing at the distal foreskin. This may be congenital/physiologic or due to scarring from infection or inflammation. Circumcision may be offered if phimosis is interfering with urination or erections.

   Paraphimosis occurs when the foreskin remains retracted over the glans for an extended period of time. This results in significant edema and pain beyond a phimotic band of the retracted foreskin and an inability to reduce the foreskin back to its anatomic position. Correction of this must be performed emergently, as prolonged paraphimosis can result in necrosis of the distal skin and glans penis.

8. **How do you treat a paraphimosis?**
   Apply gentle steady pressure to the foreskin to reduce swelling. Pain medications and ice can be used for analgesia. Once the swelling is reduced, push the glans penis with the thumbs while pulling the foreskin forward over the glans with the rest of the fingers. If this is not possible then an emergent dorsal slit or circumcision may be required.

9. **What is a penile fracture?**
   Traumatic rupture of the tunica albuginea of the corpus cavernosum.

10. **What is the typical presentation of a penile fracture?**
A "pop" sound following blunt trauma to the erect penis followed by pain, immediate detumescence, and swelling. The typical appearance is described as the "eggplant deformity" due to significant penile swelling and purple discoloration caused by the underlying hematoma. The penis may curve away from the side of the injury.

11. **What is the most common cause of a penile fracture?**
In the United States, penile fractures are most often sustained because of coital trauma. In the Middle East, the most common cause is self-inflicted snapping of the penis while bending it in an attempt to achieve immediate detumescence, a practice known as *taghaandan*.

12. **How is a penile fracture managed?**
Prompt surgical repair of the tunical injury results in lower future rates of erectile dysfunction and Peyronie's disease. Patients with blood at the meatus, hematuria, or voiding issues after penile fracture should be assessed for a urethral injury with retrograde urethrogram. Any urethral injuries should also be repaired at the time of the tunical repair.

13. **What is the differential diagnosis of an acute scrotum?**
    a. Ischemia: Testicular torsion, torsion of appendix testis or appendix epididymis, or other vascular insult such as thrombosis
    b. Infection: Infection of testis or epididymis (orchitis, epididymitis, or epididymoorchitis), abscess, or infections of skin and subcutaneous tissues (cellulitis, Fournier's gangrene)
    c. Inflammatory condition: Henoch-Schönlein purpura (scrotal wall vasculitis)
    d. Trauma: Testicular rupture, intratesticular hematoma, or testicular contusion
    e. Hernia: Incarcerated or strangulated inguinal hernia
    f. Acute on chronic events: Spermatocele, hydrocele, or testicular tumor with rupture, hemorrhage, or infection

14. **Beyond severe scrotal pain, what other findings may be present in patients with testicular torsion?**
The testicle may demonstrate a horizontal lie. In addition, the cremasteric reflex may be absent. Patients may have nausea and emesis.

15. **What anatomic variant predisposes patients to developing testicular torsion?**
The bell clapper deformity. The testis is normally fixed to the scrotum posterolaterally at its mesentery and at the lower pole by the gubernaculum. When the mesentery and gubernaculum are deficient, this predisposes a testicle to torsion. This is called a bell clapper deformity because the deficiency in attachments allows the testicle to "swing" like a clapper in a bell.

16. **What is the optimal window in which a torsed testicle must be surgically corrected?**
Suspicion for testicular torsion warrants immediate scrotal exploration to be performed. Irreversible testicular injury may occur as early as 4 hours after initiation of ischemia.

17. **What surgical intervention is performed for testicular torsion?**
Scrotal exploration and detorsion. If the testis appears viable then an orchiopexy is performed. If the testis is not viable despite restoration of blood flow, an orchiectomy is performed. An orchiopexy should be performed on the contralateral testis to prevent future episodes of torsion.

18. **What is Fournier's gangrene?**
It is a rapidly progressive necrotizing infection of the male genitalia characterized by erythema, pain, rapid extension, and crepitus. Mortality can range from 7% to 75% but averages around 20%.

19. **What are predisposing factors for Fournier's gangrene?**
Diabetes mellitus; local trauma; periurethral extravasation of urine from instrumentation; urethral strictures; or urethrocutaneous fistulas, perirectal/ perianal infections, and surgery of the genitalia such as circumcision

20. **What is appropriate treatment for Fournier's gangrene?**
Cardiovascular support and hydration, prompt debridement with tissue culture, and broad spectrum antibiotic coverage with coverage of gram negative and gram positive aerobic and anaerobic organisms. Cultures generally result with multiple organisms.

KEY POINTS: PENILE AND SCROTAL UROLOGIC EMERGENCIES

1. Ischemic priapism requires prompt treatment with corporal body irrigation and/or injection of phenylephrine. Surgical shunting may be required if these measures fail.
2. Penile fracture requires surgical exploration and evaluation for concomitant urethral injury.
3. Suspected testicular torsion cases with supporting history and physical exam findings warrant surgical exploration. Surgery should not be delayed to obtain imaging studies in this setting.
4. A patient with Fournier's gangrene requires emergent surgical debridement, broad spectrum antibiotic coverage, and cardiovascular support. Delay in treatment increases mortality.

WEBSITE

- www.auanet.org

BIBLIOGRAPHY

1. Barthold, JS. Abnormalities of the testes and scrotum and their surgical management. In: Wein AJ, Kavoussi LR. eds. *Campbell-Walsh Urology.* 10th ed. Philadelphia, PA: Elsevier Saunders; 2012:642–645.
2. Jack GS, Garraway I. Current treatment options for penile fractures. *Rev Urol.* 2004;6(3):114–120.
3. Montague DK, Jarow J, Broderick GA, et al. American Urological Association guideline on the management of priapism. *J Urol.* 2003;170(4 pt 1):1318–1324.
4. Schaeffer AJ, Schaeffer EM. Infections of the urinary tract. In: Wein AJ, Kavoussi LR. eds. *Campbell-Walsh Urology.* 10th ed. Philadelphia, PA: Elsevier Saunders; 2012:46–55.
5. Sharp VJ, Kieran K. Testicular torsion: diagnosis, evaluation, and management. *Am Fam Physician.* 2013;88(12): 835–840.

CHAPTER 99

UROLITHIASIS

Yuka Yamaguchi, MD, Timothy K. Ito, MD, Sarah D. Blaschko, MD

1. **What is the likelihood that someone in the United States will have a kidney stone in their lifetime?**
   Approximately 1 in 11 people will have at least one kidney stone in their lifetime.

2. **Are people with kidney stones likely to have stone recurrence?**
   At least 50% of first-time kidney stone patients will have another kidney stone episode within 10 years.

3. **What are the most common types of stones?**
   a. Calcium stones: 80%
   b. Struvite stones: 7%
   c. Uric acid stones: 7%
   d. Cystine stones: 1%–3%

4. **What common medical conditions are associated with kidney stone formation?**
   Obesity, diabetes, and hypertension.

5. **What is the primary dietary adjustment a kidney stone patient can make to help prevent future stone formation?**
   Increase fluid intake to drink at least 2.5 L of water daily. Low sodium and low animal protein diets can also help prevent kidney stone formation.

6. **What is the best study to diagnose urolithiasis?**
   Noncontrast computed tomography (CT) of the abdomen and pelvis. Ultrasonography may be used; however, it is not as sensitive as CT, particularly in the diagnosis of stones in the mid- to distal ureter.

7. **What is a staghorn renal calculus?**
   A branched kidney stone that occupies at least two areas of the kidney (two or more renal calices, the renal pelvis and at least one renal calyx, etc.).

8. **What is the most common stone composition for staghorn renal calculi?**
   Struvite (magnesium, ammonium, phosphate) or calcium carbonate apatite. These stone types are often called "infection stones" because they are associated with urease splitting organisms in the urinary tract.

9. **Why is surgical management of staghorn renal calculi recommended?**
   If left untreated, these stones place patients at risk for urosepsis and for loss of functional renal parenchyma.

10. **What is the recommended surgical treatment for staghorn renal calculi?**
    Percutaneous nephrolithotomy, which is endoscopic removal with direct access into the kidney. If someone has a poorly functioning kidney with a large staghorn renal calculus and evidence of chronic infections, a nephrectomy may also be considered.

11. **What is the typical presentation for a patient passing a stone?**
    Passage of renal calculi into the ureter is typically associated with severe colicky pain, beginning in the flank area. This pain may radiate to the ipsilateral groin. Microscopic or gross hematuria are commonly present (90%), as are nausea and vomiting.

12. **For ureteral calculi, what is the likelihood of spontaneous stone passage?**
    Stones that are 5 mm in size or less have an estimated approximately 70% chance of spontaneous passage, while stones that are 6–9 mm in size have an estimated approximately 50% chance of spontaneous passage.

13. In some studies, what class of medication increases the likelihood of spontaneous stone passage?
Alpha blockers (tamsulosin).

14. What are indications for intervention for a ureteral stone regardless of stone size?
a. When the patient has signs of systemic inflammatory response syndrome (SIRS) or sepsis
b. If the patient has a solitary kidney or minimally functional contralateral kidney
c. Acute kidney injury
d. Intractable nausea/vomiting or pain

15. In what situation must you place a ureteral stent rather than removing or treating the stone itself?
If the patient has signs of a urinary tract infection, SIRS, or sepsis. Manipulation of the stone can cause urosepsis or worsen it if it is already present. The treatment recommendation in this setting is to place a ureteral stent or nephrostomy tube to allow for drainage of the infected urine, to obtain urine and blood cultures, and to treat with broad spectrum antibiotics.

16. What are the two main surgical approaches for treatment of ureteral stones?
Ureteroscopy and shock wave lithotripsy. Ureteroscopy has a higher stone-free rate with a single procedure than shock wave lithotripsy but also has a slightly higher complication rate than shock wave lithotripsy.

17. When is open surgery recommended for treatment of urolithiasis?
In general, endoscopic treatments are recommended for urolithiasis. One may consider open surgery if a reasonable number of endoscopic/percutaneous treatments will not render the patient stone free.

KEY POINTS: UROLITHIASIS

Patients should have prompt surgical management for ureteral stones in the setting of the following:
1. SIRS or sepsis
2. Solitary kidney or solitary functional kidney
3. Acute kidney injury
4. Intractable nausea and emesis or intractable pain

WEBSITE

- www.auanet.org

BIBLIOGRAPHY

1. Scales Jr CD, Smith AC. Prevalence of kidney stones in the United States. *Eur Urol.* 2012;62(1):160–165.
2. Uribarri J, Oh MS. The first kidney stone. *Ann Intern Med.* 1989;111(12):1006–1009.
3. Taylor EN, Stampfer MJ. Obesity, weight gain, and the risk of kidney stones. *JAMA.* 2005;293(4):455–462.
4. Borghi L, Meschi T, Guerra A, et al. Essential arterial hypertension and stone disease. *Kidney Int.* 1999;55(6): 2397–2406.
5. Taylor EN, Stampfer MJ. Diabetes mellitus and the risk of nephrolithiasis. *Kidney Int.* 2005;68(3):1230–1235.
6. Segura JW, Preminger GM, Assimos DG, et al. Ureteral Stones Clinical Guidelines Panel summary report on the management of ureteral calculi. The American Urological Association. *J Urol.* 1997;158(5):1915–1921.
7. Surgical management of stones: American Urological Association/Endourological Society guideline. <https://www.auanet. org/guidelines/surgical-management-of-stones>; Accessed 06.04.17.
8. Medical management of kidney stones: AUA guideline. <https://www.auanet.org/guidelines/medical-management -of-kidney-stones>; Accessed 06.04.17.

XI
UROLOGY

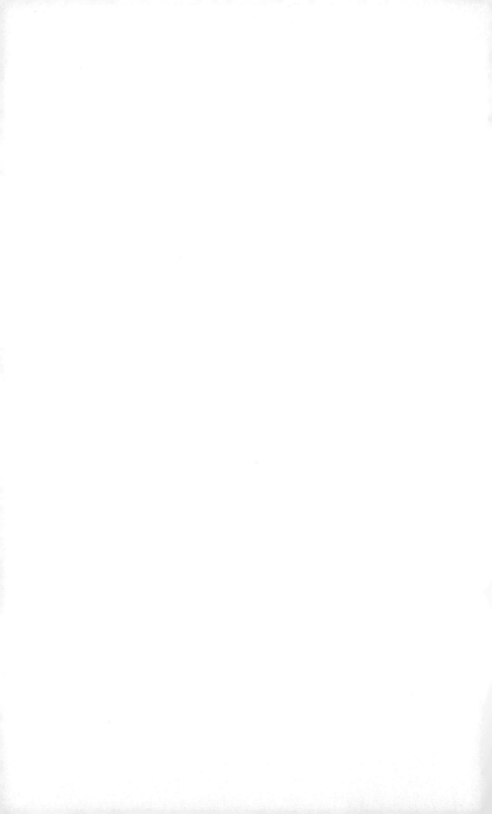

CHAPTER 100

RENAL CANCER

Rodrigo Pessoa, MD, Fernando J. Kim, MD, MBA, FACS

1. **How common is renal cell carcinoma (RCC)?**
   All solid renal masses and cystic lesions with solid components are suspicious for RCC, which affects approximately 65,000 new patients each year and has a 5-year mortality rate of 35%.

2. **What is the etiology of RCC?**
   The etiology is unknown, but cigarette smoking is a well-known risk factor. Recurrent RCC is a common manifestation in patients with von Hippel-Lindau disease.

3. **What are the signs and symptoms of RCC?**
   The most common presenting signs and symptoms are gross or microscopic hematuria. The classic triad of hematuria, flank pain, and an abdominal mass is found in only about 10%–15% of RCC cases. Patients with metastatic disease may present with symptoms of lung or bone metastasis, such as dyspnea, cough, or bone pain. About 20% of RCCs are associated with a paraneoplastic syndrome. Many solid renal tumors are detected incidentally by a computed tomography scan of the abdomen performed for another reason. Stauffer's syndrome is diagnosed with elevated liver function tests (LFTs) in the presence of RCC that normalize after nephrectomy and tumor removal; it is thought to be a type of paraneoplastic syndrome.

4. **Are all solid masses in the kidney RCC?**
   No. Other solid masses include angiomyolipomas, oncocytomas, sarcomas, and metastatic lesions. However, all solid masses should be presumed to be RCC until proven otherwise.

5. **What is the unique relationship between RCC and its vasculature?**
   RCC has a tendency to invade its own venous drainage. Tumor thrombus may extend along the renal vein into the inferior vena cava and even to the right atrium.

6. **How should suspected involvement of the vena cava be evaluated?**
   Magnetic resonance angiography.

7. **How is RCC treated?**
   Surgery is the optimal treatment for localized RCC. Based on current available oncological and quality of life outcomes, localized renal cancers are better managed by organ-sparing therapy whenever possible and for small renal masses (<4 cm) rather than radical nephrectomy (RN), irrespective of the surgical approach. Both procedures can be performed by open, laparoscopic, or robotic-assisted surgery.

8. **When is nephron-sparing nephrectomy indicated in cases of RCC?**
   Partial nephrectomy (laparoscopic assisted) is recommended in patients with T1a tumors (<4 cm). Partial nephrectomy should also be favored over RN in patients with T1b tumors (4–7cm), whenever feasible. Ablative technology (i.e., cryoablation and radiofrequency ablation) is a good option to nephron-sparing surgeries with equivalent midterm oncological outcomes.

9. **How is metastatic RCC treated?**
   Chemotherapy has been disappointing. Historically, encouraging results were achieved with cytoreductive RN and interleukin-2 (IL-2) treatment. Currently, targeted therapy with tyrosine kinase inhibitors offers some evidence of definite durable responses. Research is ongoing using different targeted therapy strategies.

10. **What are the common sites of metastatic renal cancer?**
    The overall distribution of metastatic sites is lung (45.2%), bone (29.5%), lymph nodes (21.8%), liver (20.3%), adrenal (8.9%), and brain (8.1%).

KEY POINTS: RENAL CANCER

1. The classic triad is hematuria, flank pain, and an abdominal mass, usually found in advanced cases of RCC.
2. Surgery is the optimal treatment for localized RCC.
3. Stauffer's syndrome is diagnosed with elevated LFTs in the presence of RCC that normalize after nephrectomy and tumor removal; it is thought to be a type of paraneoplastic syndrome.

WEBSITE

- www.auanet.org
- www.cancer.org/research/cancerfactsstatistics/cancerfactsfigures2014/

BIBLIOGRAPHY

1. Kim FJ, Rha KH. Laparoscopic radical versus partial nephrectomy: assessment of complications. *J Urol*. 2003;170(2 pt 1): 408–411.
2. Greenlee RT, Hill-Harmon MB. Cancer statistics. *CA Cancer J Clin*. 2001;51(1):15–36.
3. Figlin RA. Renal cell carcinoma: management of advanced disease. *J Urol*. 1999;161(2): 391–387.
4. Pierorazio PM, Johnson MH, Patel HD, et al. Management of renal masses and localized renal cancer: systematic review and meta-analysis. *J Urol*. 2016;196(4):989–999.
5. da Silva RD, Jaworski P, Gustafson D, et al. How I do it: laparoscopic renal cryoablation (LRC). *Can J Urol*. 2014;21(6):7574–7577.

BLADDER CANCER

Rodrigo Pessoa, MD, Fernando J. Kim, MD, MBA, FACS

1. **What is the incidence of transitional cell carcinoma (TCC) of the bladder?**
   Bladder cancer accounts for about 5% of all new cancers in the United States. The American Cancer Society's estimates for bladder cancer in the United States are 79,030 new cases (60,490 in men and 18,540 in women) and 16,870 deaths for 2017. Recently, the overall rates of new bladder cancers and of cancer deaths have been dropping slightly in women. In men, incidence rates have been decreasing and death rates have been stable.

2. **What are the risk factors associated with bladder TCC?**
   Age (peak incidence in seventh decade), cigarette smoking, occupational exposure to aniline dyes or aromatic amines, phenacetin abuse, and chemotherapy with cyclophosphamide.

3. **What are the signs and symptoms of bladder TCC?**
   Painless hematuria (gross or microscopic) is the most common finding and is present in up to 90% of patients. Frequency, urgency, and dysuria also may be presenting symptoms, especially for carcinoma in situ (CIS).

4. **What is the most common histologic type of bladder cancer?**
   TCC makes up >90% of bladder cancers. Other histologic types include adenocarcinoma, squamous cell carcinoma, and urachal carcinoma.

5. **How do you evaluate a patient with hematuria and bladder mass?**
   Complete workup for hematuria includes (1) urine analysis, culture and bladder washings for cytology; (2) upper tract imaging study to rule out concomitant upper tract disease with computed tomography intravenous pyelogram (IVP) or MRI IVP or IVP; and (3) cystoscopy, which will define further studies (bladder biopsy).

6. **How do you manage bladder TCC?**
   Initial management includes endoscopic transurethral resection and fulguration of bladder lesion. Further treatment is determined by the pathologic stage of the disease.

7. **What is the recurrence rate of TCC after initial transurethral resection of bladder tumor?**
   Approximately 45% of patients will have tumor recurrence within 12 months of transurethral resection of bladder tumor (TURBT) alone.

8. **How often do you expect to see a high-grade muscle invasive bladder TCC?**
   The vast majority (70%–75%) of bladder TCC present as superficial (nonmuscle invasive) lesions. Furthermore, the greater part of lesions is categorized as low grade, with only 2%–4% categorized as high grade.

9. **How often should superficial lesions be followed with surveillance cystoscopy and urine cytology?**
   Every 3 months in the first 3 years after initial diagnosis, followed by every 6 months for the subsequent 2–3 years, and then annually thereafter. Surveillance includes periodic upper tract imaging, especially for high-risk patients.

10. **Is there a chance of concurrent urothelial cancers?**
    About 5% of patients with bladder cancer will have urothelial carcinoma outside the bladder (i.e., renal pelvis, ureter, or urethra).

11. **Is CIS a less aggressive type of bladder cancer?**
    No. CIS is a flat but poorly differentiated tumor. It can metastasize and should be treated as an aggressive form of bladder cancer.

12. **How do you manage bladder CIS?**
    Immunotherapy with intravesical bacillus Calmette-Guerin (BCG) is the first-line treatment. Response rates to BCG approach 70%. Other intravesical agents, such as mitomycin C, are generally less effective than BCG.

13. **What are the organs removed during radical cystectomy in males and females?**
    Radical cystectomies include an extensive pelvic lymphadenectomy and removal of the following organs:
    - Males: Bladder and prostate
    - Females: Bladder, uterus, and often the anterior wall of the vagina

14. **What are the side effects of BCG?**
    Mild symptoms of urinary frequency, urgency, and dysuria are common. Myalgia and low-grade fever (flulike symptoms) also occur. High or persistent fever suggests a more serious problem requiring antituberculous therapy. Rarely, death from BCG has been reported.

15. **When can we start the intravesical BCG treatment?**
    Initiation of intravesical BCG therapy is usually delayed for 2–3 weeks following TURBT.

16. **What is the most important pathological finding when choosing the treatment?**
    The presence of muscle invasion. Nonmuscle invasive cancers can be treated with surveillance and repeated TURBT. The presence of muscle invasive cancer mandates a more aggressive approach (i.e., radical cystectomy or cystoprostatectomy in men, with some form of urinary diversion or maximum TURBT and radiotherapy).

17. **What types of urinary diversion are used with radical cystectomy?**
    Diversion techniques require either a conduit or a continent reservoir. The most common is an ileal conduit. The stoma collection device must be worn with a conduit. Continent reservoirs can be made with either small bowel or large intestine and must be emptied via the urethra or a continent stoma.

18. **What type of chemotherapy is used for metastatic bladder cancer?**
    Most chemotherapy regimens include a platinum-based agent.

19. **In certain countries, TCC is not the predominant form of bladder cancer. What is the predominant histologic type? Why?**
    In countries such as Egypt, where schistosomiasis is endemic, squamous cell carcinoma of the bladder is common.

20. **Are there any molecular markers that can be used to predict chemo sensitivity for the treatment of bladder TCC?**
    Yes, overexpression of epidermal growth factor receptor 3 (EGFR3) is present in basal cell bladder cancer, a chemo-sensitive subtype. A subgroup of patients with the so-called luminal type that displays an overexpression of fibroblast growth factor receptor 3 (FGFR3), ERBB3, and epidermal growth factor receptor (ERBB21) may be chemotherapy resistant.

KEY POINTS: BLADDER CANCER

1. Bladder cancer presents as painless hematuria.
2. The most common histologic type of bladder cancer is TCC.
3. CIS of the bladder is treated with intravesical BCG.

WEBSITE

- www.cancer.org/acs/groups/cid/documents/webcontent/003085-pdf.pdf
- www.auanet.org

BIBLIOGRAPHY

1. Dinney CP, Hansel D, McConkey D, et al. Novel neoadjuvant therapy paradigms for bladder cancer: results from the National Cancer Center Institute Forum. *Urol Oncol.* 2014;32(8):1108–1115.
2. Hendricksen K, Witjes JA. Current strategies for first and second line intravesical therapy for nonmuscle invasive bladder cancer. *Curr Opin Urol.* 2007;17(5):352–357.
3. Soloway MS, Lee CT. Difficult decisions in urologic oncology: management of high-grade T1 transitional cell carcinoma of the bladder. *Urol Oncol.* 2007;25(4):338–340.
4. Hall MC, Chang SS, Dalbagni G, et al. Guideline for the management of nonmuscle invasive bladder cancer (stages Ta, T1, and Tis): 2007 update. *J Urol.* 2007;178(6):2314–2330.
5. Choi W, Porten S, Kim S, et al. Identification of distinct basal and luminal subtypes of muscle-invasive bladder cancer with different sensitivities to frontline chemotherapy. *Cancer Cell.* 2014;25(2):152–165.

CHAPTER 102

PROSTATE CANCER

Rodrigo Pessoa, MD, Priya N. Werahera, PhD, Fernando J. Kim, MD, MBA, FACS

1. **What is the prevalence of prostate cancer in the United States?**
   Prostate cancer is the most common cancer among men, except for skin cancer. In 2016 an estimated 180,890 men in the United States will be diagnosed with prostate cancer. Prostate cancer is the second leading cause of cancer death in men in the United States. It is estimated that 26,120 deaths from this disease will occur in 2016.

2. **Do most men die with prostate cancer, rather than from it?**
   Yes, but more than 20,000 men will die of prostate cancer annually in the United States. Thus, it should not be treated as a benign disease.

3. **What are the early symptoms of prostate cancer?**
   There are none. By the time significant symptoms develop, the disease is likely to be advanced. This is an argument for screening to detect prostate cancer.

4. **Is prostate cancer screening performed in the United States?**
   In 2012 the United States Preventive Services Task Force reviewed new evidence on the benefits and harms of prostate-specific antigen (PSA) screening for prostate cancer and recommended screening for 55- to 69-year-old patients (Grade D recommendation). Digital rectal examination (DRE) combined with serum PSA remains the best available method to recommend prostate biopsy for detection of prostate cancer. Most societies advise to not subject men to PSA testing without counseling them on the potential risks and benefits. In summary, it is only recommended to offer an individualized risk-adapted strategy for early detection to a well-informed man with a good performance status and a life expectancy of at least 10–15 years.

5. **How is prostate cancer diagnosed?**
   It is diagnosed with prostate biopsy, which is a biopsy using transrectal ultrasound (US) for guidance or incidentally after transurethral resection of the prostate (TURP) for benign prostatic hyperplasia (BPH) is performed.

6. **When is prostate biopsy indicated?**
   When either the PSA ≥4 ng/mL or abnormal DRE (palpable nodule).

7. **Does an elevated PSA level mean a man has prostate cancer?**
   No. PSA can be elevated due to BPH, prostatitis, or after prostate trauma. It is prostate specific, not prostate cancer specific.

8. **What is a PSA?**
   It means prostatic specific antigen, a protein produced exclusively by prostate cells.

9. **Are there any known risk factors for prostate cancer?**
   Yes. A first-degree relative in the family increases the risk eight times compared to the general population. African American men are also at an increased risk. A high-fat diet may play a role in increasing risk of many cancers, including prostate cancer.

10. **What is Gleason's sum?**
    The Gleason scoring system has been revised recently. Only three Gleason grades, 3–5, are currently recognized in the revised system instead of the five original Gleason grades, 1–5. Original Gleason grades 1 and 2 are now included within the Gleason grade 3 tumors and considered to be nonaggressive. Gleason grades 4 and 5 tumors are considered more aggressive with metastatic potential and worse clinical outcomes. Prostate tumors are heterogeneous in terms of grade and behave according to the composition of grades within the tumor. Thus, tumors are graded by the sum of the two most important grades present as a Gleason score (GS) ranging from 6 to 10. Tumors of GS 6 (3 + 3) are

considered low grade (LG), while GS ≥7 with Gleason grades 4 and 5 are high grade (HG). GS is currently the best prognostic variable available to predict the clinical outcome of this disease.

11. **How is clinically localized prostate cancer managed?**
Surgery (radical prostatectomy), radiation therapy by external beam or interstitial seed implant, cryotherapy, high-intensity focused ultrasound (HIFU), or active surveillance.

12. **How is advanced metastatic prostate cancer treated?**
Hormonal ablation therapy (orchiectomy or luteinizing hormone-releasing hormone agonist drugs) and/or chemotherapy.

13. **What is androgen resistant prostate cancer?**
Castrate-resistant prostate cancer is defined by disease progression despite androgen-deprivation therapy and may present as one or any combination of a continuous rise in serum levels of PSA, progression of preexisting disease, or appearance of new metastases.

14. **What are the common sites of metastatic prostate disease?**
The most frequent sites of metastatic involvement are bone (90%), lung (46%), liver (25%), pleura (21%), and adrenals (13%). Several lines of evidence suggested the existence of a backward metastatic pathway through veins from the prostate to the spine in addition to classical hematogenous tumor spread via the vena cava.

KEY POINTS: PROSTATE CANCER

1. Prostate cancer is the most common malignancy diagnosed in men in the United States.
2. Clinically localized prostate cancer is approached with surgery, radiation, cryotherapy, or active surveillance.
3. Prostate cancer screening should be discussed between patient and healthcare provider.

WEBSITES

- www.prostatecancerfoundation.org/
- www.cancer.gov/cancertopics/types/prostate
- http://www.cancer.net/cancer-types/prostate-cancer/statistics

BIBLIOGRAPHY

1. Catalona WJ. Clinical utility of free and total prostate-specific antigen (PSA): a review. *Rev Prostate.* 1996;7(suppl):64.
2. D'Amico AV, Whittington R, Malkowicz SB, et al. Biochemical outcome after radical prostatectomy, external beam radiation therapy, or interstitial radiation therapy for clinically localized prostate cancer. *JAMA.* 1998;280(11):969–974.
3. Denberg TD, Kim FJ, Flanigan RC, et al. The influence of patient race and social vulnerability on urologist treatment recommendations in localized prostate carcinoma. *Med Care.* 2006;44(12):1137–1141.
4. Greenlee RT, Hill-Harmon MB. Cancer statistics 2001. *CA Cancer J Clin.* 2001;51(1):15–36.
5. Keetch DW, Humphrey PA. Clinical and pathological features of hereditary prostate cancer. *J Urol.* 1996;155(6):1841–1843.
6. Polascik TJ, Pound CR. Comparison of radical prostatectomy and iodine-125 interstitial radiotherapy for the treatment of clinically localized prostate cancer: a 7-year biochemical (PSA) progression analysis. *Urology.* 1998;51(6):884–890.
7. Schroder FH, Hugosson J, Roobol MJ, et al. Screening and prostate cancer mortality: results of the European Randomised Study of Screening for Prostate Cancer (ERSPC) at 13 years of follow-up. *Lancet.* 2014;384(9959):2027–2035.

CHAPTER 103

URODYNAMICS AND VOIDING DYSFUNCTION

Rodrigo Pessoa, MD, Fernando J. Kim, MD, MBA, FACS

1. **What is an urodynamic study?**
   Urodynamic studies assess the functional aspects of the storage and emptying ability of the lower urinary tract (LUT). The principles of urodynamic studies originated from hydrodynamics. The components of urodynamic studies are cystometrogram, leak point pressures, urethral profile pressures, pressure-flow studies, uroflowmetry, and electromyography. These studies have evolved into videourodynamics with the addition of fluoroscopy (i.e., video).

2. **What is uroflowmetry?**
   Uroflowmetry is the measurement of voided urine (in milliliters) per unit of time (in seconds). The important elements of the test are voided volume (which should be >150 mL), maximum flow rate (Qmax), and the curve of the flow (which should be bell shaped). In men, a Qmax >15 mL/s is considered normal, whereas a Qmax <10 mL/s is considered abnormal. Assigning normal values in females is more difficult. In women, uroflowmetry is characterized by the shorter urethra and no resistance, such as that caused by the prostate gland in the male. Normal values are described as a Qmax between 20 and 36 mL/s.

3. **What is benign prostatic hyperplasia (BPH)?**
   BPH is benign enlargement of the prostate gland that may lead to bladder outlet obstructive symptoms in men. These symptoms have been termed *lower urinary tract symptoms* (LUTSs).

4. **What is an American Urological Association (AUA) Symptom Score?**
   It is a self-reported questionnaire developed and popularized by the AUA for the assessment of bothersome LUTS in men. This questionnaire has seven questions with a maximum score of 35. The higher the score, the more bothersome; the AUA Symptom Score has become an index for both the diagnosis and evaluation of treatment outcome in patients with LUTSs.

5. **What are the main functions of the LUT?**
   Storage and emptying of urine are the main functions. For practical purposes, all symptoms of LUT dysfunction can be categorized into the malfunction of either storing or emptying ability.

6. **What are the control mechanisms for LUT function?**
   The control mechanisms for LUT function are recognized as central and peripheral. The central control mechanism consists of the cortical portion of the frontal lobe of the brain and pontine micturition center. The peripheral control mechanism includes the thoracic sympathetic and lumbar parasympathetic innervations and neuromuscular apparatus of the LUT organs.

7. **What is the role of the autonomic nervous system in the function of the LUT?**
   Sympathetic fibers, which originate from the T10-L2 portion of the spinal cord, innervate the bladder neck and proximal urethra. These fibers mostly control the contraction of the proximal urethra or bladder neck and relaxation of the bladder, which results in storage of urine. The parasympathetic fibers, which originate primarily from the S2-S4 portion of the spinal cord, innervate the bladder body. The parasympathetic innervation allows contraction of the bladder smooth muscle, leading to bladder emptying.

8. **Is there a better way to memorize this function?**
   Yes. Parasympathetic: Piss; Sympathetic: Storage.

9. **What is the role of the somatic nervous system in the function of the LUT?**
   Voluntary control of the striated muscle of the external urinary sphincter is controlled by the somatic nervous system. Somatic fibers are conveyed to the sphincter by the pudendal nerve.

10. **What is the bulbocavernosal reflex?**
    Bulbocavernous reflex tests the integrity of the peripheral neurologic control of the LUT. This reflex is elicited by stimulation of the glans penis in men or clitoris in women, which causes contraction of the external anal sphincter or bulbocarnosus muscle. Alternatively, the reflex may be stimulated by pulling the balloon of a Foley catheter against the bladder neck. This reflex is present in all normal men and in approximately 70% of normal woman. Absence of this reflex in men is strongly suggestive of a sacral neurologic lesion.

11. **What is the most common cause of urinary incontinence in the geriatric population?**
    The most common are transient causes, mostly external, that disrupt the fragile balance of LUT function in elderly patients and cause urinary incontinence. These causes can be recalled with the mnemonic DIAPPERS:
    Delirium
    Infection
    Atrophic urethritis or vaginitis
    Pharmaceuticals
    Psychologic (depression)
    Endocrine (hypercalcemia, hyperglycemia)
    Restricted mobility
    Stool impaction

12. **What is spinal shock? What type of urinary dysfunction does it cause?**
    Spinal shock is the loss of contractility of the smooth muscle below the level of spinal cord injury, leading to difficulty in bladder emptying or urinary retention. This phenomenon may last from hours to several months, with a high chance of reversibility if the spinal cord injury is not permanent.

13. **What is autonomic dysreflexia? How is it treated?**
    Autonomic dysreflexia results from systematic outpouring of sympathetic discharge, as in patients with spinal cord lesions above T6 level. This dysreflexia is triggered by distention of the bladder or other stimulus of the bowel or LUT. It is manifested by hypertension, bradycardia, hot flush, sweating, and headache. Initial treatment consists of the removal of the stimulus, such as emptying the bladder and placing the patient in a sitting position. Antihypertensive drugs may be used as either prophylaxis or treatment of severe episodes. This condition may lead to significant cerebrovascular complication if untreated.

14. **What type of bladder dysfunction is frequently seen in patients with diabetes?**
    Patients with diabetes may develop diabetic cystopathy, which is a chronic complication of diabetes with a classic triad of symptoms—decreased bladder sensation, increased bladder capacity, and impaired detrusor contractility. Impaired detrusor contractility may lead to incomplete bladder empty-ing and subsequently result in voiding difficulty, urinary retention, chronic urinary tract infection, and upper urinary tract damage.

15. **What type of bladder dysfunction is frequently seen in patients with multiple sclerosis (MS)?**
    Urgency (83%), urge incontinence (75%), detrusor hyperreflexia (62%), and detrusor sphincter dys-synergia (25%) are among the most common LUT symptoms in patients with MS. The worsening of bladder dysfunction correlates with the increasing spinal cord involvement and the neurologic symp-toms in MS. Variation in symptoms depends on the site of involvement by MS. Involvement of pontine pathways (tegmentum) is associated with a much higher rate of urinary symptoms.

16. **Which sacral roots control the micturition physiology?**
    They are S2-S4.

17. **What are the causes of urinary retention after abdominal or pelvic surgery?**
    They are injuries or disruption of pelvic plexus innervation of the LUT.

18. **What is the surgical treatment for BPH?**
    Traditionally, the transurethral resection of the prostate is the gold standard surgical treatment for BPH that failed medical therapy. Other minimally invasive therapies including laser enucleation, abla-tion, and vaporization may be included in the urologic armamentarium. Open surgical approach are reserved for large prostates (>80 g) and/or BPH with associated bladder stones.

KEY POINTS: URODYNAMICS AND VOIDING DYSFUNCTION

1. Uroflowmetry is the measurement of voided urine (in milliliters) per unit of time (in seconds).
2. BPH is benign enlargement of the prostate gland that may lead to bladder outlet obstructive symptoms in men.
3. The sacral roots involved in micturition physiology are S2-S4.

WEBSITE

- www.icsoffice.org
- www.auanet.org

BIBLIOGRAPHY

1. Cole EE, Dmochowski RR. Office urodynamics. *Urol Clin North Am.* 2005;32(3):353–370.
2. de Sèze M, Ruffion A. The neurogenic bladder in multiple sclerosis: review of the literature and proposal of management guidelines. *Mult Scler.* 2007;13(7):915–928.
3. Gibbs CF, Johnson TM. Office management of geriatric urinary incontinence. *Am J Med.* 2007;120(3):211–220.
4. Hashim H, Abrams P. Overactive bladder: an update. *Curr Opin Urol.* 2007;17(4):231–236.
5. Messelink B, Benson T, Berghmans B, et al. Standardization of terminology of pelvic floor muscle function and dysfunction: report from the pelvic floor clinical assessment group of the International Continence Society. *Neurourol Urodyn.* 2005;24(4):374–380.

CHAPTER 104

PEDIATRIC UROLOGY

Rodrigo Pessoa, MD, Siam Oottamasathien, MD, FAAP, FACS,
Fernando J. Kim, MD, MBA, FACS

1. **How should we evaluate a patient with febrile urinary tract infection (UTI)?**
   After treatment of the infection, the patient should undergo a urinary tract evaluation with a renal-bladder sonogram and ± voiding cystourethrogram (VCUG). Approximately 50% of children under the age of 12 presenting with a UTI are found to have abnormalities of the genitourinary (GU) tract. The most common abnormalities identified are vesicoureteral reflux (VUR), obstructive uropathies, and neurogenic bladder. In the absence of anatomic abnormalities, the most common causes of UTI in children are constipation and dysfunctional voiding.

2. **What is VUR disease?**
   The reflux of urine from the bladder into the upper urinary tract. Primary VUR is caused by an inadequate valvular mechanism at the ureterovesical junction, presumably related to a shortened submucosal ureteral tunnel. One-half of children with culture-documented UTIs have VUR.

3. **Is VUR damaging to the kidney?**
   VUR increases the likelihood of renal scar by 2.5-fold. Reflux of infected urine can lead to pyelonephritis and subsequent renal scarring. Currently, renal scarring is the fourth leading cause for renal transplantation in children. The combination of VUR and elevated bladder storage pressures (e.g., neuropathic bladder or bladder outlet obstruction) is harmful to the kidney, and a concurrent UTI makes this situation particularly dangerous.

4. **What are the indications for surgical correction of VUR?**
   Reflux resolves spontaneously in many children; however, high-grade reflux, especially when bilateral, is unlikely to resolve. Most children with high-grade reflux or breakthrough UTIs despite antibiotic prophylaxis should be managed surgically. Surgical management may also be appropriate in children with reflux persisting into late childhood or adolescence. Bulking agents have been evaluated, but long-term results and durability remain unclear.

5. **What is the most common cause of antenatal hydronephrosis?**
   Ureteropelvic junction (UPJ) obstruction. Hydronephrosis is the most common abnormality detected on prenatal ultrasound and accounts for 50% of all prenatally detected lesions. Fifty percent of prenatal hydronephrosis, in turn, is caused by UPJ obstruction. UPJ obstruction is bilateral in approximately 20% of cases and associated with VUR in 15% of cases.

6. **What is the most common cause of UPJ obstruction?**
   Intrinsic stenosis. Less common causes include a lower pole (renal) crossing vessel, anomalous ureteral insertions (high in the renal pelvis), and peripelvic fibrosis.

7. **Can UPJ obstruction resolve spontaneously? What are the indications for pyeloplasty?**
   Yes. Ultimately, only about 25% of children with findings consistent for UPJ obstruction require pyeloplasty. The indications for surgical intervention include worsening hydronephrosis, poor or declining renal function, pain, infection, and the presence of a solitary kidney or bilateral hydronephrosis.

8. **What is the Meyer-Weigert law?**
   This law refers to the position of the ureteral orifices in patients with complete ureteral duplication. Occasionally, two ureteral buds develop independently from the mesonephric duct. As the ureteral buds are absorbed into the developing bladder, the bud located in a lower position along the duct (draining the lower pole of the kidney) is carried to a more cranial and lateral position. The ureteral bud located in a higher position along the duct (draining the upper pole of the kidney) is carried to a more caudal and medial position within the bladder. Lower pole ureters are more likely to reflux because of their lateral position within the bladder, whereas upper pole ureters are more frequently obstructed and are more often associated with a ureterocele or ectopia.

9. **What is an ureterocele?**
   An ureterocele is a cystic dilatation of the distal portion of the ureter. Ureteroceles are usually associated with the upper pole ureter of a duplicated collecting system; however, they also may develop from single system ureters. They are usually ectopic (i.e., some portion of the ureterocele is positioned at the bladder neck or urethra) and frequently cause ureteral obstruction.

10. **What is an ectopic ureter?**
    It is a ureter with an abnormal insertion site. Ectopic ureteral insertions could involve not only the bladder but many regions of the GU system (i.e., vaginal, seminal vesicle).

11. **What is the most common presenting symptom in a girl with an ectopic ureter?**
    Incontinence. In females, an ectopic ureter will usually drain into the bladder neck, proximal urethra, or vestibule. The orifice may also be located in the vagina (25%) and occasionally the uterus. When the ectopic ureteral orifice is positioned below the external sphincter or within the female genital tract, incontinence can develop. Infection is also a common presenting symptom of an ectopic ureter, occurring as a consequence of ureteral obstruction.

12. **Do boys with ectopic ureters present with incontinence?**
    No. The ectopic pathway in boys extends from the bladder neck through the posterior urethra to the mesonephric duct derivatives (i.e., vas deferens, epididymis, and seminal vesicle). Therefore, the ectopic ureteral orifice is always positioned above the continence mechanism.

13. **What percentage of full-term male infants has an undescended testicle?**
    Three percent. This number decreases to 0.8% by 1 year of age.

14. **What is the most common location of an undescended testicle?**
    The inguinal canal (72% of undescended testicles). The testicle also may be located in the abdomen (8%) or prescrotal area (20%). Twenty percent of undescended testicles are nonpalpable at presentation; of these, 20% are absent completely.

15. **Why should the testicle be brought back into the scrotum?**
    Patients with cryptorchidism have a 15- to 40-fold increased risk of germ cell cancer compared with the normal population. Although positioning of the testicle within the scrotum does not alleviate this risk, it does permit routine, thorough, testicular examination. Patients with cryptorchidism are also at risk for infertility. Histologic studies have demonstrated progressive germ cell loss in the undescended testicle beginning at 18 months of age. Early orchiopexy can minimize the extent of germ cell loss and thereby decrease the chance of future infertility. In general, the higher the testicle (i.e., within the abdomen), the greater the risk of cancer and infertility.

16. **What is the most common cause of bladder outlet obstruction in boys? In girls?**
    Posterior urethral valves and ureterocele, respectively.

17. **What are the urinary manifestations of posterior urethral valves?**
    Posterior urethral valves are congenital leaflets of tissue, which extend from the verumontanum to the anterior urethra in boys. They occur at an incidence of 1/8000 live male births. Posterior urethral valves cause bladder outlet obstruction, which in turn leads to variable degrees of bladder and renal injury. Severe obstruction may result in oligohydramnios, pulmonary hypoplasia, bladder hypertrophy, VUR, hydroureteronephrosis, and renal dysplasia. Fifty percent of affected children have reflux, and 33% progress to end-stage renal disease.

18. **What is a myelomeningocele? What are its urologic consequences?**
    A myelomeningocele is a hernia protrusion of the spinal cord and its meninges through a defect in the vertebral column. The resulting neurologic injury causes, among other problems, bladder dysfunction. Patients with myelomeningocele are usually incontinent because of detrusor hyperactivity, detrusor hypoactivity, poor bladder compliance, inadequate outlet resistance, detrusor-outlet dyssynergy, or a combination of these factors. More importantly, patients with hyperactive, high-pressure bladders may develop upper urinary tract deterioration. Lifelong follow-up is necessary for these children because the neurologic lesion can change with time. Treatment goals include maintenance of a low-pressure urinary reservoir, prevention of UTIs, prevention of upper urinary tract deterioration, and the achievement of continence.

19. **What is the most common cause of ambiguous genitalia in the newborn?**
    Congenital adrenal hyperplasia, most commonly as a result of a 21-hydroxylase enzyme deficiency.

20. **What diagnostic evaluation should be performed in any male infant presenting with hypospadias and cryptorchidism?**
    The presence of cryptorchidism and hypospadias should alert the physician to the possibility of an androgenized female. A karyotype should always be obtained before surgical intervention.

21. **What is the most common solid renal mass in infancy? In childhood?**
    In infancy: Congenital mesoblastic nephroma. This is a benign tumor of the kidney that can be managed with surgical excision alone. In childhood: Wilms' tumor. Wilms' tumor is associated with Beckwith-Wiedemann syndrome, isolated hemihypertrophy, and congenital aniridia. The most important prognostic factors are tumor stage and histology. Treatment is multimodal, consisting of surgery, chemotherapy, and radiation.

KEY POINTS: PEDIATRIC UROLOGY

1. After treatment of febrile UTI, a full urinary tract evaluation with a renal-bladder sonogram and ± VCUG should be done.
2. Approximately 50% of children under the age of 12 presenting with a UTI are found to have abnormalities of the GU tract.
3. The most common solid renal mass in infancy is congenital mesoblastic nephroma and in childhood is Wilms' tumor.

WEBSITES

- www.auanet.org/education/guidelines
- www.spuonline.org

BIBLIOGRAPHY

1. Baker LA, Silver RI. Cryptorchidism. In: Gearhart JP, Rink RC, eds. *Pediatric Urology*. 2nd ed. Philadelphia: WB Saunders; 2010:563–576.
2. Chang SL, Shortliffe LD. Pediatric urinary tract infections. *Pediatr Clin North Am*. 2006;53(3):379–400.
3. Cooper CS, Snyder HM. Ureteral duplication, ectopy, and ureteroceles. In: Gearhart JP, Rink RC, eds. *Pediatric Urology*. 2nd ed. Philadelphia: WB Saunders; 2010:337–352.
4. Diamond DA, Yu RN. Sexual differentiation: normal and abnormal. In: Wein AJ, Kavoussi LR, eds. *Campbell-Walsh Urology*. 10th ed. Philadelphia: Saunders Elsevier; 2011:3597–3628.
5. Greenbaum LA, Mesrobian HG. Vesicoureteral reflux. *Pediatr Clin North Am*. 2006;53(3):413–427.
6. Herndon CD. Antenatal hydronephrosis: differential diagnosis, evaluation, and treatment options. *Scientific World Journal*. 2006;6:2345–2365.
7. Hutson JM, Clarke MC. Current management of the undescended testicle. *Semin Pediatr Surg*. 2007;16(1):64–70.
8. Shortliff LM. Infection and inflammation of the pediatric genitourinary tract. In: Wein AJ, Kavoussi LR, eds. *Campbell-Walsh Urology*. 10th ed. Philadelphia: Saunders Elsevier; 2011:3085–3122.
9. Yeung CK, Sihoe JDY. Non-neuropathic dysfunction of the lower urinary tract in children. In: Wein AJ, Kavoussi LR, eds. *Campbell-Walsh Urology*. 10th ed. Philadelphia: Saunders Elsevier; 2011:3411–3431.
10. Yohannes P, Hanna M. Current trends in the management of posterior urethral valves in the pediatric population. *Urology*. 2002;60(6):947–953.

XII
HEALTHCARE

CHAPTER 105

CAN HEALTHCARE BE REFORMED?

John Chapman, MBA, Alden H. Harken, MD, FACS

1. **Is healthcare reform an oxymoron?**
   Yes.

2. **What is fee for service?**
   The doctor establishes the price, and the patient agrees to pay it. This traditional system of exchange has great merit if both parties understand the value of the service provided. If either party (usually the patient) cannot estimate the service value, it is possible (even likely) that the doctor will honestly escalate the service value in a fashion unchecked by the patient's perceptions. Thus, in a fee-for-service system, medical prices tend to increase.

3. **What is discounted fee for service?**
   The patient gets together with a group of friends, and they come to the doctor with the following proposition: "Hey, Doc, you can dazzle us with your fancy medical talk, but we still think that your prices are too high. How about my pals and I pay you 80% of what you charge us?"

4. **Is there a difference between hospital costs and hospital charges?**
   Absolutely. Hospital cost is the sum of the expenses (e.g., sutures, nurses' salaries, electricity, instrumentation sterilization, Band-Aids) that are expended in suturing a laceration, for example. The hospital typically charges about twice the cost (100% markup) for repairing a cut finger. This markup is highly industry specific. Thus, whereas intensely competitive food chains may make a profit of only one penny on a loaf of bread, hospitals and liquor stores usually charge twice the cost.

5. **What are fixed costs?**
   After accounting for light, heat, and staff (nurses, housekeepers, administrators) at a hospital, but before seeing a single patient, doctors and the hospital have already spent a huge amount of money. Doctors and hospitals must pay fixed costs whether or not they provide any medical services at all.

6. **What are actual costs?**
   These are the incremental costs of actually providing a service in a hospital (in addition to the fixed costs of light and heat). For example, a patient shows up in the emergency department at midnight complaining of a lump on the tip of his nose. The doctor, with characteristic erudition, says, "Yep, you have a wart on your nose," and sends the patient home with a bill for $500. The actual cost of this encounter is obviously negligible. The patient is really paying for the fixed costs of nurses and emergency resuscitative equipment should he have a cardiac arrest.

7. **Is hospital accounting a precisely scientific and objective analysis of financial data?**
   No.

8. **What is health insurance?**
   Traditionally, people can purchase insurance that may pay either all or a portion of their hospital and physician charges if they become ill. Insurance companies make a profit, therefore, only if the patient stays healthy. Insurance companies have elaborate tables to predict who will get sick, and they prefer to sell policies exclusively to young, healthy individuals. This practice is termed *skimming*. The insurance company takes all of the risk—and they like to keep it low. Conversely, hospitals must cover fixed costs—and the more expensive (and more frequent) the healthcare that physicians provide, the better it is for the hospitals.

9. **What are health maintenance organizations (HMOs)?**
   HMOs are complex systems composed, in their most comprehensive form, of hospitals, doctors plus offices, and an insurance company. HMOs contract with large groups of people (potential patients) to

maintain their health. Enrollees pay a monthly fee (just like health insurance) so that all hospital and physician charges are covered if the enrollees become ill. Unlike health insurance, however, in the HMO model, hospitals and physicians get paid whether or not the enrollee gets sick. So, it is better for everyone if enrollees stay healthy—and out of the hospital.

10. **Initially, a lot of physicians did not like HMOs. Why?**
Because physicians are fiercely independent. They did not want a bunch of business managers telling them how to manage patients.

11. **Why are physicians fiercely independent?**
We were probably born that way.

12. **Is that good?**
Probably not. Eventually, everyone will need to work together and not hit each other when they are mad.

13. **Do HMO administrators really dictate how physicians manage their patients?**
Yes and no. Physicians have developed medically effective and optimally efficient strategies—termed *clinical pathways*—for caring for many common illnesses. Although physicians must treat each patient individually, when we adhere to predetermined treatment guidelines (as encouraged by HMO administrators), patients usually get better faster and cheaper.

14. **Do physicians follow these clinical pathways?**
Traditionally, no.

15. **What do HMO managers do?**
They evaluate each physician's use of expensive resources (within the predetermined clinical pathways) relative to the health of the physician's patients.

16. **Do physicians welcome this kind of scrutiny?**
No.

17. **What is a preferred provider organization (PPO)?**
A PPO is a group of doctors who have elected to remain legally independent of a hospital and insurance company (if they joined together, they would be an HMO) and, most of all, patients. But PPOs maintain their independence as physicians, even though most PPOs require administrators to coordinate programs, keep the books, and keep the doctors from hitting each other. PPOs have the perception of independence, however.

18. **Is healthcare expensive?**
Unfortunately, yes. Physicians argue that patients pay a lot but also get a lot. In the United States, patients expect unlimited access to liver transplantation and magnetic resonance imaging (MRI) for every headache. Americans believe that fancy, expensive healthcare is not just a privilege, it is a right.

19. **So what is the problem?**
The chief executive officers (CEOs) of big United States corporations argue that the obligatory expense of healthcare is driving up the cost of United States products and making United States companies less competitive in the global market—there is more healthcare than steel in a new Chevrolet.

20. **Does big business have a solution?**
They think so. The CEOs still want unlimited access to the most modern healthcare for themselves and their families. Without sounding cynical, the CEOs want to save healthcare dollars spent on their employees and other people's families. They want to limit access to healthcare, but they do not want to wield the axe personally. So they developed the idea of capitation.

21. **What is capitation?**
The CEOs of large businesses come to hospitals, HMOs, or PPOs and say: "Why don't you provide all healthcare for all my employees at a fixed price, say, $180 per month per head?" (Hence, capitation.) In this model, physicians make the decisions about who gets how much medical care (satisfying their urge for independence), but they also promise to provide all necessary medical care for a prearranged price. Thus, they take all of the risk. CEOs like this model because they can still offer healthcare as an employee benefit and budget the cost in advance.

22. **Why do physicians not like capitation?**
All of a sudden physicians may have acquired a little more independence than they bargained for. Now they are paid in advance so that all costs of patients' healthcare are subtracted from the money they negotiated up front. Now they must advise against an MRI for every headache and break the news to Granny that she will not think better if they dialyze her blood urea nitrogen down to 50. This is the reverse of the good old days when physicians were rewarded if their patients got sick and stayed sick. Physicians could ply them with a smorgasbord of drugs and technologies. Now physicians are trying to control healthcare costs.

23. **What is ObamaCare?**
ObamaCare, officially called the Patient Protection and Affordable Care Act, is a healthcare reform law signed in 2010 by President Barack Obama. It mandates health insurance for all. It expands subsidies for middle-income families and taxes healthcare providers and higher-income earners. The law also eliminates preexisting conditions, stops insurance companies from dropping you when you are sick as well as protects against gender discrimination, expands free preventative services, expands Medicaid and CHIP, improves Medicare pharmacy subsidies, requires large employers to insure their employees, and creates a marketplace for subsidized insurance alternatives for individuals, families, and small businesses.

24. **Is all this change good?**
Absolutely. Medicine has always changed—and the faster, the better. Physicians were initially attracted to medicine as an intellectually stimulating discipline because medicine and surgery evolve rapidly.

25. **Can physicians keep up with all this change?**
Absolutely.

26. **Despite all of the medical Chicken Littles who sonorously declare that the sky is falling, is medicine (and even more clearly, surgery) still the most gratifying, stimulating, and rewarding profession?**
Absolutely.

KEY POINTS: HEALTHCARE REFORM

1. Healthcare is continuously being reformed and always will be.
2. There is a big difference between hospital costs (what the hospital pays for an item or service) and what the hospital charges the patient.
3. The evolution of clinical pathways is both good for the patient and good for the hospital.
4. Physicians and surgeons do not welcome external scrutiny.
5. Surgery is the most gratifying, stimulating, and rewarding profession, and it's a whole lot better than whatever is second best.

BIBLIOGRAPHY

1. Blumenthal D. Controlling health care expenditures. *N Engl J Med.* 2001;344(10):766–769.
2. Dudley RA, Luft HS. Managed care in transition. *N Engl J Med.* 2001;344(14):1087–1092.
3. Fuchs VR. What's ahead for health insurance in the United States? *N Engl J Med.* 2002;346(23):1822–1824.
4. Iglehart JK. Changing health insurance trends. *N Engl J Med.* 2002;347(12):956–962.
5. Schroeder SA. Prospects for expanding health insurance coverage. *N Engl J Med.* 344(11):847–852.
6. Wilensky GR. Medicare reform-now is the time. *N Engl J Med.* 2001;345:458–462.
7. Wood AJ. When increased therapeutic benefit comes at increased cost. *N Engl J Med.* 2002;346(23):1819–1821.
8. Wright JG. Hidden barriers to improvement in the quality of health care. *N Engl J Med.* 2002;346(14):1096.

CHAPTER 106

MEDICAL ETHICS

M. Kelley Bullard, MD

1. **Are there any principles of medical ethics?**
   Yes, there are four:
   a. Beneficence: The intent of doing good and offering net benefit by therapeutic intervention. This principle requires maintenance of professional knowledge and skill by ongoing education throughout one's career.
   b. Nonmaleficence: The intent of not causing harm. To exercise this principle, one must know probability of harm from a proposed intervention.
   c. Autonomy: Deliberated self-rule requires a physician to obtain informed consent, respect privacy of healthcare information, communicate in a forthright manner that promotes trust, and respect patients' wishes regardless of their alignment with the physician's own beliefs.
   d. Justice: Acknowledgment of the patient within the context of society. This principle strives to create equitable treatments for similar patients and distribute resources as evenly as possible amongst those in need.

2. **What is included in informed consent?**
   An informed consent discussion includes:
   a. Education concerning the patient's diagnosis
   b. Explanation of the planned therapy in layman's terms
   c. Disclosure of risks versus benefits of the proposed intervention
   d. Discussion of alternative therapies and their likely outcomes (including what will happen if no treatment occurs)
   e. Thorough answering of all patient questions and concerns
   Informed consent is a voluntary decision made by the patient or a surrogate decision maker if the patient is incapacitated or a minor.

3. **What is an advance directive?**
   An advance directive is a set of instructions delineated by a competent patient to determine their wishes for treatment at a time when he or she is no longer competent. It respects the patient's autonomy by allowing self-determination of their future care. It assists families and physicians in decision making based on the patient's wishes rather than a perceived sense of what is best for the patient. Advance directives may include:
   a. An informal document, such as a living will, which is a list of instructions made by a competent person about future medical treatment. It produces a preillness guideline for future caregivers in accordance with the patient's wishes.
   b. Formal legal appointment of a decision maker, such as a medical durable power of attorney (DPOA). A DPOA is a patient-appointed proxy decision maker. This decision maker becomes active as soon as the patient is no longer able to make competent medical decisions. The durable power of attorney must be established prior to the person becoming incapacitated.
   Advance directives are activated when a patient is incapacitated by illness. Laws surrounding advance directives vary by state.

4. **What is POLST?**
   Physician orders for life-sustaining therapy complements the advanced directive. It is designed for persons who are likely to die within the next year. The POLST includes physician orders for current therapies that align with the patient's end-of-life care preferences. It can guide emergency personnel and inpatient care teams. It is intended for persons of any age with serious illness. Endorsement of POLST forms currently exists in 18 states, with many more states currently developing POLST programs.

5. **What is a do-not-resuscitate (DNR) order?**
   A DNR order informs the healthcare team of a patient's resuscitation wishes. A patient or medical decision maker can determine what degree of intervention should be allowed if a patient becomes

pulseless or apneic. There is a spectrum of interventions covered by most DNR forms that allow patients or their surrogates to include or omit interventions such as:

- Intubation
- Chest compressions
- Defibrillation
- Medications for arrhythmias and/or blood pressure support

A DNR order does not have any implications on any other treatment decision. The Joint Commission for the Accreditation of Healthcare Organizations mandates that hospitals have written guidelines that promote accountability for DNR orders. All DNR orders must be documented in writing, similar to all other orders, in the appropriate section of the patient's chart.

DNR orders only apply to episodes of acute cardiopulmonary failure. They do NOT apply to withholding other forms of therapy in stable patients.

6. **What is the difference between withdrawing and withholding support?**
Withdrawing care is when all life-supporting measures are removed, whereas withholding support means no acceleration in care. Both decisions change the treatment goal from maintaining life and restoring health to maintaining comfort during the dying process. There is no moral or ethical distinction between withdrawal and withholding of support. Either of the two allows natural progression of disease without the interface of medical technology.

The decision to withdraw or withhold support does not equate with patient death, although the probability of death may be greater. After the decision has been made, appropriate management should focus on the patient's comfort and psychosocial support.

7. **What are futile care and medical futility?**
There are four main concepts of medical futility:
a. Healthcare professionals are not required to provide physiologically futile treatment.
b. Imminent demise argues against treatment if the patient has no likelihood of survival to discharge.
c. Under the concept of lethal condition, medical care is considered futile if the patient will survive temporarily but ultimately expire as a result of the ongoing disease process within that hospitalization.
d. Quality of life or qualitative futility argues against treatment if the patient's quality of life is so poor that it would be unreasonable to prolong life.

Futility of care designation routinely initiates palliative interventions to minimize suffering in modern day intensive care units.

8. **What are the clinical determinants of brain death?**
Brain death occurs when all function of the brain and brainstem ceases and is irreversible. A brain death exam includes:
a. The cause for permanent loss of brain function (e.g., computed tomography or MRI showing edema or diffuse ischemia)
b. Elimination of reversible causes of decreased neurologic function:
   - Metabolic derangements
   - Neuromuscular blocking agents
   - Anesthetics
   - Intoxication/recreational polypharmacy
   - Hypothermia
   - Hypotension
   - Hypoxia

A clinical exam that evaluates:
a. Absence of brainstem reflexes:
   - Fixed, dilated pupils
   - No corneal, gag, or cough reflexes
   - Absent oculocephalic response
   - Absent oculovestibular response
b. No motor response to noxious stimuli
c. No breathing during apnea test (i.e., CO_2 challenge)

In the event that the patient has other injuries that preclude assessment of the criteria above, tests such as cerebral angiography, transcranial Doppler, electroencephalogram, or radionucleotide scintigraphy can serve as confirmation studies.

In children, repeat studies are required after 12 hours if between ages 1 and 18. Children under 1 year of age should have 48 hours of observation with one confirmatory test.

9. **What is a persistent vegetative state?**

   In a persistent vegetative state, the patient appears to be awake but does not have awareness of his or her surroundings or higher mental activity. This is typically seen after improvement of a comatose state. Although the patient opens his or her eyes, he or she is only capable of reflexive behavior.

10. **What is euthanasia?**

    Euthanasia occurs when a physician plays an active role in assisting in the death of the patient. This highly controversial practice can take an active form, where the physician administers the life-ending medication, or a passive form, where the physician supplies the patient with a prescription for a lethal dose of medication. Oregon was the first state to have laws pertaining to physician-assisted suicide, allowing doctors to prescribe medications to terminally ill patients for the purpose of committing suicide. Since that landmark legislation, Washington, Vermont, California, and Montana have passed similar laws.

11. **Who should approach patients' families about organ donation?**

    The organ procurement organization should be the first to approach the family. This is called the decoupling principle, and it eliminates any conflict of interest.

12. **What should patients' families be told when organ donation is feasible?**

    In the event of brain death, the family is informed that once the brain death exam is performed the patient is legally dead. This can be confusing for families because the patient's heart continues beating. It is important to reassure the family that the patient is unable to feel pain because the control center for pain has ceased to function. Once the organ procurement agency has initiated the conversation, education on the general process of donation can clear up misconceptions. Families can be reassured that:

    - They can refuse donation without fear of prejudice.
    - Several patients may benefit from the donated organs.
    - There is no guarantee that the organs will be viable for donation.
    - They are not responsible for the cost of care provided after brain death is determined.

13. **What is organ donation after cardiac death?**

    This is the process in which organs are procured on a patient that has not been declared brain dead. Most of these patients have suffered catastrophic brain or spinal cord injuries, but have not met the clinical definition of brain death. The same informed consent procedure is performed as with brain-dead patients. The patient is taken to the operating room (OR) and care is withdrawn. A doctor, who is not involved in the procurement of the organs or in the transplantation of the organs, is present and declares death. After cardiac death is pronounced, the procurement team enters the OR and proceeds.

14. **What is the role of the hospital ethics committee?**

    The hospital ethics committee educates hospital staff members and provides a source of consultation. It is made up of physicians and ancillary staff with special training in medical ethics and ethics education. Education of the hospital community is accomplished through grand rounds, seminars, special lectures, and committee consultation. The hospital ethics committee should be viewed as an intrinsic part of the hospital community. Developed policies should be reviewed by other committees and divisions of the hospital to foster a better sense of cohesiveness when ethical and moral dilemmas arise.

KEY POINTS: MEDICAL ETHICS

1. Medical ethics are based on four key principles:
   a. Beneficence
   b. Nonmaleficence
   c. Autonomy
   d. Justice
2. An advance directive is a set of instructions delineated by a competent person to communicate their wishes for care and treatment at a time when they are not competent or capable of communicating such wishes.
3. POLST complement (and not replace) the advanced directive.
4. DNR orders only apply to episodes of acute cardiopulmonary failure and do NOT apply to withholding other forms of therapy in stable patients.
5. Brain death occurs when all function of the brain and brainstem ceases and it is irreversible.

BIBLIOGRAPHY

1. Luce JM, White DB. A history of ethics and the law in the intensive care unit. *Crit Care Clin.* 2009;25(1):221–237.
2. Luce JM, White DB. The pressure to withhold or withdraw life-sustaining therapy from critically ill patients in the United States. *Am J Respir Crit Care Med.* 2007;175(11):1104–1108.
3. Schmidt TA, Zive D. Physician orders for life-sustaining treatment (POLST): Lessons learned from analysis of the Oregon POLST registry. *Resuscitation.* 2014;85(4):480–485.
4. Greer DM, Wang HH. Variability of brain death policies in the United States. *JAMA Neurol.* 2016;73(2):213–218.
5. Bernat JL. How can we achieve uniformity in brain death determinations? *Neurology.* 2008;70(4):252–253.
6. Laureys S, Boly M. What is it like to be vegetative or minimally conscious? *Curr Opin Neurol.* 2007;20(6):609–613.
7. Steinbrook R. Organ donation after cardiac death. *N Engl J Med.* 2007;357(3):209–213.

CHAPTER 107

PROFESSIONALISM

U. Mini B. Swift, MD, MPH, FACP, Ghassan Jamaleddine, MD, Alden H. Harken, MD, FACS

1. **What is a profession?**
   The professions are the means by which the complex services needed by society are organized. A profession has been defined by the American College of Surgeons as:

   ...an occupation whose core element is work that is based upon the mastery of a complex body of knowledge and skills. It is a vocation in which knowledge of some department of science or learning, or the practice of an art founded upon it, is used in the service of others. Its members are governed by codes of ethics and profess a commitment to competence, integrity and morality, altruism and to the promotion of the public good within their domain. These commitments form the basis of a social contract between a profession and society, which, in turn, grants the profession a monopoly over the use of its knowledge base, the right to considerable autonomy in practice and the privilege of self-regulation. Professions and their members are accountable to those served and to society.

2. **What are the core elements of a profession?**
   All professions are characterized by four core elements: (1) a monopoly over the use of specialized knowledge; (2) in return for that monopoly that we enjoy, relative autonomy in practice and the responsibility of self-regulation; (3) altruistic service to individuals and society; and (4) responsibility for maintaining and expanding professional knowledge and skills.

3. **What is professionalism?**
   Professionalism describes the cognitive, moral, and collegial attributes of a professional. Ultimately, it is all the reasons that your mother is proud to say that you are a doctor and a surgeon.

4. **Why do physicians need a code of professional conduct?**
   Trust is integral to the practice of surgery. The code of professional conduct clarifies the relationship between the surgical profession and the society it serves. This is often referred to as a social contract. For patients, the code of professional conduct crystallizes the commitment of the surgical community toward individual patients and their communities. Trust is built brick by brick.

5. **What is the American College of Surgeons' Code of Professional Conduct?**
   The code of professional conduct takes the general principles of professionalism and applies them to surgical practice. The code is the foundation on which we earn our professional privileges and the trust of patients and the public. It is our job description.

6. **What are the responsibilities of professionalism described in the American College of Surgeons' Code of Professional Conduct?**
   During the continuum of preoperative, intraoperative, and postoperative care, surgeons have the responsibility to:
   - Serve as effective advocates for our patients' needs.
   - Disclose therapeutic options including their risks and benefits.
   - Disclose and resolve any conflict of interest that might influence the decisions of care.
   - Be sensitive and respectful of patients, understanding their vulnerability during the perioperative period.
   - Fully disclose adverse events and medical errors.
   - Acknowledge patients' psychologic, social, cultural, and spiritual needs.
   - Encompass within our surgical care the special needs of terminally ill patients.
   - Acknowledge and support the needs of patients' families.
   - Respect the knowledge, dignity, and perspective of other healthcare professionals.

7. **Do other professional societies have a code of professional conduct?**
   Yes. Several groups have created professional codes and the American College of Surgeons supports their declarations.

8. **Why do surgeons need their own code of professionalism?**
A surgical procedure is an extreme experience. We impact our patients physiologically, psychologically, and socially. When patients submit themselves to a surgical experience, they must trust that the surgeon will put their welfare above all other considerations. The written code helps to reinforce these values.

9. **What are the fundamental principles of the code of professional conduct and the codes of other professional societies?**
   - The primacy of patient welfare
   - Patient autonomy
   - Social justice

10. **What is the primacy of patient welfare?**
This means that the patient's interests always come first. Altruism is central to this concept, and it is the surgeon's altruism that fosters trust in the physician-patient relationship.

11. **What is the principle of patient autonomy?**
Patients must understand and make their own informed decisions about their treatment. This is tricky. As physicians, we must be honest with our patients so that they make educated decisions. At the same time, we must make sure that their decisions are consistent with ethical practices and do not lead to demands for inappropriate care.

12. **What is the principle of social justice?**
As physicians we must advocate for our individual patients while at the same time promoting the health of the healthcare system as a whole. We must balance our patient's needs (autonomy) and not misdirect scarce resources that benefit society (social justice).

13. **How can I apply these lofty ideas to my everyday existence on the medical-surgical unit?**
The American College of Surgeons Code of Professional Conduct lists the responsibilities of being a surgeon specifically. For all other situations, use the guiding principles to dictate your actions. A few examples include:
   - Pursuit of the **just and equitable distribution of finite resources** could mean that you do not order unnecessary tests or even give 20 units of blood to a Child's C cirrhotic.
   - **Commitment to improving quality of care** is honored by submitting ideas to improve workflow on the wards to your chief resident, program director, or even department chair.

As a student, you have a unique opportunity to spend a little extra time with a frightened patient (they are all frightened) and to help explain the nature of the disease and what the plans are to do something. Use little words—not doctor words. Patients and families will love you for doing this. And this understanding promotes patient autonomy.

14. **Should medical professionals participate in social media?**
Many do.
The constructive opportunities and dangerous challenges are very real.

15. **What are the constructive opportunities?**
It is essential that we foster interdisciplinary, interprofessional, and intergenerational dialogue. This mode of communication is here to stay. It's a formidably effective language, but fluency must be mastered carefully.

16. **What are the dangerous challenges?**
We must assume that our patients will read everything we post, and we should never submit anything that we would not be proud to see published in our local newspaper.

KEY POINTS: PROFESSIONALISM

1. Professionalism describes the cognitive, moral, and collegial attributes of a surgeon.
2. The fundamental principles of professional conduct include:
   a. The primary of patient welfare;
   b. Patient autonomy; and
   c. Social service.
3. The constructive opportunities and dangerous challenges of social media are very real. Never post anything that you would not be proud to see published in your local newspaper.

BIBLIOGRAPHY

1. ABIM Foundation, ACP-ASIM Foundation. European Federation of Internal Medicine. Medical professionalism in the new millennium: a physician charter. *Ann Intern Med*. 2002;136(3):243–246.
2. Cruess SR, Johnston S. Professionalism for medicine: opportunities and obligations. *Med J Aust*. 2002;177:208–211.
3. American College of Surgeons Task Force on Professionalism. Code of Professional Conduct. *J Am Coll Surg*. 2003;197:603–604.
4. American College of Surgeons Task Force on Professionalism. Code of Professional Conduct. *J Am Coll Surg*. 2004;199:734–735.
5. Tilbert JC, Sharp RR. Owning medical professionalism. *Am J Bioeth*. 2016;16(9):1–2.
6. Hillis DJ, Grigg MJ. Professionalism and the role of medical colleges. *Surgeon*. 2015;13(5):292–299.
7. Gholami-Kordkheili F, Wild V. The impact of social media on medical professionalism: a systematic qualitative review of challenges and opportunities. *J Med Internet Res*. 2013;15(8):e184.

CHAPTER 108

REQUIRED READING

James Cushman, MD, MPH, FACS

Unlike medical rounds, where to keep up you need to "one-up" by quoting a current journal article (preferably yesterday's), you can flourish in surgery by knowing the following references, but you need to know them cold.

1. Mangano DT, Goldman L. Preoperative assessment of patients with known or suspected coronary disease. *N Engl J Med.* 1995;333(26):1750–1756.

   This is an update of Goldman's 1977 NEJM article in which he pioneered the concept of "risk-adjusted surgical outcome." You should copy Table 2, Three Commonly Used Indexes of Cardiac Risk, and always carry it with you. Intuitively, a triathlete will weather a surgical stress better than a Supreme Court judge, but this article provides a point system with which you can calculate objective perioperative risk. Note that most of the points derive from the heart. If a patient dies within 20 days of surgery, the heart is typically the culprit.

2. Nygren J, Thacker J, Carli F, et al. Guidelines for perioperative care in elective rectal/pelvic surgery: Enhanced Recovery After Surgery (ERAS(®)) Society recommendations. *World J Surg.* 2013;37(2):285–305.

   The (ERAS(®)) Society (www.erassociety.org) is committed to improving perioperative care worldwide. This present review describes important guidelines in and presents an evidence-based consensus of optimal perioperative care in rectal and pelvic surgery. The timeframe of literature review is between 1966 and early 2012. ERAS areas of evidence-based recommendations include but are not limited to preoperative counseling, preoperative optimization, preoperative bowel preparation, abbreviated fasting, preoperative treatment with clear fluid carbohydrates, and preanesthetic medications.

3. Fleshman J, Branda M, Sargent DJ, et al. Effect of laparoscopic-assisted resection vs open resection of stage II or III rectal cancer on pathologic outcomes: The ACOSOG Z6051 Randomized Clinical Trial. *JAMA.* 2015;314(13):1346–1355.

   This is a recent multicenter randomized controlled clinical trial comparing laparoscopic resection (240 patients) with open resection (222 patients) in patients with stage II or III rectal cancer (beyond the rectal wall) for efficacy. The primary outcome was a composite of circumferential radial margin >1 mm, distal margin without tumor, and completeness of total mesorectal excision. The primary finding was that because of pathologic outcomes, this study does not support the use of laparoscopic resection in patients with stage II and III rectal cancer.

4. Dellinger RP, Levy MM, Rhodes A, et al. Surviving sepsis campaign: international guidelines for management of severe sepsis and septic shock: 2012. *Crit Care Med.* 2013;41(2):580–637.

   Mandatory reading for any physician caring for patients who may be admitted to the hospital with sepsis, severe sepsis, and/or septic shock. This 57-page document, representing the consensus of 68 international experts and 30 organizations, contains an update to the 2008 guidelines. Although a number of recommendations are acknowledged as based on weak support in the literature, strong agreement existed among these experts regarding many Level 1 recommendations for the best care of patients with severe sepsis. The reader should know what these are, and strive to incorporate them into his or her practice.

5. McClave SA, Taylor BE, Martindale RG, et al. Guidelines for the provision and assessment of nutrition support therapy in the adult critically ill patients: Society of Critical Care Medicine (SCCM) and American Society for Parenteral and Enteral Nutrition (ASPEN). *J Parenter Enteral Nutr.* 2016;40(2):159–211.

   These updated guidelines for the management of nutritional support of critically ill patients mark the continuation of definitive evidence-based nutrition and metabolic optimization from two medical organizations credentialed to do so. The guidelines are intended to help providers establish nutritional support for any adult intensive care unit (ICU) patient expected to have a length of stay >2 or 3 days. Well organized, it covers key and recent literature in nutritional assessment, initiation of enteral feeding, dosing and monitoring of enteral feeding, and parenteral nutrition, among other aspects of nutritional care. Must read for any provider who is responsible for the nutritional support and health of an ICU patient.

6. Veronesi U, Cascinelli N, Mariani L, et al. Twenty-year follow-up of a randomized study comparing breast conserving surgery with radical mastectomy for early breast cancer. *N Engl J Med.* 2002;347(16):1227–1232.

   Seven hundred women with <2 cm breast cancer were randomized to radical mastectomy or quadrantectomy and radiation therapy. After 1976, patients with positive axillary nodes also received adjuvant cyclophosphamide, methotrexate, and 5-fluorouracil. After 20 years, 30 women in the conservative treatment group and eight women in the radical mastectomy group suffered local recurrence ($P = 0.01$). Conversely, the incidence of deaths from all causes at 20 years was identical at 41%. The authors conclude that breast conservation therapy is the treatment of choice for women with "relatively small" breast cancers.

7. Fisher B, Jeong JH. Twenty-five-year follow-up of a randomized trial comparing radical mastectomy, total mastectomy, and total mastectomy followed by irradiation. *N Engl J Med.* 2002;347(8):567–575.
Clinical investigation is hard. The National Surgical Adjuvant Breast and Bowel Project Trials, initiated 25 years ago, continue to serve as the benchmark for superb prospective, randomized investigations. In this study, 1851 women were randomized after the breast tumor was excised and the nodal status was documented. The authors conclude that lumpectomy followed by breast irradiation is appropriate therapy. To appreciate the huge problems in interpreting clinical trials, you must read this article carefully. Radiation did decrease death from breast cancer, but this reduction was partially offset by an increase in deaths from other causes.

8. Barnett HJ, Taylor DW, Eliasziw M, et al. Benefit of carotid endarterectomy in patients with symptomatic moderate or severe stenosis. North American Symptomatic Carotid Endarterectomy Trial Collaborators. *N Engl J Med.* 1998;339(20):1415–1425.
This is the North American Symptomatic Carotid Endarterectomy Trial (NASCET) initiated in 1987. NASCET randomized patients with severe carotid stenosis (70%–99%) and moderate stenosis (<70%) into standard medical therapy or carotid endarterectomy (CEA). By 1991, the clear advantage of surgery in symptomatic patients with severe stenosis was so clear that the study was stopped for this group. This manuscript reports a 5-year reduction in ipsilateral stroke from 22.2% (medical) to 15.7% (surgical) ($p = 0.045$) in patients with moderate (50%–69%) stenosis. Once a patient with carotid disease becomes symptomatic, that is ominous. As you witness various diseases, you subconsciously compile a list of diseases you do not want. A big burn and a big stroke are on the top of everyone's list.

9. van de Vijver MJ, He YD, van't Veer LJ, et al. A gene-expression signature as a predictor of survival in breast cancer. *N Engl J Med.* 2002;347(25):1999–2009.
The authors postulate that 70 of our 35,000 genes dictate the character of breast cancer. So cancer, unlike cystic fibrosis and sickle cell disease, requires a constellation of genetic mutations, not just one. They followed 295 patients for 12 years and report that this "70 gene signature" predicts survival better than the classical indicators of patient age, tumor size, tumor histology, pathologic grade, hormone receptor status, and even lymph node disease. The latter is the shocker. The authors observe that distant metastasis kills you, positive lymph nodes do not. In patients with either positive or negative lymph nodes, gene profile determines survival. Each cancer does not acquire an ability to metastasize as it grows, that capability is programmed into the first neoplastic cell that establishes residence in your patient.

10. Harken AH. Enough is enough. *Arch Surg.* 1999;134(10):1061–1063.
This article explores the surgeon's responsibility to assess surgical risk, to relate risk to anticipated physiologic and psychologic benefit, and to develop common sense strategies to appreciate individual patient happiness. When benefits exceed anticipated operative risks—this is easy—proceed with surgery. When risks exceed benefits, this can be uncomfortable, but sensitive recognition of this relatively common problem by the surgeon can limit extension of the patient's and family's grief, prevent the squandering of limited resources, and appropriately divert decision-making guilt from the family to the surgeon.

11. Eatock FC, Chong P, Menezes N, et al. A randomized study of early nasogastric versus nasojejunal feeding in severe acute pancreatitis. *Am J Gastroenterol.* 2005;100(2):432–439.
Early feeding in some patients with acute pancreatitis (AP) causes pain and is traditionally believed to be the result of worsening disease produced by premature stimulation of the pancreas. Recent scientific evidence suggests that overstimulation of pancreatic acinar cells may not be the underlying cause of AP, therefore leading physicians to question the benefits of resting the pancreas. The delivery of nutrients into distal small bowel has been shown beneficial during severe AP. This study is the first randomized prospective study in which 50 adult patients with severe AP were randomized to receive early feeding by either nasogastric tubes or nasojejunal tubes. Measured endpoints included disease severity measured by how sick the patient is (acute physiology and chronic health [APACHE] II scores), the magnitude of systemic inflammation (C-reactive protein [CRP] levels), clinical progression, and pain. Overall, 24.5% mortality was observed, with no difference in mortality between the groups. No difference in complication rates, CRP changes, APACHE II changes, or pain level changes were observed. This study is significant in that it scientifically challenges the surgical bias that resting the pancreas helps patients with AP recover faster.

12. McFalls EO, Ward HB, Moritz TE, et al. Coronary-artery revascularization before elective major vascular surgery. *N Engl J Med.* 2004;351(27):2795–2804.
This is a Veterans Administration prospective randomized trial that was conducted to assess the benefits of preoperative coronary revascularization in patients undergoing major vascular surgery. Five hundred ten patients were randomized to coronary revascularization by coronary artery bypass graft, percutaneous approach, or standard medical therapy. Patient characteristics were similar in both groups: ≈40% were diabetics, 45% were smokers, 40% with history of myocardial infarction (MI), ≈30% with three-vessel coronary disease, and 20% with history of cerebrovascular accident or transient ischemic attack. Patient outcome was assessed during hospitalization and in long-term follow up. The results showed no difference in postoperative complications or in-hospital mortality rates between the treated groups. At 2.7 years after randomization, no difference in mortality was observed between the groups. Significant delays in treatment occurred in the preoperative revascularization patients (54 days versus 18 days).

These results demonstrated that unless patients exhibit acute coronary syndrome (ACS), there are no clear short-term or long-term benefits in routine coronary revascularization before major vascular surgical procedures.

13. Fitzgibbons RJ Jr, Giobbie-Hurder A, Gibbs JO, et al. Watchful waiting vs repair of inguinal hernia in minimally symptomatic men: a randomized clinical trial. *JAMA.* 2006;295(3):285–292.

    Deciding if and when to operate is one of the most important decisions you will make as a surgeon. This trial put that decision to the test as it pertains to men with minimally symptomatic inguinal hernias. Fitzgibbons is a nationally recognized expert in the field of hernia surgery and presented the results of this prospective, randomized, multicenter study in the Society of American Gastrointestinal and Endoscopic Surgeons Grand Round Master Series (to view the video go to: www. medscape.com/viewarticle/553466). In this trial, 720 men with mildly symptomatic inguinal hernias were randomized into two groups—watchful waiting versus tension-free repair. They were followed for 2–4.5 years. No significant difference between the two groups was found based on the main outcomes of the trial, pain and discomfort interfering with activity, and changes from baseline in the physical component score of the Short Form-36 health-related quality-of-life survey. Therefore, watchful waiting in this subset of patients is permissible because the risk of incarceration is rare (1.8/1000 patient years).

14. Neumayer L, Giobbie-Hurder A, Jonasson O, et al. Open mesh versus laparoscopic mesh repair of inguinal hernia. *N Engl J Med.* 2004;350(18):1819–1827.

    With the development of minimally invasive surgery in the late 1980s, many operations, including inguinal hernia repair, were adapted to the laparoscopic approach. The advantages of laparoscopic repair include significantly less postoperative pain and speedier return to usual activities. However, laparoscopy does carry risk. The best approach to repair of inguinal hernias has been controversial, multifactorial, and inconclusive. Laparoscopic operations must be performed under general anesthesia, and there is increased potential for serious complications, including but not limited to bowel perforation and major vessel injury. Many studies have proven an overall advantage of laparoscopic over open tension-free techniques, but most of these studies were done at specialized centers. This large multicenter, prospective, randomized trial, conducted at the Veterans Administration, is the notable exception and may be more representative of the general population. In this study, 2164 patients were randomized to laparoscopic versus Lichtenstein or open tension-free repair of inguinal hernias. Though patients in the laparoscopic group had less pain and returned to work sooner, recurrence was significantly more common (10.1% versus 4.9%). Based on recurrence and safety, open tension-free repair was found to be superior to laparoscopic repair. This study, and the subsequent editorial by Dr. Jacobs, raises many questions regarding the learning curves for laparoscopic procedures, surgeon skill, and future resident training.

15. Giger UF, Michel JM, Opitz I, et al. Risk factors for perioperative complications in patients undergoing laparoscopic cholecystectomy: analysis of 22,953 consecutive cases from the Swiss Association of Laparoscopic and Thoracoscopic Surgery database. *J Am Coll Surg.* 2006;203(5):723–728.

    Using a Swiss database, the authors identified a number of risk factors for local and systemic complications in patients undergoing laparoscopic cholecystectomy. There are no surprises reported during this investigation; however, the findings seem to be useful for all of us to recognize so that we can adjust and control surgeon-related variables, including skill levels of trainee and supervisor involved in the complex cases and timing of surgery for the complex patients.

16. Hébert PC, Wells G, Blajchman MA, et al. A multicenter, randomized, controlled clinical trial of transfusion requirements in critical care. Transfusion Requirements in Critical Care Investigators, Canadian Critical Care Trials Group. *N Engl J Med.* 1999;340(6):409–417.

    Red cells are responsible for the delivery of oxygen to tissues, and the augmentation of oxygen delivery is generally presumed to be beneficial in critically ill patients; therefore, a transfusion threshold of (hemoglobin) 10 g had often been deemed acceptable in the critical care setting. Both the risks and benefits of blood transfusions can be significant. Given that blood transfusions are associated with excess volume infusion, immunosuppression, and infection transmission, the benefits of a liberal transfusion strategy had not been clearly established and potentially exposed many patients who did not necessarily need a transfusion to avoidable risks. This multicenter, randomized, controlled trial randomized 838 euvolemic, intensive care patients to either a "restrictive" or "liberal" transfusion strategy. In the restrictive group, patients were given red blood cells when their hemoglobin dropped below 7 g/dL. In the liberal group, patients were transfused at hemoglobin of 10 g/dL. Patients who were less acutely ill and were younger than 55 had a much lower 30-day mortality in the restrictive arm of the study than those in the liberal group (8.7%–16.1% and 5.7%–13%, respectively). Patients in the restrictive group also received fewer transfusions (mean of 2.6 units versus 5.6 units) and experienced lower in-hospital mortality (22.2% versus 28.1%; $p = 0.05$). Cardiac events including pulmonary edema and MI occurred more frequently among the liberal transfusion patients during their ICU stay. These findings suggest that a restrictive transfusion strategy with hemoglobin values of 7.0–9.0 may be safely applied for most critically ill patients, with the exception of patients with ACS. By shining a light on traditional transfusion triggers, this trial encourages physicians to justify the use and assess the risks and the benefits of blood transfusions.

17. Clinical Outcomes of Surgical Therapy Study Group. A comparison of laparoscopically assisted and open colectomy for colon cancer. *N Engl J Med.* 2004;350(20):2050–2059.

Studies comparing laparoscopic and open abdominal operations have generally demonstrated shorter hospitalization and recovery for patients treated laparoscopically; however, as a result of concerns with inadequate oncologic resections and a potential compromise in patient survival, laparoscopic colectomy had not been widely accepted for the management of colon cancer. This randomized control trial was designed to evaluate outcomes in patients undergoing laparoscopic colectomy for colon cancer. A total of 872 patients were randomized to open colectomy or laparoscopic colectomy, with similar patient demographics and distributions of tumor locations in both treatment arms. The findings of the study indicated no difference in complication rates, 30-day mortality, and surgical margin status between the treatment arms. However, perioperative recovery was faster among the patients treated laparoscopically, with significant shorter hospital stay and reduced duration of narcotic analgesic usage reported. At 3-year follow-up, there was no difference in recurrence rates, overall survival, and disease-free survival. These results, along with similar findings reported from a European trial (*Lancet Oncol* 2005;6(7):477–484), have clearly established laparoscopic colectomy as an acceptable surgical treatment for colon cancer. To view a laparoscopic colectomy for cancer, go to www.websurg.com.

18. Lee TH, Marcantonio ER, Mangione CM, et al. Derivation and prospective validation of a simple index for prediction of cardiac risk of major noncardiac surgery. *Circulation.* 1999;100(10):1043–1049.

During the preoperative evaluation the risks and benefits of the operation should be established and discussed with the patient. The cardiovascular system is challenged during the perioperative period and cardiac complications carry significant morbidity. Therefore, risk stratification for cardiac complications is essential for each patient. Historically, guidelines including Goldman's criteria and the Cardiac Risk Index were devised to determine cardiac risk. The use of these systems has been limited by their complexity. This study proposed a much simpler Revised Cardiac Risk Index (RCRI) to predict the risk of cardiac complications in major elective noncardiac procedures. The study was performed at a highly reputable academic hospital and included 4315 patients. The main outcome measures were cardiac complications. Six independent, equal predictors of complications were identified including high-risk type of surgery, history of ischemic heart disease, history of congestive heart failure, history of cerebrovascular disease, preoperative treatment with insulin, and a preoperative serum creatinine >2 mg/dL. The RCRI can be calculated quickly and is a valuable tool currently used to accurately risk-stratify patients for cardiac complications in major elective noncardiac procedures.

19. Gurm HS, Yadav JS, Fayad P, et al. Long term results of carotid stenting versus endarterectomy in high-risk patients. *N Engl J Med.* 2008;358(15):1572–1579.

The authors note that there is a direct relationship between the degree of carotid stenosis and ipsilateral stroke. In the hands of experienced vascular surgeons and interventionalists, this disease can be managed and patients can anticipate extraordinarily good results. The morbidity and mortality of a surgical CEA, even in debilitated patients, is quite low. When an angioplasty catheter is inflated in the cerebral circulation, there is a risk that a tiny bit of crumbled plaque floats north, causing memory loss. So, a fishing net that is placed distal to the deployment of the angioplasty balloon and stent was developed (the first two authors acknowledge that they are the inventors and hold patents on the emboli protection device). In a prospective randomized trial of 260 patients, the authors conclude that carotid artery stenting with protection by the emboli protection device is "not inferior" to CEA at 1 month, 1 year, and 3 years.

20. Giuliano AE, Hunt KK, Ballman KV, et al. Axillary dissection vs no axillary dissection in women with invasive breast cancer and sentinel node metastasis: a randomized clinical trial. *JAMA.* 2011;305(6):569–565.

The American College of Surgeons Oncology Group 2011 Trial targeted enrollment of 1900 patients with clinical T1–T2 invasive breast cancer, no palpable axillary adenopathy, and 1–2 sentinel lymph nodes containing metastasis identified by frozen section. All patients underwent lumpectomy and tangential whole-breast irradiation. Patients with metastases in 1–2 sentinel lymph nodes were randomized to undergo either a completion (median number 17), axillary node dissection (ALND), or no further axillary treatment. Further chemotherapy was at the discretion of the treating physician. The 5-year overall survival was 91.8% in the ALND group and 92.5% in the sentinel lymph node alone group, and the 5-year disease-free survival was 82.2% versus 83.9%, respectively. So, the study was stopped due to no difference or "lack of inferiority" in the sentinel lymph node alone group.

21. Shander A, Javidroozi M, Gianatiempo C, et al. Outcomes of protocol-driven care of critically ill severely anemic patients for whom blood transfusion is not an option. *Crit Care Med.* 2016;44(6):1109–1115.

All blood components are associated with some level of risk; therefore, it is reasonable to minimize the transfusion of blood in patients who are not actively bleeding. In this study, 178 bloodless and 441 transfused consecutive severely anemic critically ill patients with hemoglobin levels under 8 gms% within 24 hours of admission were compared. The transfused patients were older and had a higher APACHE II score. Hospital mortality rates were 24.7% in the bloodless and 24.5% in the transfused patients. ICU readmission and new electrocardiogram/cardiac enzyme changes were also similar.

22. Rivers E, Nguyen B, Havstad S, et al. Early goal-directed therapy in the treatment of severe sepsis and septic shock. *N Engl J Med*. 2001;345(19):1368–1377.
These authors defined a sequential strategy of treating all shock as:
Step 1: Give volume
Step 2: Pressors
Step 3: Increase oxygen carrying capacity.
They then enrolled 263 patients in "septic shock" within 6 hours of arrival in their single-center emergency department. Half these patients were randomized to "the way we've always treated shock" and the other 130 patients were treated with early goal-directed therapy (EGDT):
a. Infuse 500 mL lactated Ringer's q30 minutes until the central venous pressure (CVP) reached 12 cm H2O.
b. If the mean arterial pressure remained <65 mm Hg, start either Levophed or dobutamine (a beta-1 agonist, or norepinephrine, a pure alpha agonist).
c. If the mixed venous oxygen saturation remained below 70%, transfuse blood to a hematocrit of 30%. These patients were sick, and 46.5% of the "we've always done it this way" patients died, while only 30.5% of the goal-directed therapy patients succumbed. Big difference (*P* < 0.009)!
23. ProCESS Investigators, Yealy DM, Kellum JA, et al. A randomized trial of protocol-based care for early septic shock. *N Engl J Med*. 2014;370(18):1683–1693.
Critical care physicians who read the Rivers trial (see reference 22) questioned whether a central venous catheter was mandatory in all patients. They had also finally read the Canadian Transfusion Requirements in Critical Care trial and were worried that transfused blood up to a hematocrit of 30% might not be all good. So, 31 emergency departments ganged up and randomized 1341 septic patients into (1) the standard early goal-directed therapy protocol, (2) "modified" EGDT, and (3) "What we've learned in the past 13 years about the necessity of a central venous catheter and transfusing patients to a hematocrit of 30%" groups. In group 1, all patients had central venous monitoring and a hematocrit of 30%; in group 3, very few patients got a central venous catheter, but, perhaps surprisingly, these patients received a similar volume of fluid as the EGDT (group 1) patients. The "what we've learned" group 3 patients did receive less transfused blood, with a target hemoglobin of 7–9 gms%. So, critical care physicians can learn, and we can apply that knowledge in the care of our patients.

INDEX

Note: Pages followed by "*b*", "*t*", and "*f*" refer to boxes, tables, and figures respectively.